Third Edition

DePalma's

THE MANAGEMENT OF FRACTURES AND DISLOCATIONS

an atlas

Edited by

JOHN F. CONNOLLY, M.D., F.A.C.S.

W. B. SAUNDERS COMPANY
Philadelphia   London   Toronto   Mexico City   Rio de Janeiro   Sydney   Tokyo

W. B. Saunders Company: West Washington Square
Philadelphia, PA 19105

1 St. Anne's Road
Eastbourne, East Sussex BN21 3UN, England

1 Goldthorne Avenue
Toronto, Ontario M8Z 5T9, Canada

Apartado 26370 — Cedro 512
Mexico 4, D.F., Mexico

Rua Coronel Cabrita, 8
Sao Cristovao Caixa Postal 21176
Rio de Janeiro, Brazil

9 Waltham Street
Artarmon, N.S.W. 2064, Australia

Ichibancho, Central Bldg., 22-1 Ichibancho
Chiyoda-Ku, Tokyo 102, Japan

Library of Congress Cataloging in Publication Data

De Palma, Anthony F.

De Palma's The management of fractures and dislocations.

Second ed. published in 1970 under title: The management of
fractures and dislocations.

1. Fractures — Atlases.   2. Dislocations — Atlases.
   I. Connolly, John F.   II. Title.   III. Title: The
management of fractures and dislocations.

RD101.D29 1980   617'.15   79–64588

ISBN 0–7216–2666–1

Listed here is the latest translated edition of this book
together with the language of the translation and the publisher.

Spanish (*1st Edition*) (2 Volumes) — Ateneo, Buenos Aires, Argentina

Japanese (*2nd Edition*) (2 Volumes) — Hirokawa Publishing Co., Tokyo, Japan

De Palma's the Management of Fractures
and Dislocations

Volume 1: ISBN 0-7216-2702-1
Volume 2: ISBN 0-7216-2703-X
Complete Set: ISBN 0-7216-2666-1

Last digit is the print number: 9   8   7   6   5   4   3

The *Third Edition* of this textbook is dedicated to the seven ladies who light up my life—Anne, Mary Regina, Katie, Edna, Jeanine, Anne McGrath, and Claire.

PREFACE

The original concept for *Management of Fractures and Dislocations* was the brainchild of Mr. John L. Dusseau, then Vice President and Editor-in-Chief, and of Mr. Robert Rowan, former Executive Vice President of W. B. Saunders Company. They recognized the teaching effectiveness of the fracture clinics that have been held annually at the American Medical Association Meeting. They also realized that such an approach to the teaching of fracture management might effectively be duplicated in an atlas-textbook and exercised the good judgment of asking Dr. Anthony DePalma, who was then Professor of Orthopaedic Surgery at Jefferson Medical College, to write the text. The result proved to be a valuable and ready reference and a guide past the pitfalls of fracture management for many physicians, including myself. The text has served well the young physician seeking to learn standard methods as well as newer techniques of fracture management. It has also proved to be a challenge for the experienced surgeon who wishes to continue to learn and improve, in that it documents and demonstrates better ways. I have been extremely pleased to be asked to write the Third Edition of the text and have tried to follow carefully the format and thoroughness of the first two editions.

This edition represents my efforts to present techniques of managing fractures and dislocations that work best for me. It is presented in the same manner as I would offer my ideas to residents and students. It is not to be considered an all-inclusive survey of the literature or a complete review of different methods. I have added bibliographies at the end of each chapter to provide the reader with a more complete guide to the techniques described. The references are also included to support statements in the text that might be regarded as controversial but nevertheless must be made. The text is didactic and I offer no apologies for this; however, the reader should keep this in mind. He should also remember that not all the possible ways of treating fractures or dislocations have been presented, only the techniques that are most effective in my experience.

A recurring dilemma in managing fractures and dislocations is the choice between operative and nonoperative treatments. It may seem obvious but nevertheless must be reiterated in this modern technologic age that when results can be anticipated to be equal with either closed or open treatment, the closed method is advocated. Certain surgeons experienced in various operative methods may occasionally improve on the usual results from surgery. The majority of us, however, are most consistently of benefit to our patients when we skillfully apply effective closed treatment. We still serve our patients better as physicians helping them to avoid surgery than as surgeons convincing them that we must operate.

All texts such as this one are merely guides, not bibles. All fracture texts quickly become outdated but the basic principles tend to prevail. When possible in this guide through the pitfalls of fracture management, I have emphasized and pointed out what I consider to be basic concepts. However, even basic concepts change and every textbook is subject to revision. It has been my pleasure and my education to revise this one.

JOHN F. CONNOLLY

Omaha, Nebraska
November, 1980

ACKNOWLEDGMENT

I want to acknowledge my sincere appreciation for all the many skilled people at W. B. Saunders Company and at the University of Nebraska who have helped me so generously.

Particularly, I extend my thanks to Carroll Cann, Medical Editor, and Brian Decker, former Medical Editor, for their encouragement and thoughtful editorial advice and to Janet Macnamara for her persistent and consistent care in editing the entire text. Bob Butler, Production Coordinator, has maintained and controlled all the many facets and pieces of the manuscript and illustrations, and Rita Ann Conte has worked with the innumerable illustrations and synchronized the details necessary for such a combined text and atlas. Nina McDaid Ikeda has guided us through the design and arrangement problems of this work, and Terry Russell has compiled the index, which is always an important part of a textbook of this nature. Patti Maddaloni deserves recognition for her hard work and thought in doing the layout.

Steve McCoy, who has contributed more than 2,000 new illustrations to this edition, deserves considerable credit for the three years he has been a willing and capable co-worker. Finally to Liz Tretter, our Administrative Assistant, I owe and acknowledge my deep gratitude for her consistently accurate and effective help and support in the numerous manuscript revisions, reviews and retypings.

To these and to so many other skilled people who have given freely of their time and advice goes my sincere thank you.

JOHN F. CONNOLLY, M.D., F.A.C.S.

A series of audiovisual programs covering particular pitfalls in fracture management are available in slide tape and videocassette format. The topics covered and based on the content of this book are:

1. General Principles, Part I

2. General Principles, Part II

3. Pitfalls of Epiphyseal and Physeal Fractures

4. Pitfalls of Fractures and Dislocations of the Cervical Spine

5. Pitfalls of Fractures and Dislocations of the Thoracic and Lumbar Spine

6. Pitfalls of Fractures and Dislocations of the Pelvis

7. Pitfalls of Fractures and Dislocations of the Clavicle and Shoulder Girdle

8. Pitfalls of Subluxations and Dislocations of the Shoulder

9. Pitfalls of Humeral Fractures

10. Pitfalls of Elbow Fractures and Dislocations

11. Pitfalls of Forearm Fractures

12. Pitfalls of Fractures in the Region of the Wrist

13. Pitfalls of Fractures, Dislocations, and Other Injuries to the Metacarpals and Phalanges

14. Pitfalls of Dislocations and Fracture Dislocations of the Hip

15. Pitfalls of Femoral Fractures

16. Pitfalls of Injuries to the Soft Tissues and Bone Elements of the Knee

17. Pitfalls of Tibia Fractures

18. Pitfalls of Ankle Injuries

19. Pitfalls of Foot Injuries

20. Pitfalls of Pathologic Fractures

Further information on the audiovisual instructional programs is available from: Media Librarian, Biomedical Communications Center, University of Nebraska Medical Center, 42nd and Dewey Avenue, Omaha, NE 68105.

CONTENTS

VOLUME 1

Principles

Injuries to Physes and Epiphyses

Injuries of the Cervical Spine

Dislocations, Fractures, and Fracture-Dislocations of the Thoracic and Lumbar Spine

Fractures and Dislocations of the Pelvis

Injuries to the Thoracic Cage

Volume 2

Fractures and Dislocations in the Region of the Wrist

Fractures and Dislocations of the Hand

Dislocations and Fracture-Dislocations of the Hip and Acetabulum

Fractures of the Femur

Injuries of the Soft Tissues and Bony Elements of the Knee Joint

Fractures of the Tibia and Fibula

Injuries of the Ankle: Sprains, Dislocations, and Fractures

Fractures and Fracture-Dislocations of the Bones of the Foot

Birth Fractures and Pathologic Fractures

Appendix

PRINCIPLES

DEFINITIONS AND CAUSES

Fracture

DEFINITION

A fracture is a complete or incomplete break in the continuity of a bone.

1. Complete break in the continuity of the shaft of the femur.
2. Greenstick fracture, or incomplete break in the continuity of the shaft of the radius and the ulna.

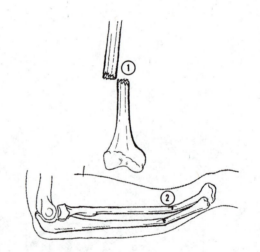

Factors Responsible for Fractures

A. Direct violence applied to the bone also damages surrounding soft tissue.
  1. A tapping force applied to the tibia produces an oblique fracture.
  2. A crushing injury results in a fragmented fracture of the tibia and fibula.
  3. A penetrating direct injury from a high-velocity gunshot blast destroys bone and soft tissue.

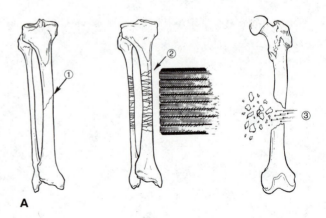

A

B. Indirect violence applied to the bone produces significantly less damage to soft and hard tissues.

1. An abduction force applied to the knee causes a compression of the external tibial condyle.
2. A forceful contraction of the rotator muscles of the shoulder avulses the greater tuberosity of the humerus.
3. Falling on the outstretched hand causes a fracture of the head of the radius.

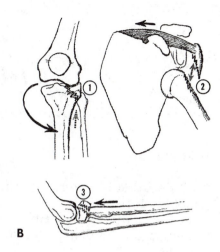
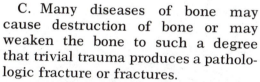

B

C. Many diseases of bone may cause destruction of bone or may weaken the bone to such a degree that trivial trauma produces a pathologic fracture or fractures.

1. Fracture of the femur invaded by an osteogenic sarcoma.
2. Fracture of the humerus through a bone cyst.
3. Fracture of the tibia and fibula in a case of osteogenesis imperfecta.
4. Fracture of the shaft of the femur in a case of bone metastasis from a breast cancer.

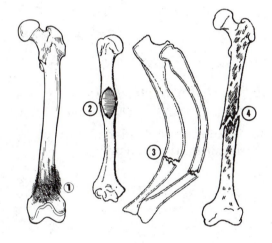

D. In repeated stresses, which cause fatigue fractures, no bone disease is demonstrable; these stress fractures are most frequently encountered in bones of the lower extremity.

1. Fatigue fracture of the three middle metatarsal bones.
2. Fatigue fracture of the shaft of the tibia.
3. Fatigue fracture of the neck of the femur.

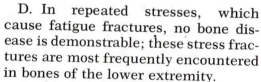
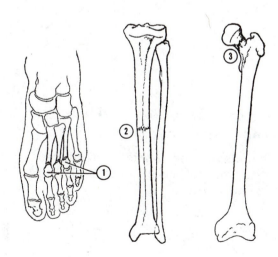

3

Dislocation

DEFINITION

A dislocation is a complete (luxation) or partial (subluxation) separation of a joint.

The dislocation is described as anterior, posterior, medial, or lateral, depending on the displacement of the distal bone relative to the proximal bone.

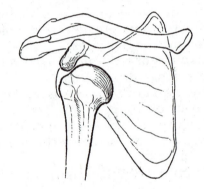

Anterior Dislocation of the Shoulder

The humerus is displaced out of, and anterior to, the glenoid.

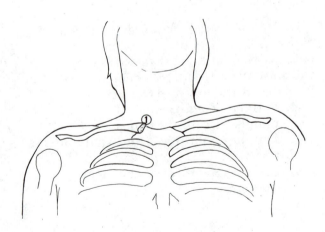

Anterior Subluxation of the Sternoclavicular Joint

The clavicle is partially displaced anterior to, and out of its articulation with, the sternum.

MECHANISMS PRODUCING DISLOCATION

In contrast to fractures, dislocations result most often from indirect mechanisms when the force is transmitted along the bone to its articulation. Only rarely is the joint dislocated by a direct blow.

Indirect Mechanism

1. A posterior hip dislocation results from a forceful blow to the distal femur.

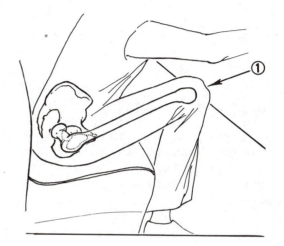

Direct Mechanism

1. A direct blow to the front of the joint produces a posterior dislocation of the shoulder. This is much less frequent than an anterior dislocation resulting from an indirect mechanism.

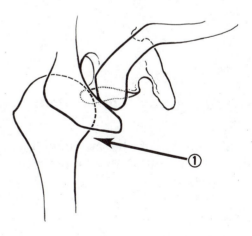

SUBLUXATION

Subluxations or partial dislocations result from laxity of the supporting structures surrounding the joint. This may be from congenital or traumatic conditions or from joint effusions or disuse atrophy.

Voluntary Subluxation

1. A voluntary posterior subluxation of the shoulder is due to congenital or acquired laxity of the capsular support and voluntary muscle contraction.

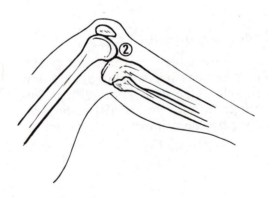

Subluxation from Ligamentous Injury

2. Disruption of the cruciate ligament produces posterior subluxation of the knee.

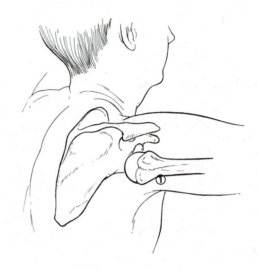

Subluxation from Joint Effusion

1. Pus accumulating from sepsis in an infant's hip joint readily causes subluxation of the joint.

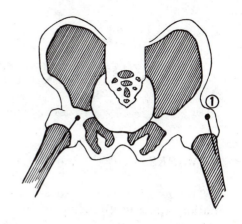

Subluxation from Disuse Muscle Atrophy

2. Prolonged immobilization for a humeral fracture and failure to exercise the support muscle results in inferior subluxation of the injured shoulder.

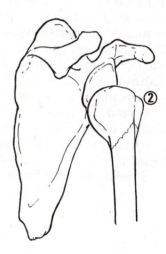

7

TYPES OF FRACTURES

The general pattern of a fracture is determined by the point of application and the direction of the causative violence as well as the intensity of the force. Other factors play a role, such as the age, the resiliency, and the structure (e.g., compact or cancellous) of the bone.

The type of fracture often gives a clue to the method of reduction and the techniques of immobilization that are most likely to give the maximal result.

In addition to the break in bone, there is always associated injury to surrounding soft tissues structures and quite frequently, injury to tissues and organs distant from the bone lesion.

The soft tissues in close proximity to the fracture site, particularly the periosteum, muscles, tendons, arteries, and nerves, are all likely to be injured. Evaluate the CMS, the circulation, and motor and sensory functions distal to the fractures as well as the fracture itself.

In certain fractures, such as surgical neck fracture of the humerus and open fracture of the tibia, treatment of the soft tissue wound is the key to success. Always evaluate the status of soft tissues and check to determine whether the fracture is open to the external environment or closed before embarking on treatment.

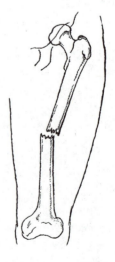

Closed Fracture

The fracture does not communicate with the external environment.

Open Fracture

The fracture site communicates with the external environment and is treated from the beginning as an infected wound. The size of the wound is no sure indication of the degree of contamination. Some of the worst infections occur from puncture wounds or following open fractures sustained in water.

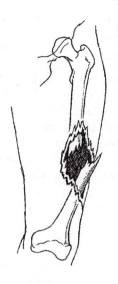

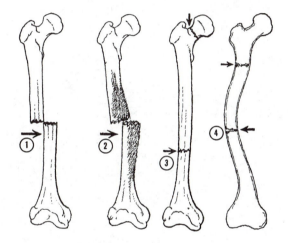

Transverse Fracture

1. Usually produced by a bending force applied directly to the fracture site with associated soft tissue injury. This is also the usual pattern noted in pathologic fractures that occur with
2. Paget's disease,
3. Osteomalacia or Milkman's syndrome, and
4. Osteogenesis imperfecta.

Oblique Fracture

Usually produced by a torsional force with an upward thrust.

The fracture ends are short and bluntly rounded and tend to slip by each other unless the surfaces interlock.

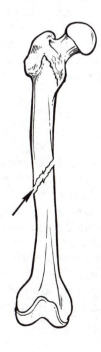

Spiral Fracture

Produced by a twisting or rotatory force, usually an indirect violence, which results in less soft tissue injury. The fracture ends are long, sharp, and pointed like a pen nib.

Because of the indirect nature of this injury, with less damage to circulation, healing is rapid and bony union is the rule.

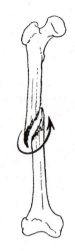

Compression Fractures

IN CHILDREN

These occur in children under the age of ten, in whom bone is more likely to fail when compressed than when bent.

1. Greenstick fracture occurs when the bone is bent and fails on the side subjected to compression.

2. Bone remains intact on the side subjected to tension force. This intact fracture should be completed or the deformity will spring back like a green stick.

3. A torus or buckle fracture is caused by compression force in the long axis of the bone.

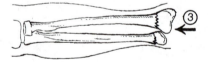

IN ADULTS

1. A compression fracture is usually produced by indirect violence applied to bone that is mostly cancellous. In this instance, the lateral femoral condyle is driven into the lateral tibial condyle.

2. Another common site for compression fracture is the vertebral body. Generally, one or more of the lower dorsal or upper lumbar bodies are compressed.

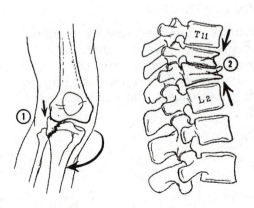

10

IN DISEASED BONE

When the bone is diseased, trivial trauma may produce severe compression of the bone. In most instances, anatomic reduction is impossible.

1. Osteomalacia or osteoporosis.

2. Myeloma or metastasis to bone from visceral carcinoma.

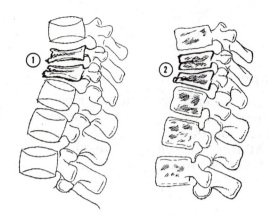

Comminuted Fracture

1. Produced by severe direct violence.

2. There are always more than two fragments.

3. Associated soft tissue injuries are frequently severe.

Reduction is difficult to achieve and maintain.

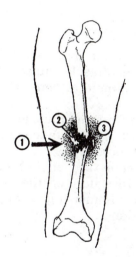

Segmental Fracture

1. Severe direct violence at several locations on long bone

2. Results in fractures in proximal and distal segments of the bone with a long, devascularized segment between.

Reduction is difficult and union is slow.

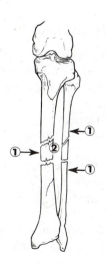

11

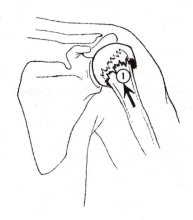

Impacted Fracture

1. Produced by indirect violence, which drives the bone fragments firmly together.

All fragments move in unison.

Union is rapid.

Avulsion Fracture

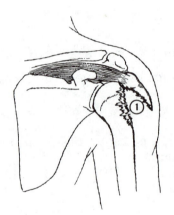

Produced by forcible resisted contraction of a muscle mass, which pulls off a fragment of bone at its site of insertion.

1. Here the rotator muscles (chiefly the supraspinatus) have pulled off the greater tuberosity.

Similar lesions are encountered at the site of insertion of the patellar tendon, the hamstrings, and the Achilles tendon.

Fracture-Dislocations

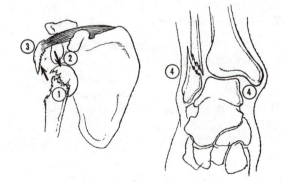

In addition to a fracture of one or more of the bony components of a joint there is subluxation or dislocation of the joint.

Here, in addition to:

1. Fracture of the upper end of the humerus.

2. There is a dislocation of the glenohumeral joint and

3. Avulsion of the greater tuberosity.

4. These are common lesions in the region of the ankle joint.

12

REPAIR OF FRACTURES

Repair of a fracture is primarily a local function of the tissues involved, but such factors as a patient's age, the character of the fracture, and the presence of systemic disorders or bone disease may affect the rate and effectiveness of the repair process significantly.

Fracture repair is a unique body process, since normal bone is regenerated rather than healed by scar.

New bone forms either through appositional ossification without initial cartilage formation or by enchondral ossification of a preliminary fibrocartilage callus. In both instances, the ossification process is intimately related to revascularization, and the active osteoblasts appear to be derived from either the walls of the small vessels or from circulating blood cells.

Bone repair takes place in the periosteal, cortical, and medullary regions, but most of the revascularization of a fracture is from medullary circulation. Which of these areas predominates in the repair process depends on the nature of the bone, the degree of initial injury, and the amount of fracture immobilization during healing.

The most rapid of all the processes of healing is the external or periosteal callus, which predominates in fractures treated nonoperatively and with early muscle function. It depends primarily on surrounding soft tissue blood supply. This callus is quite tolerant of controlled fracture motion; in fact it is most in evidence when fracture motion occurs, e.g., in rib fractures.

A second process is late medullary callus, which predominates when the external callus has failed. It is assisted by rigid immobilization and is the predominant healing process with compression plate fixation. Intramedullary callus, as McKibbon has pointed out, is not an evanescent burst of activity but a process that seems to pursue its goal of fracture bridging relentlessly.

The third process is that of primary bone union that explains the rare phenomenon of healing without external callus. It depends on the mechanism of bone turnover, which is occurring at all times and which can respond to bridge fractured bone cortices, provided that they are rigidly immobilized. By this process the dead cortical bone immediately adjacent to the fracture is invaded by new, longitudinally oriented osteones from the neighboring live bone. The major disadvantage of primary bone union is its great slowness and its dependence on rigid immobilization.

In most instances with compression plating, the fracture gap is sufficiently large that it fills first by bone formed through appositional growth inward from the external periosteal source. This primary bone forms rapidly in the first 4–6 weeks but has relatively poor attachment to the avascular bone ends. This primary callus must be remodeled and replaced at 6–8 weeks by secondary osteones bridging the fracture gap longitudinally.

The entire process of healing in bone as well as in soft tissue is dependent on the process of revascularization. This has been well-described by Rhinelander.

Examples of Fracture Healing Processes

Initial Injury

1. The continuity of the periosteum, cortical bone, and medullary trabeculae is broken.

2. Injured muscle and surrounding soft tissue.

3. Hematoma must be infiltrated or eliminated to allow bridging of the gap.

4. Dead osteocytes.

5. Empty haversian canals.

Note: Osteocytes and osteogenic cells in the vicinity of the fracture die.

6. Undamaged haversian canals from which vascular osteogenesis begins.

7. Cambium layer of periosteum, which forms primary intramembranous bone as well as fibrocartilage callus.

8. Fibrous layer of periosteum seals off callus from external soft tissues.

Note: This fracture may be treated with or without internal fixation.

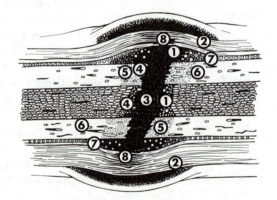

HEALING BY EXTERNAL CALLUS FORMATION AND NONOPERATIVE FIXATION

Four to Six Weeks after Injury

1. The fracture gap is still open but has been filled with cartilage.

2. Some bone has been formed on the cortical fragments by appositional ossification.

3. The haversian canals are slowly being revascularized.

4. Medullary revascularization is occurring rapidly.

5. Bone spicules promote appositional new bone formation.

6. The fibrous layer of periosteum has sealed off the calus.

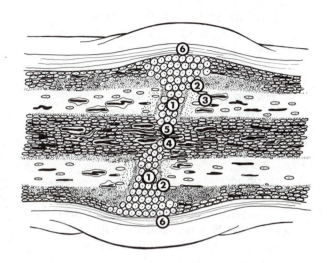

Healing at Eight to Twelve Weeks

1. Vascular bridging of the external cartilage has produced endchondral ossification and an external callus. This callus is oriented perpendicular to the fractured cortices.

2. The longitudinal bridging of the fracture occurs in the medullary canal.

3. Some bridging through the fracture cortices is occurring as a result of haversian remodeling.

4. Remodeling will continue to form longitudinal osteones and increase the bone strength.

Note: This is in contrast to the remodeling process with plate fixation, which tends to resorb and weaken the cortices (see page 17).

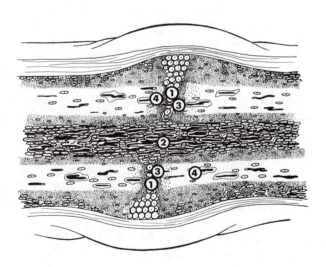

HEALING AFTER COMPRESSION PLATING

1. The fracture gap is closed by the rigid compression plate.

2. The irregular areas of dead cortical bone adjacent to the fracture must be replaced.

3. Periosteal ingrowth forms appositional bone paralleling the fracture.

4. Haversian canals are revascularized by new vascular ingrowth.

5. Cutting cones of vessels slowly channel through the area of dead bone.

Note: The cutting cones are the mechanisms of normal bone turnover occurring all the time in the skeleton.

6. Appositional bone is being laid down on the fractured trabeculae.

7. Medullary revascularization is proceeding rapidly.

8. Osteoblasts associated with the capillary endothelium form osteoid.

9. Osteoclasts in the cutting cones resorb dead bone and make room for further capillary invasion.

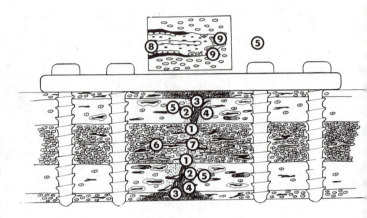

Secondary Osteon Formation Six to Ten Week After Plating

1. The medullary osteons and vessels have bridged the fracture gap longitudinally.

2. The appositional bone formed by periosteal ingrowth is resorbed as the cutting cones bridge the fractured cortices longitudinally.

3. Healing is occurring with no or minimal external callus.

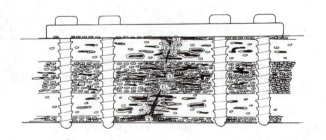

Remodelling Ten Weeks and Later

1. Some residual primary bone persists.
2. Longitudinal reorientation predominates.
3. Bone integrity is restored, but the porosity will increase and the bone strength will decrease if the rigid plate continues to absorb the forces of loading.

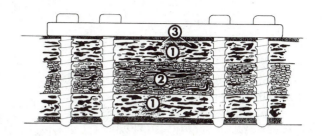

Circulation in Bone and Fracture Healing (after Rhinelander)

REMARKS

Fracture healing is utterly dependent on the process of revascularization. To appreciate the fracture healing processes one must first comprehend the normal and the altered circulatory hydrodynamics.

The major blood supply to bone is from the medullary canal and flows centrifugally. Arterioles from the medullary circulation supply the inner two thirds of the cortex.

Periosteal arterioles supply the outer third of the cortex. Periosteal circulation is intimately involved with the circulation of muscles, and muscular pumping is important for revascularization of external callus in displaced fractures.

Revascularization of the cortex and longitudinal osteon formation across the fracture gap depends primarily on medullary circulation.

1. Medullary arteries supply the inner two thirds of the cortex.

2. The outer third of the cortex is supplied by periosteal vessels.

3. An intimate anastomosis exists between muscle and periosteal vessels and becomes important for revascularization of a healing fracture.

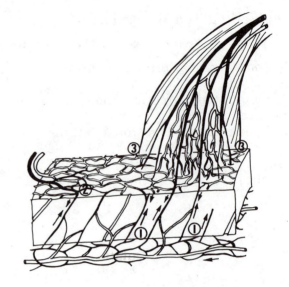

4. A microangiogram of a slightly displaced fracture shows longitudinal bridging by medullary vessels, which are responsible for the new osteon formation.

5. Periosteal vascular pattern is perpendicular to the cortical surface and is limited to external callus.

6. Cortical revascularization and longitudinal bridging are the products of the medullary inflow into the fracture gap.

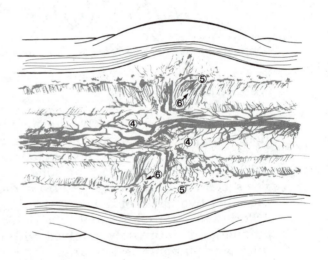

Fracture Healing After Intramedullary Nailing

REMARKS

Medullary blood supply is vital for revascularization of the fracture gap. So resilient, however, is the medullary circulation that even after intramedullary reaming and nailing the centrifugal flow pattern is restored rapidly.

1. Healing is occurring six weeks after intramedullary nailing.

2. The fracture line is still evident.

3. Union is primarily by external callus.

4. New bone is formed appositionally from periosteum directly onto fracture fragments.

5. Enchondral ossification of fibro-cartilage slowly fills in the fracture.

6. Remodeling and longitudinal reorientation of the osteons depend on revascularization by medullary circulation.

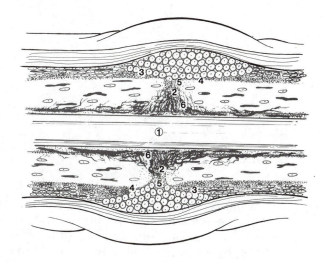

Delayed Union and Nonunion (Twelve Weeks)

1. Fracture gap is still open and is filled with fibrocartilage.

2. External callus is pronounced.

3. Some bone has formed in the external callus but has not bridged the fracture gap.

4. Intramedullary vessels form a border trying to penetrate the fibro-cartilage and lay down bridging osteons.

5. Cortical bone has become porotic from resorption, but longitudinal bridging has not been effected.

Note: Union is still possible if longitudinal revascularization occurs. This may require more time, more rigid fixation, or the use of bone grafts to aid in revascularization and osteon formation.

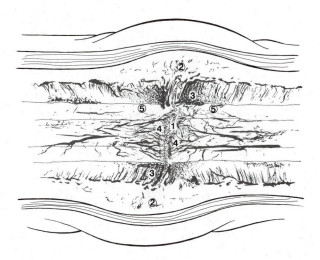

Rate of Union

REMARKS

The rate of union is influenced by the bone fractured, the type of fracture, the method of treatment, the general health of the patient, and, especially, the patient's age. Infants heal most fractures in four to six weeks. Adolescents heal most fractures in six to ten weeks. Adults heal more slowly, and in any patient older than 20 years, age makes little difference in the rate of healing. Some fractures in adults may require 16 to 20 weeks to heal without being considered delayed union.

CONDITIONS INFLUENCING RATE OF HEALING

Favorable Conditions

Fracture at ends of bone where bone is cancellous and blood supply is excellent.

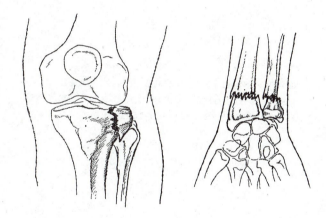

There is adequate blood supply to both fragments.

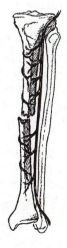

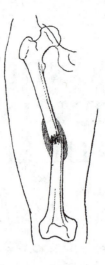
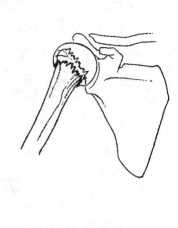

Soft tissue injury is minimal, and fracture reduction is end to end.

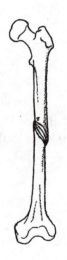

Long spiral fracture has been caused by indirect torsional loading with minimal soft tissue damage.

Fracture of the neck of the femur:

1. The femoral head is in valgus sufficient to make all stresses at the fracture site the compression type and never the shearing type. This is true in both anteroposterior and lateral views.

2. The Knowles pins are parallel to the inferior cortex of the neck of the femur and penetrate the head as far as the subcortical bone.

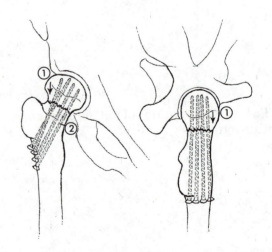

Fracture site is free of infection.

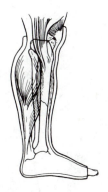

Muscle function is encouraged by weight bearing, which also promotes impaction and contributes to extra-osseous revascularization of the fracture site.

Unfavorable Conditions

Wide separation of fractured ends.

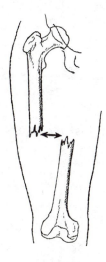

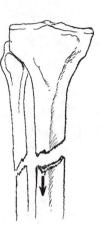

Distraction of bone ends by traction.

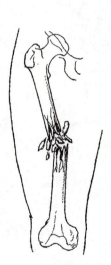

Severe comminution of the affected bone and damage to surrounding soft tissues.

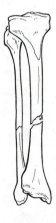

Bone has been lost by injury or surgical excision.

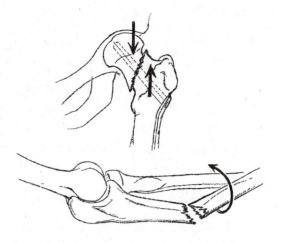

Inadequate fracture fixation has allowed rotary forces to act at the fracture site.

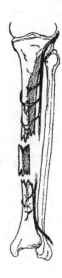

Impairment or loss of blood supply to one or both fragments.

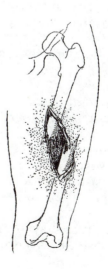

Infection.

Note: Repair may be delayed by such systemic disorders as diabetes, alcoholism, and malnutrition.

COMPLICATIONS OF FRACTURES

REMARKS

Complications will occur with any injury. They may be limb-threatening or life-threatening. By his awareness and anticipation of these numerous complications, the physician may prevent or significantly mitigate them.

Complications may result from the trauma to the bone itself, the disruption of surrounding soft tissue structures, or injury to tissues and organs at a distance from the fracture. Complications may also arise from the fracture treatment, either closed or open.

Common complications from the fracture itself include:
1. Delayed union.
2. Nonunion.
3. Ischemic necrosis.
4. Angular deformities or malunion.
5. Shortening.
6. Growth arrest.
7. Growth stimulation.
8. Infection.

Common complications from disruption of adjacent soft tissues and viscera include:
1. Injuries to blood vessels.
2. Injuries to nerves.
3. Injuries to tendons.
4. Injuries to lung, bowel, bladder, spinal cord, and associated structures.

Complications in tissues and organs at a distance from the fracture include:
1. Shock.
2. Fat embolism.
3. Malignant hyperthermia.
4. Joint stiffness.
5. Sympathetic reflex dystrophy (Sudeck's atrophy).
6. Myositis ossificans.
7. Post-traumatic arthritis.

Complications to be avoided with either closed or open treatment include:
1. Tight cast syndrome.
2. Loose cast syndrome.

3. Cast-induced injuries to neurovascular structures.
4. Traction-induced injuries to neurovascular structures.
5. Postoperative wound necrosis and infection.
6. Bone loss or excision.
7. Inadequate internal fixation.

Delayed Union and Nonunion

REMARKS

Rate of healing is governed by many factors, such as the patient's age, the bone involved, the constitution of the patient, the site of the fracture, the prevailing local conditions, the method of management, and, most important, the degree of initial injury.

In a state of delayed union, the process of repair, although slower than average, is still active.

In an established nonunion the reparative process has terminated and union is not possible without intervention.

Systemic disorders play a very minor role in the type and outcome of the reparative process.

Although the reparative process is most active in the young, the aged are very capable of adequate fracture healing; most nonunions occur in the long bones of persons less than 40 years of age.

Multiple injuries may give priority of treatment to systems other than the skeletal system; this should not prevent adequate fracture treatment nor enhance the likelihood of nonunion.

LOCAL FACTORS INFLUENCING FRACTURE HEALING

Uncontrollable Factors

Bone fractured. Some bones, such as the carpal scaphoid, are more prone to develop delayed union or nonunion than others.

Site of fracture. Certain sites in a given bone, such as the diaphysis of the tibia, heal less readily than others.

Degree of displacement of the fragments. Wide separation is indicative of much periosteal stripping and rupture of the vascular channels to the fragments.

Severe damage of soft tissues surrounding the fragments.

Open fracture. This is usually associated with severe soft tissue damage.

Infection. Usually infection is superimposed on an open fracture or on a closed fracture that has been opened surgically.

Controllable Factors

This is where the physician may inadvertently become part of the patient's disease. Anticipating the complications is safer than meeting them head-on.

Select appropriate treatment for a given fracture; for example, closed methods are preferable to open procedures if results of the two methods are comparable.

Achieve adequate reduction with good apposition of fracture fragments and elimination of shear and rotatory forces on the fracture. The femoral neck fracture fixed in a varus position is an excellent example of how this principle may be violated.

Fix the fracture until it heals, either with an adequately applied plaster cast or mechanically sound internal fixation.

Encourage impaction of the fracture and active muscle function during healing. Avoid distraction of the fracture either from excessive traction or from internal fixation that holds the fracture ends apart.

Respect soft tissues as well as bone, and prevent infection. The policy of leaving open fractures open if there is any doubt about the degree of contamination or the adequacy of debridement is the best insurance against infection.

CLINICAL FEATURES OF DELAYED UNION OR NONUNION

Pain at the fracture site is the most significant indicator that the fracture has not united. The patient who can bear weight or gentle stress at the fracture is well on his way to healing.

Tenderness can always be elicited over a site of delayed union or nonunion.

Motion, either in the form of obvious free movement or a rubbery spring when gentle stress is applied, attests to the failure of union. Frequently, this motion should be confirmed radiographically.

Radiographic Features

DELAYED UNION

1. Ends of fragments exhibit slight bone resorption and have a woolly appearance; there is no evidence of sclerosis.

2. The medullary canal is open at ends of both fragments.

3. Fracture line is wide and clearly visible.

4. External and internal callus is absent or minimal.

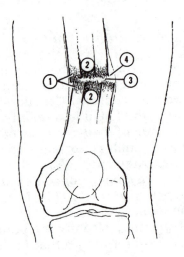

Nonunion

REMARKS

Always take anteroposterior, lateral, and oblique projections.

Serial x-rays over several months are essential to show the progress of fracture healing.

If fracture bridging is accomplished in the medullary region, the amount of external callus is not significant. External callus is needed if medullary bridging is slow.

Stress views showing fracture motion are necessary to confirm the impression of a nonunion.

1. Marked sclerosis and rounding of the bone ends.

2. Proximal fragment is convex and the distal is concave.

3. Medullary canal in each fragment is closed.

4. Fracture bridging is unsuccessful, so the gap persists between fragments.

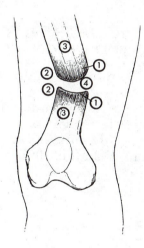

1. Large gap between bone ends from loss of bone.

2. Diffuse osteoporosis of both fragments.

3. Conical shape of the bone ends caused by absorption.

4. External callus is abundant, but fracture gap has not been bridged.

5. When nonunion is questionable, observe the effect of stress on the fracture by means of the fluoroscope. Demonstration of motion is diagnostic.

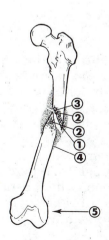

29

Nonunion (*Continued*)

1. Angulation at the fracture site.
2. Fracture of the bone plate and loose screws.
3. Wide, irregular gap between the bone ends and external callus.
4. Sclerosis of the bone ends.
5. Large amount of external callus without medullary bridging of the fracture.

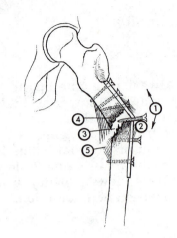

SITES OF PREDILECTION FOR DELAYED UNION

1. Fracture through shaft of humerus.
2. Fracture of lower third of ulna.
3. Fracture of scaphoid.
4. Fracture of femoral neck.
5. Fracture of shaft of tibia.

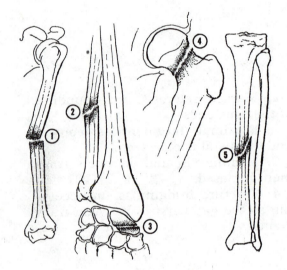

MANAGEMENT OF DELAYED UNION AND NONUNION

REMARKS

In addition to the severity of initial injury, the most common causes of delayed union are lack of muscle function or of active weight bearing necessary to impact the fracture and vascularize the callus, inadequate fracture fixation, fracture distraction, bone loss or excision, and infection.

If the diagnosis of delayed union is made early (at least before four months), elimination of the causes may avoid the need for operative treatment.

Surgical treatment becomes necessary in all cases of established nonunion, which usually should be determined by six months. However, electrical bone growth stimulation may be considered prior to surgical intervention.

TYPES OF PROBLEMS ASSOCIATED WITH NONUNION

Inadequate Muscle Function and Fracture Impaction

1. Shaft of the humerus was at one time a prime candidate for delayed union when shoulder spicas and other devices were used in attempted rigid fracture immobilization.

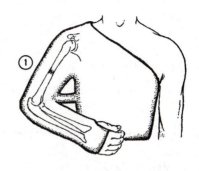

2. More success has resulted from allowing muscle contraction and fracture impaction by less restrictive but adequate fracture casts.

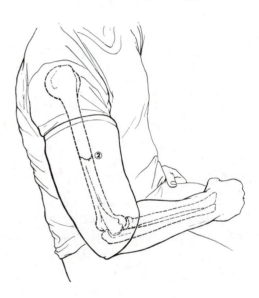

Incomplete Fracture Fixation

1. A loose-fitting intramedullary nail after open reduction inhibits medullary healing as well as periosteal callus.

2. Weight bearing with additional external cast brace fixation encourages fracture impaction and bridging of the fracture.

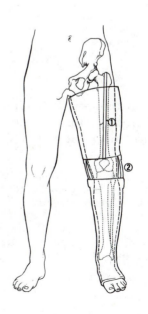

Fracture Distraction

1. Gaps created by bone loss should not be maintained by treatment.

2. Avoid continuous distraction by pin in plaster or

3. By internal fixation.

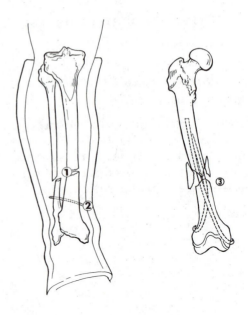

Bone Loss

Avoid surgical excision of bone. If bone gap has been created by the injury, plan early bone grafting.

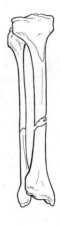

Infection

1. Infection frequently begins with wound necrosis from excessively tight closure necessitated by plate fixation.

Note: Early use of antibiotics, prompt wound treatment and debridement, and avoidance of primary closures of open fractures are the most effective ways to prevent fracture infection. If plates are used, they should be applied away from the side of the incision.

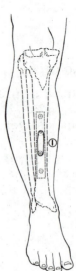

Operative Management of Delayed Union and Nonunion

REMARKS

A state of delayed union persisting for six months and established nonunions require intervention to stimulate osteogenesis.

Each case must be treated individually depending on the nature of the underlying problem and the skills of the physician. For example, fractures with initial extensive bone loss may need bone graft as a primary procedure.

Delayed union and nonunion may be treated by electrical bone growth stimulation, bone grafting, rigid internal fixation, or a combination of these methods.

ELECTRICAL BONE GROWTH STIMULATION

Electrical bone growth stimulation is a new but fairly well proven technique of inducing osteogenesis by applying direct current to the fracture site.

The current is applied to the bone by electrodes placed percutaneously (semi-invasive technique), or by pulsing electromagnetic fields that are inductively coupled across the skin to the bone (noninvasive technique).

Whether the mechanism of action is to decrease local oxygen or increase local pH, the result of the stimulation is vascular osteogenesis at the fracture site and intramedullary callus formation.

Semi-invasive Method of Electrical Bone Growth Stimulation (After Brighton and Coworkers)

This technique has been most widely reported but is still subject to review and modification.

It is especially effective in the early stages of delayed union and nonunion, from six to ten months, and entails much lower morbidity for the patient than standard bone grafting.

Note: This procedure should be done in the operating room with surgical preparation and fluoroscopic guidance.

1. With the patient under local anesthesia, four insulated 1.2-mm stainless steel Kirschner wires are placed in holes drilled into the proximal and distal fracture fragments.

2. The cathodes are connected with a battery, which includes field effect transistors and resistors in circuit to deliver a constant 20-microampere current to each cathode.

3. The anode is applied externally to the patient's skin.

4. Monitoring leads allow measurement of the current for the twelve weeks of stimulation.

5. A cast is used for fracture immobilization and is changed as necessary until the fracture is healed.

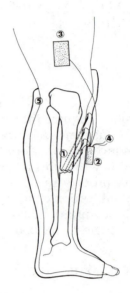

AUTOGENOUS BONE GRAFTING PROCEDURES

REMARKS

Autogenous bone grafts promote bony union of ununited fractures by introducing viable bone-forming cells and by providing the small vessels at the fracture site with a matrix across which the fracture may be bridged and vascular osteogenesis may occur. Transfer of the bone graft to the prepared bed without intermediate storage or prolonged exposure to air maximizes the graft's viability and effectiveness.

The fracture site should not be resected, but the bed for the graft should be made sufficiently vascular to allow vascular ingrowth into the graft.

The bone graft should be matchstick in size and cancellous in structure to allow most rapid vascular ingrowth.

Technique of Obtaining Graft

1. The graft is obtained from just beneath the patient's iliac crest.

2. The iliac crest is turned superiorly.

3. Multiple cortical-cancellous strips are cut with a bone gauge.

4. The iliac crest is returned to the normal position so that closure will not leave a palpable defect.

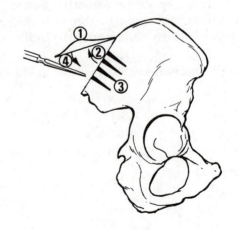

Nonunion of the Tibia

This fracture accounts for the majority of cases of nonunion requiring electrical stimulation or bone graft.

1. Fibrous tissue between the bone ends.

2. Sclerosis of the bone ends.

3. Obliteration of the medullary canal.

4. Exuberant external callus.

Note: A fracture with a large gap or bone defect is more suitable for bone graft than for electrical stimulation.

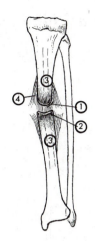

Application of Cancellous Bone Graft

1. The fracture site is not disturbed but cortical bone is shingled to encourage vascular ingrowth into the graft.

2. Fibula is osteotomized to allow fracture apposition.

3. Cancellous bone graft is packed about the fracture.

Note: Weight-bearing ambulation promotes fracture impaction and helps vascularize the graft after the procedure.

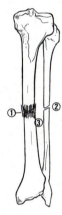

Inlay and Sliding Inlay Grafts

REMARKS

The chief advantage of these methods is simplicity. They are especially suited for nonunions of the tibia and femur.

Inlay and Sliding Inlay Grafts *(Continued)*

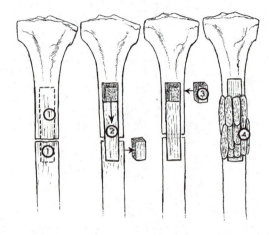

INLAY GRAFT

1. A trough is made across the non-union.

2. A graft of same dimension as the trough is removed from the opposite tibia.

3. Graft is in trough and spans the nonunion.

4. Surround the site of nonunion with cancellous matchstick grafts.

SLIDING INLAY GRAFT

1. Parallel cuts are made through the cortex of both fragments with a double-bladed bone saw.

2. Remove the short graft and push the longer graft across the non-union into the trough of the shorter fragment.

3. Place short graft in the remaining defect.

4. Surround the nonunion with cancellous bone.

Dual Onlay Graft

REMARKS

This graft is useful for (1) bridging of large defects, (2) nonunion in osteoporotic bones, (3) nonunion near a joint, and (4) nonunion with severe sclerosis of the bone ends. When the method is used for bridging defects, the trough made by the graft should be packed with cancellous chip grafts.

1. Cortical grafts span the defect and extend from good bone above to good bone below.

2. The screws traverse both grafts.

3. The defect is packed with endosteum from the grafts and cancellous chip grafts.

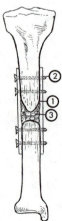

Bone Peg Grafts

REMARKS

These are most useful for nonunion in small bones such as the scaphoid and metacarpals.

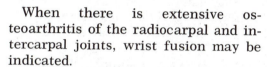

OPERATION FOR DELAYED UNION AND NONUNION OF THE CARPAL SCAPHOID

When there is no evidence of osteoarthritis at the radiocarpal and intercarpal joints:

1. Bone peg traverses and fixes both fragments.

2. Skin-tight plaster cast includes the thumb and extends from the hand to just below the elbow.

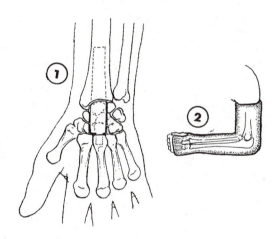

When there is extensive osteoarthritis of the radiocarpal and intercarpal joints, wrist fusion may be indicated.

1. Large tibial cortical graft extends from the radius into the base of the third metacarpal bone.

2. A circular plaster cast is applied from the hand to the upper arm.

For the individual who must retain joint mobility, a Volz wrist arthroplasty is indicated when post-traumatic arthritis is extensive.

1. The scaphoid, lunate, and proximal capitate are resected.

2. The Volz wrist joint is cemented into the second and third metacarpals and the distal radius.

3. Distal 2.5 cm (1 in) of the ulna is removed.

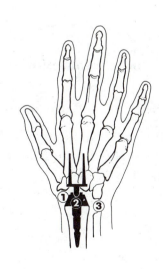

TREATMENT OF NONUNION BY RIGID FIXATION

REMARKS

When fracture bridging has failed because of incomplete immobilization, the addition of rigid fixation will promote healing.

Internal fixation with bone graft is indicated when the nonunion results from fracture distraction or excessive bone loss or is associated with malposition of the fracture that must be corrected.

Internal fixation by intramedullary nail is most useful for nonunion in the lower limb, whereas compression plating is applicable to nonunion of the arm and forearm.

A history of recent infection is a caution sign, but frequently the rigid internal support and adequate drainage eliminate the infection.

Nonunion of Tibia with Fracture Distraction

1. Fibula is healed but tibial fracture is distracted.

2. Valgus angulation has occurred.

3. There is no infection at the fracture.

4. After the tibial canal and the fracture site are reamed, a Lottes nail is inserted without excising the fracture callus.

5. 1.5 cm of fibula is resected.

6. Autogenous cancellous bone is packed at the fracture site.

Note: A weight-bearing cast is used for external immobilization until the fracture consolidates.

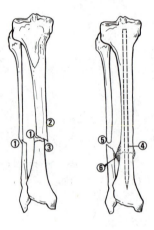

Delayed Union or Nonunion of the Femur

1. Fragments are aligned by intramedullary nail.

2. Cancellous matchstick grafts are placed around the fracture site.

Note: External support with a cast brace is useful for supplemental fixation until the fracture consolidates.

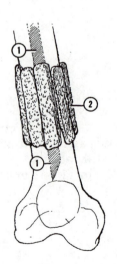

Delayed Union or Nonunion of the Neck of the Femur

RIGID FIXATION

1. Subtrochanteric osteotomy and abduction of the shaft of the femur.
2. Forces now acting at the fracture site are of the compression type.
3. Bone graft, triflanged nail, and plate.

Note: This method is of particular value in young patients; in elderly and debilitated patients, replacement of the femoral head by a prosthesis is the procedure of choice.

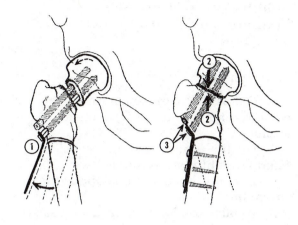

REPLACEMENT OF THE FEMORAL HEAD BY A PROSTHESIS

1. Vitallium prosthesis is used to replace the head and neck of the femur.
2. Methyl methacrylate cements the stem to stabilize its fit in the canal.

Note: This method is of special value in cases of delayed union or nonunion in the elderly.

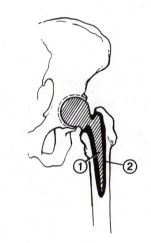

Compression Plating for Nonunion of Forearm Fractures

PREOPERATIVE X-RAY

1. Fibrous tissue between fragments of radius and ulna.
2. Defects in radius and ulna.
3. Sclerosis of bone ends.

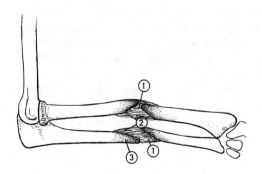

Compression Plating for Nonunion of Forearm Fractures (Continued)

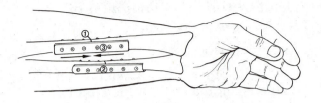

POSTOPERATIVE X-RAY

1. Callus and bone ends are resected only enough to allow application of plates.
2. On the ulna, a six-hole, tension-band straight plate is applied.
3. A semitubular plate is applied to the radius.
4. Application of a long arm cast for six weeks is followed by use of a short arm cast until union has occurred.

Note: Autogenous bone graft may be added if rigid compression does not close the fracture gap.

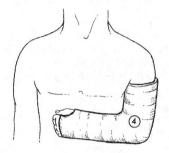

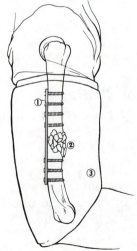

Nonunion of the Humerus

PREOPERATIVE X-RAY

1. Defect between bone ends.
2. Sclerosis of bone ends.
3. Fibrocartilage forms between bone ends.

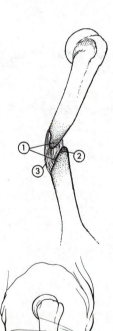

POSTOPERATIVE X-RAY

1. Alignment of the fragments is maintained by an eight-hole plate with good screw purchase on both cortices of the proximal and distal fragments. The plate is applied posteriorly to neutralize the bending moment on the nonunion.
2. Cancellous bone is placed around the nonunion.
3. A humeral cast allows active muscle contraction.

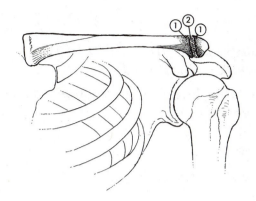

Nonunion of the Outer Quarter of the Clavicle

PREOPERATIVE X-RAY

1. Site of nonunion.
2. Fibrocartilage between fragments.

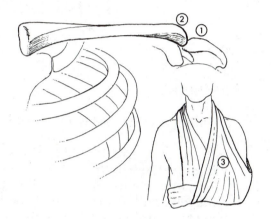

POSTOPERATIVE X-RAY

1. Excision of distal fragment.
2. Outer end of proximal fragment is rounded, and any disruption of the coracoclavicular ligament is repaired.
3. A sling is applied for postoperative immobilization.

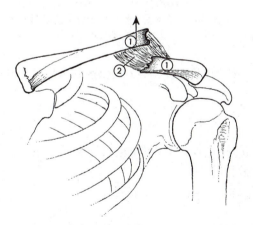

Nonunion of Other Parts of the Clavicle

PREOPERATIVE X-RAY

1. Site of nonunion with displacement of fragments.
2. Fibrocartilage between fragments.

POSTOPERATIVE X-RAY

1. The area of nonunion has been resected, and the bone fragments have been rongeured into small pieces.
2. The small bone pieces are reapplied to the area of nonunion, and the periosteum is closed over them.

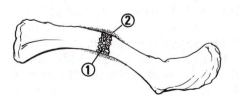

41

Nonunion of Other Parts of the Clavicle (Continued)

3. The clavicle is immobilized in a plaster velpeau.

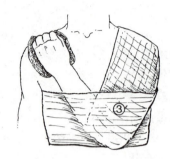

Infected Nonunion

REMARKS

The first objective is to control the infection while immobilizing the fracture.

If internal fixation has already been achieved by intramedullary nail, infection control is frequently possible without removing the nail.

Usually, when infection follows plating, the fixation device must be removed to allow drainage of the infection sequestered in the bone cortex. Open drainage and cast immobilization are then necessary to control the infection and permit future bone graft.

The methods of managing these serious complications vary, depending on the fracture and the degree of infection.

INFECTED NONUNION OF TIBIA

Posterolateral Autogenous Bone Grafting

PREOPERATIVE X-RAY

1. The fracture results from high-energy impact such as a motorcycle injury that leaves a defect in the tibia.

2. The fibula may or may not heal.

3. Drainage persists indefinitely from the injured tibia until union is achieved.

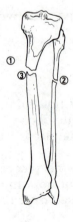

SURGICAL APPROACH

1. The fracture site is approached through the uninfected posterior compartment via an 18-cm (7-in) skin incision along the posterolateral border of the fibula.

2. The posterior compartment is entered, and the posterior tibial muscle is elevated along the intermuscular septum.

3. Cancellous grafts are applied subperiosteally to the tibia across the interosseous membrane to the fibula.

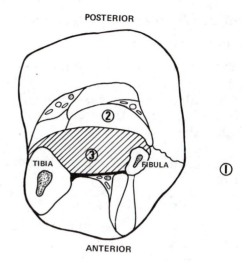

POSTOPERATIVE X-RAY

1. After the initial postoperative splints, a walking cast is applied until the graft bridges the posterior tibia and fibula.

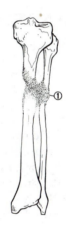

Bone Peg Operation

REMARKS

This procedure may be employed if posterolateral autogenous bone grafting is not feasible.

The bone pegs used may be cortical bank bone prepared to fit in 1-cm drill holes.

The pegs are placed close to the nonunion above and below.

A weight-bearing cast is applied until the union of the tibia occurs or the fibula hypertrophies sufficiently to take the stress of weight bearing.

Bone Peg Operation *(Continued)*

POSTOPERATIVE X-RAY

1. The site of nonunion is not disturbed.

2. Cortical bone pegs pass through the fibula and into the tibia above and below the nonunion.

3. At least four pegs above and four pegs below the nonunion should be used.

Note: The direction of the pegs.

4. The fibula is reinforced with strips of cortical bank bone.

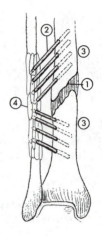

INFECTED NONUNION OF THE FEMUR AFTER PLATING

REMARKS

Single-plate fixation of femoral fractures is mechanically inadequate, and failure occurs when the screws pull out.

If infection is present, the plate should be removed to allow drainage of the infected cortical bone, and bone grafting should be delayed until the infection is controlled.

Because of the damage two procedures would inflict on cortical circulation, intramedullary nailing should be avoided after plating has failed.

PREOPERATIVE X-RAY

1. The plate has failed when the screws have loosened.

2. An infected nonunion exists and should be treated by removal of the plate and open drainage.

Note: A cast brace is used for external immobilization after plate removal.

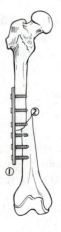

POSTOPERATIVE X-RAY

1. When the infection is controlled, the fracture site is approached laterally.

2. Cortical-cancellous sliding graft from the proximal femur is laid into the bed previously formed by the plate (see page 36).

3. Cancellous graft fills the fracture gap.

Note: External immobilization is continued with a cast brace until the fracture unites.

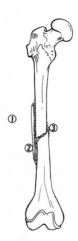

ONE-BONE-FOREARM TREATMENT FOR INFECTED NONUNION OF THE RADIUS AND ULNA

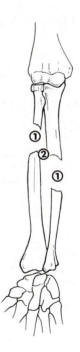

PREOPERATIVE X-RAY

1. Infection has left nonunion with 2-cm gaps in both the radius and the ulna.

2. The proximal ulna fragment is adjacent to the distal radius.

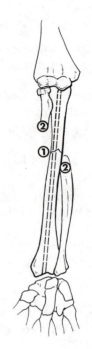

POSTOPERATIVE X-RAY

1. Rather than bone grafting both defects and producing an ankylosis of the bones, the proximal ulna is aligned to the distal radius and is fixed with intramedullary pins.

2. The remaining radial and ulnar fragments are left free.

INFECTED NONUNION OF THE ULNA

REMARKS

Grafting of large defects in the ulna may be unnecessary because of the stability from the interosseous membrane.

Forearm rotation may be diminished by attempted bone grafts. Allow the patient to use the forearm with the ulnar defect to determine what his range of motion and pain symptoms are before embarking on operative grafting of the defect.

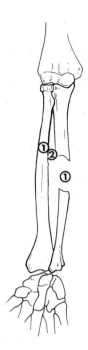

X-RAY

1. The ulna is frequently smashed by a high-energy injury, and an extensive gap may be produced.

2. The radius may be undamaged or may heal without a defect.

Note: Operative repair is usually not necessary. Forearm strength and motion may be quite satisfactory despite ulnar defect.

Ischemic Necrosis of Bone

REMARKS

Ischemic necrosis of bone implies death of bone resulting from impairment or total loss of its blood supply.

This disorder is a common cause of delayed union and nonunion, and when one surface of the bone constitutes an articular surface of a joint, osteoarthritis is a frequent sequela. Occasionally union may occur between dead and living fragments of bone.

Trauma is the most common cause of ischemic necrosis of bone, which is a frequent complication of (1) fracture of a bone close to its articular end, (2) dislocation, if the blood supply to the end of the bone is disrupted, and (3) infection, which occasionally may deprive the bone of its vital blood supply. In all instances there is serious disruption of the blood supply to the implicated bone.

Ischemic necrosis may be associated with metabolic disorders, alcoholism, infection, hematologic disorders such as sickle cell disease, and high-dose cortisone therapy.

PATHOLOGY

The problem begins most typically in the femoral head, with local stasis of flow to subchondral bone and death of the cellular elements within the compromised bone segment. This area of dead bone is frequently wedged-shaped and extends up to the articular cartilage.

The hyaline articular cartilage, which is nourished by synovial fluid, remains viable. When vascular ingrowth into the subchondral dead bone weakens the subchondral support, the viable articular surface collapses inward and becomes arthritic.

An early radiographic sign of ischemic necrosis is a crescent-shaped radiolucency beneath the articular cartilage produced by collapse of the subchondral bone.

Subsequent radiographic changes reflect mechanical alterations in the strength of the dead bone but are quite similar to changes seen in traumatic arthritis. The only true radiographic sign of dead bone is failure to change in density in comparison with surrounding bone, which increases or decreases in density.

Increased bone density occurs from impaction fractures of the fatigued, weakened ischemic bone and from new bone being laid down on dead trabeculae (creeping substitution).

Bone resorption occurs with vascular invasion, and the radiographic appearance of the femoral head becomes irregular, mottled, and cystic.

During the stage of revascularization, pressure on the affected fragment may produce marked distortion of the joint surface.

Radiographic changes may be confused with traumatic arthritis, although traumatic arthritis may be evident within 6 to 12 months, whereas ischemic necrosis tends to evolve 9 to 36 months after injury.

Complete replacement and restoration of normal density to the ischemic bone fragments requires many months or years. Generally, some distortion of the articular surface persists, and osteoarthritis is a common sequela.

COMMON SITES OF ISCHEMIC NECROSIS

Head of Femur

FRACTURE OF THE NECK OF THE FEMUR

1. Femoral head is dense and sclerotic.
2. Neck of femur is shortened by bone resorption.

Note: In high subcapital fractures such as this there is complete disruption of the capsular vessels; this sequela is also common in fractures of the neck in children when severe violence causes marked impairment of the blood supply.

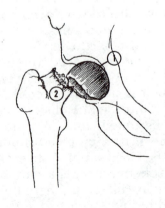

48

22 MONTHS AFTER FRACTURE OF THE NECK

There is ischemic necrosis of the femoral head.

1. Marked irregularity of the articular surface.

2. Fragmentation and collapse of the head.

3. Narrowing of joint space.

4. Site of neck fracture, which is now healed.

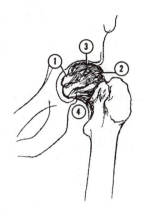

WITHOUT FRACTURE OR DISLOCATION

Sometimes necrosis is idiopathic, occurring with no history of injury to the head or neck.

1. A wedge-shaped segment of the femoral head has become ischemic.

2. Surrounding zone of viable bone is invading the ischemic bone and contributing to its fragmentation and collapse.

3. A crescent-shaped radiolucent zone follows collapse of dead subchondral bone.

4. The articular cartilage at the junction of the viable and dead bone becomes distorted and forms osteophytes.

Note: This condition is frequently bilateral and is associated with metabolic and hematologic disorders, alcoholism, and cortisone therapy, which increase intramedullary fat and impede bone blood flow.

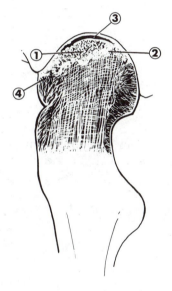

Proximal Half of the Scaphoid

1. Fracture through the waist of the scaphoid.

2. Proximal fragment is dense and sclerotic.

3. Distal fragment and other carpal bones are porotic.

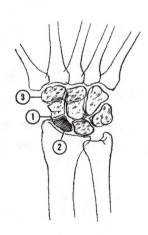

Body of the Talus

1. Fracture through the neck of the bone.
2. Body is dense and sclerotic.
3. Remaining tarsal bones are porotic.

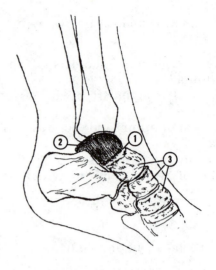

Lunate

Ischemic necrosis frequently follows dislocation of this bone.

1. Entire bone is dense, irregular, and fragmented.
2. Remaining carpal bones are porotic.

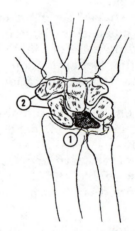

Tibia

Ischemic necrosis has occurred after segmental fracture of the shaft of the tibia.

1. Marked increased density of triangular free fragment indicates aseptic necrosis.

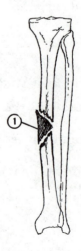

50

Patella

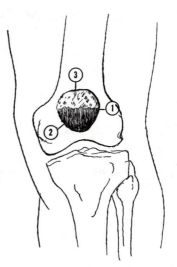

1. Fracture site is healed.
2. Increased density and sclerosis of lower half of patella.
3. Upper half is porotic.

Note: In this instance the blood supply to the distal half of the patella was disturbed during the operative procedure of wiring.

Malunion and Angular Deformities

REMARKS

Proper management of fractures should anticipate and prevent most residual deformities.

In some instances, however, deformities are unavoidable. This is particularly true after crushing injuries to epiphyseal plates or fractures with extensive bone loss.

Some deformities of the upper limb may be accepted, whereas deformities of a similar degree in the lower limb may severely interfere with function.

Injuries implicating epiphyseal plates of growing children frequently produce angular deformities or shortening. These limbs must be kept under observation for several years after the injury.

Malunion of the shafts of long bones in children often will diminish with growth. However, rotational deformities correct very little.

51

TYPICAL DEFORMITIES OF MALUNION

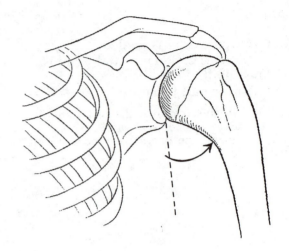

Varus deformity of the upper end of the humerus.

Note: This deformity produces little or no functional disability.

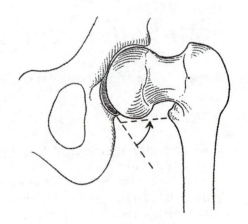

Varus deformity of the femoral neck.

Note: This deformity produces severe dysfunction and should be corrected.

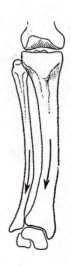

Severe angular deformity of both bones of the lower leg.

Note: This deformity causes marked dysfunction; the knee and ankle joints now perform in different planes. This deformity must be corrected by osteotomy.

1. Marked shortening of the radius.
2. Radial deviation of the hand.
3. Dislocation of the distal end of the ulna.

Note: This deformity produces marked dysfunction and should be corrected by an osteotomy of the radius and resection of the end of the ulna.

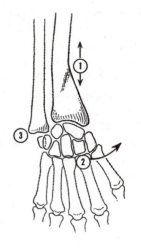

Severe valgus deformity of the elbow after lateral condylar fracture of the humerus.

This lesion, in addition to producing restriction of motion, may also cause a late ulnar nerve neuritis. In young patients the deformity should be corrected by osteotomy.

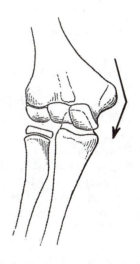

Varus deformity of the knee after fracture of the distal femur is actually a rotational malalignment produced by internal rotation of the distal fragment relative to the externally rotated proximal fragment. This is frequently caused by skeletal traction rotating the distal fragment inward and osteotomy may be needed to correct the deformity.

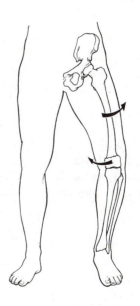

Rotational deformity of finger after phalangeal or metacarpal fracture.

1. This appears to be a varus angulation causing fingers to overlap on making a fist. It is actually a rotational malalignment at the fracture site.

2. To prevent the deformity, treat the fractured phalanx or metacarpal with the fingertips aligned toward the tuberosity of the navicular.

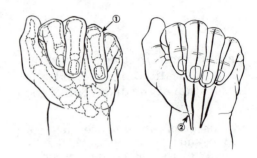

Shortening

REMARKS

Shortening of a bone following fracture occurs when:
1. The fragments unite with overlap.
2. The fragments unite with pronounced angulation.
3. A piece of the bone is lost.
4. A bone is compressed.
5. An epiphyseal plate is crushed and undergoes premature closure.

Except in cases of extensive bone loss and crushing injury to epiphyseal plates, most causes of shortening can be minimized.

EXAMPLES OF BONE SHORTENING

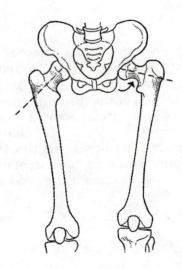

Shortening of the femur due to malunion of an intertrochanteric fracture; head and neck have united to the shaft in a position of marked varus.

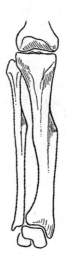

Shortening of the lower leg.
Fragments of both bones have united, with marked overlap.

Shortening of the humerus.
A large segment of the shaft was lost following a gunshot wound.
Shortening causes less significant functional disability in the upper limb than in the lower limb.

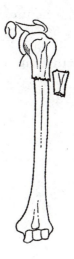

Shortening of the lower leg.
Severe comminution and compression of the calcaneus produces marked reduction of its height.

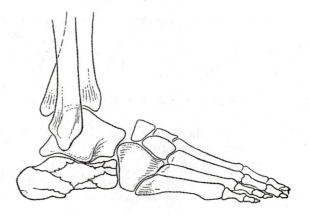

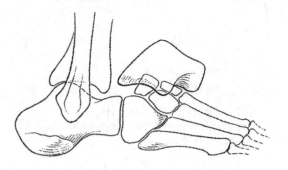

Shortening of the lower leg.
Complete extrusion of the talus.

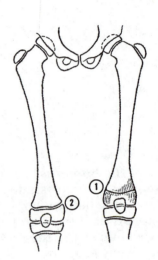

Shortening of the femur.
1. Premature closure of the distal femoral epiphyseal plate.
2. Compare with length of the opposed femur.

Stimulation of Growth

REMARKS

In young children fractures of the shafts of the long bones may stimulate growth.

For this reason it is wise to accept some overlap of the fragments in cases of fractures of the femoral shaft in children from two to ten years of age.

No dysfunction or residual deformities occur in these children provided that normal alignment of the fragments is restored.

Overgrowth of the Femoral Shaft

1. Fracture of the femoral shaft was allowed to heal with fragments in perfect end-to-end position.

2. Two years later there was an increase of 2.5 cm (1 in) in length of the femur. (Compare with opposite femur.)

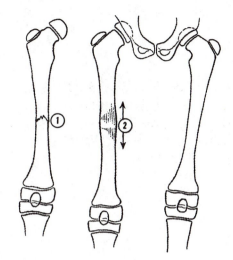

Infection

REMARKS

Introduction of pyogenic organisms from outside the body to a fracture site generally occurs in open fractures.

Only rarely are closed fractures infected; when this occurs the organisms are circulating in the blood, or they may be implanted at the site of fracture during an operative procedure.

Infection is a serious complication and as a rule implicates the fractured bone, producing localized osteomyelitis.

Once the infection is established it is difficult to eradicate: it destroys bone-forming elements; it delays or in some instances precludes osteogenesis, thereby becoming a major factor in the production of delayed union and nonunion.

Generally there is marked fibrosis and scarring of the surrounding soft tissues, further impairing the blood supply to the fractured bone.

Eradication of an established infection can be achieved only by:

1. Removal of all dead bone (sequestra).
2. Adequate drainage of the area.
3. Complete and sustained immobilization of the fracture.
4. Antibiotic therapy; this is a valuable adjunct to treatment but does not replace the first three principles.

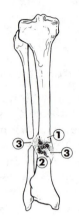

Infected Fracture of the Tibia

1. Increased density of bone ends.
2. Dense sclerotic piece of bone well delineated (a sequestrum).
3. Delayed union.

Injuries to Large Blood Vessels

REMARKS

Injuries to major blood vessels are likely with any musculoskeletal trauma, but the frequency is especially high with femoral fractures (3 per cent), supracondylar humeral fractures (10 per cent) and knee dislocations (30 per cent).

These complications may be life-threatening because of extensive hemorrhage or limb-threatening because of neuromuscular damage. Prompt recognition and repair of the arterial injury may save life as well as limb.

Post-traumatic ischemia may result from:
1. Direct arterial laceration, either partial or complete.
2. Arterial occlusion from internal thrombosis.
3. Compartmental syndromes from crush injury or swelling in restricted muscle compartments.

ARTERIAL LACERATION

Partial Laceration

Partial laceration can occur as a result of a penetrating wound.

1. Gunshot wound to the thigh fractures the femur.

2. Adjacent femoral artery sustains multiple partial lacerations.

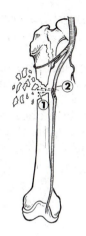

It can also result from operative treatment:

1. Skeletal traction pin inserted for a fractured femur partially injured the femoral artery near the adductor canal.

2. One month later, a massive swelling occurred from arterial aneurysm.

Note: Partial lacerations are likely to cause fatal hemorrhage, since completely lacerated vessels can occlude spontaneously by intense vasospastic reaction, whereas partially lacerated arteries cannot.

Partial laceraterions of arteries and adjacent veins can also result in expanding aneurysms and arterial fistulas as delayed complications of the injury.

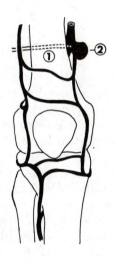

Complete Laceration from Arterial Avulsion

1. Anterior dislocation of the shoulder in an elderly patient with fixed atherosclerotic vessels.

2. Anterior humeral circumflex branch is avulsed off the axillary artery, producing complete laceration and extensive hemorrhage.

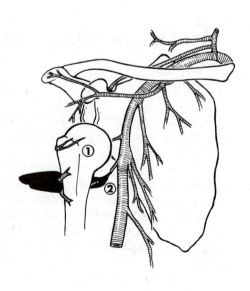

Complete Laceration from Arterial Avulsion (Continued)

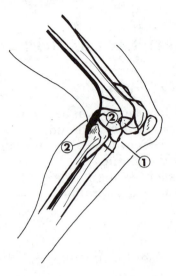

1. Posterior dislocation of the knee produces a posterior thrust on the popliteal artery.
2. Geniculate branches and fascial tunnels fix the popliteal artery, and the injury results in complete arterial laceration.

Diagnosis of Arterial Laceration

Evaluate all long bone fractures and dislocations with the assumption that circulation is disrupted until proven otherwise.

The most common sign of arterial laceration is loss of the distal pulse, but collateral circulation can maintain distal flow despite complete or partial laceration of the proximal artery.

When the integrity of the distal circulation cannot be proved with certainty, flowmeter measurements and arteriographic studies should be used liberally. This is especially true with high-risk injuries such as penetrating wounds and knee dislocations.

The most specific signs of arterial laceration are rapid swelling after injury and pulsatile bleeding after penetrating wounds. Do not interpret sudden swelling in a fractured limb as phlebitis or an infection; it most often indicates arterial injury.

ARTERIAL OCCLUSION FROM INTERNAL THROMBOSIS

REMARKS

This is a treacherous problem in that initially the flow to the injured vessel may be only partially occluded and can temporarily sustain limb viability.

As the arterial thrombosis enlarges, especially if a cast or dressing diminishes collateral circulation, distal anoxia may develop many hours or days after the initial injury.

Since this potential and limb-threatening occlusion may be delayed until after initial evaluation, neurocirculatory checks should be made regularly, especially following high-risk injuries about the knee and elbow.

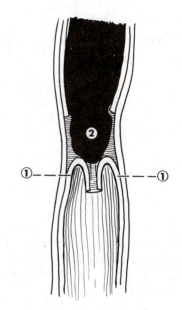

1. Blunt trauma disrupts intimal lining without lacerating the arterial wall.

2. Ball valve effect of the intimal tear leads to proximal thrombosis of the contused vessel.

Diagnosis of Arterial Thrombosis

Prompt diagnosis depends on a strong suspicion aroused by the location of the fracture.

Diminished or absent distal pulse is the most common finding, but this depends on the extent of the thrombosis and the contribution of collateral circulation.

Pain out of proportion to the injury, especially if increased after cast application or by passive stretching of the fingers or toes, is an important early sign of ischemic muscle.

Ultrasonic flowmeter measurement is a new and useful tool to evaluate distal flow.

Arteriograms should be obtained often if there is any question of arterial damage, especially after high-risk injuries such as close-range shotgun fractures and fractures or dislocations about the knee. Arteriograms are less reliable in the upper limb injuries and a normal arteriogram should not overrule clinical suspicion of arterial injury.

Management of Suspected Arterial Thrombosis in the Upper Limb

If signs of vascular occlusion occur following reduction and cast immobilization:

1. Bivalve the cast and remove the upper half.

2. Divide the underlying padding to the skin.

3. In elbow fractures, reduce the amount of flexion.

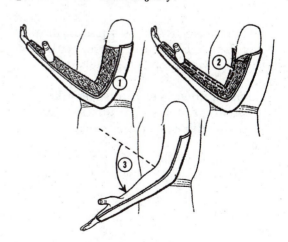

Management of Suspected Arterial Thrombosis in the Upper Limb (Continued)

If loss of distal circulation is evident at initial evaluation:

1. Gently correct any gross displacement of the fragments.

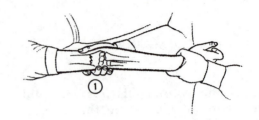

2. Elevate the fracture in side-arm traction to distinguish arterial injury from antecubital swelling, which is the usual cause of impaired distal flow in these injuries.

Note: Do not wallow in indecision. Restoration of flow is best accomplished within 8 hours to prevent significant neuromuscular damage and limb loss. If elevation does not restore distal flow within 45 to 60 minutes, explore the forearm and area of injury for supracondylar fracture. Arteriograms in children are usually not useful because vasospasm from the arterial puncture will confuse the picture.

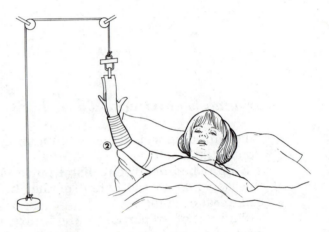

1. Free vessel from its surrounding areolar tissue. Flush the vessel with a solution of warm saline. Apply papaverine locally.

Spasm is, however, much less likely to be causing the vascular obstruction. Intimal thrombosis is more often the cause.

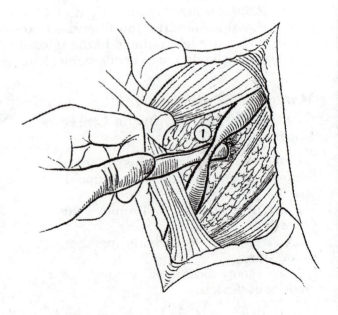

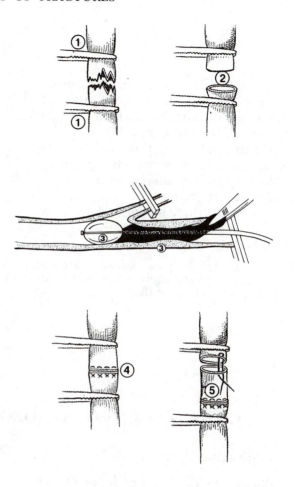

In cases of thrombosis, perforation, or rupture (with severe contusion of the vessel wall):

1. Clamp the vessel above and below the implicated segments.

2. Excise the traumatized segment.

3. Remove distal clots with balloon-tipped catheter until back-bleeding is brisk.

4. Do end-to-end anastomosis, or

5. When a longer segment is involved, replace it with a reversed saphenous vein graft.

Note: Forearm fasciotomy is often necessary if there is impending Volkmann's ischemia (see page 66).

COMMON SITES OF ARTERIAL LACERATION AND ARTERIAL THROMBOSIS

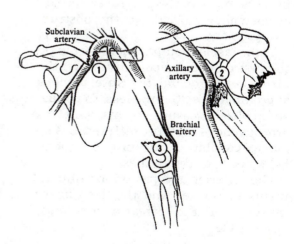

1. Subclavian artery — by fracture of the clavicle.

2. Axillary artery — by dislocation or fracture-dislocation of the head of the humerus.

3. Brachial artery — by supracondylar fracture of the humerus.

63

4. Popliteal artery injury causes the greatest loss of limb and may follow supracondylar fracture of the femur or dislocation of the knee.

5. Bifurcation of the popliteal artery into the anterior and posterior tibial vessels is disrupted by proximal tibial fractures.

6. Crush injury to the foot with extreme swelling occludes the vessels intrinsic to the foot.

Note: Blunt trauma causes arterial thrombosis, except about joints where arterial avulsion is most likely.

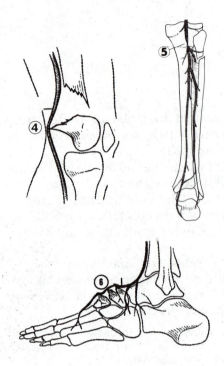

COMPARTMENTAL SYNDROMES

Mechanism

Rapid swelling of the forearm and leg muscles resulting from blunt trauma or successful arterial repair produces muscle ischemia by shutting off venous outflow and then arterial inflow.

Histamine-like substances released by ischemic muscles increase capillary permeability and add to the obstructive problem.

Tight fascial compartments strangle the neuromuscular contents when the intracompartmental pressure reaches approximately 20 mm less than diastolic blood pressure. At this point, the arteriovenous pressure difference is no longer capable of meeting the metabolic needs of the tissues.

The anterior and posterior compartments of the leg and the deep flexor muscles of the forearm are most susceptible.

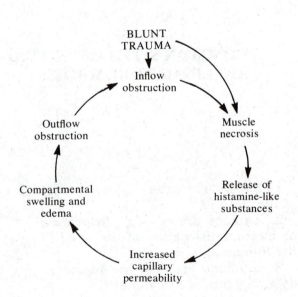

Measurement of Intracompartmental Pressure (Whitesides' Technique)

1. An 18-gauge needle attached to plastic tubing, which is half-filled with saline, is inserted into the muscle compartment.

2. A 20-cc syringe filled with air is connected to the tubing.

3. A second extension tubing is connected to a mercury manometer.

4. The syringe is opened to both extension tubes by means of a "T" connector.

5. The pressure in the system is increased by slowly depressing the plunger of the syringe while watching the saline column. The mercury manometer rises with any increase in pressure within the system. When compartmental pressure is reached, the saline is injected into the tissue and the saline meniscus moves. The level of the manometer at this point measures the muscle compartment pressure.

Note: Muscle compartment pressure measuring 20 to 30 mm Hg less than diastolic pressure indicates impending need for decompression by fasciotomy.

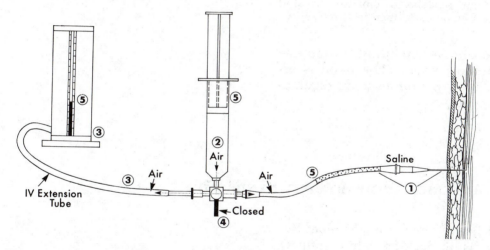

VOLKMANN'S ISCHEMIC CONTRACTURE

REMARKS

Volkmann's contracture begins usually from intracompartmental swelling.

Persistent pain, inability to passively extend the patient's fingers, sensory deficit in the hand, and loss of radial pulse should all be acted upon promptly.

Volkmann's ischemic contracture is not an "all-or-nothing" phenomenon. It may take several weeks to develop.

Contracture can begin with varying degrees of muscle and nerve injury and steadily affect all the neurovascular structures within the forearm compartment.

Forearm frasciotomy may still be effective in preventing neuromuscular damage days or weeks after initial injury.

65

Surgical Management:
Fasciotomy and Epimysiotomy

1. A longitudal incision extends from the elbow to the wrist in the midflexor surface of the forearm.

2. Antebrachial fascia is incised.

3. Epimysium of all swollen muscles is sectioned freely through its entire length. Be certain to decompress the deep compartment of the forearm.

4. The median and ulnar nerves are also explored and decompressed.

5. The pulse is monitored before and after decompression, and if it does not improve, the artery is explored proximally.

Note: The fascia and skin are not closed, but a delayed closure or skin grafting may be performed in three to five days.

Postoperative splinting to oppose thumb and prevent claw hand is essential until neuromuscular regeneration occurs.

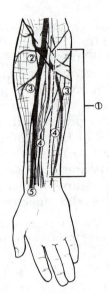

ANTERIOR COMPARTMENT SYNDROME

1. A heavy direct blow or repetitive strain, as in jogging (shin splints), causes anterior tibial muscles to swell.

2. The narrow entrance over the anterior tibial artery into the compartment becomes obstructed.

3. Distal pulses are maintained by collateral circulation despite ischemic muscle necrosis.

4. Ischemic muscle is painful and then is paralyzed and produces drop foot.

Note: This syndrome must be diagnosed promptly before the advanced clinical manifestations of muscle paralysis develop, since the prognosis for functional return is poor after ischemic paralysis occurs.

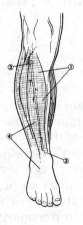

DEEP POSTERIOR COMPARTMENT SYNDROME

REMARKS

This complication occurs most often after tibial fractures but may follow an ankle sprain treated with a rigid dressing. The characteristic severe pain of muscle ischemia made worse by cast application should be distinguished from the pain of the initial injury. This syndrome may also occur in combination with ischemic muscle injury to the other compartments of the leg.

1. Ischemia of the ankle invertors and toe flexors produces an equino-varus deformity and pain on passive extension of the ankle or toes.

2. Ischemic posterior tibial nerve causes numbness along the plantar surface of the foot.

3. The distal medial part of the leg is tense to palpation.

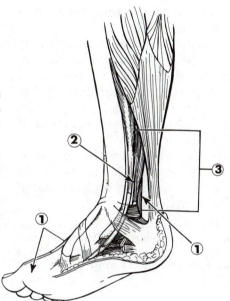

Double-Incision Fasciotomy of the Leg for Compartment Syndromes

1. A 15-cm anterolateral incision 2 cm anterior to the fibular shaft and

2. A 15-cm incision in the distal leg 2 cm posterior to the posterior medial edge of the tibia allow decompression of all four compartments.

3. The fascia of the anterior compartment is opened proximally and distally with long, blunt scissors.

4. The lateral compartment is opened in line with the fibula.

5. The deep posterior compartment is reached by undermining along the posterior tibial margin, and the fascia is opened proximally and distally beneath the soleus muscle.

6. The saphenous vein and nerve should be avoided.

7. The superficial posterior compartment is opened 2 cm posterior and parallel to the incision in the deep posterior compartment.

Note: The entire muscle compartment must be decompressed. If there is any doubt, repeat the intracompartmental pressure measurements and open skin widely.

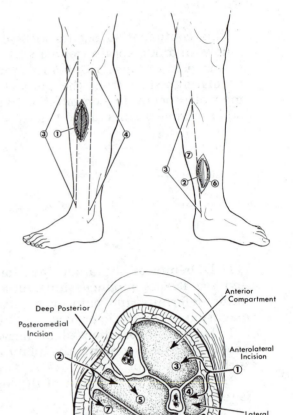

Compartmental Syndromes from Skin Traction

1. Heavy skin traction with legs elevated for a femoral shaft fracture may lower arteriovenous pressure to levels that can produce muscle ischemia.

2. Heavy skin traction raises venous pressure by means of the Chinese finger-trap effect.

Note: To prevent this occurrence, avoid using (1) heavy skin traction, more than 8 lb (3.6 Kg) and (2) elevated traction in patients weighing more than 30 lb (13.6 Kg).

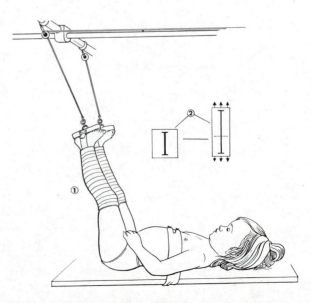

FRACTURE MANAGEMENT AFTER ARTERIAL INJURY

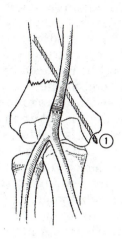

1. After vascular continuity is restored, the fracture may be fixed internally or an external splint may be used.

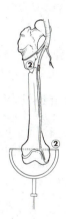

2. In the lower limb, traction may be utilized to allow the fracture to shorten slightly after vascular repair.

Note: Use of internal fixation may be necessary for extremely unstable fractures with arterial injury, but external immobilization is effective and gives generally higher salvage rates in these serious injuries.

Common Injuries to Nerves Adjacent to the Fracture Site

REMARKS

Nerves are even more likely than large vessels to be injured by a fracture, although 75 per cent of these nerve injuries recover spontaneously.

As a rule, the nerve remains intact in a closed fracture, but in an open fracture, especially a gunshot wound, the nerve is very often severed.

The degree of damage to the nerve varies in intensity:

1. A minor injury may cause only a transitory physiologic block (neuropraxia), and rapid spontaneous recovery within a few weeks is the rule.

2. More severe injuries may cause pronounced damage and interruption of the axons (axonotmesis). Here the continuity of the nerve is intact, but Wallerian (peripheral) degeneration occurs, and regeneration is slow (about 1 cm a month).

3. The nerve trunk may be completely severed (neurotmesis), or a segment may be replaced by fibrous tissue. Spontaneous recovery is impossible, and end-to-end suture of normal nerve ends is essential to recovery.

In closed injuries to the upper limb, neuropraxia is the rule and "watchful waiting" is justified. If electromyographic and clinical evidence of nerve return is lacking within three to four weeks after fracture, operative exploration of the nerve is indicated.

Radial nerves injured by fractures in the distal third of the humerus, nerves injured during fracture reduction, and nerves damaged by open fracture demand prompt exploration. Most nerves injured by fractures in the lower limb require exploration.

The earlier the injured nerve is decompressed or repaired after entrapment or laceration, the smaller the loss of distal motor function and the better the overall recovery.

COMMON SITES OF PERIPHERAL NERVE INJURIES

Injury to the brachial plexus associated with fracture of the clavicle:

1. The fracture is incidental and the plexus injury is produced by the violence of initial injury, or,

2. Delayed compression neuropathy can result from excess callus formed by a displaced clavicle fracture.

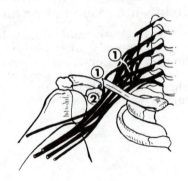

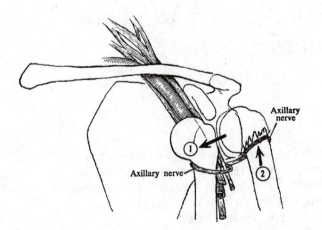

Injury to the axillary nerve by
1. Dislocation or
2. Fracture-dislocation of the humeral head.

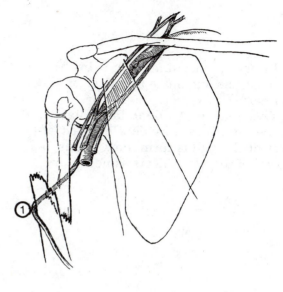

Injury to the radial nerve by fracture of the humerus:

1. Nerve injury is usually a neuropraxia with spontaneous recovery.

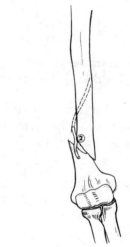

2. Fracture in the distal third, where the nerve penetrates the intramuscular septum, entraps the nerve and requires surgical decompression.

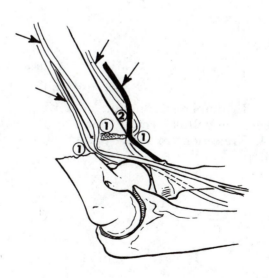

Supracondylar fracture of the humerus:

1. Contusion, compression, or laceration of the radial, median, or ulnar nerves occurs in 15 per cent of these injuries, but function should return within 3 weeks.

2. Brachial artery may also be damaged.

Injury to the ulnar nerve by fracture of the medial epicondyle of the humerus:

This may be evident immediately, or nerve injury may be a delayed effect of the callus formation. Transposition of the ulnar nerve is necessary.

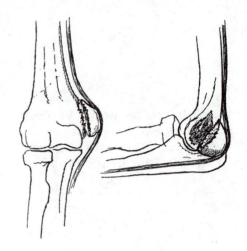

Injury to the median nerve by:

1. Fracture of the distal end of the radius or

2. Dislocation of the lunate bone.

This nerve injury may be primary or more often it is secondary to:

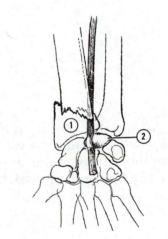

3. Incomplete reduction of a fragment and callus formation or

4. Treatment in acute palmar flexion.

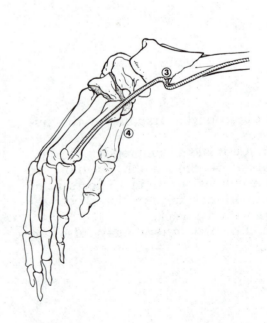

Injury to the common peroneal nerve by dislocation or transient subluxation of the knee:

This condition is so often associated with injury to the artery and ligaments that operative repair and decompression are usually necessary.

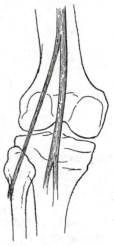

Posteroanterior

Fracture of the femur with sciatic nerve injury:

This condition should be explored promptly. The recovery period is too long for surgical repair to be effective after lack of spontaneous recovery indicates that the nerve has been transected.

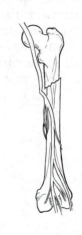

1. Injury to the sciatic nerve by dislocation of the hip is usually a stretch injury and does not require exploration.

2. Injury to the sciatic nerve by fracture-dislocation is frequently an entrapment injury and requires exploration.

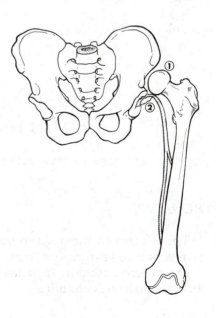

73

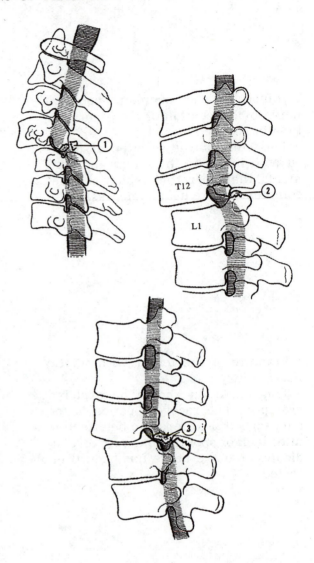

Injuries to the spinal cord in:

1. Fractures, dislocations, and fracture-dislocations of the cervical spine.

2. Fractures and fracture-dislocations of the thoracic spine.

3. Fractures and fracture-dislocations of the lumbar spine produce true peripheral nerve injuries since the cord ends at L1. Reduction and stabilization of the lumbar spine must be performed to decompress the peripheral nerve and restore function.

Injuries to Tendons

REMARKS

These injuries most often occur in the upper limb and require operative repair to restore function.

Frequently, tendon injuries in the hand will go unrecognized until functional loss is obvious.

Fracture-dislocation of the glenohumeral joint:

1. In an older patient, impaction of the humeral head against the glenoid produces a complete fracture of the greater tuberosity with displacement of the rotator cuff insertion.

2. Reduction of the dislocation should restore the tuberosity of the humerus completely. If the fracture remains displaced more than 5 mm, the rotator cuff should be repaired surgically.

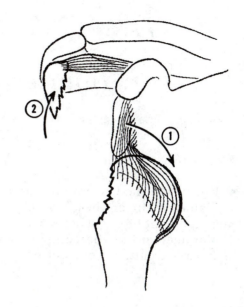

Shirt-tacklers injury occurs when:

1. An avulsion fracture of the flexor profundus is produced by the football tackler's pulling on the runner's shirt and tearing the profundus insertion from the long or ring finger.

2. Significance of the small chip fracture from the phalanx may be overlooked until the patient demonstrates inability to flex the distal interphalangeal joint. The tendon insertion should be repaired surgically.

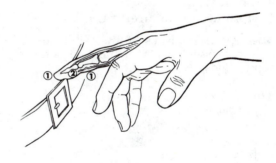

Boutonnière disruption of the extensor tendon occurs commonly with:

1. Laceration or blunt injury to dorsum of mid-phalanx, which tears central extensor slip.

2. The extension of the mid-phalanx is initially possible because of the lateral bands.

3. The lateral bands slide volarly to become flexors of the proximal interphalangeal joint and extensors of the distal interphalangeal joint (boutonnière deformity).

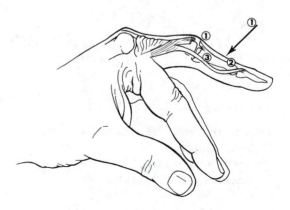

Injuries to Viscera

REMARKS

Injuries to the viscera are not uncommon with certain fractures.

Management of these complications must be considered under the management of the specific fracture.

Management of the complications frequently takes priority over the definitive treatment of fracture.

Fracture of the Pelvis

This injury may be complicated by:

1. Rupture of the bladder.
2. Laceration or perforation of the colon or rectum.
3. Rupture of the urethra.

Note: Open fractures of the pelvis are very often associated with these visceral complications.

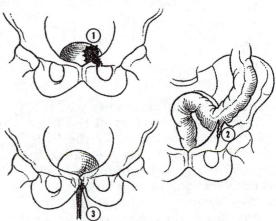

Seat Belt Fracture (Chance Fracture)

This injury causes:

1. Compression injury to the abdomen, rupturing the viscus.
2. Distraction injury to the spine, causing vertebral fracture.

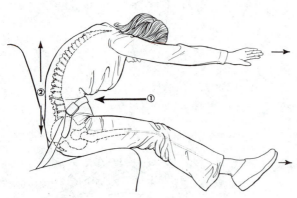

Fracture of the Chest Wall

This injury may be complicated by:

1. Hemothorax.
2. Pneumothorax.
3. Laceration of the lung.

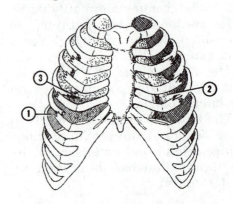

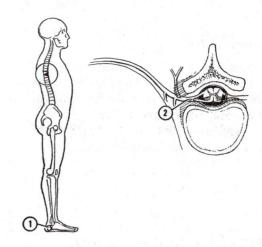

Fracture of the Spine

This injury may be complicated by:
1. Fracture of the calcanei.
2. Injury to the spinal cord, cauda equina, or nerve roots.

Shock

REMARKS

Shock is the state of impaired cellular metabolism that usually results from inadequate capillary profusion and that has many causes.

There are six general categories of shock:

1. Anaphylaxis from violent allergic reaction.
2. Obstruction of blood flow, e.g., by cardiac tamponade, massive pulmonary embolism.
3. Cellular shock or impaired cellular utilization of oxygen, e.g., from infectious toxins, drug poisoning.
4. Neurogenic, e.g., "fainting," spinal shock, shock of spinal anesthetic.
5. Cardiogenic, e.g., myocardial infarction, arrhythmia.
6. Hypovolemic, from internal or external hemorrhage, plasma loss, or loss of body fluids and electrolytes. This is by far the most common cause of shock after injury.

DEVELOPMENT OF SHOCK

The stages in the development of hypovolemic shock are: an initial generalized vasoconstriction followed by expansion of the vascular volume, progressing to problems of disseminated intravascular coagulation, and terminating in failure of the kidneys and other vital organs.

Each of these stages may be reversed by adequate fluid volume replacement.

Normal State

1. Arterioles are open wide.
2. Most of the capillaries are closed, and they open only in rotation on demand from cells.
3. Capillary flow is rapid, and pH drop along the capillary is minimal.

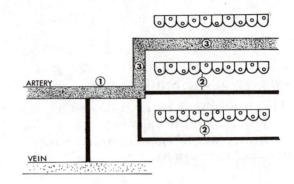

Phase of Vasoconstriction

Catecholamines released by hemorrhage and trauma cause:
1. Arteriolar constriction and
2. Arteriovenous shunt.
3. Capillary flow is slowed and cells become acidotic.

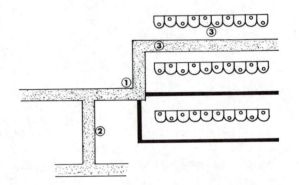

Phase of Expanded Vascular Space

1. Energy demands by cells cause capillaries to open, enlarging vascular space.
2. Blood volume is inadequate to fill vascular space, and cellular perfusion is diminished.
3. Slow capillary flow produces cellular acidosis, and acidic blood becomes hypercoagulable.

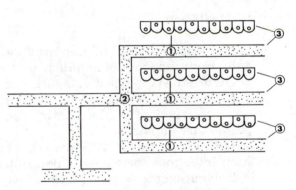

Phase of Disseminated Intravascular Coagulation (DIC)

1. Acidic blood becomes hypercoagulable and stagnant.
2. Combination of this blood and the thromboplastin from traumatized vessels produces disseminated intravascular coagulation (DIC).
3. The cells of the kidneys and other major organs become severely acidotic and die.

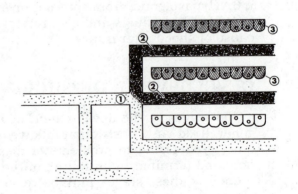

CARDINAL SIGNS OF SHOCK

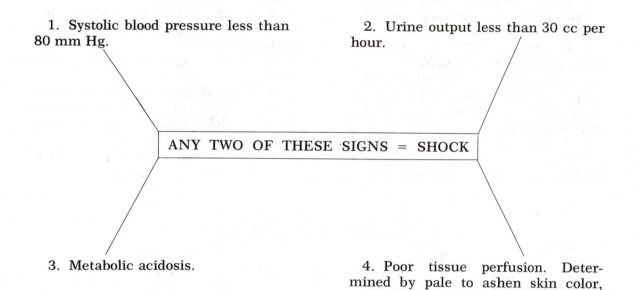

1. Systolic blood pressure less than 80 mm Hg.

2. Urine output less than 30 cc per hour.

ANY TWO OF THESE SIGNS = SHOCK

3. Metabolic acidosis.

4. Poor tissue perfusion. Determined by pale to ashen skin color, cool skin temperature, and sluggish response to pressure blanching.

Other manifestations of shock are narrowed pulse pressure, rapid pulse, shallow labored respirations, and a state of consciousness changing from anxiety to apathy to unresponsiveness. Marked thirst, nausea, and vomiting are common.

The patient who manifests any of these signs should be stabilized before diagnosis and treatment of the fractures are begun.

DO NOT SEND THE PATIENT TO X-RAY IN A STATE OF IMPENDING OR ACTUAL SHOCK.

TREATMENT FOR SHOCK

REMARKS

The prime considerations are to:

1. Restore circulating blood volume lost by the injury and accentuated by the expanded vascular space.

2. Assist respirations to help oxygenation and especially to avoid gastric aspiration in the unconscious patient.

3. Prevent further blood loss by controlling obvious external hemorrhage with voluminous pressure dressings.

4. Evaluate for internal hemorrhage by paracentesis or thoracentesis.

RESTORE NORMAL BLOOD VOLUME:

1. Blood should be typed and cross-matched immediately.

2. Up to 2000 cc of balanced electrolytes (e.g., Ringer's lactate solution) should be given rapidly.

3. Plasma or albumin may be given until blood is available.

4. Even when blood is begun, electrolyte solution must continue to be given to replace extracellular and intracellular fluid.

5. As long as volume is adequate, a fraction of the red cell mass will suffice initially for oxygen transport.

TAKE MEASUREMENTS OF PATIENT'S VITAL FUNCTIONS:

1. Arterial blood pressure and pulse should be measured.

2. Central venous pressure and pulmonary wedge pressure should be taken if possible.

3. Urine output should be measured.

4. Arterial blood should be tested for Po_2, Pco_2, pH, and lactate levels.

5. Cardiac output should be measured.

6. Hematocrit should be determined.

TREATMENT FOR SHOCK

GIVE RESPIRATORY ASSISTANCE:

1. Always try to manage the airway first without entering the patient's mouth in order to avoid aspiration. The combination of backward tilt of the head and anterior displacement of the mandible prevents obstruction by the tongue.

2. Endotracheal intubation performed by an experienced operator is essential to protect the airway of an unconscious patient against aspiration.

3. Even a conscious shock victim needs the increased level of oxygen and the minute ventilation supplied by respiratory assistance, which should *not* be delayed until the patient is obviously dyspneic.

GIVE ADDITIONAL CRITICAL SUPPORT:

1. Digitalization should be instituted for cardiac failure and anti-arrhythmic agents (Lidocaine) for dysrhythmias.

2. Steroids will stabilize cellular and intracellular membranes; they are of most benefit in septic shock.

3. Diuretics (Lasix) should be given if oliguria persists after blood volume is restored.

4. Vasopressors are contraindicated in hypovolemic shock, because they exacerbate perfusion deficiencies. Vasodilation may rarely be useful in aiding tissue perfusion if hypovolemia is corrected.

PREVENT INFECTION:

1. Promptly debride open fractures.

2. Prophylactic antibiotics should be administered for most open fractures.

3. Tetanus toxoid should be given; an immunized patient should receive 0.5 cc of toxoid intramuscularly; the unimmunized patient should receive 0.5 cc of toxoid intramuscularly and then immune globulin intravenously.

After the patient is out of shock make a meticulous assessment for injuries.

Check for:

Evidence of direct communication between fractures and the exterior.

Evidence of vascular embarrassment of the affected extremities.

Evidence of neurologic deficit.

Evidence of visceral injury.

Fracture of other bones.

Continue to monitor urine output over the next several days for signs of renal failure. This is critical if there has been a crush injury to muscle.

Increases in blood urea nitrogen and creatinine levels and a decrease in urine output to under 30 cc per hour indicate renal failure.

If the oliguria does not respond to diuretics such as mannitol or high-dose furosemide, dialysis must be instituted promptly.

Malignant Hyperthermia

Malignant hyperthermia (M.H.) is an autosomal dominant condition that exposes a number of patients (approximately 1 in 10,000) to sudden death after injury, particularly when subjected to anesthetic agents such as succinylcholine or halothane.

The condition, which has come to be studied in the past ten years, has been the cause of many "anesthetic" deaths in young adults undergoing surgery for either injury or elective procedures.

M.H. is characterized by a rapid development of severe acidosis, hypercarbia, electrolyte shift, muscle supercontractility, and rapid elevation in body temperature during anesthesia ("triggering").

The defect appears to be in the ability of the skeletal-muscle fibre to control its internal calcium concentration. The leakage of calcium into the sarcoplasm sustains the muscle supercontractility, and this in turn stimulates multiple catabolic reactions, among which is

$$ATP \rightarrow ADP + pyrophosphate + heat$$

The continual loss of ATP disrupts the integrity of the sarcolemma so that ions and molecules leak across it and worsen the intracellular disturbances.

81

The diagnosis of malignant hyperthermia should be considered in:
1. History of sudden anesthetic death in the patient's family.
2. Generalized muscle weakness or cramping, especially after exercising in hot weather.
3. Localized areas of muscle weakness such as ptosis, kyphosis, kyphoscoliosis, and joint hypermobility.
4. Abnormally elevated creatine phosphokinase levels.

SIGNS OF MALIGNANT HYPERTHERMIA

Temperature monitoring should be routine during surgery. Among the early warning signs are:
1. Tachycardia or other arrhythmias associated with instability of blood pressure.
2. Flushing or cyanosis of the skin.
3. Hyperventilation.
4. Excessive heat and blueness of soda lime cannister.

MANAGEMENT

1. Cease all inhalation anesthetics and muscle relaxants.
2. Change anesthetic tubing.
3. Hyperventilate with oxygen-enriched mixtures.
4. Cool immediately with ice baths, cold intravenous solution, and gastric, rectal, and wound irrigation.
5. Agents such as sodium dantrolene that prevent calcium release from sarcoplasmic reticulum are effective prophylactically and in the early stages of triggering.

Fat Embolism

REMARKS

This is a significant life-threatening complication of injury that in the past was considered to be caused by numerous fat droplets from the fracture acting as emboli. The basic problem is now recognized as a respiratory insufficiency sequela of injury and shock.

Mortality rate in the past from fat embolism was at least 50 per cent, and 20 per cent of all fracture deaths were attributed to this complication. Comprehension of the underlying pathophysiology has improved these statistics considerably.

A major reason for past high mortality has been failure to recognize the incipient state of the syndrome, which begins within three days after an injury.

By monitoring the injured patient for any sudden change in mental state or sudden tachycardia, tachypnea, or pyrexia, physicians and nursing personnel can detect the onset of the syndrome and confirm the diagnosis by blood gas studies.

Arterial Po_2 below 50 mm of mercury is diagnostic of a fat embolism–respiratory insufficiency syndrome and indicates the need for prompt treatment.

The objective of therapy is to restore and maintain Po_2 level above 60 mm, and in the early mild condition this can be accomplished by administration of oxygen through nasal intubation or mask.

If symptoms are severe, as manifested by significant changes in level of consciousness, by Po_2 well below 50 mm and by radiographic evidence of pulmonary edema, treatment must be prompt and vigorous. Sedation, endotracheal intubation, use of volume-limited respirators, positive end-expiratory pressure, and diuretics may all be needed to achieve and maintain Po_2 over 60 mm.

Diagnosis

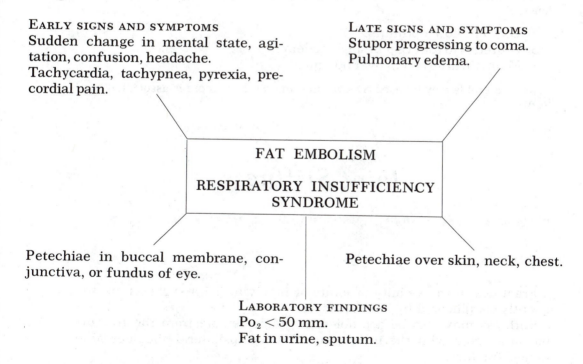

EARLY SIGNS AND SYMPTOMS
Sudden change in mental state, agitation, confusion, headache.
Tachycardia, tachypnea, pyrexia, precordial pain.

LATE SIGNS AND SYMPTOMS
Stupor progressing to coma.
Pulmonary edema.

FAT EMBOLISM

RESPIRATORY INSUFFICIENCY SYNDROME

Petechiae in buccal membrane, conjunctiva, or fundus of eye.

Petechiae over skin, neck, chest.

LABORATORY FINDINGS
$Po_2 < 50$ mm.
Fat in urine, sputum.

PREVENTIVE TREATMENT

1. Gentle handling of fractured limbs with effective fracture immobilization at site of injury.
2. Complete and prompt blood volume replacement after injury.

3. Surveillance by all personnel for any change in patient's mental status and other early signs of syndrome, especially in the first three days after injury.

TREATMENT FOR ACTUAL CASES (AFTER MURRAY AND RACZ)

Mild Cases

Mild cases may be treated with oxygen by mask to maintain arterial Po_2 over 60 mm.

Severe Cases

1. Sedate with morphine, 10 to 15 mg IV.
2. Intubate.
3. Ventilate at rate of 12/min., tidal volume $= 1000$ ml.
4. Positive end-expiratory pressure: 10 cm H_2O.

Note: Blood volume must be corrected first, or PEEP may potentiate hypotension.

5. Oxygen: 40% optimum.
6. Diuretics to relieve pulmonary edema.
7. Maintain arterial Po_2 over 60 mm.

Note: Steroids may be used (Decadron 4 mg q 6 h) if there is associated head injury.

Joint Stiffness

REMARKS

Fractures in the vicinity of joints or involving joint surfaces are frequently complicated by joint stiffness.

Stiffness may also be a problem in joints remote from the fracture but associated with the injury, such as the ipsilateral shoulder after Colles' fracture.

Joint stiffness results from the combination of muscle and joint contracture following injury and prolonged immobilization imposed by treatment.

In the upper limb, the shoulder, elbow, and finger joints are most prone to stiffening; the knee is the problem joint after fracture in the lower limb.

The major causes of joint stiffness after fracture are:

1. Inadequate functional activity of the injured limb and associated muscles as an integral part of treatment.
2. Persistent dependent edema of the hand or foot.
3. Prolonged cast immobilization of intra-articular fractures.
4. Infection.

PREVENTION OF JOINT STIFFNESS

Active functional exercise of muscles and joints of the affected limb is the single most important factor in prevention. This should be not a casual effort but a specific program laid out for the patient. Physical therapy may be helpful initially, but the patient must be educated about his responsibility to exercise by himself every hour.

Manipulation of the joint for stiffness after fracture is not necessary, but passive stretching exercise may be helpful, especially after injuries to the shoulder or knee.

Fractures about some joints, such as the surgical neck fracture of the humerus, are best treated with emphasis on the soft tissue injury and mobilization in the first few weeks without waiting for radiographic signs of complete fracture healing.

Compression dressing and limb elevation early after injury prevent problems of prolonged hand and foot edema.

Intra-articular fractures are especially prone to cause joint stiffness if immobilized for more than a few weeks in casts. These fractures are best treated with either rigid internal fixation or early active exercise to restore joint mobility.

Open fractures and penetrating wounds of joints should be treated by joint exploration and vigorous irrigation to prevent infection, followed by early mobilization of the open joint to restore maximum range.

RULES TO PREVENT JOINT STIFFNESS OF SPECIFIC JOINTS

Shoulder

Exercise the shoulder actively for any fracture of the hand, wrist, forearm, elbow, or humerus.

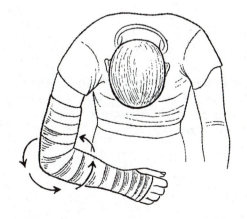

Elbow

Fractures about the elbow require rigid internal fixation or excision of loose fragments to allow for early joint mobilization.

1. Fracture of the radial head is best treated by excision of the fragments and joint mobilization.

2. Fracture of the olecranon is treated by rigid fixation and early mobilization.

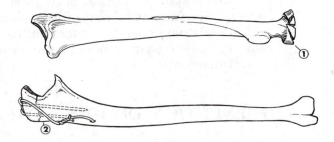

Hand

Compression dressings are necessary to combat edema and stiffness:

1. Thumb is abducted.

2. Metacarpophalangeal joints are flexed.

3. Interphalangeal joints are extended.

4. Fluffs between fingers and circumferential plaster apply even compression to hand.

5. Elevation eliminates dependent edema.

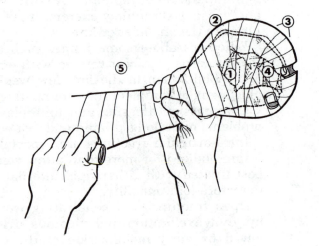

Knee

1. Active, functional weight bearing in casts is most important to prevent atrophy or contracture of quadriceps and other muscles.

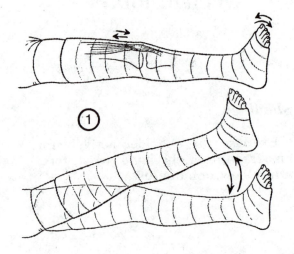

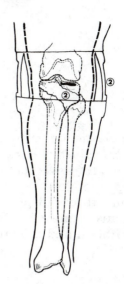

2. Cast brace permits knee joint motion while fracture is healing.

Toes

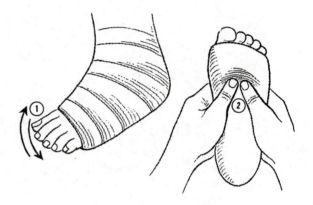

1. For any fracture of the lower limb, leave the toes free and enforce active exercises.

2. Mold the plaster well under the heads of the central metatarsal bones to preserve the transverse arch and prevent clawing of toes.

CAUTIONS

Upper Limb

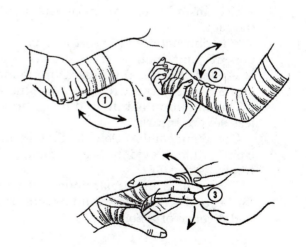

1. Never forcefully manipulate a shoulder after fracture, but insist on early active exercises.

2. Never forcefully manipulate an elbow.

3. Never forcefully manipulate fingers. Dynamic knuckle bender splints are more effective.

Lower Limbs

1. Apply an elastic support from the toes to the knee after removing a plaster cast from the lower leg for fracture of the leg or ankle.

2. Always use threaded pins where possible. Because they do not migrate, skin irritation and infection are diminished.

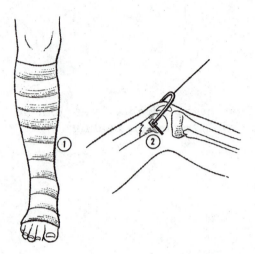

Sudeck's Acute Bone Atrophy

REMARKS

This disorder occurs most frequently in the hand but may occur in the foot.

It is characterized by intense pain and swelling and marked restriction of joint motion. The skin is glossy in appearance, smooth, and stretched. The local temperature is increased. There is extreme porosis of the bones. In severe cases, trophic ulcers may form.

The condition is initiated by trauma to the limbs, either fracture or a less severe injury.

The responsible etiologic factors are not known, but there is sufficient clinical evidence to indicate that a reflex neurovascular dystrophy is acting.

The clinical manifestations and residual dysfunction often noted are far beyond what one would expect as the result of functional inactivity and disease of a bone.

MANAGEMENT

1. Institute intensive active exercise on a regulated basis.
2. Physical therapy in the form of gentle heat and elevation of the limb is valuable.
3. Intravenous block anesthesia (see page 114) followed by gentle manipulation and dynamic splinting of the hand is helpful to regain motion in stiff wrist and fingers.
4. Parasympathetic blocks may occasionally be necessary if vasospasticity appears to be the dominant cause of the symptoms.
5. If the condition persists and symptoms are relieved by the block, a sympathectomy may be necessary.

Full recovery requires several months and patient persistence.

Post–Traumatic Ossification (Myositis Ossificans Traumatica)

REMARKS

This complication of fractures, dislocations, and soft tissue contusions can be serious because of the tendency to confuse it with osteogenic sarcoma.

Myositis ossificans occurs anywhere in the body, but in 80 per cent of cases the arms or thighs are affected.

In its mature state it is a localized lesion of heterotrophic bone and cartilage near bone and in the proximity of muscle.

The lesion is frequently the result of repeated trauma, as seen in the arms of riflemen or the thighs of football players.

The disorder is commonly encountered not only in athletes but in children, adolescents, and young adults, who constitute the population most likely to develop osteogenic sarcoma. In addition, myositis ossificans is seen about joints that are paralyzed from spinal cord or brain injury.

The histopathology of this disorder concerns the connective tissue of fascia enveloping muscle, intramuscular fibrous septa and fascial planes. The muscle tissue itself does not participate in the evolution of myositis ossificans.

The evolution of this process as seen on x-rays comprises four stages:

1. For the 2 weeks after injury, no radiographic changes are seen.
2. Calcification begins in the fascial planes 2 to 4 weeks following injury.
3. The lesion completes development and reaches maximum size by 14 weeks.
4. In 5 to 6 months the matured lesion appears to be ossified rather than irregularly mineralized and serum alkaline phosphatase is returning to normal.

DIAGNOSIS

PAROSTEAL (MOST COMMON)

Seen near shafts of long bones, such
as humerus and femur.
Occurs along the vertebral column.

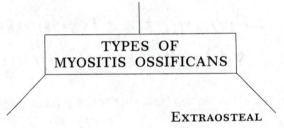

TYPES OF
MYOSITIS OSSIFICANS

PERIOSTEAL

Evolves with disruption of periosteum.
An eccentric bone mass adjacent to bone.

EXTRAOSTEAL

Rare.
Seen in tendons and ligaments such as Achilles tendon, collateral ligaments of the knee, ligaments in the sole of the foot.

Do not confuse this lesion with a juxtacortical sarcoma.

Serial x-rays will reveal the true nature of the lesion.

In the paravertebral areas, the lesion may resemble an aneurysmal bone cyst.

The age of the patient, a history of trauma, and the site of the lesion are valuable guides in establishing the diagnosis.

Even with open biopsy, myositis ossificans may be confused with osteogenic sarcoma. The biopsy specimen must be generous enough to show the zonal characteristics of myositis ossificans.

Biopsy for Myositis Ossificans

This should be done only after serial x-rays fail to show progressive ossification or maturation.

Open biopsy, rather than needle aspiration, is necessary to obtain a specimen adequate for zonal characterization.

The most important tissue involved is the connective tissue, or fascia, and the intramuscular septa, not the muscle.

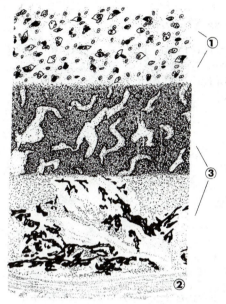

1. The central part of the lesion resembles an undifferentiated sarcoma of proliferative connective tissue.

2. Muscle may or may not be evident, but if present it is helpful in diagnosis.

3. Bone forms first in the periphery and then towards the center.

COMMON SITES OF POST-TRAUMATIC OSSIFICATION

Elbow

Ossification on the anterior aspect of the elbow joint.

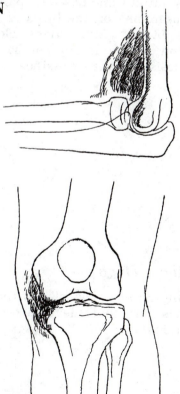

Knee

Ossification on the inner aspect of the knee implicating the medial collateral ligament (Pellegrini-Stieda disease).

91

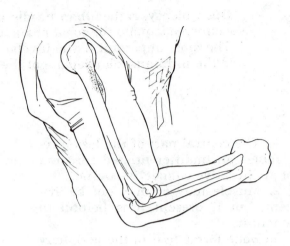

Blocker's Shoulder

Ossification in lateral deltoid region from repetitive blows, as received in football blocking.

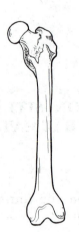

Horseback Rider's Hip

This ossification in the anterior hip capsule of a young horseback rider was initially diagnosed as parosteal osteosarcoma on the basis of incomplete biopsy. Subsequent close observation of the lesion confirmed the diagnosis as myositis ossificans.

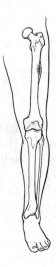

Footballer's Thigh

Football runners who play without thigh pads commonly develop ossification in thigh.

PRINCIPLES OF TREATMENT

The most effective treatment is prophylactic: Avoid repetitive soft tissue injury.

Injuries to the thigh and arm known to induce myositis should be treated with rest followed by active joint mobilization to avoid development of myositis ossificans.

Awareness of the resemblance of early myositis to sarcoma avoids tragic overtreatment.

Anticipate the tendency of myositis ossificans to recur; never excise sooner than six to twelve months after injury and wait for serum alkaline phosphatase to return to normal before excising.

Cortisone injection is rarely useful except for well-localized calcification.

Athletes who wish to remain competitive must wear arm and thigh pads to prevent myositis ossificans from developing.

Post–Traumatic Arthritis
(Osteoarthritis)

REMARKS

Following a joint fracture, any incongruity of the articular surfaces favors development of osteoarthritis.

Angular deformities resulting from healing of shaft fractures in malalignment also predispose to development of osteoarthritis in a joint; this is particularly true in weight-bearing joints.

Severe osteoarthritic alterations follow avascular necrosis, such as occurs in the hip when the femoral head is implicated or in the wrist when the scaphoid is involved.

The interval between the injury and the appearance of the clinical manifestation of osteoarthritis varies considerably. In general, the more severe the injury, the sooner the alterations in the joint and the sooner clinical manifestations appear.

COMMON SITES OF POST–TRAUMATIC ARTHRITIS

Osteoarthritis often develops after avascular necrosis of the femoral head.

1. Sclerosis and increased density of the femoral head.

2. Narrowing of the joint space.

3. Incongruity of the articular surfaces.

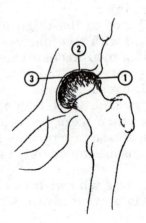

A depressed fracture of the lateral tibial cordyle can be followed by osteoarthritis of the knee.

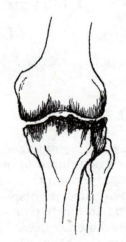

Healing of a fracture of the tibia with incongruity of the articular surfaces can result in osteoarthritis.

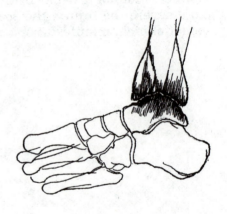

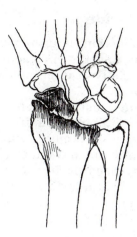

Osteoarthritis can develop after avascular necrosis of the scaphoid.

PRINCIPLES OF TREATMENT

The violence of initial injury to the articular surface is the key factor in the development of post-traumatic arthritis.

Anatomic restoration of articular surfaces and restoration of normal alignment in fractures of long bones are important in preventing the development of osteoarthritis.

In the face of osteoarthritis, further progression of the disorder can be retarded by not exceeding the functional capacity of the joint, by eliminating harmful stresses and strains, and by maintaining the muscles controlling the joint at their maximum level of efficiency.

Joints severely involved may require some form of surgical intervention such as arthrodesis or arthroplasty, and in many instances a total joint prosthesis is the preferable reconstructive approach.

Complications Associated with Treatment of Fractures

REMARKS

Complications may occur with any method of fracture treatment, either open or closed.

Before selecting treatment the physician should be aware of the potential pitfalls likely to develop.

Certain complications occur with sufficient frequency that they may be avoided by anticipation.

95

Tight Cast Syndrome

Avoid application of unpadded circumferential plaster in acute injuries, especially those about the knee or elbow.

This patient's dislocated elbow was reduced and immobilized in a long arm cast. He did not return for follow-up until ten days later, when he had developed ischemic muscle contracture (Volkmann's contracture) under the cast.

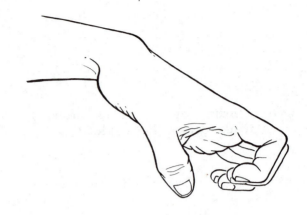

Loose Cast Syndrome

Rather than reapplying a new long leg cast, the physician rewrapped a bivalved cast. When the loose cast was changed three weeks later, the dorsal surface of the foot had sloughed.

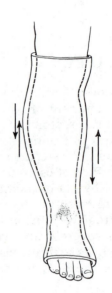

Cast-Induced Open Fracture

1. Cast was applied without complete reduction of the anterior angulation of the proximal fragment.

2. The skin caught between the cast, and the bone became necrotic, producing an open fracture.

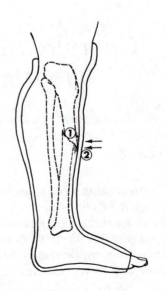

Nerve Injury

1. While in a long arm cast for a fracture of the radius this patient developed burning pain and clawing of the hand.

2. The ulnar nerve, which subluxed over the medial humeral epicondyle with elbow flexion, had been pinched between the cast and bone.

Note: This complication may also develop during or after surgery if the elbow is immobilized in hyperflexion.

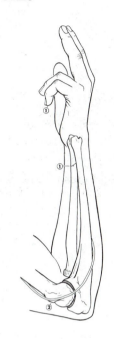

Ischemic Muscle Necrosis from Traction

1. In children, skin traction and limb elevation narrows the arteriovenous pressure significantly and can produce ischemic contracture. Avoid Bryant's traction in children weighing over 30 lb (13.6 kg).

2. Skin traction, which if heavy can narrow muscle compartments of the leg by Chinese finger-trap effect, should be no heavier than 8 lb (3.6 kg).

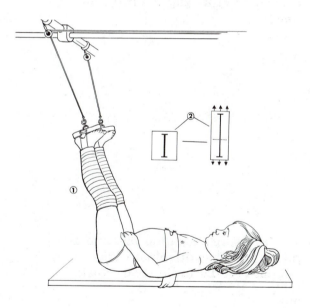

Operative Pitfalls

1. Wound necrosis was evident one week after tight closure over a tibial plate on the medial surface.

Note: Avoid tight closure and do not apply plates where skin closure will be difficult.

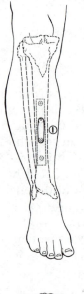

1. Excision of loose bone fragments leads to fracture gap and infected non-union.

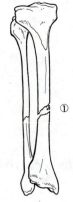

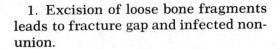

2. Pressure irrigation of bone fragments can decontaminate bone without need for discarding bone stock.

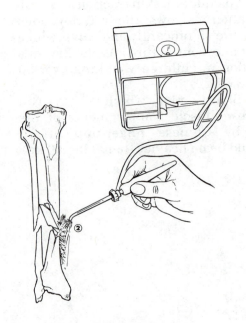

Internal fixation is only as strong as its weakest component.

1. Single plates on femoral shaft fractures frequently fail when

2. Screws pull out of cortical bone.

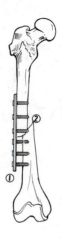

3. Fixation devices should allow fracture impaction, not distraction.

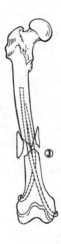

CLINICAL AND RADIOGRAPHIC FEATURES OF FRACTURES

REMARKS

A history of some form of injury is obtained in most fractures.

A history of injury in the presence of these objective signs should suggest a fracture:
1. Local swelling.
2. Deformity.
3. Ecchymosis.
4. Localized bone tenderness.
5. Loss or impairment of function.

Note: If any of these findings, especially localized bone tenderness, is elicited, treat and protect as a fracture until it is proven otherwise.

The following features are pathognomonic of fracture:
1. Crepitus.
2. Abnormal mobility.

Absence of a history of injury does not preclude fracture; this is true of most pathologic fractures and fatigue fractures.

Absence of dysfunction does not preclude fracture; this is particularly true of:
1. Greenstick fractures.
2. Impacted fractures.
3. Fatigue fractures.

Clinical evaluation of a fracture must always include:
1. The state of the soft tissue (does the fracture communicate with the exterior?).
2. The state of the circulation of the limb. Note the surface temperature, the color of the part distal to the fracture, the arterial pulses, and the capillary return when the nail bed or pulp of a digit is compressed.
3. Presence or absence of any nerve deficit.
4. Presence or absence of visceral damage.
5. Examination of other bones for fracture. Fractures of the calcaneus may be associated with a fracture of the spine; a fracture of the upper third of the ulna may be complicated by a dislocation of the radial head.

The Importance of Radiographic Examination

REMARKS

Never fail to take an x-ray of the injured part. This is especially true for lacerating and penetrating injuries to rule out the possibility of retained foreign bodies.

In all instances at least two views taken at right angles to each other are mandatory.

Always include joints proximal and distal to the fracture on the x-ray.

Lack of radiographic evidence does not overrule clinical impressions of fracture.

In certain areas, oblique views and other special views are necessary to reveal the fracture.

Remember that in some instances a fracture line may not be discernible for several weeks; hence, later x-rays are necessary; this is especially true for fractures of the carpal scaphoid, and the femoral neck and for fatigue fractures.

Cervical Spine

FRACTURE

1. An injury most commonly missed in the cervical spine is a fracture-dislocation of C6 or C7, which is frequently hidden by shoulder structures.

2. X-ray must demonstrate down to T1 and should be taken with patient's shoulders pulled caudally.

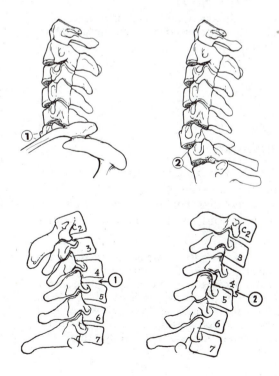

SUBLUXATION

1. No evidence of subluxation is noted when the cervical spine is held in the neutral position.

2. Forward subluxation of C4 on C5 is demonstrated when the x-ray is taken with the patient carefully flexing his neck under the physician's supervision.

Cervical Spine *(Continued)*

SHOULDER

1. Anteroposterior view reveals no obvious abnormalities.
2. Lateral view reveals a posterior dislocation.

Note: Axillary view is always possible if the cassette is held above the injured shoulder and the x-ray tube points up through the axilla.

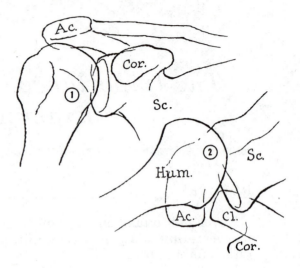

Ulna

1. Fracture of the upper third of the ulna.
2. X-ray of the elbow of the same patient showing dislocation of the head of the radius.

Note: Always insist that the x-ray include the joints proximal and distal to the fracture.

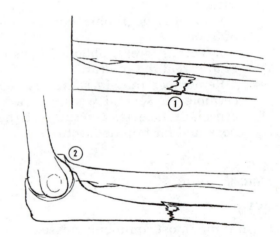

Scaphoid

1. No abnormality is noted in x-ray taken at the time of injury.
2. Fracture through the waist of the scaphoid is noted three weeks later.

Note: A negative x-ray does not preclude a fracture; if symptoms persist take another x-ray in two or three weeks. Now the fracture if present will be discernible. Also, always take oblique views of the scaphoid; conventional anteroposterior and lateral views may fail to show the fracture.

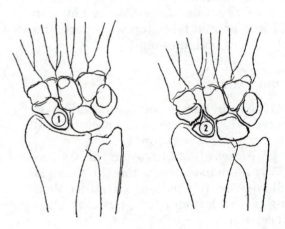

Femoral Neck

1. Anteroposterior view; fracture of the neck of the femur in "good" position.

2. Lateral view of same hip reveals marked displacement of the femoral head.

Note: Always take anteroposterior (AP) and lateral views of the hip. The AP view may fail to show a displaced femoral head. When in doubt, protect the patient's hip by having him use crutches, and take another x-ray in one to two weeks.

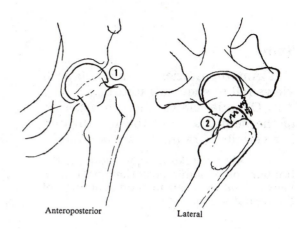

Anteroposterior   Lateral

Patella

1. Lateral view shows no fracture.

2. Axial view shows tangential fracture of the patella.

Note: Always take axial and anteroposterior views in different degrees of flexion of the knee joint; these views best reveal fractures of the patella and of the articular surfaces of the femoral condyles.

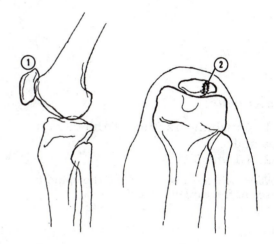

Ankle

1. Fracture-dislocation of the ankle.

2. Fracture of the neck of the fibula.

Note: In dislocations and fracture-dislocations of the ankle joint always take x-rays of the entire lower leg.

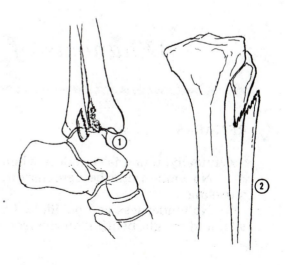

103

Spine

1. Anteroposterior and lateral views fail to show a fracture.

2. Oblique views show a fracture of the neural arch of the fourth lumbar vertebra (traumatic spondylysis).

Note: Always take oblique views of the lumbar spine; anteroposterior and lateral views alone may fail to show fractures of the neural arches.

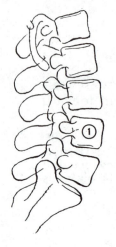
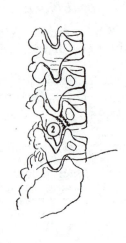

Calcaneus

1. Crushing fracture of the calcaneus and

2. L1 and T12.

Note: Always take x-rays of the spine in cases of fracture of the calcaneus.

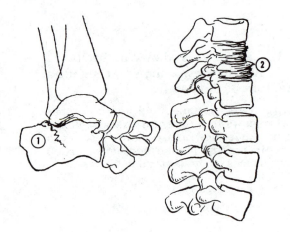

Diagnosis of Bony Union

REMARKS

Clinically, union is complete when:

1. No motion can be demonstrated at the fracture site with gentle stressing.

2. No tenderness can be elicited by direct pressure over the fracture site, and weight bearing on the fracture in the lower limb is pain free.

Clinical evaluation should always be supported by x-ray examinations, using stress films if necessary.

Demonstration of bony trabeculae across the fracture is confirmatory evidence that healing is complete and remodeling is taking place. This is seen in the late phases of union.

Caution: Overlapping fragments or impacted fragments may give the erroneous appearance on x-ray of true bony trabeculae across the fracture.

Visible external callus bridging the fragments is also evidence of bony union; this occurs in the early phases of healing.

1. Early bone union is indicated by longitudinal bridging of the fracture in the medullary region.

2. External callus bridging the fracture also signifies early union.

3. Bony trabeculae obliterate the fracture site after mature bony union.

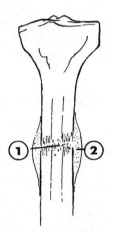
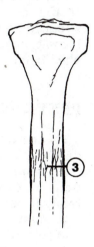

GENERAL PRINCIPLES OF FRACTURE MANAGEMENT

REMARKS

Stabilization of the injured patient begins immediately at the scene of the accident. Skillful handling in extricating the patient from wrecked vehicles or other sites of entrapment is essential. Spine boards, splints, and thoughtful precautionary measures should be applied before moving the patient.

PREVENTION AND TREATMENT OF SHOCK

1. Control hemorrhage with voluminous pressure dressings and bandages. DO NOT USE TOURNIQUETS.
2. Insure an airway and prevent aspiration in the unconscious patient by extending the head and drawing the mandible forward. Be ready to suction promptly to prevent aspiration of stomach contents.
3. Apply necessary splints or use antishock trousers to splint the limb and restore central blood volume.
4. Keep the patient warm with blankets.
5. Morphine (8 to 10 mg for adults) may be given for pain, but note the dose and inform admitting hospital personnel. Never give morphine if there are manifestations of cerebral injury.
6. Begin intravenous fluid administration if possible, during extrication and especially if anticipated time of transportation is prolonged.

For further discussion of shock, see page 77.

EMERGENCY SPLINTING

Cervical Spine

1. Protect neck at all times with cervical support.

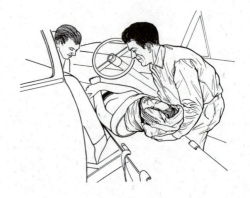

106

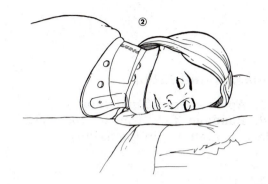

2. The unconscious patient may be turned to the side with this splint if vomiting occurs.

Thoracic and Lumbar Spine

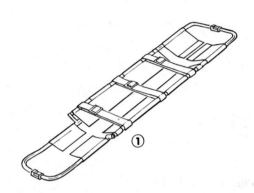

1. A scoop stretcher is most useful for extrication and transportation to avoid flexing the spine while lifting the patient.

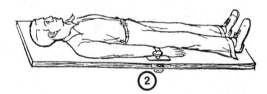

2. The patient should be kept on a firm surface with the face up.

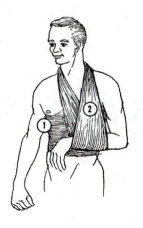

Ribs

1. Apply a swathe around the chest.
2. Support the arm in a sling.

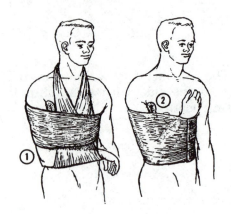

Humerus and Elbow

1. Apply a swathe and sling or
2. Bandage the arm to the side (place a small pad in the axilla).

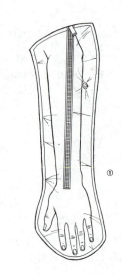

Forearm and Wrist

1. Inflatable splint is ideal.

or

1. Bandage the forearm and hand to a padded board and
2. Suspend the arm in a sling.

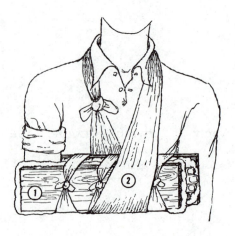

Multiple Fractures or Fractured Pelvis

1. Military antishock trousers (MAST or MAST suit) are an effective support for the victim of multiple fractures. Because the MAST forces one third of the blood volume from the lower limbs to vital organs, it can be useful and even life-saving.

Note: The MAST must be removed carefully to avoid abrupt recurrence of hypovolemic shock.

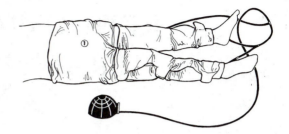

Femur

1. Apply a Hare splint.
2. Strap splint to ankle and foot over shoes.

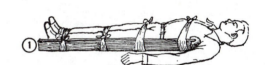

3. The ring fits comfortably against the buttock.
4. Traction is applied to the leg and the fracture.

or

1. Bandage the limbs together to a board extending from the axilla to the foot on the injured side.

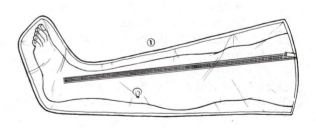

Knee and Lower Leg

1. Use inflatable splint.

or

1. Apply a pillow splint reinforced by
2. Boards placed on both sides and on the posterior surface of the limb.

Note: Pillow splint is especially useful for ankle fractures.

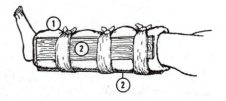

REDUCTION OF FRACTURES

REMARKS

In general the goal in the definitive treatment of a fracture is to achieve healing of the fragments with anatomic alignment and to restore normal function in the shortest possible time.

Clinical experience reveals that there are many exceptions to this rule. Many fractures need no reduction, the degree of displacement is acceptable, and normal function is the rule.

Accurate replacement of fragments is not essential for a good functional result in the following fractures:

1. Impacted fracture of the neck of the humerus.

2. Fracture of the clavicle, especially in children.

3. Fracture of the femur in children, provided that there is no angular deformity.

4. Fracture of forearm bones in children, provided that there is no angular deformity.

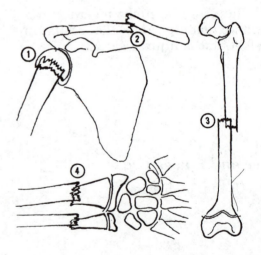

Accurate apposition of fragments is not always necessary, provided that no angular deformity exists and that the shortening is not too great. This is particularly true in children.

1. This amount of displacement is acceptable in both adults and children.

2. This angular deformity is not acceptable in either children or adults. To evaluate the true angular deformity, compare the proximal and distal joint alignment.

3. Shortening of 2 cm without angular deformity is acceptable in patients younger than 10 years because of the growth spurt that will occur after the fracture.

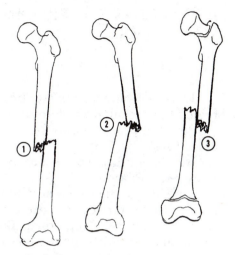

1. Bayonet apposition of forearm fractures may be accepted in children rather than employing open reduction.

2. Growth remodeling occurs as long as the epiphysial plate is open.

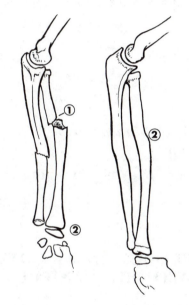

Always restore normal alignment of joints above and below a fracture; failure to do so favors development of osteoarthritis.

Perfect reposition of fractures implicating the articular surfaces is mandatory. This is especially true of weight-bearing joints; if this requisite is not fulfilled, osteoarthritis is inevitable.

Reduction should be accomplished as soon as possible after injury before tissues become infiltrated with blood and fluid and lose their elasticity. Once reduced, the fractured limb is still likely to swell; circular casts should be bivalved at the first suspicion of tightness.

111

REDUCTION BY TRACTION AND MANIPULATIVE MANEUVERS

REMARKS

Always employ an anesthetic agent. The anesthesia may be general, regional, or local. Complete muscle relaxation facilitates the procedure.

Study the prereduction x-ray films and keep them in view during the procedure.

Always confirm the position of the fragments after reduction by x-ray examination.

In most instances steady manual traction is employed while the manipulative maneuvers are executed. This is especially true in over-riding fractures of long bones and in impacted fractures.

The manipulative maneuvers must:

Restore alignment and correct angulation.

Correct all rotational displacement.

Restore length.

Place fragments in apposition.

Note: The exceptions to this goal are listed in Remarks on page 110.

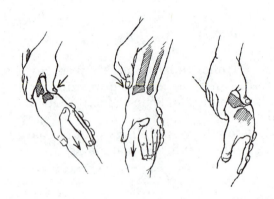

Example of Manipulative Reduction

Reduction of a Colles' fracture.

REDUCTION BY CONTINUOUS TRACTION WITH OR WITHOUT MANIPULATION

REMARKS

Injury to the soft tissue envelope around fractured long bones permits overriding of the fragments. This is particularly a problem with transverse and oblique fractures of the femoral shaft.

Continuous traction is necessary in these unstable fractures to maintain the desired fracture position.

Continuous traction is rarely employed in the upper limb except for supracondylar fractures of the humerus with circulatory impairment from swelling.

Fixed skeletal traction with pins inserted proximal and distal to the fracture and incorporated in plaster is very useful for open unstable fractures of the forearm and the tibia.

Example of Reduction by Continuous Traction

Oblique fracture of the femur. The reduction is achieved and maintained by continuous skeletal traction.

Gravity-Assisted Reduction of Trimalleolar Ankle Fracture Without Anesthetic (After Quigley)

1. A stockinet is gently rolled over the fractured ankle, and tincture of benzoin is used to make it adhere to the skin.

2. The foot is elevated by ropes and weights and the knee is supported by sling.

3. The force of gravity and the inverted position of the ankle reduce the fracture while allowing the edema to subside.

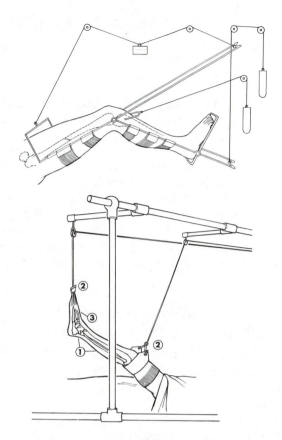

OPEN REDUCTION

REMARKS

This method is used when closed methods fail.

In some fractures operative reduction is the method of choice.

As a rule, when operative reduction is executed the fragments are stabilized by some form of internal fixation.

Fractures for Which Open Reduction is the Method of Choice

1. Transverse fracture of the femur (fixation by an intramedullary nail).

2. Fracture of the patella with separation of the fragments.

3. Fracture of the olecranon with separation of the fragments.

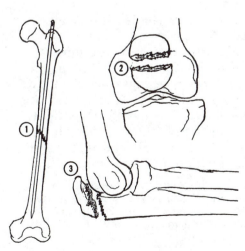

ANESTHESIA FOR FRACTURE TREATMENT

REMARKS

Immediate management and debridement of open fractures should be done with the patient under complete regional or general anesthesia.

Closed reduction of certain fractures in lower limb may be frequently accomplished without anesthetic and with the aid of gravity and steady continuous traction.

Closed reduction of upper limb fractures is effectively accomplished with intravenous anesthetic block.

Use of the intravenous anesthetic requires adequate assistance and understanding of technique and ready availability of resuscitation equipment for the infrequent adverse reaction.

Intravenous Regional Anesthetic for Fractures of the Upper Limb

1. A 0.33% solution (1 cc of 1% Lidocaine for every 2 cc saline) is used in dose of 0.5 cc per kg. of body weight.

2. Insert a small pediatric needle in the dorsal vein of the hand distal to the fracture.

3. Elevate the arm for at least 3 minutes to allow for gravity drainage of blood.

4. Using a pretested blood pressure cuff with encircling tape, inflate rapidly above 210 mm Hg.

5. Lower arm and inject Lidocaine solution.

Remove the needle and wait 10 minutes for analgesia. Then,

6. Perform fracture reduction.

7. After cast is applied and postreduction x-ray is accepted, deflate cuff to 80 mm Hg. for 10 seconds and reinflate to 210 mm Hg. If patient's status and vital signs do not change within 1 minute after this trial release, deflation may be completed.

Note: With precaution, regional intravenous anesthetic is the safest and most effective method for closed reduction of fractures distal to the elbow in both children and adults.

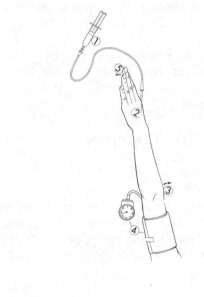

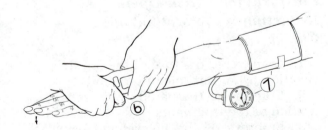

114

IMMOBILIZATION

REMARKS

Although most fractures require rigid immobilization to achieve union, some fractures are best treated without rigid fixation.

When immobilization is indicated it must be so applied that it:

1. Relieves all pain.
2. Prevents any shearing or rotatory stresses at the fracture site.
3. Maintains the desired position of the fragments and prevents displacement or angulation.
4. Permits active muscle contraction.

The method of immobilization to be utilized is dictated by the peculiar features of each fracture.

In general the method selected should permit free active movement of joints not immobilized.

Whenever possible the patient should be made ambulatory just as soon as it is safe to do so. This enhances overall functional activity and prevents atrophy of muscles and stiffness of joints.

Always strive for early use of the affected extremity without disturbance of the fracture site.

Certain joints, such as the wrist, knee, and hip, tolerate long periods of immobilization well, provided that the soft tissues around them are actively exercised.

Certain joints, such as the shoulder and the joints of the hand, tolerate prolonged immobilization poorly.

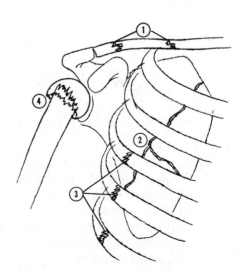

Examples of Fractures That Do Not Require Rigid Immobilization

1. Fracture of the clavicle.
2. Fracture of the scapula.
3. Fracture of the ribs.
4. Impacted fracture of the upper end of the humerus.

Examples of Fractures That Do Not Require Rigid Immobilization (Continued)

1. Undisplaced fractures of the metacarpals and metatarsals.
2. Undisplaced fractures of the phalanges of the fingers and toes.

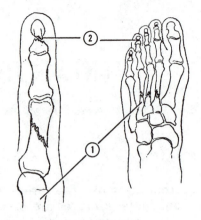

Examples of Fractures That Do Require Rigid Immobilization

1. Fracture of the scaphoid.
2. Fracture of the olecranon.
3. Fracture of the neck of the femur.

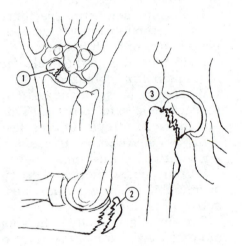

Methods of Immobilization

When immobilization must be utilized, three methods are available. The peculiarities of the specific fracture to be immobilized will dictate the method to be employed.

The three methods are:

1. Immobilization by circular plaster, splints, or fracture braces.
2. Continuous traction.
3. Internal fixation.

CIRCULAR PLASTER CAST OR EXTERNAL PLASTER SPLINT

REMARKS

In order to insure against displacement of the fragments and to attain maximum rigid fixation, the plaster cast should fit snugly and should be accurately molded to the configuration of the limb.

Padding under the cast or splint should not be excessive; however, some padding provides added insurance against damage to soft tissues, nerves, and circulation.

All bony prominences should be well padded.

Generally, a layer of stockinet or one or two layers of sheet wadding is sufficient padding, except when marked swelling is expected, as after a surgical procedure, for which more layers of sheet wadding should be used.

When there is any significant swelling about the limb, apply a bivalved cast and elevate the limb for five to seven days before applying the definitive cast.

Application of a Circular Plaster Cast: Acute Forearm Fracture

1. Apply a layer of stockinet or one or two layers of sheet wadding.

2. Immerse completely a roll of plaster bandage in lukewarm water; leave the roll immersed until bubbles cease to rise.

3. Remove excess water from the roll by squeezing the ends (do not twist the roll).

4. Prepare slabs of plaster of required length and width on a smooth surface (four to six layers are sufficient). Keep the bandage wet and sloppy and rub in each layer to produce a homogeneous plaster slab.

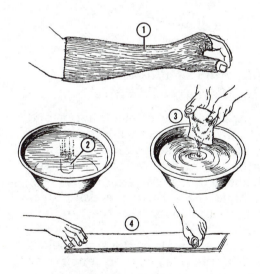

Application of a Circular Plaster Cast: Acute Forearm Fracture (Continued)

1. Apply anterior and posterior slabs and mold them accurately on the contours of the limb.
2. Then apply a circular plaster bandage.

Note: Each turn is laid on smoothly and evenly without tension.

3. Tuck in the margin of the bandage if necessary to avoid wrinkling. (Four to six layers of circular bandage usually suffice; rub in each layer.)
4. An assistant supports the patient's hand while the plaster is being rolled.

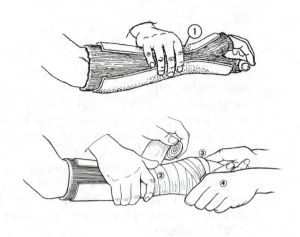

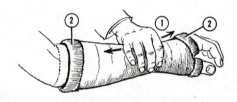

Application of Plaster Slabs — Forearm Fracture

1. Apply a layer of stockinet or one or two layers of sheet wadding.
2. Apply a plaster slab of sufficient length and width to the limb (the slab should be wet and sloppy).
3. Mold the slab to the contour of the limb and over the bony prominences.
4. Turn the ends of the slab back.
5. Fix the slab by an encircling cotton elastic bandage; this is applied snugly but without tension.

(Hold the limb immobile and in the desired position until the plaster is hard.)

Note: A cast applied for management of acute fracture should be replaced in one to two weeks by a functional cast or fracture brace.

1. While the plaster is still wet, mold the plaster to the limb with the palm of the hand.
2. Turn the ends of the stockinet or sheet wadding over the ends of the cast.

Note: Keep the limb immobile until the plaster is hard; any movement at the joints while the plaster is setting will produce ridges which may make undue pressure on the underlying soft tissues.

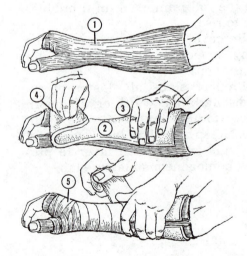

Application of a Fracture Brace

After a preliminary period with a long arm cast, the patient with a forearm fracture may be given a fracture brace.

1. The fracture is held reduced by suspension in Chinese finger traps and thermoplastic Orthoplast (Johnson & Johnson) is applied over double layered stockinet.

2. A supracondylar extension is used to prevent forearm rotation while allowing elbow flexion and extension.

3. Hinged joint permits wrist flexion and extension.

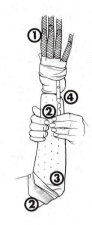

CAUTIONS

Avoid ridges and irregularities on the inner surface of the cast; these may produce pressure sores.

Protect bony prominences with adequate padding and careful molding of the plaster before it sets.

Progressive edema in a rigid encasement is capable of producing first venous and then arterial obstruction. Watch the limb carefully for the *first 36 hours.*

Persistent pain under a plaster cast is always indicative of trouble; always give the patient the benefit of the doubt and uncover the area.

Edema, pain, cyanosis, numbness, and anesthesia are clinical features signaling trouble, usually caused by circulatory impairment. When any of these is present, split or bivalve the cast promptly.

Never apply a circular cast if there is any evidence of circulatory damage.

Never apply an unpadded plaster cast after a fresh fracture or following any operative procedure.

Unpadded casts are justified only after all reactive swelling has subsided and shows no sign of recurring (usually 1 to 2 weeks after the fracture or operation).

Application of unpadded casts must be reserved for those skillful in the techniques of plaster immobilization. It is not a method of immobilization to be employed by the uninitated.

Splitting the Cast

1. Split the cast throughout its entire length.

2. Divide any padding or dressing under the cast down to the skin, or

3. Spread the margins of the split cast from top to bottom.

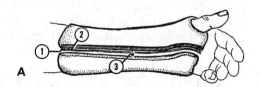

Bivalving the Cast

1. Bivalve the cast.
2. Spread the margins on both sides of the cast.
3. Fix the two halves with a cotton elastic bandage.

Note: After splitting or bivalving the cast, elevate the limb; maintain the elevation until circulation is reestablished and the edema subsides.

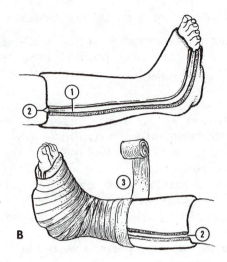

CONTINUOUS TRACTION

REMARKS

Continuous traction may be necessary to hold the fragments in the desired position. This is particularly true of spiral and oblique fractures of the long bones such as the femur and tibia.

Continuous traction balances the pull of the long muscles and thus overcomes any overriding; also, the stretched soft tissues tend to press the fragments into place, correcting anteroposterior or lateral displacement.

Traction on the distal fragment is made in the line of the proximal fragment. This corrects angulatory displacements.

Rotatory deformities are corrected by turning the distal fragments to match accurately the proximal fragment.

Countertraction is attained by the pull of the body's weight in the opposite direction.

Some form of splint or suspension apparatus is always employed to support the fragments in the desired position, e.g., a Harris-Aufranc splint for femoral shaft fractures.

Never allow distraction, because it favors delayed union and nonunion.

Do not hesitate to manipulate fragments into place if traction alone fails to correct lateral or angulatory displacement.

Perform manipulation while traction is maintained and always with the patient under anesthesia.

Continuous traction may be obtained by:
1. Skin traction or
2. Skeletal traction.

Skeletal traction is superior to skin traction in attaining and maintaining reduction in fractures of long bones.

120

Always use a threaded pin; this minimizes the chance of skin and bone infection.

Always insert the threaded pins under strict aseptic technique and in the direction which avoids adjacent nerve structures, e.g., from the medial side of the ulna to protect the ulnar nerve. Do not insert pins through or in the region of growing epiphyses.

Make repeated checks of the traction apparatus and make necessary corrections.

Skin Traction

1. Apply foam rubber traction straps to the outer and inner surfaces of the limb.
2. Place a 1 cm pad of foam rubber over the malleoli.
3. Fix the straps with 7.6-cm cotton elastic bandages applied snugly.

Note: More than 10 lbs (4.5 kg) of skin traction may blister the skin and produce circumferential constriction of muscle compartments.

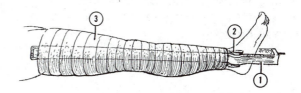

Sites for Skeletal Traction

1. Below the olecranon.
2. Pins through the olecranon and distal radius and ulna, incorporated in plaster for open forearm fractures.
3. Through the supracondylar area of the femur.
4. Through the upper end of the tibia.
5. Proximal and distal pin fixation, especially for open tibial fractures.
6. Through the lower end of the tibia and fibula.
7. Occasionally through the os calcis for comminuted ankle fractures.
8. Skull traction.
Insertion by hand-powered drill is preferable.

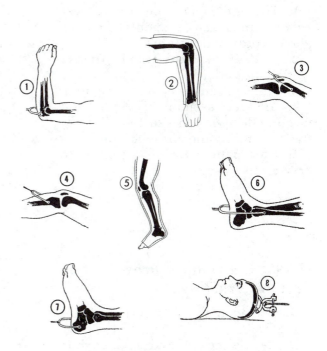

DO NOT INSERT TRACTION PINS WITH POWER DRILL WITHOUT PRE-DRILLING BONE. OTHERWISE, RING SEQUESTRUM WILL RESULT FROM BURNED BONE.

Russell Traction

Russell traction is used for fractures of the femur, especially in older children.

1. Foam rubber straps.
2. Sling under the knee (line the sling with a sheet of foam rubber).
3. The knee is flexed.
4. The hip is flexed.
5. A pillow supports the leg.
6. The foot of the bed is elevated.
7. The distal pull in the line of the femur is twice the upward pull because of the arrangement of the system of pulleys.

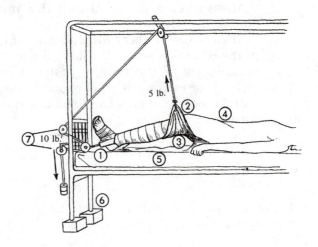

Balanced Suspension Traction Apparatus

1. The limb is suspended in perfect balance in a Harris splint by a system of cords and weights.
2. A Pearson attachment permits motion at the knee.
3. Tibial or femoral pin may be used.
4. Another system of cords and weights designed to exert continuous traction in the line of the femur.
5. Foot plate (this is essential to prevent foot drop).

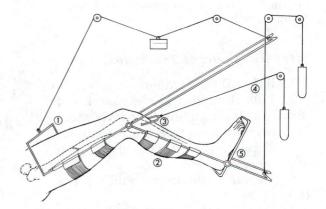

90°-90° Traction for Proximal Femoral Fractures

1. Threaded pin is inserted in distal femur.
2. Leg is flexed and abducted to align distal fragment with proximal fragment.
3. Knee is flexed 90° and leg is supported in cast.

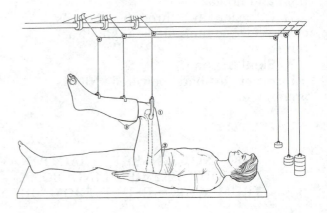

INTERNAL FIXATION

REMARKS

Internal fixation is justified in the following situations:

When it is impossible to maintain a desired reduction by closed methods such as plaster immobilization or continuous traction.

In certain fractures, it is the method of choice to obtain a satisfactory reduction and permit early functional use of the limb, particularly with fractures involving joints.

Internal fixation is occasionally useful in open fractures in which it is impossible to maintain length by any other method.

Immediate plate fixation of open fractures should be avoided, but intramedullary nailing may be helpful in providing immobilization without further damaging soft tissue.

When choosing open methods of internal fixation, one should always be aware of its dangers, i.e., contamination with possible infection and further damage to the tissues with consequent impairment of normal repair processes, either of which leads to nonunion.

For Fresh Fractures

1. Compression plates for forearm fractures provide rigid fixation of both bones and permit early functional use of the hand and limb.

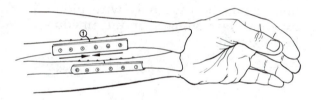

2. The intramedullary nail is useful in most long bone fractures but is especially applicable to fractures of the femur and tibia. Frequently, intramedullary nailing may be done without opening fracture site if image-intensified fluoroscopy is used to guide insertion. In order for fracture fixation to be adequate, the nail should fit firmly in the canal and should not allow rotation of fragments. Occasionally, cortical screws or circumferential wire may supplement the intramedullary fixation. Intramedullary nails are inadequate for fractures in the proximal and distal femur unless they are specially designed to accommodate the widened canal.

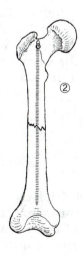

Intramedullary nailing is not without hazard and complications and should be done only when the mechanical advantages outweigh the biologic disadvantages.

For Fresh Fractures (Continued)

3. Transfixion screws are useful supplements to plate fixation, especially to butterfly fragments. By over-drilling of the proximal cortex, a lag-screw effect compresses the fracture. To accomplish this the screw is inserted at the angle halfway between lines perpendicular to the cortex and perpendicular to the fracture.

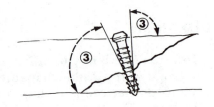

4. Circumferential wires are very useful to help immobilize open, oblique fractures of the tibia and to supplement intramedullary fixation of the long bones. Thin, strong, 18-gauge circumferential wires will not damage circulation to the bone. Circumferential wire fixation in itself is incomplete and should be used only with either external cast support or intramedullary fixation.

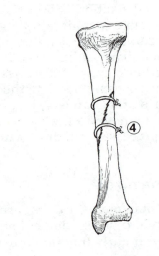

5. Tension-band cerclage wiring is effective for avulsion fracture of the olecranon or the patella. The wires are inserted so as to resist the tensile force of muscle, which would distract the fracture, and at the same time to compress the fracture towards the articular surface.

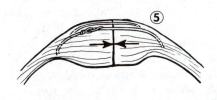

6. MOST IMPORTANT: Internal fixation of long bones, except intramedullary fixation of the femur, requires adequate external immobilization until bone healing is achieved.

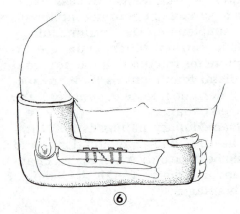

MANAGEMENT OF OPEN FRACTURES

Decisions should be made promptly about associated head, chest, or abdominal injuries. Do not delay fracture treatment to observe for "possible" head injury or abdominal injury. General anesthetic is safest for patient with cerebral concussion and open fracture.

If 8 hours or more have elapsed from the time of injury to the time of operation or the wound is extremely contaminated, infection is likely and the wound must be treated for it. Begin intravenous antibiotics in the emergency room after wound culture. Initial antibiotic therapy should be directed against Staphylococcus, the most common infecting organism. Change antibiotics subsequently according to culture and sensitivity.

The goals should be removal of all contaminated and devitalized tissue and avoidance of primary closure.

Always use a pneumatic tourniquet if any tourniquet is deemed necessary. Check distal pulses, and be sure that the fracture has not caused arterial injury before applying the tourniquet.

Operative Procedure

Operation for open fracture is performed with strict aseptic technique.

Preparation of the Field

1. Support the limb without applying traction.

2. Cover the wound with sterile gauze.

3. After shaving the skin, cleanse the limb thoroughly with Betadine solution.

Note: Do not use strong antiseptics to clean the wound.

Throughout the procedure, continue to treat for shock with blood or plasma.

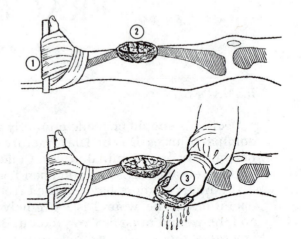

Irrigation of the Fracture Site

1. Irrigate copiously with at least 10 l of water to flush off contaminants from the skin and from the depths of the fracture.

Note: Grease and oil may be removed by special solvents.

2. While the irrigation continues, the skin is cleansed once again with Betadine antiseptic solution.

3. A drainage table is useful to keep the field dry.

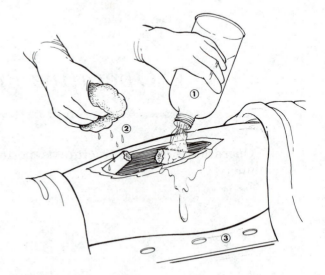

Wound Debridement (After Learmonth)

Note: *To debride* means to unbridle or to unleash tight structures. Be certain that all tight muscle compartments are released and that all potential and actual sources of infection are removed. The method is summarized by Sir James Learmonth's verse:

On the edge of the skin take a piece very thin (1);
The tenser the fascia, the more you should slash 'er (2);
Of muscles much more, 'til you see fresh gore (3)
And the bundles contract at the least impact;
Hardly any of bone, only bits quite alone (4).

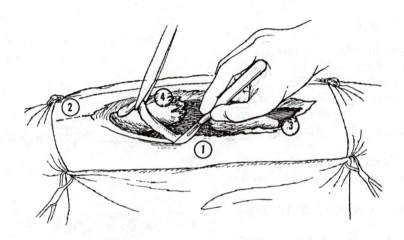

Decontamination of Bone

1. Enlarge the wound as necessary to visualize both ends of the fracture.
2. Use a curette to remove dirt from bone fragment but avoid excising bone if at all possible.

OR

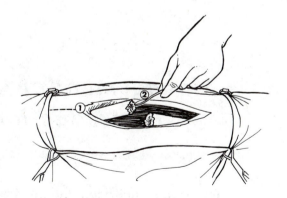

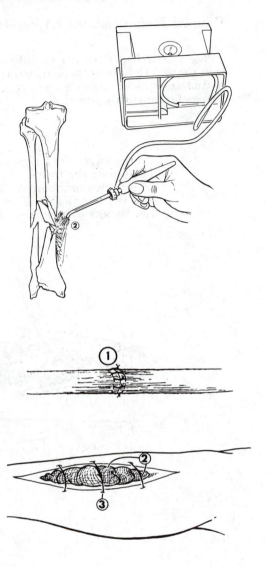

Decontamination of Bone (Continued)

2. Pressure irrigation systems are very useful to remove dirt ground in the bone.

Closure of Wound

Closure should be avoided in wounds more than 8 hours old, in high-velocity missile injuries, in mass casualties, in wounds from human bites, or whenever there is any doubt about the degree of contamination.

1. Repair simple lacerated nerves and tendons which are directly accessible.

2. Pack the wound lightly with gauze.

3. Support the wound edges with 3–0 wire sutures tied without tension.

Note: Do not use relaxing incisions to close, since these would add considerably to the risk of necrosis of traumatized skin.

Management of the Fracture and Postreduction Treatment

After wound debridement the fracture is immobilized with cast or traction.

Internal fixation is rarely necessary unless the fracture is so unstable that fracture motion would add further damage to the soft tissues or would risk disruption of a vascular repair. Proximal and distal pins incorporated in plaster are most effective for stabilizing the open fracture of the tibia or forearm.

Be sure that tetanus immunization is adequate and record this in the patient's chart.

Continue intravenous antibiotics and adjust according to wound culture and sensitivity. Antibiotic treatment is maintained until wound is healing adequately (at least five to seven days).

Reinspect and reirrigate the wound under sterile operating-room conditions in three to five days or sooner if signs of sepsis develop. Do not rely on cast windows to "peek" at the wound, since this deprives bone and soft tissue of the benefits of uninterrupted immobilization.

Secondary closure may be begun at the time of reinspection, provided that the wound edema has subsided and the wound is clean.

WHEN IN DOUBT, LEAVE THE WOUND OPEN TO CLOSE BY INTUSSUSCEPTION OF WOUND EDGES.

With any open fracture, especially when there is associated muscle damage, keep in mind the possibility of gas gangrene.

Lethal Anaerobic Infection After Open Fractures (Tetanus and Gas Gangrene)

REMARKS

Clostridial organisms are the anaerobic, gram-positive rods present all about us that frequently contaminate wounds and that, when given appropriate anaerobic wound conditions, can proliferate, secrete toxins, and kill the patient.

Clostridium tetani infections are still prevalent, with a mortality rate that remains above 50 per cent, primarily because of delayed recognition rather than difficulty of treatment.

Tetanus is a disease of the unimmunized, the elderly, and the newborn. It does not occur in patients who have been adequately immunized.

The incubation period for tetanus is 8 days but may range from 1 to 30 days. Suspect tetanus in any elderly or unimmunized patient who develops general myalgia progressing to trismus, facial muscle spasm, and convulsions after any wound, no matter how minor.

Clostridial myonecrosis, or gas gangrene, which is most often associated with Clostridium perfringens infection of damaged muscle, is among the most lethal infections of man.

Although clostridial myonecrosis has been considered a complication primarily of military wounds, it is now most common in civilian injuries, especially from mass casualties. The basic contributory factors are incomplete or delayed wound débridement and a persistent tendency to close wounds, thereby producing the anaerobic environment on which the organisms thrive.

Clostridial Tetanus Prophylaxis

FOR THE PREVIOUSLY IMMUNIZED PATIENT

1. Remove all devitalized tissue.
2. Unless patient has received a booster or completed immunization series within 5 years, give toxoid booster (0.5 cc).
3. Give the patient a written record of his immunization.

FOR THE UNIMMUNIZED PATIENT

1. If wound is clean, give initial immunizing dose.
2. Instruct the patient to complete the basic immunization.
3. If wound is neglected or otherwise tetanus-prone, give toxoid, immune globulin, penicillin, or oxytetracycline.

Clostridial Myonecrosis

1. Characteristically occurs one to three days after injury in a contaminated wound.
2. Wound becomes acutely painful and swollen, and the patient senses impending doom.
3. Pulse and temperature rise rapidly, although initially they may be normal.
4. Gas infiltrating muscle layers can be felt and frequently seen on x-ray. Muscle necrosis is widespread.

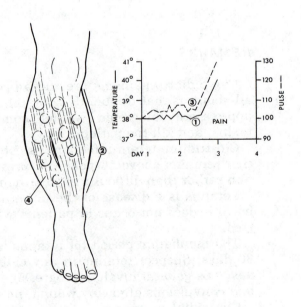

Note: Clostridial myonecrosis must be distinguished from clostridial contamination of the wound and clostridial cellulitis, neither of which causes the severe toxicity of the deep anaerobic infection in muscle. Other infections such as from Streptococcus and Bacteroides may also form gas in tissue.

Preventive Treatment of Anaerobic Myonecrosis

The best treatment is prophylactic: Completely debride all open fractures and do not close any dubious wound.

Especially avoid primary closure in:

1. Wounds about the buttocks and perineum.

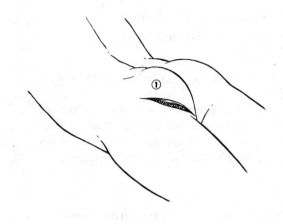

2. Close-range gunshot injuries that are contaminated by shotgun wadding or the patient's clothing.

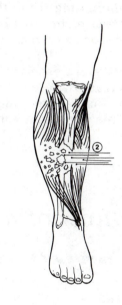

3. Wounds sustained in water that may look clean but frequently are heavily contaminated.

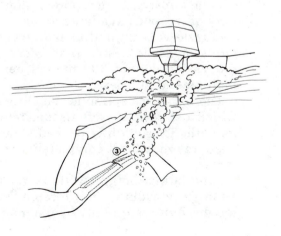

Preventive Treatment of Anaerobic Myonecrosis (Continued)

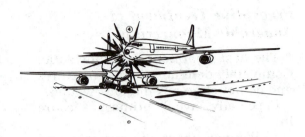

4. Wounds sustained in mass casualties.

Plan to reinspect and redebride all open fractures under sterile conditions within three to five days after the initial injury and debridement.

Treatment of Acute Anaerobic Myonecrosis

This is a fulminating, limb-threatening, and life-threatening infection for which treatment must be prompt and decisive.

Begin high-dose intravenous penicillin (at least 18 million units per day).

Hyperbaric oxygen treatment, at 2.5 atmospheres, will diminish toxicity and demarcate the area of tissue loss.

Complete excision of necrotic muscle is necessary and may mean amputation of the limb even with hyperbaric oxygen treatment.

Gunshot and Shotgun Fractures

REMARKS

Proper management of these increasingly common civilian injuries depends upon a basic appreciation of tissue damage from the wide variety of weapons available today.

Muzzle velocity and missile weight are the most important determinants of tissue destruction. Most civilian firearms do not exceed the muzzle velocity of 305 meters per second that is required to produce high kinetic injuries.

The major exception is the close-range (under 10 m) shotgun injury, which destroys all soft tissue, neurovascular structures, and bone in its path. These tightly packed shot clouds with large amounts of kinetic energy may blast completely through the limb and damage all structures.

Penetrating shotgun wounds without a wound of exit consistently leave retained wadding and foreign material that must be thoroughly sought, quite frequently by means of counter-incisions.

Major arteries in any proximity to the shotgun injury should be explored, to rule out the possibility of significant vascular damage.

Immediate internal fixation of a shotgun fracture is unwise as well as unsatisfactory, since these comminuted fractures can be treated by traction, cast, or cast braces.

The soft tissue wounds should be left open to heal secondarily, with the use of cast immobilization to aid healing of both soft tissue and bone.

The gunshot fracture from a low-velocity, small-caliber bullet, in contrast with the shotgun injury, may be treated by superficial debridement and fracture immobilization. Probing for and extrication of the bullet is not helpful, except in the hand or foot where leaving the bullet in place may cause pain. The only exception is a bullet that has penetrated a joint or seems to have damaged a major artery or nerve.

Antibiotic treatment is not necessary for the low-velocity gunshot injury but is quite necessary for the shotgun wound.

Close-Range Shotgun Fracture of Femur

1. Wound of entrance left open after debridement.

2. Fracture site explored in the operating room and thoroughly debrided.

3. Two shotgun wads removed from the medial side of the thigh.

4. Femoral artery is visualized and found intact.

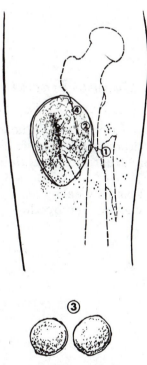

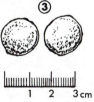

133

Close-Range Shotgun Fracture of Femur (Continued)

Fracture was treated in skeletal traction and cast brace.

Six months after injury:

1. Soft tissue wound has closed by intussusception without skin graft.

2. Comminuted fracture is healed.

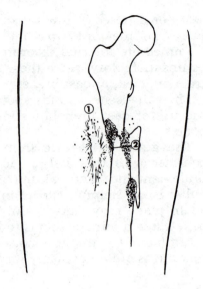

.22-Caliber Gunshot Fracture of Femur

1. Wound treated by superficial debridement without exploring fracture.

2. Fracture treated in traction and cast brace.

3. Healing at 16 weeks.

4. Bullet was not removed.

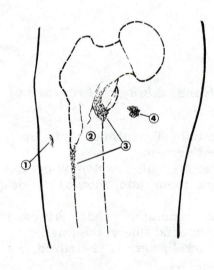

FUNCTIONAL REHABILITATION DURING AND AFTER FRACTURE HEALING

REMARKS

The objective of fracture treatment is to restore the patient to normal functional level as early and as completely as possible.

All muscle groups, including those immobilized in plaster, should be actively exercised on a regular basis.

Consider the psychological aspects: Explain to the patient what you are trying to achieve, clearly demonstrate what he is to do, and reinforce these instructions by having the patient demonstrate his progress to you at follow-up examination.

Purposeful functional exercises during fracture treatment and intensified exercises after healing are most effective. A selective combination of active and passive stretching exercises solves most of the difficult problems in joint immobilization and muscle stiffness following injury.

SPINE

Hyperextension Exercises for Fracture of the Thoracic Spine

1. The patient stands facing a corner and places one hand on each wall at shoulder level.
2. Holding head up, he leans forward to try to touch his chest to the corner while inhaling deeply.
3. He pushes back to the starting position, and repeats 30 times.

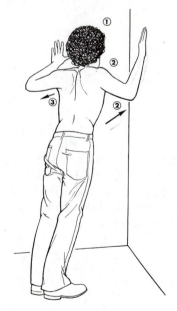

Flexion Exercises for Lumbar Spine Injury

These are very useful after extension injuries that have produced damage to the discs or posterior elements. Flexion exercises should not be employed for compression fractures or other injuries produced by flexion vectors.

1. The patient is supine with his head flat or supported by a low pillow. Both knees are pulled up simultaneously into the axilla so as to decrease lumbar lordosis.

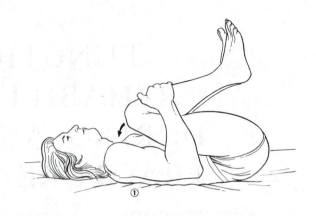

2. With hips flexed to eliminate hip flexor pull and maximize abdominal muscle function, the patient sits up, extending his arms between his legs. He may be helped in this effort by having someone hold his feet.

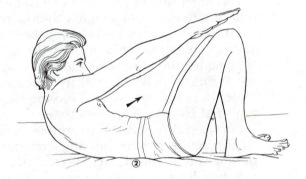

3. Sitting on a chair with thighs spread apart, the patient tries to touch the floor with his elbows. His head must hang loosely and his general muscle tone must be relaxed.

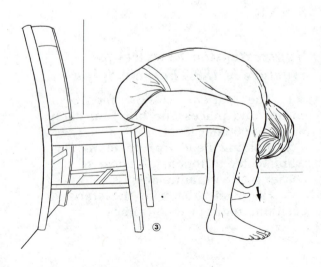

4. While holding a rail or back of a chair for support, the patient squats back with his heels flat on the floor to decrease lumbar lordosis. This is especially helpful for back pain following prolonged standing.

HIP

Passive Skateboard Exercises for Hip Injuries

These are especially useful after acetabular fractures in which joint resurfacing is encouraged by the molding effect of the femoral head in contact with the healing fracture.

1. The patient lies supine on a firm, smooth, comfortable surface with his feet on a skateboard and uses the skateboard to support the legs while passively abducting and rotating the hips.

Note: Exercises should be done hourly, if possible, during recovery from the fracture.

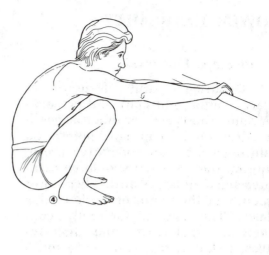

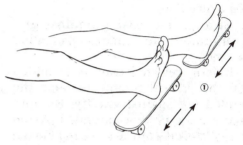

Active Exercises for Muscles Around the Hip Joint

1. The patient lies in the prone position and forcefully contracts the gluteal muscles to raise the extended limb. This position is held for a specified count and then the leg is slowly lowered; the limb is always under muscle control.

2. After the muscles improve in power the exercise is performed against increasing resistance.

3. The patient lies in the lateral position with the affected side upward. The extended leg is abducted to the maximum level and held there for a specified count; then it is lowered slowly. This is repeated a specific number of times.

4. Next, the same exercise is performed against increasing loads.

Note: A powerful quadriceps also adds to the stability of the hip joint; add quadriceps exercises to the program.

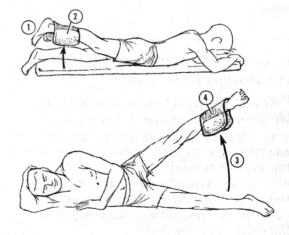

LOWER EXTREMITY

Quadriceps Exercises

1. Quadriceps drill: designed to prevent muscle atrophy and preserve its volume and power as much as possible; drill should be initiated before and continued after any operative procedure on the knee and should be instituted and maintained during healing of fracture of the femur or the lower leg bones. The patient forcefully contracts the quadriceps and then relaxes it slowly; this is done 15 to 20 times every hour.

2. Straight leg raising against gravity: initiated after quadriceps drill is mastered.

3. Elastic resisted exercises: added when the patient is able to raise the extended leg against gravity. Be sure that the knee is kept extended. Avoid resisted exercise of the knee in a flexed position, which causes patella chondromalacia.

4. Bicycling: designed to increase endurance of the quadriceps and the range of joint movement.

5. Stair-climbing exercise.

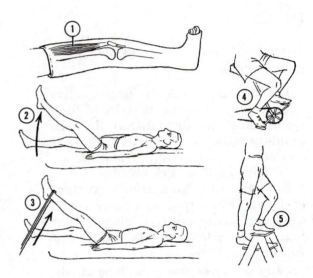

Passive Stretching Exercise for Quadriceps Contracture

This is useful when flexion is limited after distal femoral fractures or knee injuries and depends on gravity-assisted, passive stretching done by the patient himself.

1. While lying supine, the patient flexes his hip 90 degrees, flexes his knee to the maximum, and supports his thigh with his hands.

2. The patient then uses the good leg to push the stiff knee into flexion by employing quick, repetitive strokes and using gravity assistance.

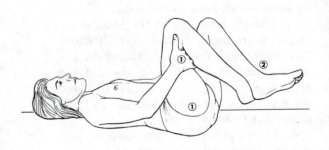

SHOULDER

Gravity Exercises

First start with gravity exercises.

1. The patient bends far forward holding shoulders and trunk immobile.

2. The arms hang loosely and swing like a pendulum (A) across the front of the body, (B) backward and forward and (C) in a circle.

Note: The arc at first is small, then is gradually increased.

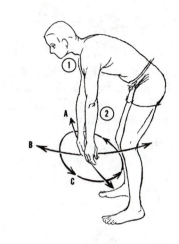

Passive Stretching Shoulder Exercises

These are most valuable for the painful stiffening of the shoulder that can occur after very minor injury and can persist for many months or years. The patient must work to regain motion in all planes, including external rotation and abduction as well as extension and flexion.

1. The patient stands with scapulae against the wall and hands clasped behind his head. He abducts and externally rotates his shoulder rapidly in order to touch elbows to wall. This may require assistance to get full external rotation and abduction.

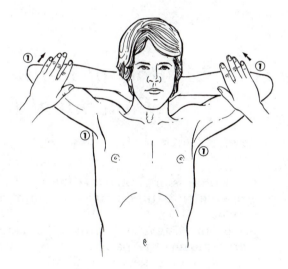

2. The patient reaches to an overhead support or door and flexes at the knee to pull with body weight on stiff shoulder.

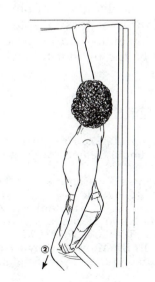

Passive Stretching Shoulder
Exercises (Continued)

3. The patient reaches behind his back, grasps the wrist on the side of the stiff shoulder, and pulls upward toward the opposite scapula.

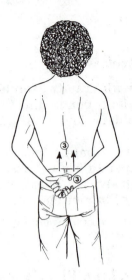

Role of Physical Therapy in Functional Rehabilitation

A professional physical therapist can make valuable contributions to the patient's functional rehabilitation during and after fracture treatment.

By applying heat, ice, and other pain-relieving techniques to the injured area during the patient's exercising efforts, the therapist can assist and speed recovery considerably.

The disadvantage of physical therapy is that it may allow the patient to assume a passive role in his rehabilitation program. The therapy then becomes counterproductive, since the primary active therapist must be the patient himself.

REFERENCES

Anderson, L. D., Hutchins, W. C., Wright, P. E., et al.: Fractures of the tibia and fibula treated by casts and transfixing pins. Clin. Orthop., 105:179–191, 1974.

Bagby, G. W.: Compression bone-plating. J. Bone and Joint Surg., 59-A:626–631, July 1971.

Brighton, C. T., Friedenberg, Z. B., Zemsky, L. M., Pollis, P. R.: Direct current stimulation of non-union and congenital pseudoarthrosis. J. Bone and Joint Surg. 57A:368–377, 1975.

Britt, B. B.: Malignant hyperthermia: a pharmacogenic disease of skeletal and cardiac muscle. New England J. of Med., 290:1140–1142, May 1974.

REFERENCES

Brown, P. W., and Kinman, P. B.: Gas gangrene in a metropolitan community. J. Bone and Joint Surg., 56-A:1445–1451, Oct. 1974.

Connolly, J. F.: Perils and pitfalls of open tibial fractures. Am. Fam. Phys., 11:64–72, Jan. 1975.

Connolly, J. F., Dehne, E., and LaFollette, B.: Closed reduction and early cast-brace ambulation in the treatment of femoral fractures. J. Bone and Joint Surg., 55-A:1581–1599, Dec. 1973.

Connolly, J. F., Whittaker, D., and Williams, E.: Femoral and tibial fractures combined with injuries to the femoral or popliteal artery. J. Bone and Joint Surg., 53-A:56–68, Jan. 1971.

Eaton, R. G., and Green, W. T.: Epimysiotomy and fasciotomy in the treatment of Volkmann's ischemic contracture. Orthop. Clin. N. Am. 3:175–186, 1972.

Hardaway, R. M., James, P. M., Anderson, R. W., Bredenberg, C. E., West, R. L.: Intensive study and treatment of shock in man. J.A.M.A. 199:779–790, 1967.

Harris, W. H., and Aufranc, O. E.: A new splint for balanced suspension. Clin. Orthop., 72:216–218, 1970.

Holstein, A., and Lewis, G. B.: Fractures of the humerus with radial-nerve paralysis. J. Bone and Joint Surg., 56-A:1338–1349, Oct. 1974.

Howland, W. S., and Ritchey, S. C.: Gunshot fractures in civilian practice. J. Bone and Joint Surg., 53-A:47–55, Jan. 1971.

McKibbin, B.: The biology of fracture healing in long bones. J. Bone and Joint Surg. 60B:150–162, 1978.

Mubarak, S. J., and Owen, C. A.: Double incision fasciotomy of the leg for decompression in compartment syndromes. J. Bone and Joint Surg. 59A:184–187, 1977.

Murray, D. G., and Racz, G. B.: Fat-embolism syndrome (respiratory insufficiency syndrome). J. Bone and Joint Surg., 56-A:1338–1349, Oct. 1974.

Olerud, S., and Danckwardt-Lilliestrom, G.: Fracture healing in compression osteosynthesis. Acta Orthop. Scand., Suppl. 137, 1971.

Paradies, L. H., and Gregory, C. F.: The early treatment of close-range shotgun wounds to the extremities. J. Bone and Joint Surg., 48-A:425–435, Apr. 1966.

Quigley, T. B.: A simple aid to reduction of abduction–external rotation fractures of the ankle. Am. J. Surg. 97:488–493, 1959.

Rhinelander, F.: Circulation of bone. In The Biochemistry & Physiology of Bone. 2nd edition, edited by G. Bourne, New York, Academic Press, 1972, Vol. 2, pp. 2–76.

Sarimento, A., Cooper, J. S., and Sinclair, W. F.: Forearm fractures. Early functional bracing — a preliminary report. J. Bone and Joint Surg., 57-A:297–303, Apr. 1975.

Schiller, M. G.: Intravenous regional anesthesia for closed treatment of fractures and dislocations of the upper extremities. Clin. Orthop., 118:25–29, 1976.

Whitesides, T. E., Jr., Haney, T. C., Morimoto, K., and Harada, H.: Tissue pressure measurements as a determinant for the need of fasciotomy. Clin. Orthop., 113:43–51, 1975.

INJURIES TO PHYSES AND EPIPHYSES

ANATOMIC FEATURES

REMARKS

Injuries to the epiphyses and physes, or epiphyseal plates, are more common than generally appreciated; they account for roughly 15 per cent of all injuries to the long bones during the period of growth.

They occur more frequently (1) in boys than in girls and (2) during the periods of rapid skeletal growth, which are the first year and the preadolescent period.

Comprehension of the nature of injuries implicating the epiphyses and epiphyseal plates permits the treating physician: (1) to institute adequate treatment, (2) to prevent shortening and angular deformities of the growing bones, and (3) to predict, in a measure, the outcome of specific injuries.

This comprehension is predicated on knowledge of the anatomic peculiarities of the epiphyses and physes.

Types of Ossification Centers

1. The epiphysis is the secondary center of bone formation that in long bones is located at the end and that determines shape and size of the articular surface.

2. The physis is the area of growing cartilage cells that remains from the embryonic primary ossification center and that is responsible for longitudinal growth.

3. The primary and secondary ossification centers remain separated by an epiphyseal bone plate.

4. Metaphysis is the area of spongiosa or new bone formed from the physis.

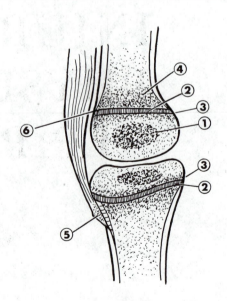

144

5. An apophysis is a secondary ossification center at the site of tendon attachment. It is extra-articular and contributes to bone contour but not to longitudinal growth.

6. The ring of Ranvier is a separate area of ossification that contributes to growth in circumference and supports and protects the physis.

Circulation to Epiphyseal-Metaphyseal Region (After Brookes)

REMARKS

Enchondral growth depends on precise integration of chondrogenesis and osteogenesis. Circulation is vital for the growth of cartilage as well as for ossification in both the secondary epiphyseal and primary physeal centers.

Throughout most of growth, the blood supplies to these two centers remain separated by the bone plate, and any significant vascular communication between them results in bony bridge formation, growth arrest, and deformity.

The ossification groove of Ranvier encircles the growth plate and forms a thin cylindrical collar of bone supporting the physeal-metaphyseal junction. This area is richly supplied by its own perichondrial circulation.

1. The vascular circle bordering the joints supplies numerous epiphyseal, metaphyseal, and perichondrial vessels.

2. The metaphyseal arteries arise directly from the vascular circle as well as from the principal nutrient artery.

3. The epiphyseal vessels enter through nonarticular surfaces and supply the bony epiphysis.

4. Epiphyseal vessels form rake-like arcades which perfuse the growing cartilage cells but do not penetrate the physis.

5. Separate perichondrial vessels give blood supply to ossification groove of Ranvier.

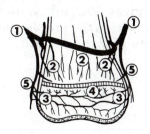

STRUCTURE OF THE GROWTH CENTER (AFTER BRIGHTON)

1. Epiphyseal bone plate separates primary and secondary ossification centers.

2. The zone of small cells also acts as a buffer between the epiphyseal circulation and the active portion of the physis below.

3. In the zone of cell columns, cells proliferate and produce matrix resulting in longitudinal growth of physeal cartilage. As long as the physis remains open, the cartilage column must grow as rapidly as new bone is formed at the bottom of the physis.

4. In zone of hypertrophic cells, the cells swell and bud off matrix vesicles, which initiate calcification; the cells then degenerate.

5. The last three or four cells in the hypertrophic zone comprise the provisional zone of calcification.

6. The metaphysis begins distal to the last intact transverse septum at the bottom of each hypertrophic cell column.

7. Where the disrupted lacuna is invaded by vascular elements, the vascularized and calcified cartilage tissue becomes the zone of primary spongiosa.

8. Osteoblasts appear on the calcified longitudinal septa and form bone. The newly formed bony trabeculae in the metaphysis are the zone of secondary spongiosa.

9. The perichondrial groove or ring of Ranvier gives circumferential mechanical support to the physis and contributes to its growth in width.

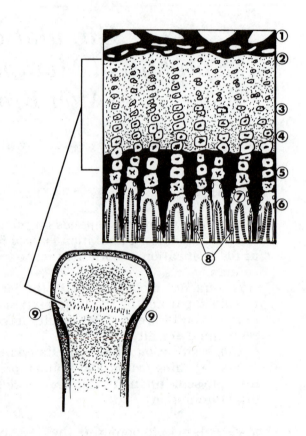

Perichondrial groove of Ranvier (after Shapiro).

1. The perichondrial groove of Ranvier is covered on the outside by a continuation of the outer fibrous layer of periosteum.

2. It is bordered on the inside by the epiphyseal cartilage.

3. Fibroblasts and fiber bundles form the roof of the groove in continuity with the outer fibrous layer of periosteum.

4. The inner portion of the groove is bone bark, which provides mechanical support for the physis while longitudinal and horizontal growth occur.

5. The area of densely packed cells in the groove of Ranvier contributes to the growth of the bone bark.

6. An area of loosely packed cells in the groove probably adds cells appositionally to the epiphyseal cartilage above the growth plate so as to increase the diameter of the cartilage epiphysis.

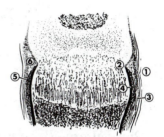

Strength of the Physis

The weakest portion of the physis when tested by tensile loading is its junction with the metaphysis or the region of primary spongiosa. The transition from calcified cartilage to immature bone makes this region structurally weak and susceptible to failure on initial loading. The failure may continue to propagate either in a direction to include other zones of the physis or in the opposite direction, toward the metaphysis.

As a whole, the physis is weaker than bone, ligaments, tendons, and the fibrous capsule.

This explains the frequency of epiphyseal separations in children and the infrequency of dislocations and of tears of tendons and ligaments.

Forces capable of producing subluxations and dislocations in the adult produce epiphyseal separations in the growing child; this is particularly true of the shoulder, knee, hip, and ankle.

MECHANISMS OF INJURIES (AFTER BRIGHT, BURSTEIN AND ELMORE)

REMARKS

Physeal growth centers are subjected to a variety of traumatic force vectors, including 1) shearing, 2) avulsion, and 3) crushing vectors, all of which may disrupt the balance between cartilage growth and ossification as well as disrupt the joint surface. If injury to the physis causes vascular ingrowth across the previously impenetrable epiphyseal bone plate, a bony bridge may form between the epiphysis and metaphysis. This produces a mechanical block or stapling effect on the cartilage columns, which prevents further growth and eventually closes part or all of the physis.

The usual mechanism of the injury is that the fracture begins in the physis along the lines of the highest shear forces produced by the injury. Most commonly, this occurs in the zone of the primary spongiosa or the junction between the physis and metaphysis. As the force vector increases, the fibers of the perichondrium (the ring of Ranvier), which are subjected to the maximum tension, may rupture and may allow complete physeal displacement. Usually the failure tends to be propagated downward toward the metaphysis, and since the resultant fracture disrupts neither the articular surface nor the cartilage columns, healing is uneventful.

The force vector may also propagate upward toward the epiphysis and the joint surface. Traumatic arthritis and growth deformity from epiphyseal-metaphyseal bone bridging are likely sequelae if this type of physeal injury is not reduced anatomically. Open reduction and careful internal fixation are required for injuries crossing the physis, epiphysis, and articular surface.

148

Growth Potential of Physes

REMARKS

In order to evaluate correctly the seriousness of epiphyseal injuries, it is essential to know the contribution of each epiphysis to the longitudinal growth of the bone to which it is attached.

The following is a comprehensive guide:

CONTRIBUTION OF EACH PHYSEAL CENTER TO GROWTH OF LONG BONES

Humerus

    Upper physis 80%
    Lower physis 20%

Femur

    Upper physis 30%
    Lower physis 70%

Radius

    Upper physis 25%
    Lower physis 75%

Tibia

    Upper physis 55%
    Lower physis 45%

Ulna

    Upper physis 20%
    Lower physis 80%

Fibula

    Upper physis 60%
    Lower physis 40%

Classification of Injuries to the Physis

REMARKS

There are five general classifications of injuries to the physis (Salter and Harris), but keep in mind that the growth effect depends more on the degree and direction of initial vectors of injury and the age of the patient than on the x-ray category.

TYPE I

REMARKS

This lesion is produced by a shearing force through the physeal-metaphyseal junction and occurs in early childhood and sometimes at birth during difficult deliveries.

Usually, the degree of trauma is not severe, the physis remains intact in the sagittal plane, and the epiphyseal vessels perfusing the cartilage cell columns are undamaged.

Occasionally, circulation to an epiphysis that is completely covered by cartilage, such as the proximal femoral epiphysis, may be disrupted by the injury, and ischemic necrosis of the bony epiphysis occurs.

Commonly, however, the vascular system remains undamaged, and healing is rapid and complete within three weeks.

The perichondrium or groove of Ranvier remains intact usually on one side and severe displacement is prevented.

Separation of Lower Femoral Physis

1. Separation through the physeal-metaphyseal junction.

2. Perichondrium on the convex side of the displacement usually ruptures in severe injuries.

3. Perichondrium on the concave side is intact and acts as a hinge. It also stabilizes the epiphysis after reduction.

4. Blood vessels to the epiphysis are not damaged.

Note: Growth prognosis based on x-ray is uncertain after injury to this most important physis of the lower limb.

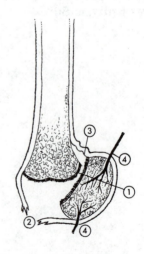

150

Separation of Upper Femoral Physis

1. Separation through junction of physis and metaphysis.

2. Blood vessels to the bony epiphysis may rupture at the point of entry.

Note: The prognosis in this lesion may be poor. The intra-articular bony epiphysis can undergo avascular necrosis. Clinically, this may follow separation of the upper femoral epiphysis and, less frequently, separation of the proximal radial epiphysis.

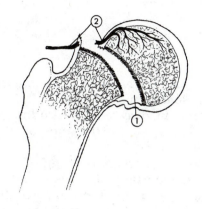

TYPE II

REMARKS

The physis is separated along with a triangular segment of the metaphysis. The type II injury is produced by shearing or avulsion force vectors. It is rarely encountered in children under ten years of age. The perichondrium is torn on the convex side and is preserved on the concave side. The intact portion of the perichondrium stabilizes the physis following reduction.

Generally, the blood supply to the epiphysis is undamaged, and the physis remains intact. Therefore, the prognosis is good.

1. Separation of the physeal-metaphyseal junction. The major portion of the physis is uninjured.

2. Ruptured perichondrium on the convex side of the deformity.

3. Metaphyseal triangular fragments.

4. Intact perichondrium.

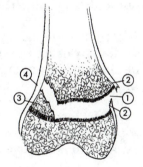

TYPE III

REMARKS

A type III fracture results when the force vector is directed first transversely and then longitudinally across the physis and epiphysis. This may occur, for example, with a valgus injury to the knee when the force runs transversely across the physis and then is directed toward the articular surface by the pull of the cruciate ligaments.

It is essential to restore the joint congruity as well as reduce the physis and epiphysis anatomically to prevent bony bridging and traumatic arthritis.

The prognosis with this injury depends on whether perfusion of the physis is impaired and whether bony bridging is prevented by anatomic reduction.

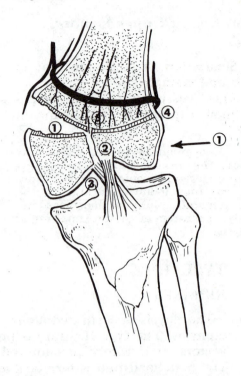

1. Valgus strain to the knee causes shearing load across physis.

2. Force is directed longitudinally toward the knee by the pull of the cruciates.

3. Articular surface is disrupted.

4. Perichondrial support is intact.

5. Vascular penetration across the physis will lead to metaphyseal-epiphyseal bony bridge formation unless the fracture is reduced anatomically.

TYPE IV

REMARKS

The fracture line traverses the full thickness of the growth apparatus, crosses the physis, and splits off a portion of the metaphysis.

Generally, there is an upward displacement of the epiphyseal-metaphyseal fragment that produces incongruity of the articular surface.

Complete anatomical reduction of this lesion is essential in order to realign the physis and restore a smooth articular surface.

Some form of internal fixation is necessary to maintain the desired position.

Fracture of the lateral condyle of the humerus is a typical example of the type IV lesion.

This lesion usually results from severe abduction or adduction force vectors, and physeal arrest is common if reduction is not anatomic.

1. The fracture line traverses the epiphysis, physis, and a portion of metaphysis.

2. The epiphyseal-physeal-metaphyseal fragment is displaced upward.

3. Failure to reduce the physis will permit bony bridging and growth arrest.

4. The articular surfaces are incongruous.

5. The periosteum is slack but intact.

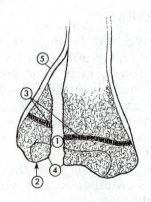

TYPE V

REMARKS

A portion of the physis is compressed by the force vectors acting across it through the epiphysis, and the circulatory arcade to the proliferating cells of the physis is damaged.

This lesion is encountered in joints moving in one plane such as the knee and ankle.

Displacement of the epiphysis is rare, but it may occur with severe abduction or adduction injuries.

Radiographs, as a rule, give no clue to the extent of the injury.

Premature closure of the plate with loss of growth and angulatory deformity is common in this rare injury.

1. Injury to the physis.

Note: No disruption of the physis is evident initially. The major damage is probably sustained by the epiphyseal vascular arcade perfusing the physeal zone cell columns. The lesion manifests itself only after a period of delayed growth.

2. A portion of the physis has closed prematurely, causing an angular deformity.

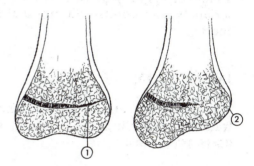

Factors Governing Prognosis of Injuries to the Physes

REMARKS

Certain abnormal conditions, such as endocrine disorders, rickets, scurvy, and osteomyelitis, render the epiphyseal plates vulnerable to even minor injuries.

AGE

In the face of an epiphyseal injury, the younger the child the greater the probability that shortening, angular deformity, or both are likely to occur.

NATURE OF THE LESION

a. Type I lesions have a good prognosis provided that the blood supply to the epiphysis and physis is not disrupted.

b. Prognosis for other types of injuries depends on the degree of initial injury and displacement, the adequacy of reduction, and particularly the growth center involved. Growth effect from fractures of the distal femoral growth center is notoriously unpredictable.

BLOOD SUPPLY TO THE EPIPHYSIS

Normal longitudinal growth depends on the ability of the cartilage cells in the physeal columns to proliferate at the same rate as angiogenic ossification occurs on the metaphyseal side. Disruption of the arcade of epiphyseal vessels that perfuse these cartilage columns may seriously compromise the physeal balance of cartilage cell growth and death.

INFECTION

Pyogenic infections destroy the epiphyseal plate; therefore, open fractures involving the plate, in which infection may occur, carry a grave prognosis.

ADDITIONAL TRAUMATIC INSULTS

The delicate plate may be further traumatized by forceful manipulative maneuvers during closed reduction and by instrumentation during open reduction.

Gentleness in reduction of epiphyseal fractures is most essential in all instances.

Management of Injuries to the Physis

REMARKS

Management of any physeal injury must never be taken lightly, since growth disturbances may occur even under the most favorable conditions.

Parents should be warned of the possibility of growth disturbances but should not be alarmed.

Growth disturbances may not be apparent for six to twelve months; therefore, all epiphyseal injuries should be carefully observed for at least one year.

Healing processes at the site of physeal injury are very active in children; reduction of a fracture becomes more difficult with the passing of each day. Reduction should be performed the same day the injury occurs. After ten days it is practically impossible to achieve a reduction unless unusual force is employed. This is dangerous to the plate.

If the physis is not disrupted, as in type I and type II injuries, considerable displacement may be corrected by growth, and open reduction to achieve anatomic positioning is not indicated.

If the physis is disrupted and the joint surface is incongruous, as in type III and type IV injuries, anatomic reduction is essential and is best accomplished by open reduction.

Try to place pins and wires for internal fixation in the bony epiphysis without crossing the physis. If fixation across the physis is necessary, use smooth Kirschner wires rather than screws or threaded pins so as to avoid compressing the zone of cartilage columns in the physis.

SEPARATION OF THE UPPER EPIPHYSIS OF THE HUMERUS

Epiphyseal Separation at Birth and in Children Younger than Six Years

REMARKS

At birth, the lesion may be associated with a dislocation that generally reduces spontaneously.

When the lesion is present at birth, frequently an erroneous diagnosis of brachial palsy is made and an abduction splint is applied. This favors redislocation.

Because in children under one year of age the epiphysis is entirely cartilaginous, it may be impossible to make a diagnosis by x-ray. However, the relationship of the metaphysis to the center of the glenoid cavity may be a clue.

Lateral projections may be helpful in determining the presence of a dislocation.

In the infant, clinical features should be depended on to establish the diagnosis — swelling, pain, dysfunction, pseudoparalysis, and evidence of callus within five to ten days.

In children under six years of age, the epiphyseal lesion is usually type I, whereas the older child sustains a type II injury.

Anatomic restoration of the epiphysis is not essential; in time, remodeling of the upper end of the humerus will restore the anatomic position of the epiphysis.

156

EPIPHYSEAL SEPARATION AT BIRTH AND IN INFANTS

Appearance on X-Ray

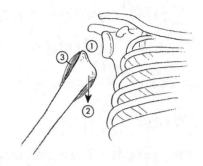

1. Ossification center of the epiphysis has not appeared.
2. Metaphysis of the humerus is displaced downward in relation to the glenoid cavity.
3. Callus formation is evident (ten days after injury).

Management

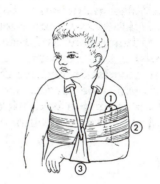

1. Place wad of cotton in the axilla.
2. Fix the arm to the chest with a bias-cut cotton bandage.
3. Suspend the forearm with a collar and cuff.

Note: Keep the arm immobilized for two to three weeks. Manipulation for reduction is not necessary.

EPIPHYSEAL SEPARATION IN CHILDREN YOUNGER THAN SIX YEARS

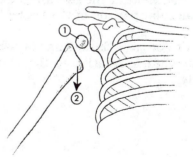

Prereduction X-Ray

1. Epiphysis is centered in the glenoid cavity.
2. Metaphysis is displaced downward by the type I physeal fracture.

Management

Exact reduction is not necessary, and administration of general anesthetic is not justified. Use the simplest immobilization possible, such as the Velpeau dressing described above, and maintain immobilization for two to three weeks. Any malalignment or angulation will be corrected with remodeling from growth.

Epiphyseal Separation in Children Older Than Six Years

REMARKS

The proximal humeral epiphyseal separation is most frequently a type II lesion in a child older than six years.

Complete reduction of the epiphysis is not essential, since correction of the deformity by remodeling is the rule.

If displacement and fracture angulation is less than 20 degrees, reduction is unnecessary.

For angulation greater than 20 degrees, gentle manipulation and reduction may be carried out under general anesthetic.

Open reduction is not indicated unless the epiphysis has been dislocated out of the glenohumeral joint as well as fractured.

Prereduction X-Ray

1. Epiphysis together with the triangular fragment of the metaphysis.

2. Triangular portion of the metaphysis.

3. Shaft of the humerus is displaced upward in relation to the glenoid cavity.

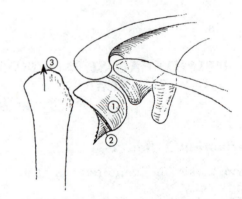

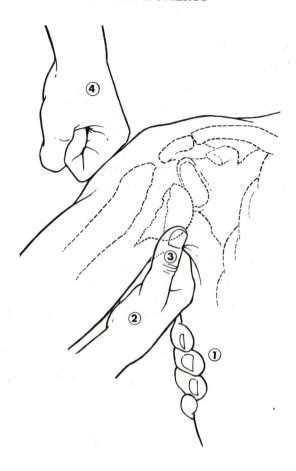

Manipulative Reduction

Complete muscle relaxation is essential. Use a general anesthetic so that the distal fracture fragment can be brought down into alignment with the epiphysis.

1. An assistant stabilizes the scapula by reaching under the child's back and holding the axillary border.

2. The operator maintains steady traction while slowly abducting and externally rotating the arm to the overhead position.

3. The operator places his thumb in the axilla and pushes the epiphyseal-metaphyseal fragment upward.

4. The shaft fragment is pushed downward while the shoulder is abducted.

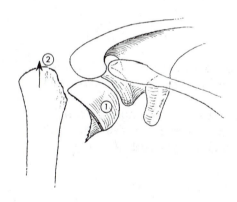

Postreduction X-Ray

1. The epiphysis with the triangular metaphyseal fragment is in normal alignment with the shaft of the humerus.

2. Fracture line through the metaphysis.

Postreduction Management

Apply a shoulder spica holding the arm abducted 70 degrees and externally rotated 30 degrees.

The shoulder is maintained in its reduced, abducted, externally rotated position by means of the shoulder spica for four to five weeks. Remove the spica after five weeks.

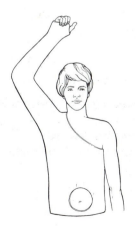

159

Postreduction Management
(Continued)

Now apply a triangular sling and institute exercises to restore motion at the shoulder, elbow, wrist, and hand.

Discard the sling seven to ten days after removal of the plaster spica, and allow free use of the arm.

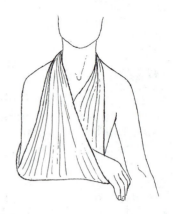

Unreducible Epiphyseal Separations with Severe Displacement or Dislocation

REMARKS

In rare instances, a severely displaced or dislocated upper humeral epiphysis in a young adult cannot be reduced by the manipulative maneuvers just described.

The most common cause is a displacement of the biceps tendon between the fragments. This is an indication for open reduction, but only if the patient is a young adult in whom remodeling is unlikely.

Prereduction X-Ray

1. Epiphysis with a triangular fragment of the metaphysis is displaced downward and backward.

2. The shaft of the humerus is displaced upward.

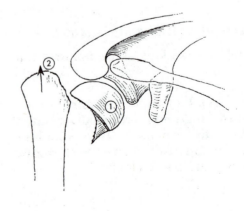

Operative Reduction

1. Fracture is exposed through an incision splitting the anterior deltoid.

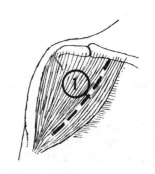

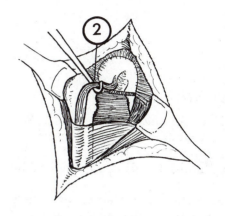

2. Expose the biceps tendon and disengage it from between the fragments.

3. Make downward traction on the arm to restore length, then
4. Push the shaft under the epiphysis.

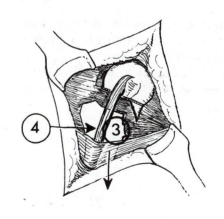

5. If the reduction is not stable, pass a smooth stout wire through the epiphysis and into the shaft. (The wire is cut just below the level of the skin.)

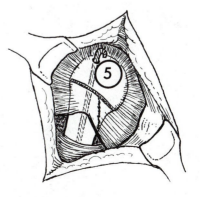

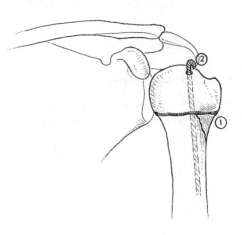

Postreduction X-Ray

1. Epiphysis is in alignment with the shaft of the humerus.

2. Smooth wire passes through epiphysis and into the shaft.

Postoperative Management

Apply a shoulder spica that keeps the arm abducted 45 to 60 degrees.

After four weeks remove the wire, which should be directly under the skin.

Remove the plaster spica after five weeks and place the arm in a triangular sling.

Institute exercises to restore normal motion in the shoulder, elbow, wrist, and hand.

Discard sling after another week and allow free use of the arm.

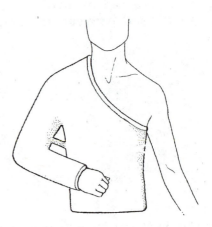

FRACTURE OF THE EPIPHYSIS OF THE LATERAL CONDYLE OF THE HUMERUS (CAPITELLUM)

REMARKS

This lesion is relatively common in children up to the age of 15 years.

It usually is caused by severe varus forces acting on the elbow or by a force directed upward through the radius against the capitellum, shearing it off.

The resulting lesion is usually a type IV injury of the physis, which carries a grave prognosis.

The fragment usually comprises the epiphysis of the capitellum, a small portion of the trochlea, and a small portion of the metaphysis of the capitellum.

The degree of displacement of the fragment varies from no displacement or simple lateral displacement to wide lateral displacement with rotation of the fragment. Rotation occurs in both the horizontal and vertical axis.

Slight lateral displacement without rotation of the fragment does not preclude good bony union. However, displacement tends to increase during the period of immobilization, and some of the worst results are from relatively undisplaced fractures treated without complete reduction.

Healing with rotation of the fragment inevitably results in fibrous union and premature closure of the affected portion of the physis. This in turn produces progressive cubitus valgus and, later, implication of the ulnar nerve.

Every effort should be made to achieve and maintain reduction of the displaced fragments. Open reduction with internal fixation is the safest way to insure the desired result.

Simple Lateral Displacement
Without Rotation of the Fragment

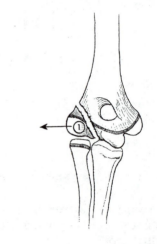

Prereduction X-Ray

1. The lateral condyle, with a small portion of the trochlea and a small portion of the metaphysis of the capitellum, is displaced directly laterally.

Manipulative Reduction

1. The forearm is flexed and supinated.
2. With both hands make firm pressure on the condyles.

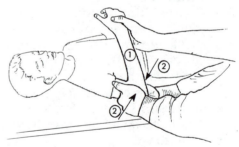

Postreduction X-Ray

1. The lateral condyle is restored to its anatomic position.

Note: If any displacement persists, open reduction should be performed, since growth deformity and nonunion are frequent.

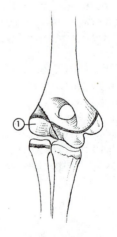

Immobilization

1. Apply a posterior plaster slab directly to the skin of the arm and forearm, extending to the base of the fingers.

2. The elbow is flexed 90 degrees. (Further flexion may displace the fragment laterally). Mold the plaster well around the condyle and fix the plaster slab with a cotton elastic bandage.

3. Support the arm with a collar and cuff.

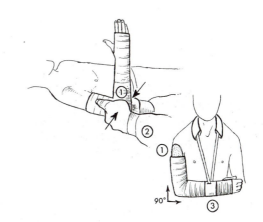

Postreduction Management

Reduction must be anatomic.

Check position of the fragment with frequent x-rays, because reduction may be readily lost in the first week.

Any fracture displacement is indication for internal fixation of the fragment.

Remove the plaster splint after three weeks. Place the arm in a triangular sling.

Institute a regimen of graduated active exercises for the elbow.

Do not forcefully stretch the elbow.

Lateral Displacement and Rotation of the Lateral Humeral Epiphysis

REMARKS

This lesion (type IV) is relatively common.

Accurate reduction is essential to prevent a progressive cubitus valgus deformity and a late ulnar nerve palsy.

Manipulative reduction occasionally succeeds in early cases, but there is a tendency for redisplacement. Operative intervention is the procedure of choice to achieve an adequate reduction and prevent future growth disturbances.

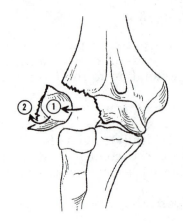

Prereduction X-Ray

1. The lateral epiphysis is displaced laterally and backward.

2. The fragment is rotated so that the fractured surface is outward. It is also rotated around its vertical axis.

Operative Reduction

1. Make a lateral incision 8.75 to 10 cm. long.

2. Identify the capitellum and attached muscle mass.

3. With a curette remove all tissue debris and bone spicules from the bed of the epiphysis.

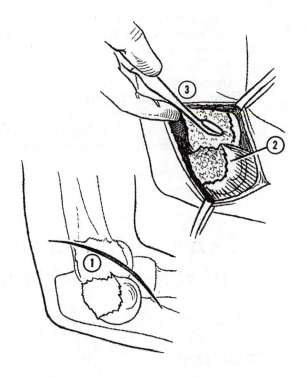

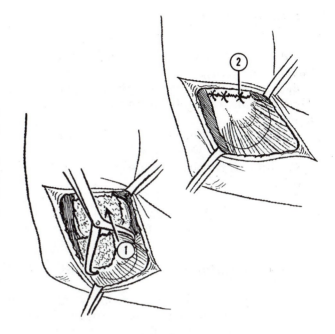

1. Grasp the fragment with a forceps, derotate it, and pull it into its anatomic position.

2. Fix the fragment in place with interrupted sutures passed through the adjacent soft tissues (or through two or three drill holes in the bone), and

3. Secure fixation with two smooth, fine Kirschner wires passed through the metaphysis, if possible. (Cut them below the level of the skin.)

Note: Obtain intraoperative anteroposterior and lateral x-rays to insure fracture reduction and correct placement of pins.

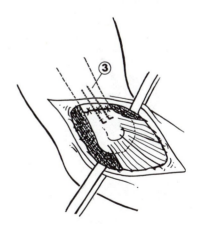

Immobilization

1. Apply a posterior plaster slab to the arm and forearm, extending to the base of the fingers.

2. The elbow is flexed 90 degrees. Mold the plaster well around the condyles.

3. Fix the plaster slab with a cotton elastic bandage.

4. Support the arm with a collar and cuff.

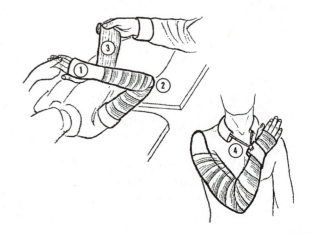

Postreduction Management

Remove the plaster slab after three weeks; also remove the wires.
Place the arm in a triangular sling.
Institute a regimen of graduated active exercises for the elbow.
Do not forcefully stretch the elbow.

APOPHYSEAL SEPARATION OF THE MEDIAL EPICONDYLE OF THE HUMERUS

REMARKS

The medial epicondyle is an apophysis for the origin of the common flexor muscles of the forearm.

In patients younger than 18 years, avulsion of the medial epicondyle following abduction strains of the elbow is relatively common. Since the apophysis does not contribute to longitudinal growth, its fracture does not produce a growth deformity.

Accurate replacement is followed by union of the epicondyle to the shaft of the bone. However, a displaced apophysis becomes attached only by fibrous tissue.

When the injury occurs before the cartilage of the apophysis becomes ossified (in children younger than 4 years), x-rays provide little or no information. Diagnosis must be made on the basis of clinical evidence, i.e., swelling and tenderness over the epicondyle and, in severe lesions, instability of the elbow joint.

The avulsed fragment assumes various positions depending on the severity of the abducting force.

Separation may be minimal, the fragment being displaced slightly laterally, or the fragment may be pulled down to the level of the joint and even rotated, or it may be trapped in the joint with or without a lateral dislocation or subluxation of the elbow joint.

Severe lesions are frequently associated with traction injury of the ulnar nerve. Usually, rapid and complete recovery follows.

The severity of the injury, particularly if there is gross displacement of the medial epicondyle, can best be evaluated by testing stability of the elbow joint under general anesthetic, applying abduction force to the extended elbow joint.

If the joint is stable, closed treatment should be instituted, but if instability is demonstrated, operative repair should be carried out.

With Minimal Displacement

REMARKS

Complete anatomic restoration of the fragment is not essential for complete restoration of function.

Operative intervention is not indicated.

Prereduction X-Ray

1. The epicondyle is avulsed and is displaced laterally.

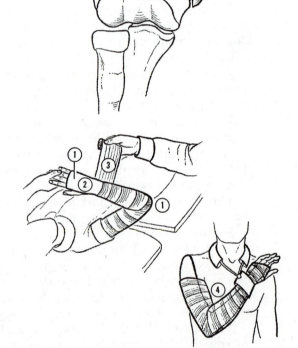

Immobilization

1. Apply a posterior plaster slab holding the arm in acute flexion.

2. The forearm is in full pronation to relax pronator teres muscle.

3. Fix the slab with a 7.5-cm bandage.

4. Support the arm with a collar and cuff.

Management

Remove the posterior plaster slab after two weeks.

Place the arm in a triangular sling.

Institute active graduated exercises for the elbow joint.

Avoid forceful measures.

Complete restoration of function is slow.

With Gross Displacement

REMARKS

This lesion may or may not heal by bony union.

Immediate results are excellent, but in many instances late ulnar neuritis results from incongruity of the groove of the nerve behind the epicondyle.

Anatomic restoration of the fragment is essential to prevent this late complication.

Prereduction X-Ray

1. The internal epicondyle is displaced outward and downward.
2. The fragment lies at the level of the joint space.

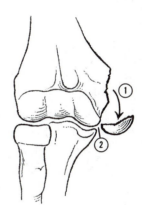

OR (IN CHILDREN YOUNGER THAN FOUR YEARS):

1. Forearm is abducted at the elbow joint.
2. Marked widening of the medial joint space indicates displacement of epicondyle into joint.
3. Medial epicondyle is not visible.

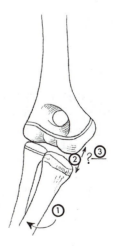

Manipulative Reduction

1. The arm is acutely flexed and the forearm is pronated.

2. The operator pushes the fragment upward and inward with his thumbs.

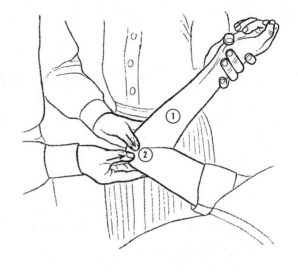

POSTREDUCTION X-RAY

The fragment is restored to its normal anatomic position.

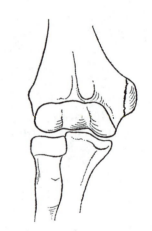

IMMOBILIZATION

1. Apply a posterior plaster slab holding the arm in acute flexion.

2. The forearm is in full pronation to relax pronator teres muscle.

3. Fix the slab with a 7.5-cm cotton bandage.

4. Support the arm with a collar and cuff.

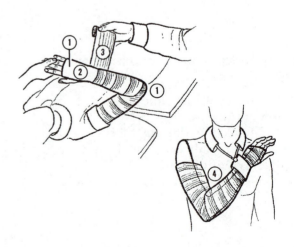

POSTREDUCTION MANAGEMENT

Remove the posterior plaster slab after two weeks.
Place the arm in a triangular sling.
Institute active graduated exercises for the elbow joint.
Avoid forceful measures.
Complete restoration of function is slow.

Alternate Method

Operative treatment is indicated if manipulative reduction fails or if marked lateral instability of the joint exists. Approach the fracture antero-medially and protect the ulnar nerve at all times.

OPERATIVE REDUCTION

1. Make a curved incision 8.75 to 10 cm long on the inner aspect of the elbow joint in front of the epicondyle.
2. Divide the deep fascia.
3. Identify the raw surface on the inner side of the humerus. (This is the bed of the epicondyle.)
4. Identify the displaced fragment with attached muscles.

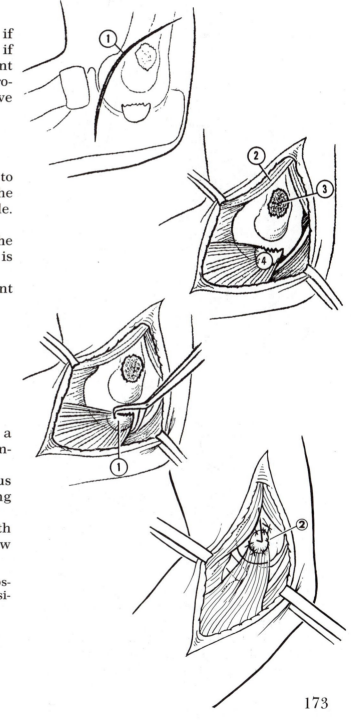

1. Grasp the loose fragment with a towel clip and pull it into its anatomic position.
2. Anchor the bone to the humerus with interrupted sutures passing through the adjacent soft tissues, or
Fix fragment with one or two smooth Kirschner wires and cut them below the level of the skin.

Note: Obtain intraoperative anteroposterior and lateral x-rays to evaluate positions of the fragment and the pin.

Alternate Method (Continued)

IMMOBILIZATION

1. Apply a posterior plaster slab holding the arm in acute flexion.
2. The forearm is in full pronation.
3. Fix the slab with a 7.5-cm cotton bandage.
4. Support the arm in a collar and cuff.

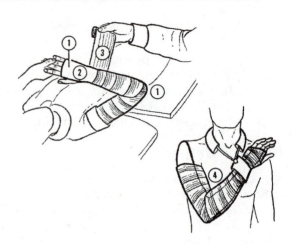

POSTOPERATIVE MANAGEMENT

Remove the posterior plaster slab and Kirschner wires after two weeks.
Place the arm in a triangular sling.
Institute active graduated exercises for the elbow joint.
Avoid forceful measures.
Complete restoration of function is slow.

Displacement of Medial Epicondyle into the Elbow Joint

REMARKS

This lesion results from severe abduction forces sufficient to dislocate the elbow and is frequently associated with traction injury to the ulnar nerve, which usually heals completely. However, the nerve may be pulled into the joint with the fragment.

Conservative measures occasionally achieve an acceptable reduction and may be tried; however, most lesions require surgical repositioning of the avulsed fragment. In all instances in which marked instability is demonstrable or the ulnar nerve is injured, open reduction should be carried out.

If the patient is an older child, or the fragment is severely traumatized, the fragment can be removed and the muscle mass can be sutured directly to the humerus.

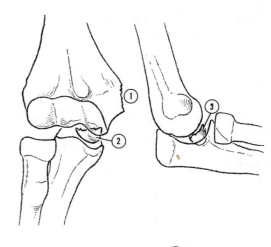

Prereduction X-Ray

1. The defect on the inner side of the humerus is apparent.

2. The medial epicondylar fragment lies in the joint.

3. The fragment is readily seen in the lateral views.

Manipulative Reduction

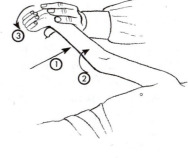

With the child under general anesthesia:

1. The forearm is forcefully abducted, and at the same time

2. The forearm is supinated, and

3. The wrist is extended to extract the fragment by its muscle attachments.

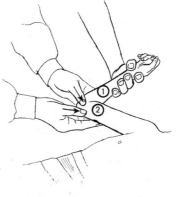

1. The arm is acutely flexed and the forearm is pronated.

2. Operator pushes the fragment upward and inward with the thumbs.

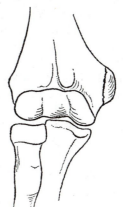

Postreduction X-Ray

The fragment is restored to its normal anatomic position.

Note: This fortunate reduction is rare. If the fragment is displaced, test elbow stability, and repair if it is unstable.

Manipulative Reduction (*Continued*)

IMMOBILIZATION

1. Apply a posterior plaster slab holding the arm in acute flexion.

2. The forearm is in full pronation to relax the pronator teres muscle.

3. Fix the slab with a 7.5-cm cotton bandage.

4. Support the arm with a collar and cuff.

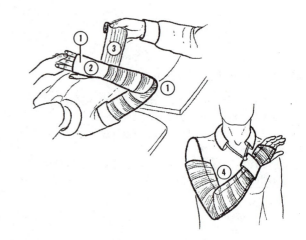

POSTREDUCTION MANAGEMENT

Remove the posterior plaster slab after two weeks.

Place the arm in a triangular sling.

Institute active graduated exercises for the elbow joint.

Avoid forceful measures to restore motion.

Complete restoration of function is slow, especially if the lesion is associated with dislocation, and some permanent limitation of motion may result.

Operative Reduction

1. Make a curved incision just in front of the epicondyle.

2. Divide the deep fascia.

3. Identify the raw epicondylar bed on the inner aspect of the humerus.

4. Open the inner aspect of the joint by forcing the elbow into valgus.

5. Now grasp the muscle mass with the attached epicondylar fragment and remove it from the joint space.

6. The ulnar nerve is identified and is protected at all times.

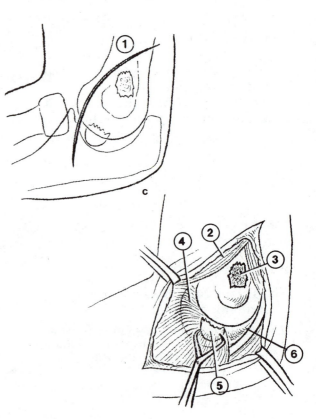

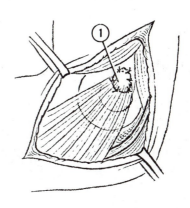

1. Replace the fragment in its normal anatomic position.

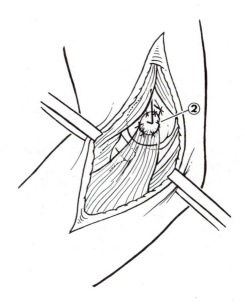

2. Anchor the fragment to the humerus by interrupted sutures through the surrounding soft tissues, or

Fix fragment with one or two smooth, fine Kirschner wires.

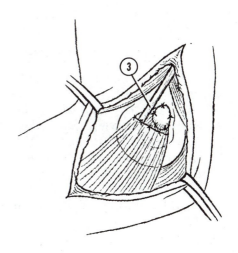

3. The ulnar nerve, if injured, should be transposed anteriorly beneath the flexor muscles.

Note: If the patient is an older child or the fragment is severely injured, excise it and attach muscle mass directly to the humerus.

Operative Reduction (*Continued*)

POSTREDUCTION X-RAY

1. The epicondylar fragment is in its normal position.

2. The lateral view shows the joint space to be free of the displaced fragment.

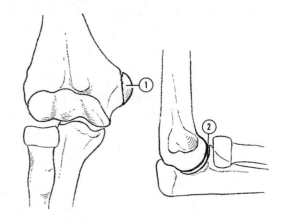

IMMOBILIZATION

1. Apply a posterior plaster slab holding the arm in acute flexion.

2. The forearm is in full pronation.

3. Fix the slab with a 7.5-cm cotton bandage.

4. Apply a collar and cuff.

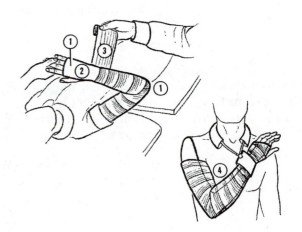

POSTOPERATIVE MANAGEMENT

Remove the posterior plaster slab after two weeks; also remove wires if used.

Place the arm in a triangular sling.

Institute active graduated exercises for the elbow joint.

Avoid forceful measures.

Complete restoration of function is slow, especially if the lesion is associated with a dislocation.

Some permanent restriction of motion is quite possible, and parents should be warned of this beforehand.

AVULSION OF THE LATERAL EPICONDYLE OF THE HUMERUS

Without Inclusion of the Fragment in the Elbow Joint

REMARKS

This is a rare lesion, but it is encountered occasionally in patients between the ages of 13 and 15 years.

Generally the fragment is very small and is avulsed by an adduction strain at the elbow joint.

Anatomic reduction is not essential.

Appearance on X-Ray

1. The external epicondyle is avulsed and is displaced outward and slightly downward.

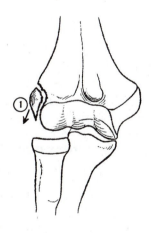

Immobilization

1. Apply a posterior plaster slab.
2. The elbow is flexed acutely.
3. The forearm is in full supination.
4. Support the arm with a collar and cuff.

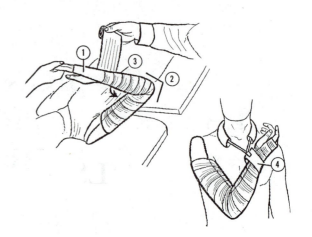

Management

As in other fractures about the elbow joint in children, the splint should be discarded as soon as possible within the limits of the patient's pain (usually by the end of the second week).

Active range-of-motion exercises can then be instituted.

Forceful passive movements should be avoided.

With Inclusion of the Fragment in the Elbow Joint

REMARKS

The lesion results from severe varus strains at the elbow in patients between 13 and 15 years of age.

The lesion is very rare.

Operative intervention is indicated to restore the fragment to its normal position.

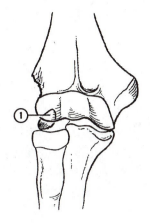

Prereduction X-Ray

1. The lateral epicondyle lies in the lateral compartment of the elbow joint.

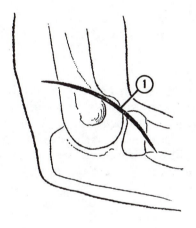

Operative Reduction

1. Make a curved incision over the lateral epicondylar area.

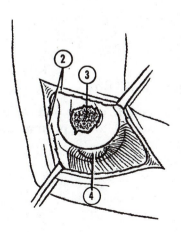

2. Divide the deep fascia.
3. Identify the raw surface on the lateral aspect of the humerus and
4. The fragment with the extensor muscle mass in the lateral joint compartment.

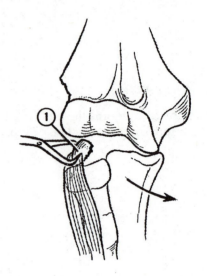

Operative Reduction (Continued)

1. Adduct the elbow and remove the fragment with the attached muscle mass.

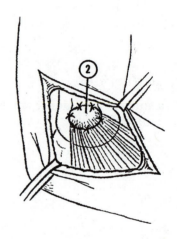

2. Anchor the fragment to its bed by interrupted sutures through the surrounding soft tissue *or*
Fix the fragment with one or two smooth, fine Kirschner wires. (Cut them below the level of the skin.)

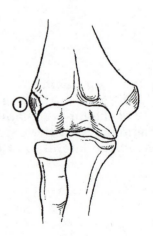

Postreduction X-Ray

1. The fragment of the lateral epicondyle is restored to its normal anatomic position.

Immobilization

1. Apply a posterior plaster slab holding

2. The elbow flexed acutely.

3. The forearm is in full supination.

4. Support the arm with a collar and cuff.

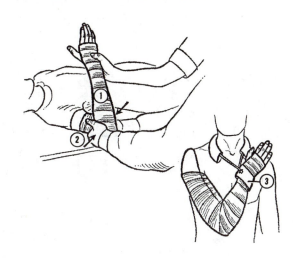

Postoperative Management

As in other fractures about the elbow, the splint should be removed as soon as possible within the limits of the patient's pain (usually by the end of the second week).

Active range-of-motion exercises can then be instituted.

Forceful passive movements should be avoided.

EPIPHYSEAL SEPARATION OF THE LOWER END OF THE HUMERUS

At Birth

REMARKS

The diagnosis is established by the clinical features: pain, swelling, and dysfunction.

Early x-rays are of no help because the center of ossification has not as yet appeared; after 10 to 14 days x-ray evidence of callus formation is evident.

Check the circulatory status of the limb. If there is severe swelling, elevate the limb in sidearm traction.

Look for any nerve deficits by observing the infant's hand function.

Generally, the epiphysis is displaced backward.

Manipulative Reduction

1. Steady traction is maintained on the arm.

2. An assistant makes counter traction on the upper arm.

3. While traction is maintained, the surgeon's thumb forces the distal fragment into normal position, and at the same time

4. The elbow is flexed to just beyond a right angle.

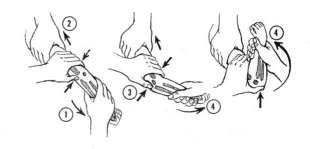

Immobilization

1. Apply a collar and cuff.

Note: Perfect anatomic reduction is not essential. The process of remodeling eventually corrects most angulation. Occasionally, some limitation of elbow motion or angulation of the humerus persists.

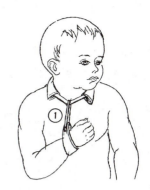

In Childhood

REMARKS

In these lesions the distal fragment comprises the entire lower end of the humerus and the physis.

Depending on the mechanism, the distal fragment may be displaced anteriorly or posteriorly.

The lesions are either type I or type II. A portion of the plate may be severely damaged, resulting in a valgus or varus angular deformity.

These injuries usually occur in children under five years of age and are frequently associated with severe soft tissue damage.

Management of these lesions is similar to supracondylar fractures of the humerus and therefore is considered in Fractures of the Lower End of the Humerus.

SEPARATION OF THE UPPER RADIAL EPIPHYSIS

REMARKS

This lesion is caused by an abducting force that forces the capitellum against the radial epiphysis, driving it downward and outward so that the fragment assumes varying degrees of angulation.

This is usually a type II lesion, in which a triangular portion of the metaphysis remains attached to the epiphysis.

Considerable angulation of the radial epiphysis can be accepted without impairment of function. This is true because of the great remodeling potential of the upper radial shaft.

As a rule, remodeling with growth will correct angulation up to 30 degrees; however, an attempt should be made to reduce this angulation.

Angulation greater than 30 degrees generally will result in some loss of pronation and a valgus deformity of the elbow, especially in children older than 8 years.

Open reduction is indicated when manipulative measures fail to reduce the angulation of the epiphysis to less than 30 degrees and when the epiphysis is severely or completely displaced.

The radial epiphysis in children should never be removed; excision results in loss of longitudinal growth of the radius, radial deviation of the hand at the wrist, prominence of the distal end of the elbow, and a valgus deformity at the elbow.

In late cases with severe or late displacement of the radial epiphysis, it is best to accept the deformity.

In severe displacements of the epiphysis, even when adequately reduced, premature closure of the physis may ensue, resulting in varying degrees of restriction of pronation and supination.

Prereduction X-Ray

1. The radial head in the lateral view is tilted forward.
2. The radial head in the anteroposterior view is tilted outward.

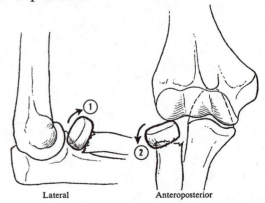

Lateral   Anteroposterior

Manipulative Reduction

1. An assistant steadies the arm.
2. The operator grasps the wrist of the extended forearm with one hand and the elbow with the other.
3. The thumb is placed over the anterior aspect of the displaced radial epiphysis. The forearm is rotated so that the most prominent portion of the displaced head is in a lateral position and superfascial (between the extensor muscles and the anconeus).

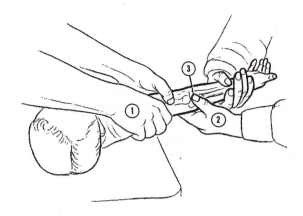

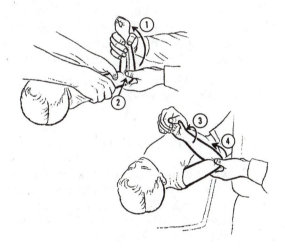

1. While the forearm is adducted.
2. The thumb makes firm pressure upward and inward on the radial epiphysis.
3. Next, the forearm is supinated and
4. Is flexed acutely.

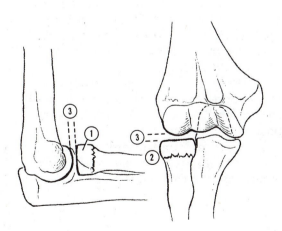

POSTREDUCTION X-RAY

1. In the lateral view, the forward tilt of the epiphysis is corrected.
2. In the anteroposterior view, the outward tilt of the epiphysis is corrected.
3. In both views, the articular surface of the epiphysis is parallel to that of the capitellum.

Manipulative Reduction
(Continued)

IMMOBILIZATION

1. Apply a posterior plaster slab from the axilla to the base of the fingers.
2. The forearm is moderately flexed and in midposition.
3. Suspend the arm with a collar and cuff or a sling.

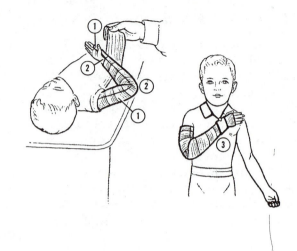

POSTREDUCTION MANAGEMENT

Discard the posterior plaster slab after two weeks.

Apply a triangular sling for one week.

After removal of the plaster, institute active progressive motion within the patient's tolerance of pain to restore flexion, extension, pronation, and supination.

Avoid forceful stretching of the joint.

Note: Maximal restoration of function is attained only after many months. Progress is usually very slow.

Operative Reduction

Operative reduction is justifiable in all instances in which manipulative attempts fail to restore an acceptable alignment of the displaced fragments. The angulation of the epiphysis should not exceed 30 degrees in children over 8 years of age. In younger children, more angulation may be accepted.

1. Make an oblique incision extending downward from the lateral epicondyle to the ulna in the interval between the anconeus and the extensor carpi ulnaris.
2. Deepen the incision through the fascia and between the anconeus and the extensor carpi ulnaris. This exposes the capsule.
3. Make a longitudinal incision in the capsule to expose the radial epiphysis and the capitellum.

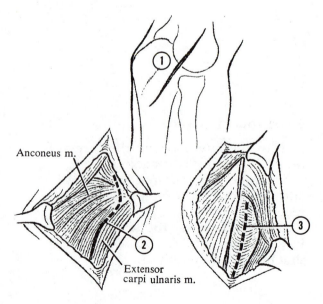

Anconeus m.

Extensor carpi ulnaris m.

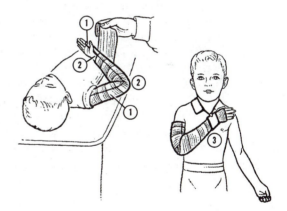

THEN:

1. The surgeon places his thumb over the displaced radial epiphysis and pushes upward and inward until the articular surface of the epiphysis is parallel to that of the capitellum.

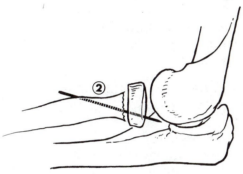

2. Insert a smooth Kirschner wire obliquely in a posterior to anterior direction through the radial epiphyseal fracture to hold reduction. Bury the pin beneath the skin.

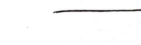

IMMOBILIZATION

1. Apply a posterior plaster slab from the axilla to the base of the fingers.
2. The forearm is moderately flexed and in midposition.
3. Suspend the arm with a collar and cuff or a sling.

POSTREDUCTION MANAGEMENT

Discard the posterior plaster slab after three weeks and remove the pin.

Apply a triangular sling for one week.

After removal of the plaster, institute active progressive motion within the patient's tolerance of pain to restore flexion, extension, pronation, and supination.

Avoid forceful stretching of the joint.

Note: Maximal restoration of function is attained only after many months. Progress is usually very slow.

SEPARATION OF THE
LOWER RADIAL EPIPHYSIS

REMARKS

Separation of the lower radial epiphysis is the most common epiphyseal injury in children between the ages of six and 10 years.

The radius may be involved alone or in combination with a fracture through the distal end of the ulna.

In general, two types of epiphyseal fractures are encountered:

1. Epiphyseal separation occurs on the metaphyseal side of the epiphyseal plate; invariably in this lesion a triangular segment of the metaphysis is displaced with the radial epiphysis.

2. The radial epiphysis is crushed. Crushing of the radial epiphysis may lead to premature closure of the physis, and shortening and angular deformities of the radius. Always check for these complications and warn the parents of the possibility of their development.

Minor displacements need no correction; with growth, remodeling and resorption will restore normal anatomic alignment.

Minor displacements should be accepted after attempts at reduction. Forceful manipulations may cause severe trauma to the physis; therefore, they should be avoided.

These fractures can be reduced under intravenous regional anesthetic, which gives excellent muscle relaxation and pain relief and avoids the complications of a general anesthetic (see page 121).

Open reduction is rarely indicated and should be avoided.

Occasionally these lesions are complicated by fracture of the scaphoid or dislocation of the semilunar bone.

Prereduction X-Ray

Note: This type of lesion rarely causes premature closure of the physis.

1. The radial epiphysis is displaced dorsally and radially. Its articular surface is directed dorsally.

2. The distal ulnar epiphysis is separated.

3. Triangular segment of the metaphysis is displaced with the radial epiphysis.

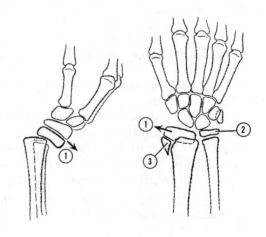

190

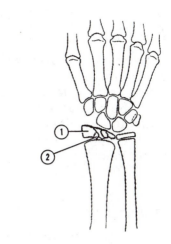

Or:

Note: This type frequently causes premature closure of the physis.

1. There is minimal displacement of the radial epiphysis.
2. The radial epiphysis is fragmented (The physis must be damaged.)

Manipulative Reduction

Reduction is performed with the patient under intravenous anesthesia (see page 121).

To reduce epiphyseal fracture of the right radius:

1. Grasp the distal fragment with the right hand.
2. Grasp the wrist above the level of the fracture with the left hand.
3. Make steady traction in the line of displacement of the distal fragment and disimpact the fracture by hyperextending the wrist.

While traction is maintained:

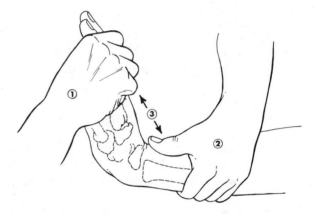

4. Flex and pronate the distal fragment with the right hand.
5. The index finger of the left hand on the volar surface acts as the fulcrum; at the same time,
6. Push the distal fragment forward and downward with the thumb of the left hand.
7. Take a new grip on the wrist with the right hand; the thenar eminence is placed against the radial styloid.
8. Grasp the forearm with the left hand.
9. With the right hand, push the distal fragment toward the ulna.

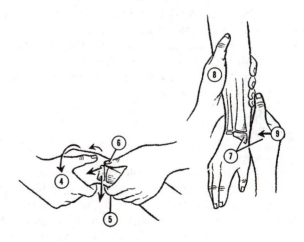

Postreduction X-Ray

1. The radial epiphysis is restored to its normal anatomic position.

2. The normal radial length has been restored. The radial styloid is now distal to the ulnar styloid.

3. The articular plane of the radius is now projecting volarly.

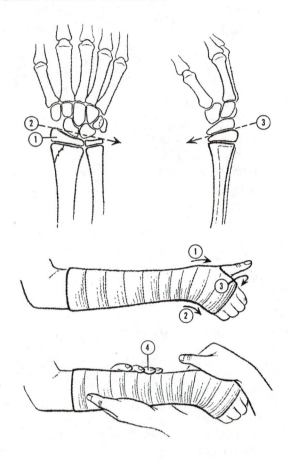

Immobilization

While an assistant maintains traction on the thumb and fingers:

Apply a plaster cast over very little padding from just below the elbow to proximal to the metacarpal heads.

While the plaster is setting, hold the position of

1. Flexion,
2. Ulnar deviation, and
3. Pronation.
4. Mold the plaster along the radial concavity.

Postreduction Management

Take x-ray immediately after application of cast, and before releasing tourniquet if intravenous anesthetic has been employed. Accept minor displacement. Only gross displacements justify another attempt at reduction.

The cast should be well molded to the wrist but not so tightly as to embarrass the circulation.

Check constantly for circulatory embarrassment, especially for the first 24 or 48 hours. If any is manifested, split the cast along its dorsum for its entire length.

Elevate the arm with the fingers pointing toward the ceiling for the first 24 hours; apply ice bags.

Take more x-rays on the fifth and tenth days. Check for maintenance of position.

If the cast becomes loose after about 10 to 14 days, apply a new plaster cast.

During the healing period, allow free use of the arm. No sling is necessary.

Remove the cast after 6 weeks.

No special physical therapy is needed in children.

If physeal damage has occurred, premature closure will become manifest clinically, and the parents should be advised of the possibility of its occurring over the year or two following the fracture.

192

SEPARATION OF THE PHALANGEAL EPIPHYSIS

REMARKS

Separation of the phalangeal epiphysis is a fairly common childhood injury, and when it occurs, considerable deformity can ensue if adequate reduction is not achieved.

The epiphyses most commonly involved are those at the base of the proximal phalanges, but any phalangeal epiphysis is vulnerable to injury.

Separation of the Epiphyses at the Bases of the Proximal and Middle Phalanges

REMARKS

The lesion is usually of type II, in which a small triangular portion of the metaphysis is displaced with the epiphysis.

The shaft of the phalanx rotates on the epiphysis.

Manipulative measures readily restore normal anatomic alignment of the shaft in relation to the epiphysis.

Prereduction X-Ray

1. Separation through epiphyseal plate.

2. Triangular segment of the metaphysis still attached to the epiphysis.

3. Rotational deformity of the phalanx in relation to adjacent metacarpals.

Note: Overlapping of fingers will occur on flexion if rotation is not corrected.

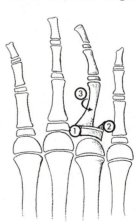

Manipulative Reduction

1. While steady traction is applied to the finger, a solid object like a pencil is placed between the fingers to hold the epiphyseal fragment, while

2. The distal phalangeal fragment rotation is corrected.

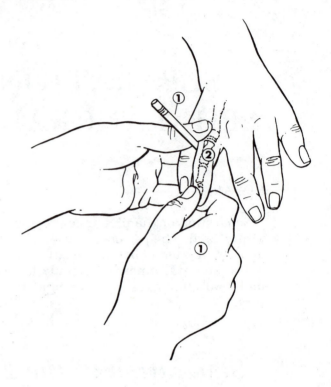

3. Finger is in normal relation to the adjacent fingers in flexion and extension after reduction.

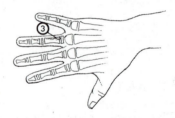

Postreduction X-Ray

1. Rotation of the finger is corrected.

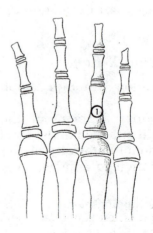

194

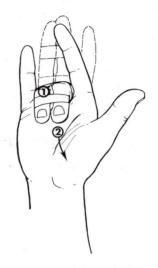

Immobilization

1. The fractured finger is immobilized by "buddy taping" to the uninjured finger.

2. Rotational malalignment is prevented by directing the fingers toward the scaphoid tuberosity.

Postreduction Management

Remove the tape at the end of two weeks.

Institute a regimen of active exercises to restore normal function in the joints of the affected finger.

Separation of the Epiphysis of the Distal Phalanx

REMARKS

Separation of the epiphysis of the distal phalanx is usually the result of a flexion injury.

The clinical features are those of a mallet finger in the adult.

Lateral x-rays show the lesion best.

Reduction is readily achieved and must be done to avoid deformity.

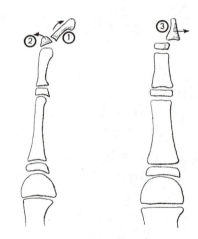

Prereduction X-Ray

1. The phalanx is flexed.
2. The epiphysis is extended in relation to the phalanx.
3. The phalanx is displaced laterally.

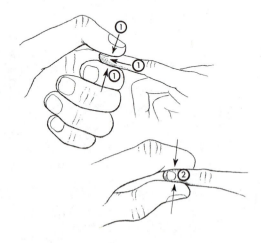

Manipulative Reduction

1. Make traction and mold the fragments by squeezing the end of the finger between the index finger and the thumb.
2. Correct any lateral displacement by compressing the lateral borders of the terminal phalanx between the index finger and the thumb.

Immobilization

Apply a cast over a single layer of cast padding using tincture of benzoin or some adherent.

1. The patient hyperextends his distal interphalangeal joint by pushing upward with the thumb while the cast is drying.
2. The proximal interphalangeal joint is flexed slightly.

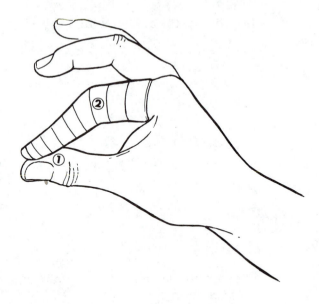

Postreduction Management

Allow free use of the uninvolved fingers.

The plaster cast may need to be changed several times during treatment.

Remove the plaster at the end of three weeks and evaluate the ability of the patient to extend the distal interphalangeal joint. If the patient can maintain active extension, institute exercises to restore joint function.

196

AVULSION OF TRACTION APOPHYSES OF THE PELVIS

REMARKS

This injury results from powerful contracture of muscles, especially in adolescents engaged in strenuous activity.

Bony union is the rule, with complete restoration of function.

Restoration of fragments to their anatomic position is not essential.

Appearance on X-Ray

1. Avulsion fracture of anterior superior iliac spine (by action of sartorius).

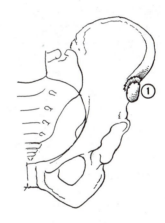

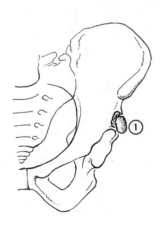

OR:

1. Avulsion fracture of anterior inferior iliac spine (by action of rectus femoris).

Management

Treatment is mainly to relieve pain symptoms and includes:

Rest in bed with hips slightly flexed for one to two weeks until symptoms diminish.

Followed by restricted activity for two to three more weeks and Complete restoration to normal function in six to eight weeks.

Avulsion of Tuberosity
of Ischium

REMARKS

This injury results from powerful contractions of the hamstring muscles, as in athletes who run the high hurdles.

Amount of separation of fragments varies.

Bony union is the rule. Occasionally, fibrous union occurs (especially if fragments are widely separated).

Repositioning of fragments is not necessary for a good result.

Normal function is the rule in all cases of bony union and in most cases of fibrous union with pain.

Excision of the fragments is indicated only in old cases of fibrous union with pain.

Appearance on X-Ray

1. Avulsion of the tuberosity of the ischium with minimal displacement.

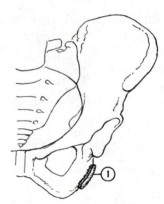

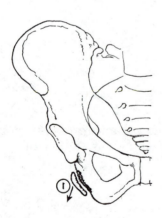

Or:

1. Avulsion of the tuberosity of the ischium with excessive displacement.

Management

Treatment is mainly to relieve pain symptoms and includes:

In acute cases, rest in bed for one to two weeks and restriction of activity for ten to twelve weeks.

Note: In case of fibrous union, if pain persists, the avulsed fragments should be excised.

198

SEPARATION OF THE UPPER FEMORAL EPIPHYSIS

In Infants

REMARKS

This injury may occur rarely at birth or in an infant who has been abused or run over by a car.

It may also be associated with underlying problems of bone metabolism such as scurvy and renal rickets.

The epiphyseal injury is type I, and since the epiphysis is entirely covered with cartilage and the nutrient vessels enter it at the rim of the physis, the blood supply is frequently disrupted by the mechanism producing the separation.

At birth, the diagnosis is extremely difficult to make because the epiphysis is entirely cartilaginous. A diagnosis can be made only on clinical findings: pain, dysfunction, and crepitus. However, within five to ten days, x-rays show new bone formation at the upper end of the femur, establishing the diagnosis.

In the infant more than four months old, the diagnosis is readily made, provided that there is marked displacement of the epiphysis. When displacement is minimal, the x-ray diagnosis is very difficult, but within two to three weeks the signs of fracture healing become evident, and within ten weeks x-rays will demonstrate whether there has been vascular damage to the bony epiphysis.

Because of the risk to circulation, the likelihood of secondary avascular necrosis is high after these injuries. However, the infant's ability to recover from these complications is also high if overly vigorous treatment is avoided.

Reduction of the injury is accomplished by immobilizing the hip in internal rotation and abduction. The remodeling and growth potential is so great that minimal reduction effort is necessary.

Prereduction X-Ray

1. The epiphyses are entirely carti-laginous and therefore are not visual-ized on x-ray.

2. Occasionally there may be a slight increase in the interval be-tween the metaphysis and the center of the acetabulum and some malalign-ment of the metaphysis compared with the normal side, suggesting dysplasia of the hip joint.

3. Ten days later there is evidence of new bone formation along the upper end of the femur.

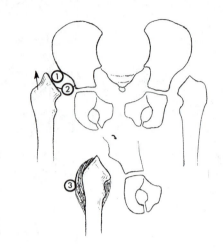

Management

1. Make gentle traction on the leg in line with the trunk.

2. While traction is maintained ab-duct and internally rotate the leg.

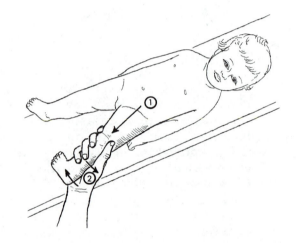

Immobilization

1. Apply a single hip spica.

2. The leg is abducted 30 to 45 de-grees.

3. The leg is slightly internally ro-tated.

Note: The cast is discarded after three weeks. Take x-rays of the hip every eight to ten weeks to determine the fate of the epiphysis.

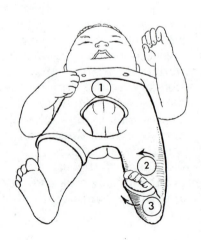

Acute Separation in Children Younger than Nine Years

REMARKS

In a young child, this epiphyseal injury is the result of severe violence such as a fall from a height or being run over by a car.

The patient exhibits all the signs and symptoms of a fracture of the neck of the femur. There is complete loss of function, pain, shortening, and external rotation deformity of the limb. However, since these children may have multiple injuries, the epiphyseal injury may be missed initially and for some time after the injury.

X-rays of the hip usually show considerable displacement of the femoral epiphysis. Rarely, it may be completely dislocated. Fortunately, acute separation of the upper femoral epiphysis is extremely rare in young children, because trauma is more likely to dislocate the child's hip than to fracture the epiphysis.

Occasionally, the only sign of epiphyseal injury is widening of growth plate.

This type I epiphyseal injury in young children frequently results in premature closure of the physis, avascular necrosis, and resultant shortening of the femoral neck with coxa vara. Functional results may be quite good despite these radiological changes.

Treating acute epiphyseal fracture in a child under nine years of age by reduction in traction assures the best chance for continued growth of the physis. Operative treatment should be avoided, because pin fixation required after operative reduction insures premature closure of the physis, does not utilize the natural remodeling capabilities of the femoral head and neck, and increases the risk of avascular necrosis.

Even an unrecognized traumatic slipped epiphysis in a child less than nine years old, which cannot be reduced by traction, should be left unoperated until the result of natural remodeling is manifest. Appropriate osteotomies or ostectomies may be carried out, if necessary, when the child is older.

Prereduction X-Rays

1. Severe displacement of the epiphysis.
2. No evidence of healing in metaphysis.

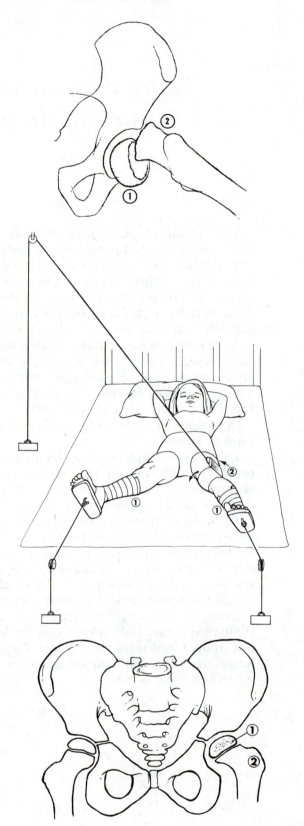

Reduction by Traction

1. Bilateral Buck's traction with legs abducted 30°.
2. Internal rotation strap lines up metaphyseal fragments with epiphyseal fragments.

Note: Traction was maintained for four weeks and followed by spica cast immobilization for an additional six weeks.

Postreduction X-Ray at Ten Years

1. Articular surface and femoral head are normal.
2. Neck has shortened slightly due to physeal injury.

Unreducible Separation

Appearance on X-Ray Six Weeks After Injury

1. Severe displacement of the epiphysis.
2. Callus along the femoral neck and prominence on the anterosuperior metaphysis indicate relative chronicity of this injury.

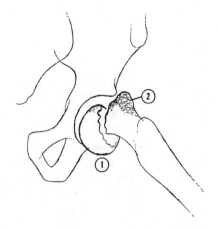

Management

Accept the displacement rather than attempting open surgical reduction and pin fixation in this young child.

Potential for remodeling of these displaced injuries in children younger than nine years is remarkable, and results of surgical intervention are generally inferior to those of natural healing.

Appearance on X-Ray Three Years after Displacement Was Accepted

1. Bony epiphysis is slightly altered and dense.
2. Some coxa vara is still present.
3. Physis is still open. It would be closed and growth would be arrested if surgical fixation had been employed.

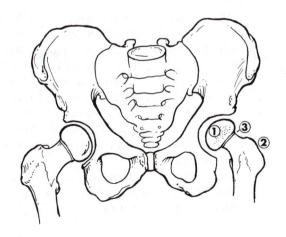

Separation of the Upper Femoral Epiphysis in Adolescents

REMARKS

In most instances, a slip of the proximal femoral epiphysis in an adolescent is gradual, but in 15 per cent of patients the condition occurs acutely, much like a fracture.

The etiology of this lesion is debated, but a major underlying factor is mechanical fatigue of the physis, which is changing from a horizontal to an oblique orientation in the adolescent.

The condition occurs most often in obese, active boys with clinical evidence of slow sexual maturation. However, it may also occur in rapidly growing adolescents with sexual precocity.

The proximal femoral epiphyseal slip is three to five times more common in boys 12 to 16 years old than in girls this age. In one fourth of cases, both hips are involved. Involvement of the second hip may occur while the first hip is under treatment, and the patient's parents should be warned of this possibility.

Acute sudden slip may occur at any time during the course of the disease. The predisposition to further slipping, gradual or acute, is only halted by natural or surgical closure of the physis.

Fusion or closure of the physis eventually occurs but should be enhanced by surgical intervention.

The displacement of the femoral epiphysis most often is posterior and inferior, resulting in anterior and superior bony prominence of the metaphysis.

Treatment depends on the acuteness as well as the degree of slippage.

Prognosis is always guarded because of the risk of avascular necrosis and of chondrolysis with complete loss of the joint space, which may follow both treated and untreated conditions. The incidence of these complications, however, is directly proportional to the aggressiveness of surgical treatment. Some of the worst results in children's orthopedics arise from surgical treatment of slipped femoral epiphysis.

For the acute slip, reduction by careful closed manipulation followed by two or three pin fixations across the physis gives most satisfactory results. Open reduction of the acute slip is too risky to be of benefit in most cases.

Acceptance of displacement and pinning in situ is safest for chronic slips and takes advantage of the vast remodeling capabilities of the adolescent femoral neck.

204

If remodeling does not occur in subsequent years, corrective osteotomy or ostectomy may be employed.

Rarely, if pinning in situ is impossible because of the degree of displacement, osteotomy may be chosen as a primary procedure.

It is essential to make a diagnosis early. Always suspect the lesion in an adolescent who complains of pain in the knee, walks with a limp, and has an external rotation deformity of the hip.

Typical Deformity

1. The patient is a rather obese adolescent male.
2. The limb is externally rotated.
3. The limb is slightly abducted at the hip.
4. The limb is slightly shortened.

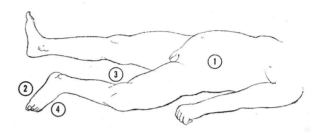

5. In full flexion:
    The affected knee lies at the side and is externally rotated.
    The normal knee touches the chest near the midline.

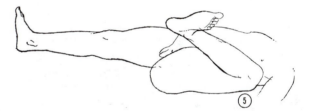

Prereduction X-Ray

"Frogleg" lateral position gives the best lateral view of the femoral neck. Obtain x-rays in this position for all suspected cases.

1. The thigh is flexed 45 degrees.
2. The thigh is abducted 45 degrees.
3. A tube is centered directly over the capital epiphysis.

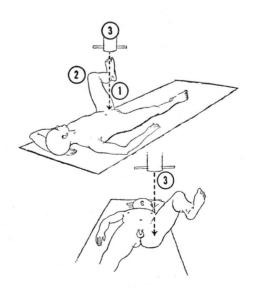

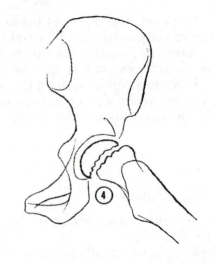

Prereduction X-Ray (Continued)

4. The femoral head and neck are shown in profile.

Evaluating Slippage

Measure the angle of the slip on lateral views of both hips (after Southwick):

1. Line A is drawn between the superior and inferior margins of the metaphyseal surfaces of the epiphysis.

2. Line B is drawn at right angles to A and through the center of the femoral neck.

3. Line C is drawn parallel to the shaft.

Note: The angle formed by the interception point of these three lines is compared with the same angle on the contralateral side. The difference is the degree of slippage.

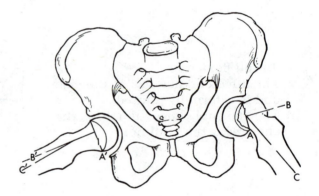

SLIPPED CAPITAL FEMORAL EPIPHYSIS

Acute Slip With Symptoms of Less than Three Weeks' Duration

REMARKS

This is usually an acute injury superimposed on a pre-slip or slowly progressing slip.

The young patient presents with acute pain after a fall or injury to the hip. The involved limb is slightly shortened and externally rotated.

Frequently, the pain is referred to the knee. Failure to recognize this common referral pattern delays diagnosis.

The position of epiphyseal slips of less than two or three weeks' duration can be significantly improved by gentle manipulation. The sooner this is carried out after injury, the better.

Fixation of the slip is then best achieved with two or three (Knowles) pins. Use of a triflanged nail for fixation may displace the epiphysis during insertion and also carries a greater risk of avascular necrosis.

Prereduction X-Ray

1. The depth of the capital epiphysis is less than that of the opposite side.

2. The superior portion of the metaphysis is uncovered.

3. The epiphyseal line is widened and irregular.

4. The beak of the epiphysis projects posteriorly and inferiorly.

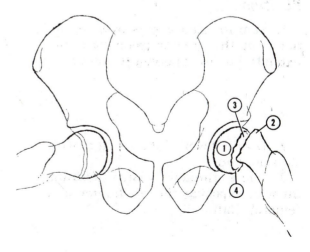

207

Technique of Closed Reduction

1. The patient is anesthetized on a fracture table.

2. Image-intensified fluoroscopy expedites the procedure, but be sure that the unit gives an adequate lateral view as well as an anteroposterior view of the hip.

3. With the patient's muscles relaxed, flex the hip to 90° in the direction of the deformity and then extend the hip while internally rotating and abducting the leg. Do not perform the maneuver repeatedly if reduction is incomplete, but pin in situ if possible.

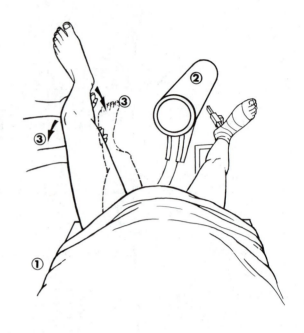

POSTREDUCTION X-RAY

1. Lateral view shows restoration of the relationship of the femoral epiphysis to the neck.

2. Widening of the physis is evident, and pin fixation is necessary to prevent recurrence of the slip.

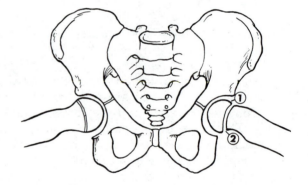

Technique of Multiple Pin Fixation

1. Skin incision begins over prominence of the greater trochanter and extends 8 to 10 cm down the shaft.

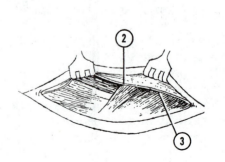

2. Divide fascia lata in line with skin incision.

3. Incise through vastus lateralis muscle, exposing the trochanter and femoral shaft.

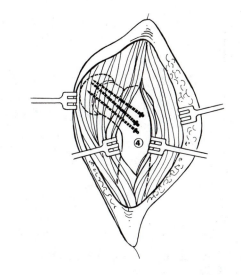

4. Insert the three partially threaded Knowles pins beginning at the level of the lesser trochanter, and evaluate the direction and depth of the pins using fluoroscopy.

POSTOPERATIVE X-RAY

1. Knowles pins need not be parallel but should cross the epiphyseal plate and enter well up into the femoral head.
2. The pins do not penetrate the articular cartilage of the femoral head.

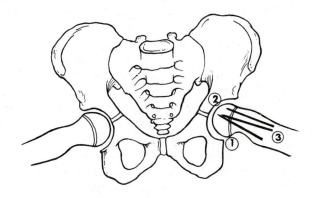

POSTOPERATIVE MANAGEMENT

Place the patient in Buck's traction to help support the limb for three to five days.

Begin quadriceps exercises within one to three days after operation. After three to five days, allow the patient up on crutches with toe-touch weight bearing on the operated limb.

Full weight bearing is not allowed for four to six months after the operation, until x-rays reveal evidence of closure of the physis.

Always check the opposite hip on a follow-up x-ray for signs of impending slip.

Subacute or Chronic Slip: In Situ Pinning, Open Reduction, or Osteotomy?

REMARKS

Selection of treatment for these serious problems should consider the following facts:

Open reduction or osteotomy to correct slipped femoral epiphysis is associated with complications of avascular necrosis or chondrolysis in one third of patients.

Conversely, remodeling of the femoral neck after pinning of a slipped epiphysis in situ can correct for displacement up to 60°. Remodeling of the femoral metaphyseal fragment in relationship to the acetabulum is especially effective if the triradiate acetabular cartilage is open at the time of the slip.

If the epiphyseal slip cannot be reduced, pinning it in situ prevents further slip and allows the natural remodeling processes to work.

Should the superolateral metaphyseal prominence cause significant symptoms or limitation of motion, the prominence may be corrected surgically when the adolescent patient matures with minimal risk of avascular necrosis or chondrolysis.

For the acute, subacute, or chronic slip, the risk of significant damage to the femoral head or its articular surfaces after open reduction or osteotomy of the slip greatly exceeds the risk of functional limitation likely to follow pinning in situ.

Preoperative X-Ray

1. Advance slipping in a 13-year-old boy that measures close to 60 degrees.
2. Triradiate cartilage is open.
3. The anterosuperior aspect of the femoral neck is prominent, but remodeling should occur because the triradiate cartilage is open.

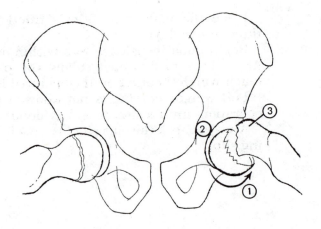

Technique of Pinning In Situ

Use a fracture table but drape the limb free so a frog-leg lateral view can be obtained. Image-intensified fluoroscopy is helpful but be sure that the lateral view of the hip is adequate before draping.

1. Skin incision begins over the greater trochanter and extends 8 cm down the shaft.

2. Divide the fascia lata in line with the incision.

3. Expose the greater trochanter and femoral shaft by incising through the fibers of the vastus lateralis.

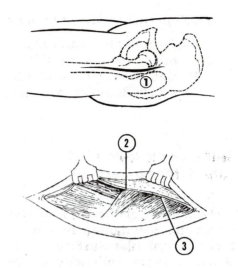

1. Use two or three partially threaded pins and begin insertion anteriorly in order to enter the epiphysis, which is displaced posteriorly.

2. Pins may pass out through the posterior cortex of the neck and then reenter the epiphysis.

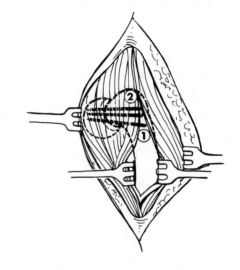

Postoperative X-Ray

1. The depth of insertion of the pins should be determined accurately by x-ray, especially if the pins are in the peripheral part rather than the center of the epiphysis.

2. Pins need not be parallel, but they should cross the plate and penetrate into the bony epiphysis.

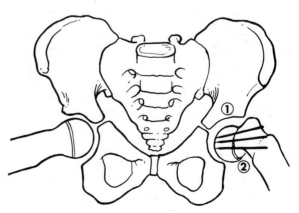

Postoperative Management

Early function encourages remodeling. Allow the patient up on crutches as soon as possible.

By four to six weeks, weight bearing as tolerated may be allowed.

Routinely, Knowles pins need not be removed.

Appearance on X-Ray Ten Months After Surgery

1. The physis has closed.

2. The portion of the neck in contact with the acetabulum becomes a part of the articular surface of the head and restores sphericity of the head.

Note: On long-term follow-up, the minimal residual of the slip caused only 15-degree limitation of internal rotation with a 1.3-cm shortening and no pain.

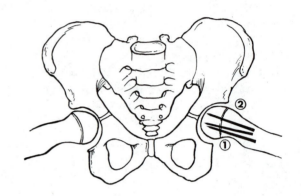

MALUNITED UPPER FEMORAL EPIPHYSEAL SLIPS GREATER THAN 60 DEGREES

REMARKS

Subtrochanteric osteotomy may be useful for the rare slipped capital femoral epiphysis that exceeds 60 degrees and cannot be pinned succesfully in situ.

The patient whose physis closes without remodeling of the femoral metaphysis may benefit from excision of the superolateral metaphyseal fragment if it restricts motion.

Malunited slipped upper femoral epiphysis with marked limitation of motion and pain from avascular necrosis or chondrolysis should be treated by arthrodesis if one hip is involved.

If both hips are severely involved, total joint replacement may be considered, and the patient should understand that revision may be necessary later.

Appearance on X-Ray

Malunited slipped upper femoral epiphysis not exceeding one third of the diameter of the neck. This lesion needs no treatment unless the prominence restricts motion, in which case it can be excised.

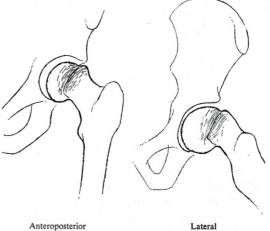

Anteroposterior   Lateral

Appearance on X-Ray
(Continued)

Malunited slipped capital femoral epiphysis with neck shaft angle exceeding 60 degrees. Motion is good except for limitation of internal rotation. Coxa vara deformity produces limp.

This lesion is treated by subtrochanteric osteotomy (Southwick type) to correct angulation in the anteroposterior and mediolateral planes.

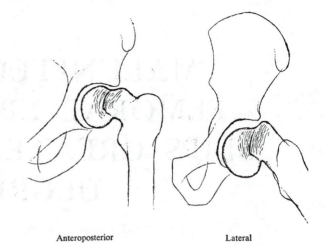

Anteroposterior   Lateral

Preoperative X-Ray Evaluation

Measurement by Southwick technique shows that an anterior wedge of 40 degrees would correct the posterior angulation and a lateral wedge of 70 degrees would correct the inferior angulation.

Osteotomy Technique

1. With a reciprocating motor saw, remove the wedges as outlined.
2. When wedges are cut, the distal thigh fragment is abducted, flexed, and internally rotated and is then affixed with a nail plate.

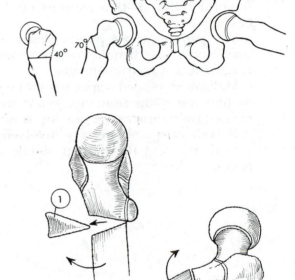
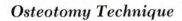

Postoperative X-Ray

1. Subtrochanteric osteotomy is held with internal fixation.
2. Angle of the neck of the femur in relation to the femoral shaft has been restored.

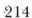

Malunited Upper Epiphyseal Slip Involving One Hip

Preoperative X-Ray

1. Malunited slipped femoral epiphysis exceeding one third of the diameter of the femoral head.
2. The joint space is narrowed from chondrolysis.

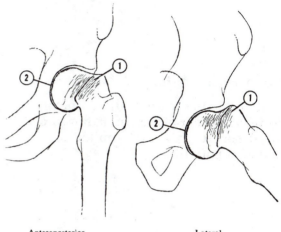

Anteroposterior   Lateral

X-Ray After Arthrodesis of the Hip (DePalma)

1. One third of the femoral head is resected.
2. Intramedullary spline is anchored to the side of the ilium.
3. Cancellous bone grafts from the greater trochanter to the side of the ilium.

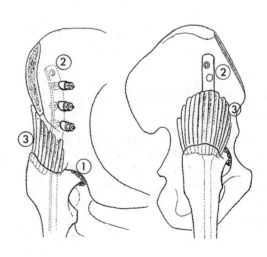

Malunited Upper Femoral Epiphyseal Slip Involving Both Hips

Preoperative X-Ray

Bilateral slips with cartilage necrosis in a 20-year-old woman has produced severe pain and limitation of motion of both hips.

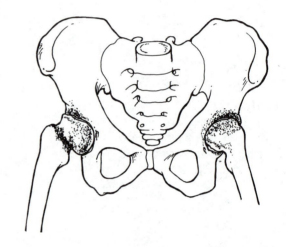

X-Ray After Total Hip Replacement

Total hip joint replacement may be offered this seriously disabled patient provided that she understands that revisions may well be necessary in later life for loosening or wearing of the prosthesis.

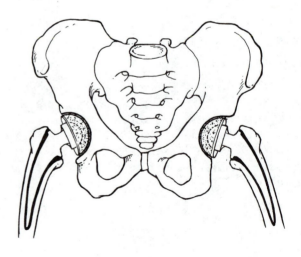

SEPARATION OF THE EPIPHYSIS OF THE LESSER TROCHANTER

REMARKS

The epiphysis of the lesser trochanter is a traction epiphysis to which the iliopsoas muscle is attached.

Because the insertion of the iliopsoas extends on to the shaft of the femur, in isolated lesions, the displacement of the epiphysis is not great.

The epiphysis is avulsed by powerful contraction of the iliopsoas muscle.

No growth disturbance follows this injury.

Prereduction X-Ray

1. The epiphysis is displaced upward and inward by the iliopsoas muscle.

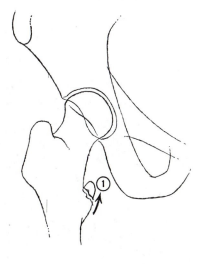

Reduction and Immobilization

1. Flexing the hip relaxes the ilop-soas muscle.

2. This position is maintained by placing the limb on pillows or in balanced suspension.

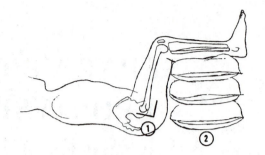

Postimmobilization Management

The position of flexion is maintained until pain and discomfort subside, usually within one to two weeks.

Then allow the patient to resume crutch walking within the limits of pain tolerance.

Prevent forceful abduction and hyperextension movements of the limb for several months.

SEPARATION OF THE DISTAL FEMORAL EPIPHYSIS

REMARKS

This lesion may occur at birth during difficult breech delivery, but most often it results from severe violence to the knee in a child more than seven years of age.

The birth injury, which is a type I epiphyseal fracture, is usually manifested as a painful swollen knee in the newborn. X-ray changes may not be evident for one to two weeks, until callus forms.

Birth fractures in this region generally have a good prognosis. Anatomic reduction is not vital, since remodeling during growth corrects most deformity.

The injury in the older child carries a guarded prognosis regardless of the type of fracture, and approximately 30 per cent of these injuries will produce significant shortening or angular deformity.

The distal femoral epiphysis contributes 70 per cent of the growth of the femur and 40 per cent of the overall growth of the lower limb. Any injury that displaces this epiphyseal center or that is not completely reduced can affect growth.

The distal femoral epiphyseal fracture is most often the result of a hyperextension force that displaces the metaphysis posteriorly and frequently compresses popliteal vessels and nerves. Vascular impairment that does not improve with reduction of the epiphyseal fracture demands surgical exploration of the popliteal space.

Rarely, a hyperflexion injury will displace the epiphysis posteriorly to the metaphysis rather than anteriorly.

The epiphysis may also be fractured by a valgus knee injury, usually in sports, which in the older patient causes ligamentous rather than epiphyseal disruption. The differential diagnosis between these two injuries depends on stress x-rays.

Type III or type IV epiphyseal fractures, which can produce bone bridging across the physis, are best treated by open reduction and internal fixation.

Always warn the parents and the patient of possible growth defects, especially if there has been significant epiphyseal displacement in the skeletally immature child.

Take follow-up x-rays for several years after the fracture and during growth spurts, and be prepared to excise any bony physeal bridges that develop.

Separation at Birth

REMARKS

The center of ossification is readily discernible at birth; therefore, the lesion is detectable by x-ray.

Displacement is usually backward.

Correction of the displacement is not necessary except in extreme cases. Formation of a new lower end of the femoral shaft and remodeling eventually result in a normal femur and knee.

Check for evidence of circulatory embarassment.

Appearance on X-Ray

1. Posterior displacement of the lower femoral epiphysis.

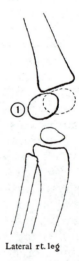

Lateral rt. leg

Management

1. Apply a single hip spica.
2. The knee is slightly flexed.

Note: The cast is discarded after three weeks.

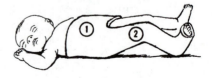

Alternate Method (Bryant Traction)

1. Apply skin traction to both legs (use strips of foam rubber for traction on the skin).

2. Make vertical traction; the feet are in a symmetrical position.

3. Use weights and pulleys; the buttocks must clear the mattress.

4. Hold child in a fixed position with a wide binder.

Note: Traction is removed after three weeks.

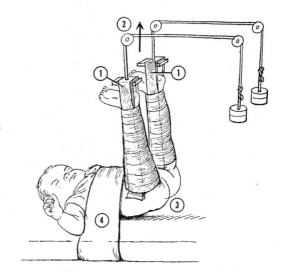

Type I Separation in Older Children

Prereduction X-Ray

1. The femoral epiphysis is displaced forward.

2. The end of the diaphysis is displaced into the popliteal fossa.

Note: The degree of displacement may vary from minor to complete separation.

Manipulative Reduction

Note: Whenever a massive hemarthrosis is present, the joint should be aspirated before reduction.

1. Place the patient on a fracture table.

2. Fasten the unaffected foot to a foot plate.

3. With the knee flexed 30 to 45 degrees, make strong manual traction in the long axis of the thigh.

4. Correct any lateral displacement by making pressure on the epiphysis and the lower end of the shaft in opposite directions.

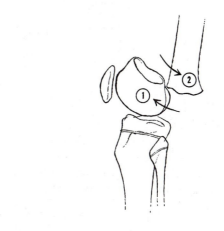

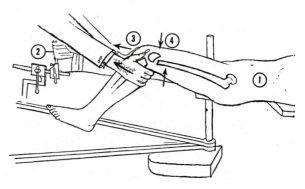

Manipulative Reduction
(Continued)

1. While an assistant makes upward pressure on the lower end of the thigh,
2. Reduce displacement by flexing the knee beyond a right angle. (Now check position by x-ray.)

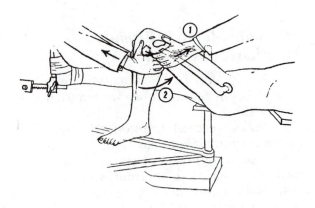

Postreduction X-Ray

The epiphysis is restored to its normal anatomic position.

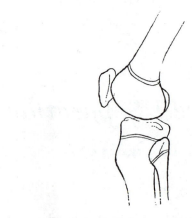

Immobilization

1. Apply long leg cast with knee flexed 70 degrees to maintain the reduction.
2. Split the cast to accommodate the swelling and to permit monitoring of the patient's pulses.

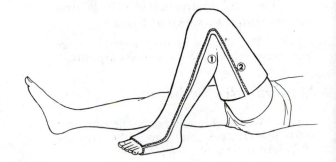

Postreduction Management

The fracture reduction may be lost as limb swelling subsides. Be sure to take x-rays several times in the first week to evaluate the reduction.

At the end of three weeks, remove the plaster cast and prescribe progressive flexion and extension exercises to regain quadriceps strength. The patient should continue partial weight bearing with crutches until quadriceps is sufficiently strong to stabilize the knee. This usually requires about four weeks of crutch walking.

Irreducible Displacement

REMARKS

This method is used in late cases in which some healing has occurred or in unstable injuries in which reduction is lost.

A threaded Steinmann pin is inserted into the bony epiphysis under image-intensified fluoroscopic guidance to avoid the physis.

Once the distal epiphysis is controlled, steady traction will permit reduction.

Skeletal Fixation of a Displaced Epiphysis

1. Reduction was lost in a displaced, unstable epiphyseal fracture.

2. Under image-intensified fluoroscopic guidance, a 3-mm threaded Steinmann pin was drilled from the medial to the lateral aspect of the distal femoral epiphysis, with care taken to avoid the physis.

3. Steady traction with the knee extended and then flexed pulled the epiphysis distally and posteriorly in line with the metaphysis.

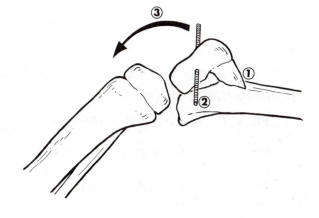

4. Pin was incorporated in plaster with the knee flexed and was removed after three weeks.

Note: The knee was allowed to regain extension and subsequent management was the same as with fresh fractures.

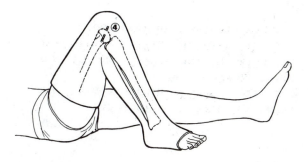

223

Backward Displacement

Prereduction X-Ray

1. The femoral epiphysis is displaced backward.
2. The distal end of the shaft of the femur is displaced forward. (Varying degrees of lateral displacement of the epiphysis may be present.)

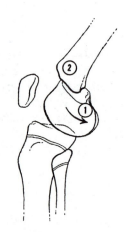

Manipulative Reduction

1. Place the patient on a fracture table.
2. Fasten the unaffected foot to a foot plate.
3. Make straight traction on the limb to restore length.

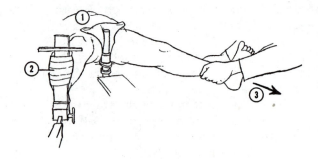

While traction is maintained,
1. An assistant makes downward pressure on the distal end of the shaft, while
2. The operator hyperextends the knee, effecting the reduction.

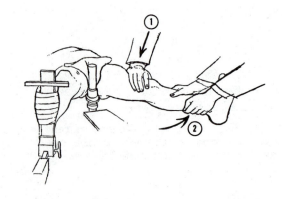

Immobilization

1. Apply a plaster cast from the groin to the toes.
2. The knee is in full extension.
3. The foot is at a right angle.

Note: Mold the plaster well around the condyles of the femur.

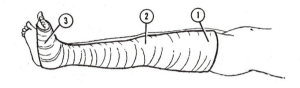

Postreduction Management

Remove the plaster cast after four weeks.

Institute graduated exercises to restore power to the quadriceps and motion at the knee joint.

Allow the patient on crutches with protected weight bearing.

Discard the crutches when the quadriceps is powerful enough to stabilize the knee joint adequately.

Type IV Separation in Older Children

REMARKS

In this lesion anatomic alignment of the physis and the articular surfaces of the epiphysis is most essential to prevent growth disturbances and later osteoarthritis. This can only be achieved by open reduction and internal fixation.

Preoperative X-Ray

1. The fracture line traverses the epiphysis and physis and splits off a triangular segment of the metaphysis.
2. The physis is not in alignment.
3. The articular surfaces are not congruous.

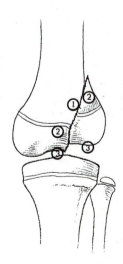

225

Operative Reduction and Internal Fixation

1. Make a 12.5-cm to 15-cm incision on the anterolateral aspect of the thigh in the interval between the rectus tendon and the vastus lateralis muscle. Continue the incision downward around the patella.

Note: For medial injuries a similar approach is made on the medial aspect of the joint between the rectus tendon and the vastus medialis.

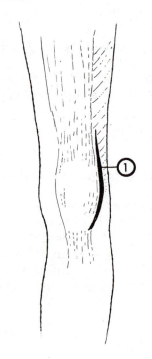

2. Divide the fascia lata, the lateral aponeurosis, and the joint capsule in the line of the incision.

3. Proximally develop the interval between the rectus femoris and the vastus lateralis.

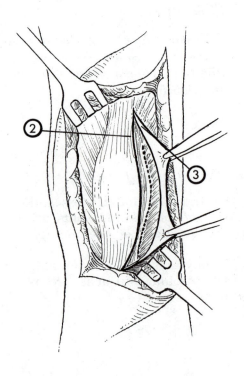

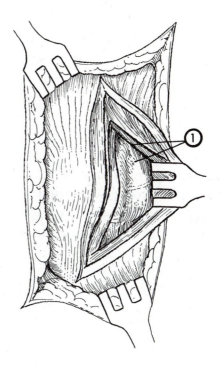

1. Split the vastus intermedius longitudinally and expose the distal end of the femur and the displaced epiphysis with the attached metaphyseal fragment.

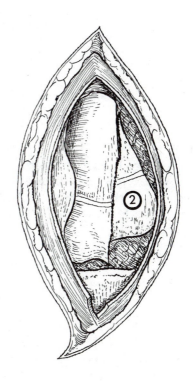

2. Divide the synovial membrane, exposing the knee joint and fracture.

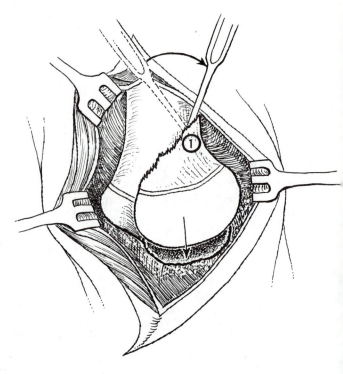

Operative Reduction and Internal Fixation (Continued)

1. Under direct vision lever the epiphysis into its anatomic position.

Then:

1. Secure the fragment with two Kirschner wires passing through the metaphysis into the femur. Cut the wires below the level of the skin and bend the ends.

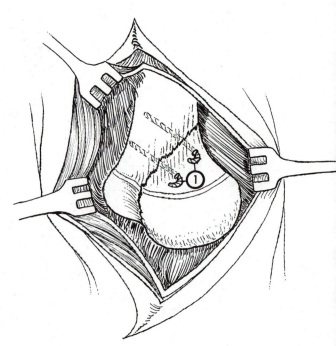

Postreduction X-Ray

1. The alignment of the physis is restored.
2. The articular surfaces are congruous.

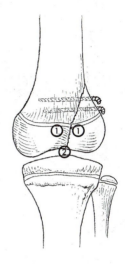

Immobilization

1. Apply a plaster cast from the groin to the toes.
2. The knee is slightly flexed.
3. The foot is at a right angle.

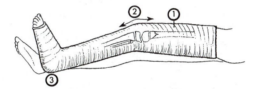

Postoperative Management

Encourage static contractions of the quadriceps and exercise for the toes.

Remove the plaster cast and wires at the end of six weeks.

Institute a regimen of progressive active exercises for the quadriceps, knee, and foot. The patient should perform the exercises under supervision, if possible.

When the patient has achieved good quadriceps power, allow him out of bed on crutches without bearing weight on the affected leg.

After two weeks begin partial weight bearing on crutches.

Generally, after two more weeks, the crutches can be discarded.

Growth Deformities Following Distal Femoral Epiphyseal Fractures

Approximately 30 per cent of these fractures will produce shortening or angular deformities sufficient to require operative correction.

If the shortening is 4 cm or less, epiphysiodesis of the opposite femoral physis may be all that is necessary.

Usually the deformity is a combination of shortening and angulation due to physeal bridging, which may be efficiently treated by resection of the bridge and physeal distraction.

Preoperative X-Ray

1. Lateral physeal bridging following a type II fracture three years before has produced a 25-degree valgus deformity and a 5-cm shortening.

2. Physis will continue to grow on the open medial side, producing more valgus deformity.

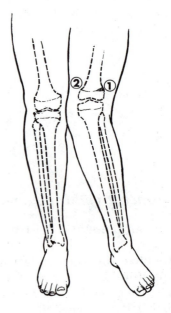

Technique of Physeal Distraction Treatment

1. The physeal bony bridge is resected.

2. Under image-intensified fluoroscopic guidance, a 4-mm Steinmann pin is drilled into the epiphysis, from medial to lateral.

3. A turnbuckle distraction apparatus is attached to the epiphyseal pin and is used as a guide to drill two other pins into the diaphysis.

4. The distraction apparatus is locked onto the pins and turned to distract the metaphyseal-physeal junction. The lateral side is distracted further than the medial side to correct the valgus deformity. The distraction apparatus is turned approximately 1 mm per day until the desired correction is achieved.

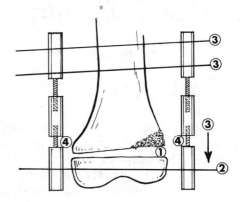

Postoperative Treatment

1. The distraction apparatus is removed when the callus is evident in the metaphysis.

2. The epiphyseal and metaphyseal pins are incorporated in plaster for eight to ten weeks until the callus solidifies in the lengthened area.

Note: After removing the pins, protect the area of lengthening for four to six weeks more with plaster.

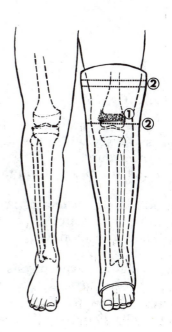

231

Occult Femoral Epiphyseal Injuries

REMARKS

Valgus injury to the skeletally immature knee may produce a type III epiphyseal fracture, which can be mistaken for a ligamentous injury. This epiphyseal injury has occurred in patients as old as 17 years in whom the physis appeared almost completely closed. Even at this late stage, however, the physis is still weaker in certain respects than the ligaments.

Unless the articular fracture is displaced, operative reduction is not necessary.

It is important to evaluate the unstable knee in the adolescent and teenager by means of stress x-rays.

Mechanism of Injury

1. The knee is subjected to a valgus stress injury while the foot is planted on the ground.

2. The force fractures through the physis.

3. The pull of the cruciates results in the valgus strain being directed toward the knee and producing a type III epiphyseal fracture.

4. Bony bridging of the physis may occur, but the growth effect is minimal because of the relative skeletal maturity in most of these patients.

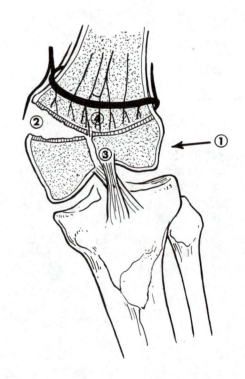

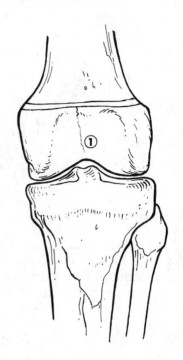

Appearance on X-Ray

1. Standard x-rays do not demonstrate the fracture, and the laxity of the knee joint might be attributed to ligamentous injury.

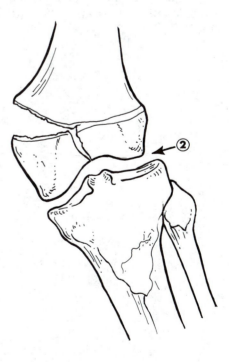

2. A stress x-ray will show the true nature of the epiphyseal fracture.

Note: This is usually a stable injury in an adolescent close to skeletal maturity. Immobilization using a long leg cast for four to six weeks is adequate treatment.

FRACTURES OF THE
TIBIAL SPINE

REMARKS

This injury occurs most often in children from 8 to 13 years of age as the result of sudden extension and internal rotation of the knee, most characteristically incurred in falling from a bicycle.

The injury, when it occurs in adults, results from more violence to the knee and produces greater disruption of the joint support structures.

The prognosis for complete recovery after this injury is much better in children than in adults.

Fractures of the tibial spine in children that maintain contact with the tibial surface are treated by aspiration of the hemarthrosis and cast immobilization with the knee in slight flexion.

Fractures that are completely dislodged should be treated by open reduction and suturing of the fragment down to its bed.

Open reduction and fixation should also be done for an old fracture with displaced fragments that cause catching and locking of the knee joint.

234

Slightly Displaced Tibial Spine Fracture

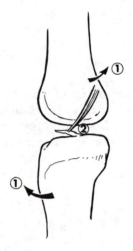

1. Injury typically occurs in a fall from a bicycle in which the knee is forcefully extended and internally rotated.

2. The attachment of the spine to the tibial surface is still evident.

Management

Aspirate the knee joint for the hemarthrosis and then immobilize the knee in slight flexion.

Cast immobilization is continued for eight to ten weeks until healing is evident.

Acute or Chronic Complete Displacement of a Tibial Fragment

1. No attachment of the fragment to the tibial surface is evident, and the fragment is completely rotated. Impingement and locking of the knee will occur during knee motion.

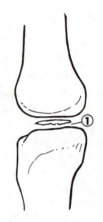

2. The fragment is visualized at arthrotomy and is reattached to the edge of the meniscus by simple absorbable suture.

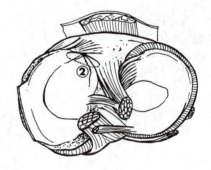

Postoperative Management

Cast immobilization with the knee in slight flexion is maintained for eight to ten weeks.

The patient is then allowed to regain range of motion with protected crutch walking for an *additional* three to four weeks more.

236

SEPARATION OF THE PROXIMAL TIBIAL EPIPHYSIS

REMARKS

This is one of the most uncommon fractures of childhood, because the absence of ligamentous attachments to the proximal tibial epiphysis makes it relatively immune to injury.

Most injuries result from a hyperextension injury to the knee that produces posterior displacement of the shaft and consequently a high incidence of damage to the popliteal vessels.

Occasionally, severe valgus injury to the knee will produce this physeal fracture and may be confused with ligamentous injury. Stress x-rays distinguish the two injuries.

Reduction should be performed immediately, especially after hyperextension injuries, so as to relieve any popliteal vascular compression.

It may be quite difficult to maintain reduction of these unstable fractures; occasionally, proximal and distal transfixion pins are necessary.

Open reduction and internal fixation are necessary only for the rare type III or type IV fracture of the proximal tibial epiphysis.

Careful follow-up is necessary to evaluate and treat for any growth arrest or deformity.

Hyperextension Injury

Prereduction X-Ray

1. Separation of the epiphysis from the metaphysis.

2. Posterior displacement of the shaft of the tibia.

Note: This displacement may injure the popliteal vessels.

3. The tibial epiphysis includes the tibial tubercle.

4. The shaft is displaced laterally.

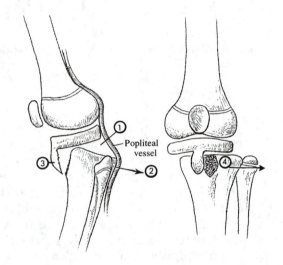

Manipulative Reduction

Note: Whenever massive hemarthrosis is present, the joint should be aspirated before reduction.

1. Place the patient on a fracture table.

2. Fasten the unaffected foot to a foot plate.

3. With the knee flexed 30 to 45 degrees, an assistant grasps the forefoot with one hand and the heel with the other and makes strong traction on the lower leg.

4. While traction is maintained, correct any lateral displacement by making pressure with the heels of the hand on the epiphysis and the upper end of the shaft of the tibia in opposite directions.

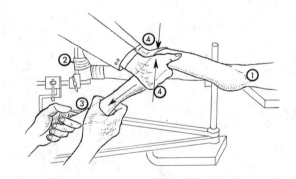

238

1. While the thigh is supported on the table, allow the knee of the affected leg to bend to 90 degrees.

2. Place thumbs on either side of the tibial tubercle and encircle the upper end of the calf with the fingers of both hands.

3. While an assistant steadies the lower leg by moderate traction toward the floor,

4. Forcefully pull forward on the upper end of the shaft of the tibia as the thumbs make strong backward pressure on the epiphysis.

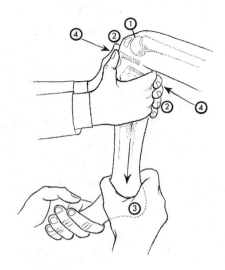

Postreduction X-Ray

1. The epiphysis is in normal alignment with the metaphysis.

2. Lateral displacement of the diaphysis is corrected.

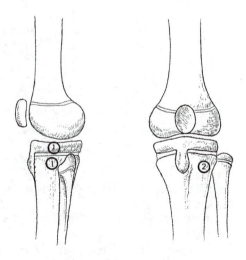

Immobilization

1. Apply a plaster cast from the groin to the toes.

2. The knee is flexed 30 degrees.

3. The foot is at a right angle.

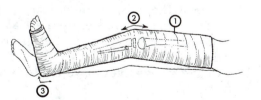

239

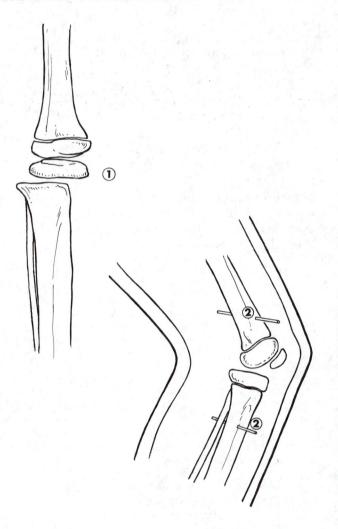

Transskeletal Pin Fixation for Unstable Fracture

If the fracture cannot be stabilized after reduction:

1. Transverse 3-mm skeletal pins are inserted in the distal femur and proximal tibia to maintain reduction.

2. Pins are incorporated in plaster, and the foot of the cast is windowed to allow monitoring of pulses.

Postreduction Management

Encourage static contractions of the quadriceps and exercise the toes.

Remove the plaster at the end of three weeks and remove any pin fixation that might have been used.

Note: If a portion of the metaphysis was displaced with the epiphysis or if pin fixation was necessary, reduce the amount of flexion 10 to 15 degrees and apply another cast for three more weeks.

Institute a program of progressive active exercises for the quadriceps, knee, and foot.

Allow the patient up on crutches without weight bearing.

After three weeks allow partial weight bearing.

Generally after one to two more weeks the crutches can be discarded.

Take x-rays every two or three months to note behavior of the epiphysis.

Adduction, Abduction, and Crushing Injuries

REMARKS

Generally there is only minimal displacement.
A portion of the physis is most likely damaged.
Protect these lesions for at least three months before permitting weight bearing.

Prereduction X-Ray

Note: There may be no x-ray evidence of displacement or the epiphysis may be displaced minimally.

1. There is no anteroposterior displacement.
2. The metaphysis is displaced slightly laterally in relation to the epiphysis.

Manipulative Reduction

Note: No manipulative maneuvers are employed for undisplaced separations.

1. Place the patient on a fracture table.
2. Fasten the unaffected foot to a footplate.
3. With the knee flexed 30 to 45 degrees, an assistant grasps the forefoot with one hand and the heel with the other and makes steady traction in the line of the lower leg.
4. While traction is being maintained, correct any lateral displacement by making pressure with the heels of the hands on the epiphysis and on the upper end of the shaft of the tibia in opposite directions.

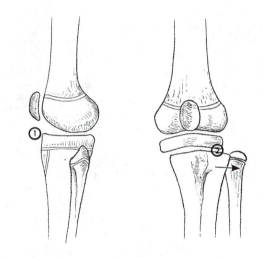

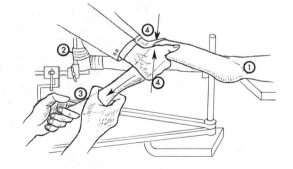

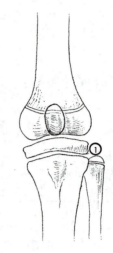

Postreduction X-Rays

1. Lateral displacement is corrected.

Immobilization

1. Apply a plaster cast from the groin to the toes.
2. The knee is flexed 10 to 15 degrees.
3. The foot is at a right angle.

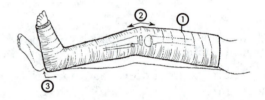

Postreduction Management

Encourage static contractions of the quadriceps and exercises for the toes.

Allow the patient up on crutches.

After three weeks remove the cast.

Allow the patient up on crutches without weight bearing.

Protect the physis from weight bearing for three months.

During this period institute a program of progressive active exercises for the quadriceps, knee, and foot.

Take x-rays every two or three months to determine the fate of the physis.

COMPLETE AVULSION OF
THE TIBIAL TUBERCLE

REMARKS

This lesion is the result of violent contracture of the quadriceps with the knee flexed.

Complete extension is not lost because the lateral expansions of the quadriceps apparatus are not completely torn from the tibia.

The lesion is most common in patients younger than 18 years, in whom the epiphysis is not as yet fused to the head of the tibia.

Operative repair is the treatment of choice because the extent of injury is greater than is evident on x-ray.

Types of Fracture

A. PREREDUCTION X-RAY

1. The entire anterior prolongation of the tibial epiphysis is pulled away from the anterior surface of the tibia; the base of the prolongation is intact.

B. PREREDUCTION X-RAY

1. The anterior prolongation is pulled away from the anterior surface of the tibia.

2. The base of the epiphyseal prolongation is fractured.

C. PREREDUCTION X-RAY

1. A small separate epiphysis of the tubercle is avulsed and is pulled upward.

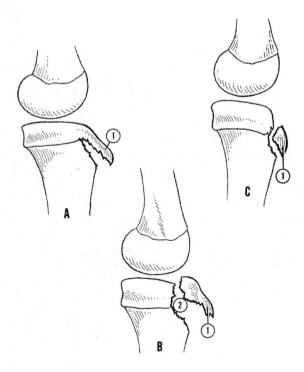

243

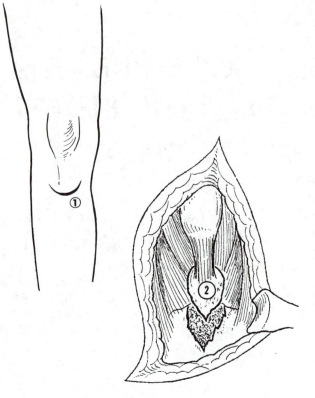

Operative Reduction

1. Make a curved "smile" incision from the medial aspect to the lateral aspect of the injury. This incision may be closed by subcuticular suture and gives the least prominent scar about the knee joint.

2. Reflect the skin and the deep fascia outward, exposing the patellar tendon and the avulsed epiphysis.

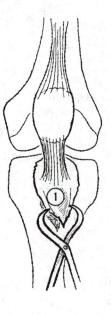

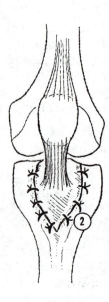

1. Grasp the epiphysis with a towel clip and place it in its anatomic position on the anterior surface of the tibia.

2. Anchor the epiphysis in this position by interrupted sutures passing through surrounding soft tissues. Cancellous screw fixation may also be necessary in muscular individuals.

Postoperative Management

1. Apply a compression bandage around the knee.
2. Place the limb on a posterior plaster splint extending from the upper third of the thigh to the toes.
3. The knee is extended fully and the foot is at a right angle.

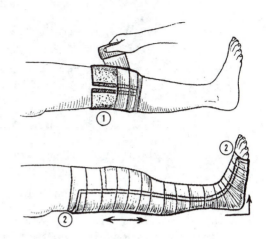

After ten days remove the splint and:

1. Apply a plaster cylinder from the groin to just above the malleoli.
2. The knee is extended.

Note: Cylinder may become loose in some individuals and a long leg cast may be preferable.

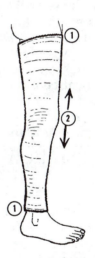

Now institute a program of progressive quadriceps exercises.

Remove the cast at the end of five to six weeks and permit protected weight bearing with crutches. Now increase the intensity of the quadriceps and flexion exercises.

After eight or nine weeks permit unprotected weight bearing; continue the exercises until maximum restoration of quadriceps power and extension and flexion of the knee are achieved.

INJURIES OF THE DISTAL TIBIAL EPIPHYSIS

REMARKS

Just as the most frequently injured epiphysis of the body is the distal radial epiphysis, the most frequently injured epiphysis in the lower limb is the distal tibial.

These injuries occur most often in patients older than 8 years, the average patient being 12 years old.

Since the contribution of the distal epiphysis to growth after this age is minimal, growth deformities are infrequent, except for adduction injuries that crunch the medial side of the physis.

These epiphyseal fractures are produced by the same mechanisms that cause ankle fractures and fracture dislocations in adults.

The most common mechanism of injury is abduction, which is characterized by lateral displacement of the epiphysis along with a lateral metaphyseal fragment.

External rotation injury, the second most common mechanism, displaces the epiphysis posteriorly along with a fractured fibula.

Plantar flexion injury is the third most common mechanism and is recognized by a posteriorly displaced epiphysis without a fractured fibula.

Axial compression injuries may also be caused by direct violence, which displaces the epiphysis either posteriorly or anteriorly and may comminute the metaphysis in multiple areas.

The most treacherous of these fractures and the type most likely to produce growth arrest and angular deformity is the adduction injury. It is frequently mistaken for a simple fracture of the medial malleolus. This is actually a type IV epiphyseal fracture, which closes the medial side of the physis and often produces a severe varus deformity of the ankle. It is essential to perform open reduction and fixation after this type of injury so as to achieve anatomic position and minimize the risk of future deformity.

Except for adduction injuries, the majority of these fractures can be treated by closed reduction and cast immobilization with the anticipation of normal subsequent growth. Repeated manipulation to achieve perfect reduction is not wise for most of these problems. Valgus deformity of the ankle of up to 15 degrees will correct with growth. Varus deformities tend to worsen and should be prevented.

246

Types of Physeal Fractures and Separation

ABDUCTION INJURIES (MOST COMMON)

1. Separation of the distal tibial epiphysis.
2. Small triangular lateral metaphyseal fragment.
3. Epiphysis and metaphysis fragments are displaced backward and laterally.
4. Fracture of the shaft of the fibula.

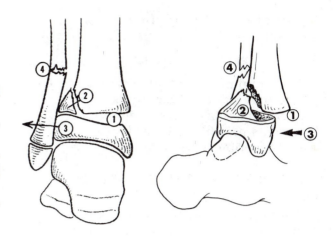

EXTERNAL ROTATION INJURY

1. Triangular fragment from medial metaphysis.
2. The epiphysis with metaphyseal fragment is displaced backward and medially.
3. Fracture of the shaft of the fibula.

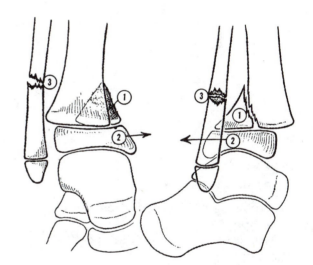

PLANTAR FLEXION INJURY

1. Separation of distal tibial epiphysis.
2. Posterior metaphyseal fragment.
3. Plantar flexion force vector displaces epiphysis backward.
4. Intact fibula indicates that the injury was not extremely violent.

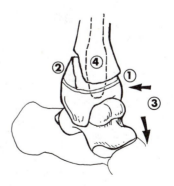

Types of Physeal Fractures and Separation (Continued)

AXIAL COMPRESSION INJURY

1. Comminution of metaphysis.
2. Comminution of epiphysis.
3. Metaphyseal and epiphyseal fragments are displaced anteriorly or may sometimes be displaced posteriorly.
4. Fracture of the shaft of the fibula.

Note: This type usually occurs in children near skeletal maturity, and growth deformities are relatively infrequent.

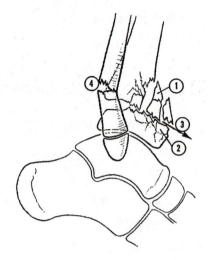

ADDUCTION INJURY

1. Crushing of the medial aspect of the metaphysis.
2. Crushing of the medial portion of the epiphysis.

Note: This lesion occurs frequently in relatively young children and is very likely to produce growth arrest and varus ankle deformities.

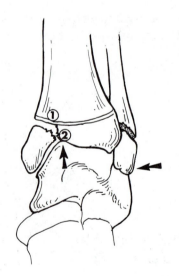

Manipulative Reduction

Note: Choice of manipulative maneuvers depends on the direction of the displacement of the epiphysis; the following method is employed for posteromedial displacements.

With the patient under general anesthesia:

1. The leg hangs over the end of the table.
2. Place one hand over the lateral aspect of the leg.
3. Place the other hand over the medial aspect of the foot and the medial malleolus.
4. Push the foot strongly outward. (This corrects the medial displacement.)
5. Place one hand on the anterior aspect of the lower leg.
6. Grasp the heel with the other hand.
7. Pull the foot strongly forward. (This corrects the posterior displacement.)

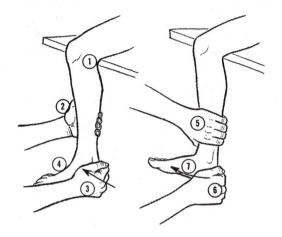

1. While an assistant holds the limb by the toes and the thigh,
2. Apply a circular cast from behind the metatarsal heads to the upper thigh.
3. The foot is in a neutral position.
4. The knee is flexed 45 degrees.

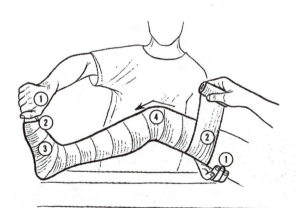

Manipulative Reduction (Continued)

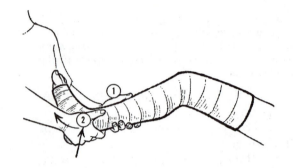

While the plaster is setting:

1. Steady the limb with one hand on the lateral aspect of the leg.

2. Make strong lateral and forward pressure on the foot with the other hand.

Note: Mold the plaster well around the malleoli. Maintain outward and forward pressure until the plaster has set.

Postreduction X-Ray

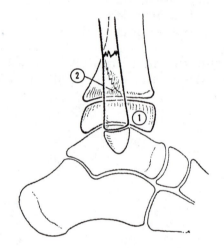

1. The epiphysis is restored to its anatomic position.

2. The triangular metaphyseal fragment is restored to its normal relation to the rest of the metaphysis.

Note: Do not try repeated manipulations. Valgus angulation up to 15 degrees will correct with growth. Varus angulation should not be accepted, because it tends to worsen.

Postreduction Management

Remove the plaster cast at the end of six weeks.
Now allow free use of the limb.

Note: If there is evidence of crushing of the epiphyseal plate, protect the limb in plaster for ten to twelve weeks.
Check for growth disturbance by x-ray every four to six months for the first two years.
Do not permit an arrest of growth with angular deformities to produce secondary changes in the joint; correct the deformity by osteotomy.

250

Adduction Fractures of the Malleolus in Children

REMARKS

These are the most treacherous injuries and most likely to produce unanticipated deformities from growth arrest.

They result from adduction forces that fracture the medial malleolus (epiphysis as well as physis) and produce a type III or type IV fracture.

Their innocuous appearance on x-ray frequently results in inadequate treatment, so that subsequent asymmetric growth arrest causes varus deformity sufficient to require osteotomy.

Open reduction with internal fixation is the preferred treatment, but even with anatomic reduction growth deformity is possible.

TYPE IV FRACTURE

Appearance on X-Ray

1. Vertical fracture through the medial portion of the distal tibial epiphysis without displacement.

2. Chip fracture of the metaphysis indicates that this is a type IV fracture, which has crossed the physis and can cause bony bridging. Operative fixation will minimize the risk of bony bridge formation.

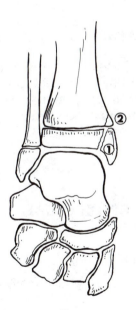

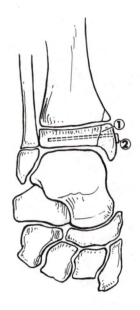

Postreduction X-Rays

1. Epiphyseal fragment is in normal position.

2. Epiphyseal fracture has been closed by smooth Steinmann pin to minimize physeal bridging.

Technique of Operative Reduction and Internal Fixation

REMARKS

Any adduction injury to the distal tibial epiphysis is generally best treated by open reduction and internal fixation.

Closed treatment is usually associated with varus growth deformity, which must be corrected by a supramalleolar osteotomy as soon as it becomes evident.

TYPE III EPIPHYSEAL FRACTURE

Preoperative X-Ray

1. Fracture through the body of the epiphysis.

2. Separation through the medial portion of the plate.

3. Medial displacement of the epiphyseal fragment.

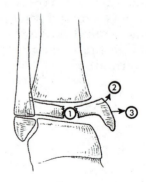

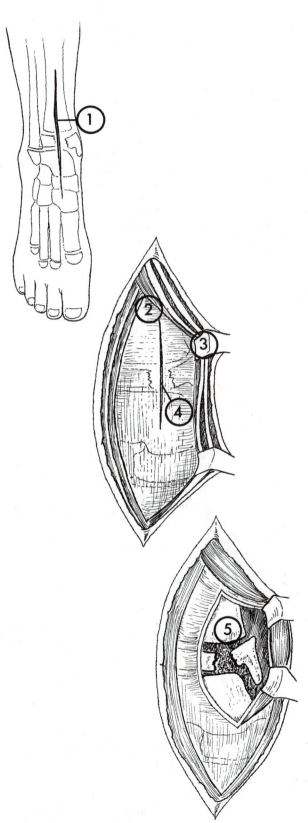

Operative Reduction

1. Make a vertical incision on the anterior aspect of the ankle; it begins 9 cm above and terminates 2.5 cm below the ankle joint.

2. Divide the deep fascia in the line of the skin incision and develop the interval between the extensor hallucis longus and the extensor digitorum longus tendons.

3. Identify the neurovascular bundle and retract it medially with the extensor hallucis longus.

4. Incise the periosteum and capsule in the line of the skin incision.

5. Expose the anterior surface of the tibia and ankle joint by subperiosteal and subcapsular dissection.

Operative Reduction (Continued)

1. Identify the fracture line in the epiphysis and the plate.

2. With a curette gently lever the fragment into its anatomic position; fix with transverse Kirschner wires or a screw.

Note: Do not insert a curette between the fragments; this inflicts damage to the physis.

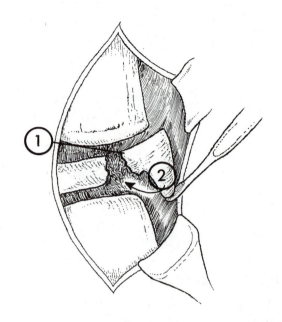

Postreduction X-Ray

1. Fragment is in its normal position.

2. Alignment of the physis has been restored and likelihood of physeal bridging is minimized by internal fixation.

3. The articular surface has been restored.

Note: Fixation pins need not be routinely removed.

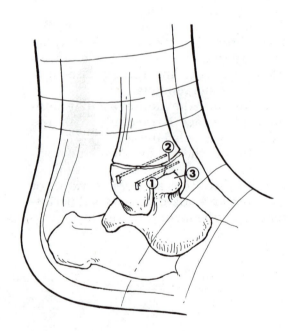

Immobilization

1. Apply a plaster cast from behind the metatarsal heads to below the knee.

2. The foot is at a right angle.

3. The foot is in a neutral position.

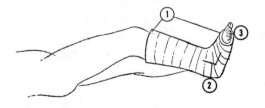

Postoperative Management

For the first four to six weeks, the limb is in the cast and must not bear weight.

With the cast still on, partial weight bearing may be allowed for four to six weeks more.

Ten to twelve weeks after the operation, remove the cast. Weight bearing should be progressive and should be determined by clinical and radiographic signs of healing.

Evaluate the effect on growth with periodic x-rays for at least two years after injury.

Internal fixation pins need not be removed unless they produce local symptoms.

Correction of Varus Deformity

REMARKS

Ankle varus of more than 5 to 10 degrees following distal epiphyseal injury requires correction. This is usually necessary as an individual nears skeletal maturity, and it can best be done by an opening osteotomy to correct shortening as well as varus angulation.

Preoperative X-Ray

1. An adduction fracture 3 years before has produced a 20-degree ankle varus deformity and 2-cm shortening in a 15-year-old boy.

2. Overgrowth of the fibular has contributed to the deformity and should be corrected.

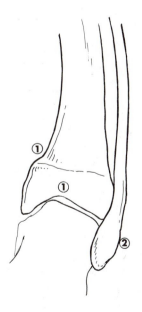

Postoperative X-Ray

1. An opening supramalleolar wedge osteotomy has corrected the varus deformity as well as the shortening.

2. Autogenous iliac graft filled the opening.

3. The tibial position has been maintained by internal fixation.

4. The overgrown fibular has been shortened and fixed with a heavy screw, which inhibits further over-growth.

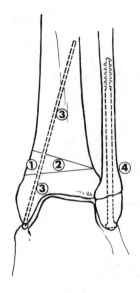

SUMMARY: PITFALLS IN MANAGING EPIPHYSEAL FRACTURES

Pitfalls in managing injuries to growth centers of bone may be created by both overtreatment and undertreatment. Comprehending the types and significance of epiphyseal fractures, particularly from the standpoint of potential effects on future growth, is the key to the most appropriate management.

Fractures of the proximal humeral epiphysis tend to be overtreated because of their alarming appearance on x-ray. Since these are generally a type II fracture, their remodeling potential is great and operative intervention is rarely necessary.

Fractures of the distal humeral epiphysis, which are frequently type IV, tend to be undertreated because their radiographic appearance is deceptive. Bone that forms after these fractures causes bridging of the physis and asymmetric growth unless prevented by anatomic reduction and internal fixation.

Proximal radial epiphyseal fractures are generally type II. Reduction by closed methods is usually satisfactory, except for persistent displacement that is likely to block forearm rotation.

Distal radial epiphyseal injuries, the most common epiphyseal fractures, almost always are type I or II. These can be treated by closed methods even though reduction may be incomplete, because the remodeling potential is considerable.

Phalangeal epiphyseal fractures tend to be undertreated, not because of their effect on growth but because of their mechanics. Malrotation must be corrected to prevent overlapping finger.

Injuries to the proximal femoral epiphysis can be quite destructive to hip joint function. Treatment by internal fixation after gentle closed reduction of the acute slip, or pinning in situ for chronic slip, gives the most satisfactory result. Attempted operative reduction of these epiphyseal injuries can produce further damage that can become a serious complication from overtreatment. Pinning the slipped capital femoral epiphysis in situ permits normal femoral head remodeling, particularly if the acetabular triradiate cartilage is open at the time of pinning.

Distal femoral epiphyseal injuries, like distal humeral injuries, are most often undertreated. These fractures frequently result in growth arrest and deformity from bone bridge formation. Accurate anatomic reduction is essential in managing injuries to this most rapidly growing area in the lower limb.

Injuries to the proximal tibial epiphysis are rare. Careful evaluation must distinguish these injuries from ligamentous injuries and must determine whether the closely adjacent popliteal artery has been damaged.

Fractures of the distal tibial epiphysis are the most common epiphyseal fracture in the lower limb. Most are type I or II injuries and respond well to closed reduction. Adduction injuries that fracture across the medial physis or medial malleolus are most treacherous and can produce significant varus growth deformities. They should always be reduced anatomically and fixed internally.

The physician who undertakes treatment of these injuries to growth centers should anticipate the common pitfalls so as to avoid overtreatment and undertreatment.

REFERENCES

Bright, R. W., Burstein, A. H., and Elmore, S. M.: Epiphyseal-plate cartilage. A biomechanical and histological analysis of failure modes. J. Bone and Joint Surg., 56-A:688–703, June 1974.

Brighton, C. T.: Clinical problems in epiphyseal plate growth and development. In Instructional Course Lectures, American Academy of Orthopaedic Surgeons, 23:105–121, 1974.

Brookes, M.: The Blood Supply of Bone. An Approach to Bone Biology. London, Butterworth & Co. (Publishers) Ltd., 1971.

Canale, S., and Bourland, W.: Fracture of the neck and intertrochanteric region of the femur in children. J. Bone and Joint Surg., 59-A:4, 1977.

Crenshaw, A. H.: Injuries of the distal tibial epiphysis. Clin. Orthop. 41:98–107, 1965.

Edelshteyn, B. M., Udalova, N. F., and Bochkarev, G. F.: Dynamics of reparative regeneration after lengthening by the method of distraction epiphyseolysis. Acta Chir. Plast (Praha), 15:149–153, 1973.

Fahey, J. J., and O'Brien, E. T.: Acute Slipped Capital Femoral Epiphysis. J. Bone and Joint Surg., 47-A:1105–1127, Sept. 1965.

Jones, E. R. L., and Esah, M.: Displaced fractures of the neck of the radius in children. J. Bone and Joint Surg., 53-B:429–439, Aug., 1971.

Lombardo, S. J., and Harbey, J. P.: Fractures of the distal femoral epiphyses. Factors influencing prognosis: a review of thirty-four cases. J. Bone and Joint Surg., 59-A:742–751, 1977.

O'Brien, E. T., and Fahey, J. J.: Remodeling of the femoral neck after in situ pinning for slipped capital femoral epiphysis. J. Bone and Joint Surg., 59-A:62–68, Jan., 1977.

Ratliff, A. H.: Traumatic separation of the upper femoral epiphysis in young children. J. Bone and Joint Surg., 50-B:757–770, Nov., 1968.

Salter, R. B., and Harris, W. R.: Injuries Involving the Epiphyseal Plate. J. Bone and Joint Surg., 45-A:587–622, Apr. 1963.

Shapiro, F., Holtrop, M. E., and Glimcher, M. J.: Organization and cellular biology of the periochondrial ossification groove of Ranvier. A morphological study in rabbits. J. Bone and Joint Surg., 59-A:703–722, Sept., 1977.

Southwick, W. D.: Osteotomy through the lesser trochanter for slipped capital femoral epiphysis. J. Bone and Joint Surg., 49-A:807, 1967.

Trueta, J., and Amato, V. P.: The vascular contribution to osteogenesis. III. Changes in the growth cartilage caused by experimentally induced ischaemia. J. Bone and Joint Surg., 42-B: 571–587, Aug., 1960.

INJURIES OF THE CERVICAL SPINE

EPIDEMIOLOGY

REMARKS

The annual occurrence rate for fractures and dislocations of the entire spinal column is approximately 230 per million people.

The overall probability of neurologic damage from a spinal column injury is 10 to 15 per cent, or 30 new cases of paraplegia and quadriplegia per million. This probability increases to 40 per cent if the injury involves the cervical spine and to 70 per cent if there is a dislocation associated with a fracture.

By far the major portion of these injuries result from motor vehicle accidents, and if paralysis occurs, the victim is most likely to be an adult less than 25 years of age.

Fracture of the arthritic spine in an elderly patient who has fallen represents the second most frequent spinal injury.

Diving injuries with resultant quadriplegia produce a third major category.

Penetrating injuries from firearms, the fourth most common cause of cervical spine fracture, often produce neurologic damage.

Because of the severity of injury, 50 per cent of patients with spinal cord damage die prior to arrival at the hospital or shortly after hospitalization.

Effective care of the patient who survives depends on comprehension of the anatomic susceptibility of the cervical vertebrae to injury, mature judgment regarding the various options for surgical and nonsurgical treatment, and a real appreciation of the rehabilitation as well as the immediate care needs of the patient with cervical spine injury.

PERTINENT ANATOMIC FEATURES

The cervical spine is a flexible, compact column of seven distinct units (vertebrae) situated between the head and the relatively fixed thorax.

In order to accommodate the special senses located in the head, the cervical column has developed extreme flexibility at the expense of stability.

Great mobility is possible because of the special arrangement of the articulations between the vertebrae.

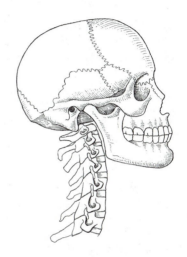

Between every two vertebrae below C2 there are five articulations:

1. A pair of posterolateral articulations.

2. A pair of lateral articulations (joints of Luschka).

3. An intervertebral disc.

Note: The articular facets between the atlas and axis approach the horizontal, whereas those below C2 progressively approach the vertical.

4. Articular facets between the atlas and the axis.

5. Articular facets below C2.

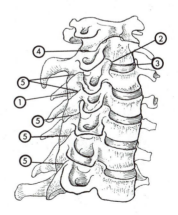

Stability of the cervical spine depends on the intervertebral disc and particularly on the system of ligamentous supports and articulations.

Intervertebral Disc

REMARKS

The disc structure is an important stabilizer and shock absorber for the vertebrae to which it attaches. Severe injuries that displace the vertebral bodies invariably implicate the disc.

Displacement of the disc may cause instability of the cervical vertebrae as well as pain and neurologic deficits from dural and nerve root impingement.

The intervertebral disc structure may be injured by either flexion overload or extension overload.

Cross Section of a Vertebral Disc

1. The annulus fibrosus is a stout structure at the peripheries and

2. Its fibers are attached to the bone and blend with the cartilaginous plate of the vertebra above and below.

3. The nucleus lies in the central portion of the disc and is in contact with the cartilaginous plate above and below.

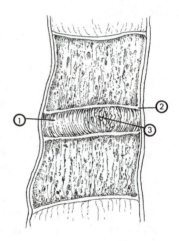

Ligamentous Apparatus

REMARKS

The ligaments provide considerable stability to the entire cervical spine and particularly to the occiput–C_1–C_2 articulations, which are more horizontally oriented than the lower cervical spine articulations. This horizontal orientation is particularly true in children and less true in adults, who tend to develop greater vertical inclination of the upper cervical facet joints.

The occiput is supported by ligaments to the atlas as well as to the axis, but the major support for the occipito-atlantal motion is the tectorial membrane, an upward extension of the posterior longitudinal ligament.

The alar ligaments from the sides of the dens to the occipital condyles restrict the amount of rotation that can occur around the dens.

The transverse ligament, which lies deep to the tectorial membrane and attaches to both ends of the arch of the atlas, limits forward displacement of C_1 on C_2.

Ligaments provide considerable stability to the lower cervical spine. Disruption of the posterior longitudinal ligament occurs primarily with flexion-rotation injuries whereas the anterior ligament is disrupted with hyperextension.

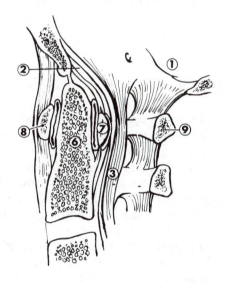

Articulations of the Occiput, Axis, and Atlas

1. Occiput is supported by
2. Tectorial membrane, which is an upward extension of
3. Posterior longitudinal ligament.
4. Alar ligaments limit rotation of
5. Atlas around
6. Odontoid.
7. Transverse ligament prevents forward shift of
8. Anterior arch and
9. Posterior arch of C_1.

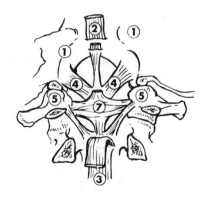

Articulations of Lower Cervical Spine

1. Anterior longitudinal ligament is firmly attached to the bone and annulus fibrosus.

2. Posterior longitudinal ligament is not as strong as the anterior ligament.

3. Capsule of the posterior lateral joint is a loose, relaxed structure.

4. Interspinous ligaments.

5. Supraspinous ligament.

6. Disc.

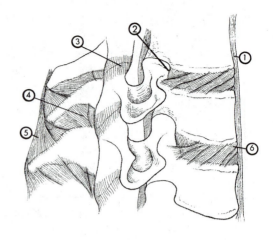

Contents of the Cervical Column

REMARKS

The most important function of the cervical spine is protection of the soft tissue structures traversing it.

Although the cervical spine is very flexible, its contents are contained in relatively rigid bony canals, so that any displacement of the bony elements may compromise the important soft tissue elements by direct injury, stretching, or angulation.

The cord and its blood supply lie in the cervical canal, fixed in position by the dentate ligaments.

The nerve roots lie in oval rigid bony canals.

The vertebral arteries and the accompanying sympathetic chains also are held in rigid bony canals.

1. Cervical portion of spinal cord.
2. Nerve roots.
3. Vertebral arteries.
4. Sympathetic nerve fibers.

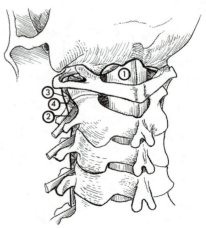

Motion of the Cervical Spine

REMARKS

Comprehension of the limits of the arcs of motion at specific levels is necessary to understand the different mechanisms responsible for injuries of the cervical spine.

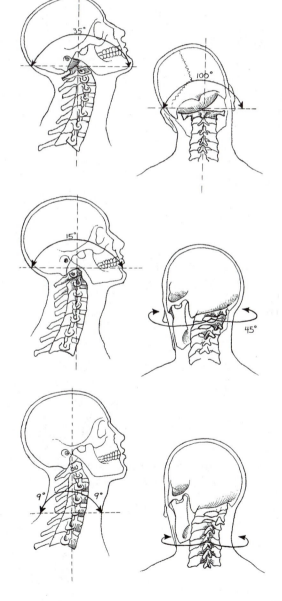

Atlanto-Occipital Joint

1. Flexion-extension motion is approximately 35 degrees.
2. Side-to-side motion is about 100 degrees.

Note: There is no rotation at this joint.

Atlanto-Axial Joint

1. Flexion-extension is approximately 15 degrees.
2. Rotation is approximately 45 degrees.

Note: During rotation the atlas rises vertically on the axis. This phenomenon is caused by the convexity of the articular surfaces of the joints between the atlas and the axis.

Motion from C2 to C7

1. Flexion-extension about 9 degrees at each level.
2. Only a few degrees of lateral and rotatory motion.

FACTORS INFLUENCING NORMAL MOTION

REMARKS

Certain existing abnormalities in the cervical spine cause varying degrees of restriction of motion of the levels affected. Essentially these are congenital or degenerative in origin.

Such abnormalities render the cervical spine vulnerable to even minor trauma.

1. Cervical spine with congenital failure of segmentation of two vertebrae.

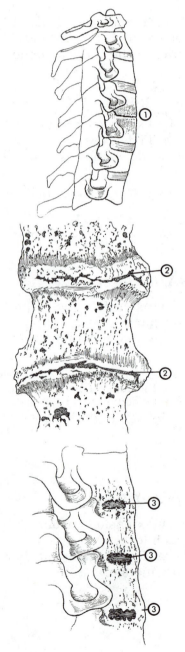

2. Advanced degenerative changes of the intervertebral discs.

3. Fusion of the cervical vertebrae in rheumatoid arthritis or spondylitis.

266

MECHANISMS OF INJURY

REMARKS

Knowledge of the various mechanisms of cervical spine injury is essential for rational treatment.

The vector of forces applied to the cervical spine and the head, and the position of the neck at the time of injury determine to a great extent the nature and location of the spinal column injury.

External evidence of violence to the face, head, or chin may be valuable in judging the mechanisms of injury. Hematoma and areas of tenderness over the spine are also warning signs of significant injury.

The cervical spine and head may be subjected to six general types of injuries:

1. *Pure flexion* violence is expended on the vertebral body, and since the posterior ligament complex can absorb the longitudinal pull, the result is usually a stable wedge fracture of the vertebral body.

2. *Flexion with rotation* causes posterior ligaments to rupture. Since the facet joints of the cervical spine are small, flat, and almost horizontal, dislocation frequently results from such an injury.

Because the majority of fractures and fracture dislocations are from flexion or flexion and rotation forces, treatment with traction to extend the neck is usually effective (except for extension injuries).

3. *Hyperextension* violence applied to the upper cervical spine, particularly the large second cervical spine, produces a comminuted fracture of the posterior ring. Hyperextension loading of the lordotic lower cervical spine ruptures the disc and anterior longitudinal ligament, causing a dislocation that may reduce spontaneously. The resultant quadriplegia may follow no apparent skeletal injury, and approximately 17 per cent of patients with spinal cord paralysis have no x-ray evidence of either fracture or dislocation.

4. *Hyperextension with rotation* fractures the articular pillars of the lower cervical spine, producing fractures or dislocations.

5. *Vertical compression* injury occurs most frequently from striking the head while diving into shallow water, so that compression is superimposed on a flexion moment. The vertical load shatters the vertebral endplates and forces the nucleus of the disc into the vertebral body, causing it to explode. Vertical loading of the head may also compress the occipital condyles on the ring of the first cervical vertebra and cause them to shatter.

6. *Lateral flexion* injuries occur frequently from football tackling or falls from motorcycles, in which the shoulder and neck are driven in opposite directions. The resultant stretch injury of nerve roots may or may not be associated with unilateral compression fractures of the vertebrae.

Hyperflexion Mechanisms

REMARKS

Simple hyperflexion of the cervical spine without an externally applied force to the head rarely causes severe injury because the chin strikes the anterior chest wall, thus preventing further flexion.

This range of motion is within normal range of the cervical spine.

If an external force is acting on the back of the head, the damage is determined by the intensity and direction of the applied force.

If the externally applied force is not severe, the injury is usually limited to the posterior soft tissues, occasionally avulsing one or more spinous processes.

A severe flexion force combined with rotational injury can produce unilateral or bilateral facet fractures, dislocations, or fracture-dislocations.

Flexion-rotation injuries may crush or disrupt the disc or may detach it from the vertebrae above or below and produce severe damage to cord and nerve roots.

Hyperflexion of the Cervical Spine with a Moderate External Force Acting

1. Rupture of the supraspinous ligament.

2. Rupture of the interspinous ligament.

3. Avulsion of the spinous process.

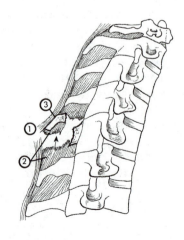

OR:

If the posterior ligaments hold:

Note: The force is now expended on the vertebral body, producing a wedge compression fracture.

1. Supraspinous ligament is intact.
2. Interspinous ligament is intact.
3. Ligamentum flavum is intact.
4. Capsular ligaments are intact.
5. Vertebral body is wedged anteriorly.
6. Disc may be injured.

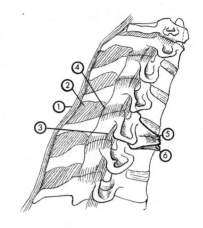

Hyperflexion of the Cervical Spine with a Greater External Force and a Rotation Force Acting

1. Rupture of the supraspinous ligament.
2. Rupture of the capsular ligaments.
3. Rupture of the interspinous ligament.
4. Rupture of ligamentum flavum.
5. Rupture of the posterior longitudinal ligament.
6. Subluxation or dislocation of the facets (unilateral or bilateral).
7. Compression of intervertebral disc.

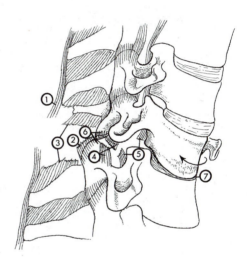

OR:

8. Fracture of the facets with unilateral or bilateral dislocation and with or without fractures of the laminae.
9. Chip of bone off the anterior superior margin of the vertebra below.
10. Disruption of the intervertebral disc.

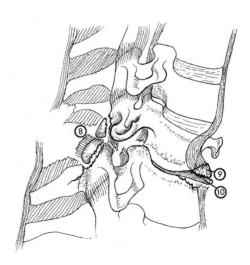

HYPERFLEXION WITH COMPRESSION — THE TEARDROP FRACTURE-DISLOCATION

REMARKS

The usual mechanism of this severe injury is striking the head while diving into shallow water or, occasionally, while tumbling in gymnastics.

The violence of the injury smashes the endplate of the fifth cervical vertebra, (usually) producing a burst fracture with fragmentation that compresses the cord and results in anterior cord syndrome. This is characterized by 1) motor paralysis, 2) loss of pain and temperature sensation, and 3) preservation of vibration, touch, and position.

Anterior decompression and fusion of these incomplete cord lesions are frequently the indicated treatment, provided that the posterior elements and support ligaments are not disrupted.

Usually, the anterior longitudinal ligament and the interspinous ligaments remain intact to stabilize the spine, but if these structures are damaged the result is an extremely unstable injury.

Mechanism

1. With the head slightly flexed, as in diving, the cervical spine is straight.

2. Striking the head in shallow water produces a burst fracture of the vertebral body.

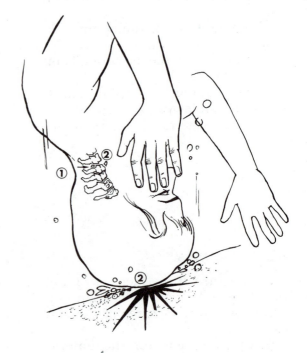

Result

1. Crushed vertebral body.
2. Anterior teardrop fragment is displaced forward, but anterior longitudinal ligament remains intact.
3. Posterior fragment is displaced backward into the canal.
4. Anterior cord syndrome results from cord compression and damage to anterior spinal artery.
5. Intervertebral disc is disrupted and extruded into vertebral body.
6. Direction of forces.

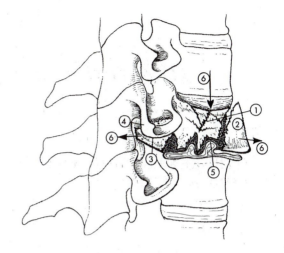

COMPRESSION FRACTURE OF THE ATLAS (BURSTING OR JEFFERSON'S FRACTURE)

REMARKS

The most common fracture of the atlas is produced by a severe compression force directed vertically downward while the spine is straight.

The force is usually the result of a blow on the top of the head; the force is transmitted through the atlanto-occipital articulations, which force the lateral masses of the atlas outward.

The fracture usually occurs through the posterior arch of the atlas but may occur through both the anterior and the posterior arches.

Generally there is no damage to the cord.

The anterior and posterior ligaments are intact; this is a stable fracture.

1. Force applied to the top of the head.
2. The cervical spine is straight.
3. Fracture through the posterior and anterior rings of the atlas produced by the condyles of the occiput splitting the ring.
4. Spreading of the lateral masses indicates fracture, which may be visualized only on an anteroposterior tomogram or CT (computed tomography) scan.

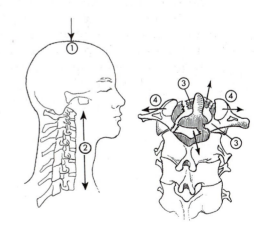

271

Hyperextension Mechanisms

HYPEREXTENSION WITHOUT A COMPRESSIVE FORCE ACTING

REMARKS

This injury, which occurs when an auto strikes the rear of the auto in which the patient is a driver or passenger, represents a virtual pandemic in the urban population. The incidence in some areas is 6 to 14 per 1000 people.

More than 40 per cent of patients with hyperextension injury have persistent symptoms that tend to be attributed by observers and some physicians to psychoneurosis or motives of monetary or other gain rather than to actual physical disorder. Electroencephalography may reveal changes due to damage sustained when the head pursued a backward and then a downward movement during the auto collision.

The forces acting are hyperextension and prolongation of the neck, which may damage the intervertebral disc and detach it from its vertebral attachments.

In severe hyperextension injuries, especially in elderly patients, the anterior longitudinal ligament may rupture, allowing the upper facet to slide downward on the lower. The infolding of the ligamentum flavum consequent to this injury may damage the cord and even cause death.

X-rays may show no fracture or dislocation, and even at postmortem no disc protrusion may be found.

Most often the injury produces head, neck, shoulder, and interscapular pain consistent with disc protrusion on the dura.

The absence of x-ray changes, the sometimes bizarre pain symptoms, and the impending compensation claims may result in biased attitudes on the part of the patient's physician, employer, family, and acquaintances if the underlying disc problem goes unrecognized.

1. Hyperextension and prolongation of the neck.

2. Hyperflexion — chin strikes the anterior chest wall or the windshield, preventing further flexion.

3. Head returns to neutral position.

Note: Stiff neck and pain from the disc injury may not develop for several days.

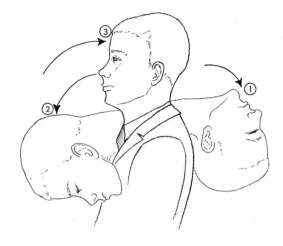

OR:

1. Severe hyperextension and prolongation of neck.

Note: These are the forces responsible for soft tissue injuries as well as disc disruption.

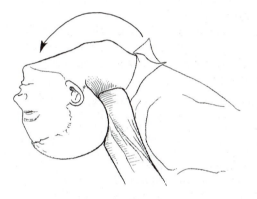

Hyperextension Injuries of the Intervertebral Discs

REMARKS

The structures most frequently injured are the intervertebral discs.

Implication of the intervertebral discs may occur in any age group.

The most common lesions are crushing of the discs and avulsion of the discs from their attachments to the vertebra above or below.

Detachment of the disc is associated with rupture of the anterior longitudinal ligament and may permit a momentary subluxation of the cervical spine.

No gross disruption of the bony elements occurs except, in some instances, avulsion of a small chip of bone from the anterior rim of one of the vertebral bodies associated with disruption of the anterior longitudinal ligament.

These patients, especially older patients, may present with severe neurologic deficit but little demonstrable damage to the spinal column itself.

Hyperextension Injuries of the Intervertebral Discs (Continued)

BULGING DISC

1. Wedging of the disc.
2. Anterior bulging of the disc.
3. Thin and attenuated anterior longitudinal ligament.

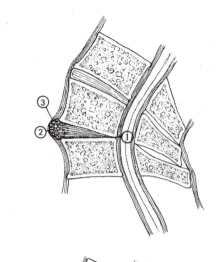

SEPARATION OF THE DISC

1. Separation of disc from caudal articular plate.
2. Separation of disc from cephalic articular plate.
3. Separation of disc through cancellous bone of caudal vertebral body.
4. Rupture of the anterior longitudinal ligament.

Note: Extreme hypermobility of a cervical vertebra approaching subluxation is a frequent finding in the upper cervical spine of children (C2 on C3); ten per cent of children under the age of nine years show this abnormality.

In the absence of any injury or symptoms, do not interpret this finding as pathologic.

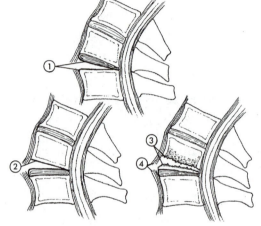

POSTERIOR DISLOCATION FOLLOWING DETACHMENT OF THE DISC

1. Cervical spine severely hyperextended.
2. Detachment of disc from inferior articular plate.
3. Tear of the anterior longitudinal ligament.
4. Chip of bone off the anterosuperior surface of the caudal vertebra.
5. Stripping of the posterior longitudinal ligament.
6. Compression of the cord between
7. The posteriorly displaced vertebra and
8. The ligamentum flavum and lamina of the subjacent vertebra.

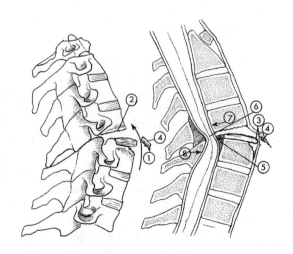

274

Hyperextension Injuries in the Presence of Posterior Osteophytes Causing Central Cord Syndrome

REMARKS

Severe cord damage may occur from hyperextension injury in a cervical spine with osteoarthritic changes.

During hyperextension, the ligamentum flavum bulges into the spinal canal, reducing its diameter.

The cord is pinched by the bulging ligament and the posterior osteophytes.

A characteristic neurologic pattern results from damage to the central portion of the cord.

The pathologic condition responsible for the syndrome is hemorrhage, edema, or vascular insufficiency affecting the central portion of the cord, particularly the region of the lateral corticospinal tracts.

X-rays fail to show any fractures or dislocations of the vertebrae.

There may be a chip of bone off the anterosuperior rim of the inferior vertebra, indicating a rupture of the anterior longitudinal ligament.

The acute central cord syndrome is characterized by the following:

1. There is a history of a hyperextension injury.

2. Paralysis may be complete, involving both upper and lower extremities, or varied patterns of paresis of the upper and lower extremities may exist.

3. The sensory pattern is bizarre.

4. Urinary control is lost.

5. Recovery may begin within a few hours to several days.

6. Occasionally, partial neurologic lesions may rapidly progress to total paralysis before recovery starts.

7. In general, neurologic involvement is greater and appears earlier in the upper extremities than in the lower.

8. Recovery of the cord lesion begins in reverse order from that in which it appeared: first, return of motor power in the lower extremities; next, return of bladder control; and then, return of motor power in the arms and hands. Sensory recovery appears prior to motor recovery and improves more rapidly.

9. This is the most common incomplete lesion of the cord; more than half the patients with central cord syndrome regain significant neurologic function.

10. Surgery is contraindicated initially because spontaneous recovery is so frequent and because the shock of surgical procedure may increase the ischemic damage to an already questionable cord.

Hyperextension Injuries in the Presence of Posterior Osteophytes Causing Central Cord Syndrome (Continued)

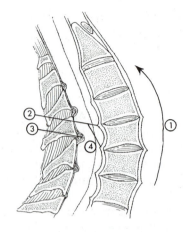

1. Hyperextension of the cervical spine.
2. Posterior osteophytes.
3. Bulging ligamentum flavum.
4. Pinched spinal cord.

Note: This may occur at several levels.

Hyperextension Injuries in the Presence of Degeneration Causing Damage to the Nerve Roots

REMARKS

In the presence of osteoarthritic changes in the region of the intervertebral foramina, the diameter of the foramina is reduced in size.

The contents of the foramina (nerve root) are crowded.

Even minimal hyperextension injuries may severely compress the already compromised nerve roots.

Crushing and tearing of soft tissues in the region of the foramina (annulus fibrosus, capsules of the posterolateral joints and the intervertebral disc) produce hemorrhage and edema, which further constrict the nerve roots.

This chain of events frequently initiates the symptoms characteristic of the cervical syndrome observed following acceleration and deceleration mechanisms of the cervical spine.

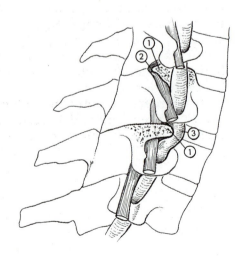

1. Osteophytes surrounding the foramen.
2. Cervical nerve root.
3. Vertebral artery.

Note: The vertebral artery and its investing sympathetic chain may also be involved because of their proximity to the foramen.

276

HYPEREXTENSION-COMPRESSION INJURIES

REMARKS

In these injuries, in addition to hyperextension, compression forces are acting from above. Injuries to the chin, face, or head indicate the sites at which these forces have been applied.

Sudden hyperextension and compression from a blow to the forehead or under the chin produces a comminuted compression fracture of the prominent posterior element of C2, the so-called "hangman's fracture." This is similar to the injury produced in execution by hanging, during which the submental knot hyperextends the head. The cause of death is not fracture but the sudden distraction of the cord resulting from the six-foot fall from the gallows platform.

Today, the usual mechanism of this fracture is a sudden striking of the head against an auto roof or windshield.

The upper cervical spine is sufficiently large that neurologic damage infrequently follows the hyperextension-compression fracture of C2.

In the lower cervical spine, hyperextension and compression forces are expended on the posterior bone elements, the base of the spinous processes, the articular facets, the pedicles, and the laminae. Here, neurologic damage is much more likely to occur.

The injury is best treated by forms of external immobilization that do not reproduce the mechanism of the original trauma, i.e., hyperextension.

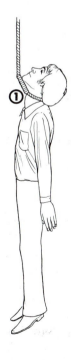

Hyperextension-Compression Fractures of the Upper Cervical Spine — The "Hangman's Fracture"

1. Submental knot forcefully hyperextends and fractures C2.

Hyperextension-Compression Fractures of the Upper Cervical Spine — The "Hangman's Fracture" (Continued)

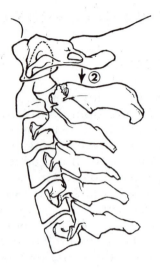

2. The long fall from the gallows platform avulses the posterior elements and destroys the cord, causing instantaneous death.

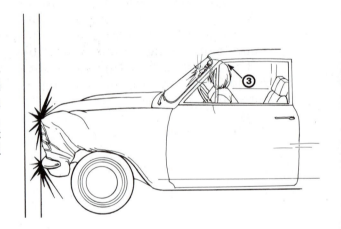

3. Present-day "hangman's fracture" is produced by auto windshield or roof. This sudden hyperextension disrupts the posterior elements of C2, but neurologic damage is infrequent because of size of the cervical canal at this level.

Hyperextension Fracture-Dislocation

REMARKS

This lesion occurs more frequently than is generally realized.

It is often mistaken for an anterior flexion fracture-dislocation because the vertebral body may be displaced forward.

It is caused by a severe hyperextension compression mechanism in which the forces are primarily expended on the posterior bony elements.

There is a fracture of the articular processes, with or without a fracture of the pedicles or laminae.

The characteristic x-ray features are (1) upward displacement of the inferior articular processes and (2) forward displacement of the vertebral body. Wide separation of the bodies does not occur.

There may be a fracture at the base of the spinous process with upward displacement.

The anterior longitudinal ligament may rupture and avulse a chip of bone from the vertebra above or below.

Fractures of the posterior bony elements may occur at several levels, such as a fracture through the posterior arch of the atlas, a fracture at the pedicles of C5, and a fracture of the spinous process of C7.

These fracture-dislocations are unstable, and often they are responsible for severe neurologic lesions.

1. Severe hyperextension of the cervical spine, and direction of the force.

2. Approximation and impingement of all the posterior elements.

3. Fracture through the pedicle of C5.

4. Fracture at the base of the spinous process of C7.

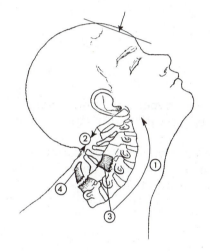

5. Anterior displacement of C5 on C6.

6. Upward displacement of the inferior articular mass of C5.

7. Upward displacement of the spinous process of C7.

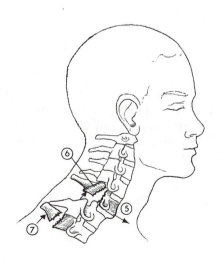

279

Rotatory Hyperextension Fracture-Dislocation

REMARKS

In this lesion a rotatory force is added to the hyperextension-compression forces, as when one is struck on the side of the skull.

The forces are expended on the posterior bony elements on the opposite side from which the force is applied.

The lesion usually occurs in the most mobile portion of the cervical spine (C4–C5, C5–C6).

The inferior articular process is fractured and is displaced upward, outward, and backward.

The body of the vertebra is displaced slightly forward.

The fractured facet may injure the cord, producing unilateral neurologic damage.

This is an unstable fracture.

1. Severe hyperextension, compression, and rotation of the cervical spine.

2. Impingement of posterior bony elements on the side opposite from the application of the force.

3. Fracture of the articular process of C5.

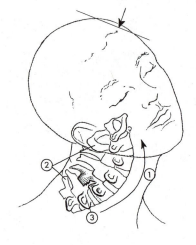

4. Upward displacement of the inferior articular process of C5.

5. Slight anterior displacement of the body of C5 on C6.

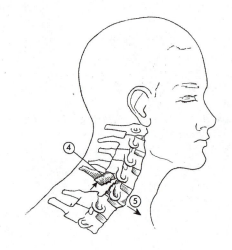

Lateral Flexion Injuries of the Cervical Spine

REMARKS

Severe lateral flexion may cause distraction of the cervical vertebra at one or more levels, stretching nerve roots in the process. This injury occurs most often from football and motorcycle accidents, in which the head and shoulder are driven in opposite directions.

1. Head tackling drives head and shoulder in opposite directions causing "nerve pinch." This is especially likely if shoulder pads are too low.

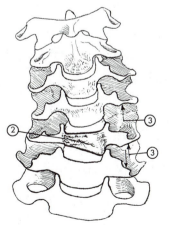

2. Lateral wedging of the body of C5 may rarely occur.
3. Separation between C4–C5, and C5–C6.

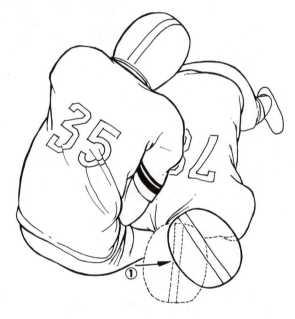

Injuries Peculiar to Occiput–C1–C2 Articulations

The upper cervical spine is designed to allow nodding and rotational motions, and facet joints are more horizontal than those in the lower cervical spine. This horizontal orientation makes the occiput–C1–C2 articulations susceptible to dislocations, especially in young people.

The tectorial membrane, the transverse and the alar ligaments, and the articular capsular structures provide strong support (see p. 263).

The spinal instability incurred when these structures are damaged may be considerable.

The neurologic damage, should the patient survive the initial injury, may be minimal because of the size of the spinal canal at this level.

Occiput–C1 Dislocation

Dislocation of the occiput on the atlas is rare, but some patients, especially young ones, have survived this injury without neurologic damage.

Initial treatment should be directed at prompt respiratory assistance.

Cervical traction should not be utilized, since it may increase the distraction. Immobilization is best achieved with a halo, which permits later posterior fusion.

Skull traction increases the displacement of the
1. occiput from
2. C1, and should be avoided.

Note: After an open airway is insured, occipitocervical fusion should be carried out using halo apparatus.

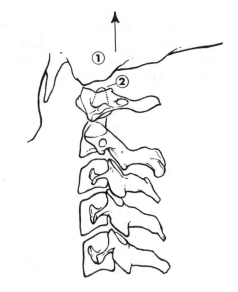

Traumatic Forward Atlanto-Axial Dislocation

REMARKS

Severe trauma causing hyperflexion and forward shift of C1 on C2 ruptures the transverse ligament.

Normally, the transverse ligament stabilizes the ring of C1 on the odontoid and limits anterior shift to less than 3 mm.

If the transverse ligament ruptures, the atlas dislocates forward, while the odontoid displaces backward occupying the neural canal.

Severe cord damage may be immediately evident, or the patient may manifest neurologic symptoms only intermittently with forward flexion of the head, i.e., "fall-out spells."

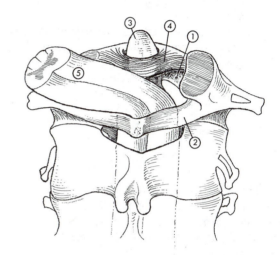

NORMAL ANATOMY

1. Anterior arch of the atlas.
2. Posterior arch of the atlas.
3. Odontoid process of C2.
4. Transverse ligament holding the odontoid against the anterior arch of the atlas.
5. Cervical cord.

ANATOMY AFTER A SEVERE HYPERFLEXION INJURY

1. The transverse ligament ruptures.
2. The atlas is displaced forward.
3. The odontoid is displaced backward in the neural canal.
4. The cord may be severely damaged or the patient may have neurologic symptoms only with neck flexion.

Note: Surgical fusion of C1 and C2 is necessary to protect the patient in whom instability is causing neurologic symptoms.

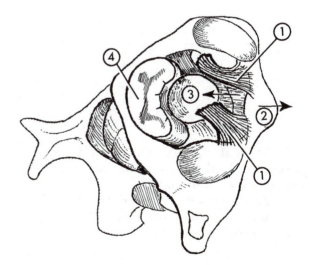

Dislocation of the Atlas Associated with Rheumatoid Arthritis

REMARKS

This lesion is so frequent that it must be considered in any patient with rheumatoid arthritis with or without injury.

Rheumatoid arthritis involves the C1–C2 articulation in 25 per cent of patients with generalized disease. Damage to the joints and transverse ligaments allow progressive subluxation of C1 on C2 with either horizontal displacement compressing the cord or vertical displacement compressing the brainstem.

The ring of C1 is 3 cm in diameter; 1 cm is taken up by the odontoid process and 1 cm by the cord, and there is usually 1 cm for allowable displacement.

Myelopathy and weakness resulting from C1–C2 instability occurs in 5 per cent of these patients and may be confused with a worsening of their peripheral arthritis unless the problem in the cervical spine is considered.

Patients with rheumatoid arthritis should always be evaluated for this cervical condition, especially prior to any surgery requiring endotracheal intubation.

C1–C2 fusion relieves myelopathy caused by this cervical instability.

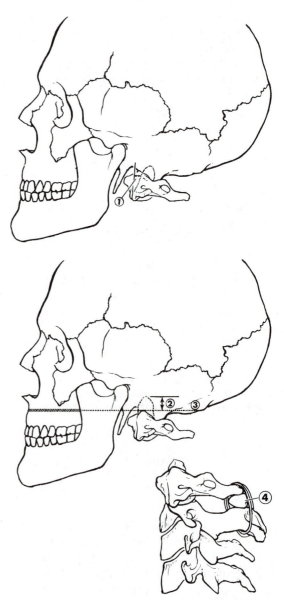

1. Horizontal subluxation, the most common type, is present if the distance from the anterior surface of the odontoid to the posterior surface of C1 arch exceeds 3 mm.

2. Vertical subluxation should be suspected if the tip of the odontoid measures 4.5 mm above

3. McGregor's line from the posterior margin of the hard palate to the caudal part of the occiput.

4. Fusion should be done if neurologic symptoms occur.

Dislocation of the Atlas Associated with Congenital or Acquired Abnormalities of the Odontoid

REMARKS

The odontoid may be absent either congenitally or because of trauma, or it may have a separate ossicle (os odontoideum).

Abnormalities of the C1–C2 articulation are relatively common in conditions such as spondyloepiphyseal dysplasia, Morquio's syndrome, and Down's syndrome.

These patients are exposed to neurologic catastrophe with any sudden flexion of the neck, and a C1–C2 fusion is indicated.

1. Hyperflexion of the cervical spine causes instability.

2. Absence of the odontoid is congenital, secondary to trauma, or associated with an os odontoideum.

3. The capsules of C1–C2 are the only supporting structures and may be damaged.

4. Forward displacement of the atlas is greater than 1 cm.

5. Cord damage may cause sudden and severe neurologic deficit or progressive myelopathy.

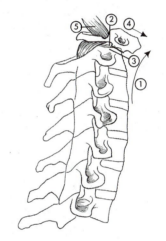

1. The odontoid process is hypoplastic.

2. Transverse ligament is intact.

3. The odontoid process has slipped under and behind the ligament.

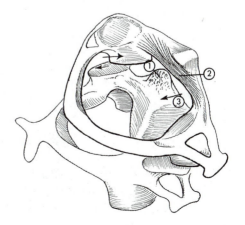

285

Rotatory Subluxation of the Atlanto-Axial Joint

REMARKS

Flexion and forced hyperrotation beyond 65 degrees will cause subluxation of C1 on C2. This rotatory deformity is usually shortlived and easily corrected.

Acute torticollis is the most common lesion of the cervical spine in children and may follow an upper respiratory tract infection or trivial injury or may be spontaneous.

The typical deformity is the "cock robin" position, in which the patient's head is tilted like that of a robin listening for a worm. The head is tilted 20 degrees to one side and rotated 20 degrees to the opposite side. Chronic maintenance of this position may cause facial flattening.

If the deformity persists for longer than three months, it is considered fixed. Treatment then is skull traction to correct rotation and atlanto-axial fusion if symptoms warrant.

Neurologic injury is infrequent, but sudden death may occur, especially in adults in whom rotational deformity is associated with anterior displacement of the atlas because of transverse ligament rupture.

ACUTE TORTICOLLIS

1. Forward and slight rotary displacement of the inferior articular facet of C1 on the superior articular facet of C2.

2. Flattening of the normal cervical curve.

3. Deviation of the spinous process of C1 to the same side as the chin.

4. Typical deformity of torticollis is corrected with rest and immobilization. The shortened sternomastoid muscle is a deforming force.

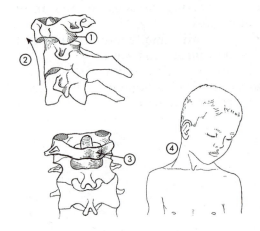

Atlanto-Axial Rotatory Fixation

REMARKS

Persistent C1–C2 subluxation for longer than three months may require surgical stabilization.

Rotatory fixation is diagnosed on the basis of asymmetric relationship of the dens to the articular masses of the atlas that persists on either right or left rotation. This is best seen on cineradiography.

TYPICAL DEFORMITY

1. "Cock robin" position with facial asymmetry from prolonged abnormal positioning.

2. Forward displacement of head.

3. A lengthened sternomastoid is in spasm from attempting to correct the deformity. This contrasts with shortened sternomastoid in acute torticollis (see above).

APPEARANCE ON X-RAY

1. Atlas and axis move as a unit with rotation. This is best seen on cineradiography.

2. Spinous process of C1 rotates to the same side as the chin.

3. Anterior displacement of C1 relative to the rest of the canal may cause neurologic damage.

Note: Rotatory fixation, especially with anterior displacement of C1, requires atlanto-axial fusion.

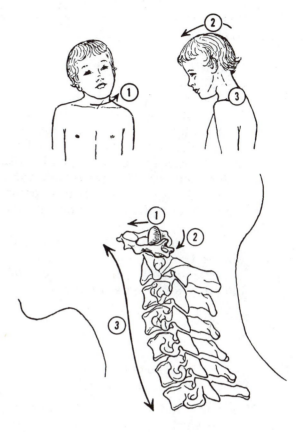

Fractures of the Odontoid Process without Displacement

REMARKS

Anterior sheering thrust of C1 on C2 ruptures the transverse ligament and produces forward dislocation of C1 and C2.

A posterior thrust of the ring of C1 on C2, when combined with an avulsion pull by the alar ligament, is most likely to fracture the odontoid process.

Ordinarily, no neurologic damage results from this injury.

The most common associated injury is a fractured mandible produced by the force vector that also fractures the odontoid.

1. Fracture line at the base of odontoid process, no lateral displacement. This most often results from a

2. Posterior thrust on C1 combined with

3. Avulsion by the alar ligaments due to hyperrotation.

4. Posterior thrust of the ring of C1 contributes to the fracture.

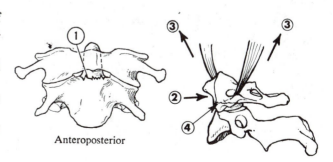

Anteroposterior

Fracture of the Odontoid with Dislocation of the Atlanto-Axial Articulations

REMARKS

Depending on the moment of force and the pull of the alar ligaments, the odontoid may fracture and displace anteriorly or posteriorly. Anterior displacement is far more common.

Displacement of the fractured odontoid process with the ring of C1 allows room for the cord, and these lesions are less lethal than acute dislocations of C1 from transverse ligament rupture. However, significant neurologic damage may result in sudden death, and the potential for such complications from an odontoid fracture should not be taken lightly.

Since the mechanism of this injury includes an avulsion force, the use of traction adds to the risk of nonunion. Halo cast devices that avoid traction are ideal methods of minimizing C1–C2 rotation without causing fracture distraction.

WITH ANTERIOR DISLOCATION OF THE ATLAS (MOST COMMON INJURY)

1. The atlas and the odontoid are displaced forward.

2. Atlas shows some rotatory displacement; this is the usual finding.

3. Spinous process of C2 is unusually prominent.

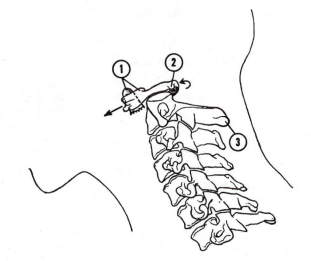

WITH POSTERIOR DISLOCATION OF THE ATLAS

1. Atlas and odontoid are displaced backward.

2. Tips of the spinous processes of C1 and C2 are almost in the same plane.

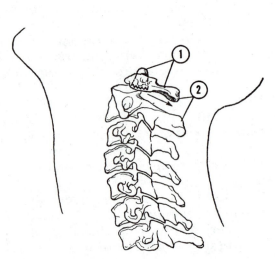

3. There may be a fracture of the posterior ring of the atlas or the odontoid or both.

Note: If this fracture is treated with traction, the odontoid process will be distracted and union will be delayed.

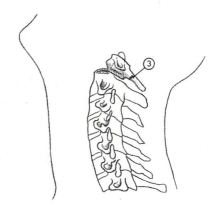

Iatrogenic Causes of Cervical Instability

REMARKS

Spontaneous subluxation or dislocation may occur after extensive laminectomies, which should be avoided in managing cervical injuries.

This is particularly true if the integrity of the posterolateral articulation is impaired.

When the posterior elements are sacrificed, the disc may not be able to withstand the forward thrust of the head and thus gradually gives way.

This mechanism produces a swanlike deformity of the neck with varying degrees of anterior displacement of the cervical vertebrae involved and worsening neurologic symptoms.

1. Extensive laminectomies at C4–C5–C6.

2. Swanlike deformity of the cervical spine.

3. Anterior displacement of C6 on C7.

4. Thinning of the disc at C6–C7.

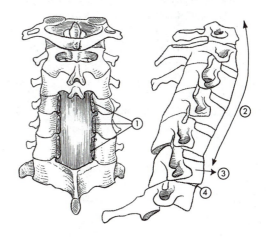

EMERGENCY TREATMENT OF CERVICAL SPINE INJURIES

REMARKS

Any patient suspected of having a cervical spine lesion should be handled with the utmost care from the moment of injury to the moment that definitive care is instituted.

Failure to observe this rule may result in catastrophic consequences that could have been avoided.

Always keep in mind the possibility of cervical spine injury in the unconscious patient, and check for facial fractures or cervical hematomas indicating forceful injuries to the neck.

Following an accident, the diagnosis of cervical cord injury in a paralyzed patient is obvious but:

Remember that in some cervical cord injuries symptoms may come on insidiously; failure to recognize cervical spine damage at this time may allow inadvertent motion, such as sitting or standing up, which may result in irrevocable cord damage.

At the scene of the accident don't move the patient until an evaluation is made.

If the patient is conscious the first question before any examination should be "Where do you hurt?"

Always suspect a cervical spine injury in accident victims who complain of severe occipital, shoulder, and arm pain.

Suspect a cervical spine injury, in a patient complaining of any weakness, numbness, or tingling in the arms or legs.

The patient who supports his head with his hands because of sensation of looseness or loss of control has a serious cervical injury until proven otherwise.

Before extricating patients with suspected neck injuries, apply a spine and neck board to assure maximum protection.

Emergency Splinting of Cervical Spine

1. If the patient complains of any neck or back pain apply a spine board prior to extrication to prevent further injury or

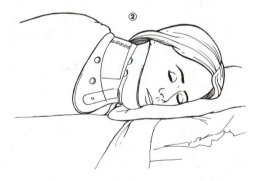

2. Transport the patient with a Philadelphia collar, immobilizing the neck rather than applying traction to an uncertain injury.

Note: For the unconscious patient, the cervical spine is protected while the patient is transported in the side-lying position to prevent aspiration.

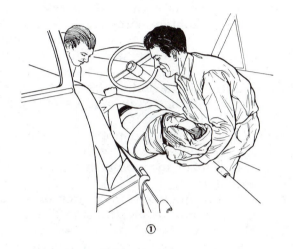

In the Emergency Room

All patients with suspected cervical spine injury should have a thorough evaluation without moving the head.

From history and local evidence of violence such as facial fractures or soft tissue contusions, the mechanism of injury and the type of cervical lesion may be suspected.

Determine whether the patient has any motor or sensory loss in the limbs and the trunk, and carefully document the level of sensory loss by pinwheel testing.

In the paralyzed patient, evaluate for paradoxical breathing or respiratory distress that will require respiratory assistance.

The following points are helpful in determining the extent of the cord damage:

1. In complete transsection of the cord, paralysis is immediate, with a sharp line of anesthesia. There is total areflexia with paralysis of bladder and bowels, loss of sweating, and loss of perianal sensation.

2. Spinal shock from injury lasts no longer than 24 hours. The return of the bulbocavernosus reflex (anal sphincter contracts when urethral catheter is tugged) indicates spinal shock is over. If no sensory or motor function is evident at this time, the cord lesion is complete.

3. Do not mistake hypotension from spinal shock with normal pulse and skin temperature for surgical shock, which is relatively infrequent in cord injury and presents with tachycardia and cool, clammy skin.

4. Be sure to check for sacral nerve function by testing perianal sensation, and toe flexion, which if present may be the only indicators of an incomplete lesion.

5. Presence of priapism and pathologic Strümpell reflex (slow plantar flexion of the hallux on plantar stimulation) indicates a complete lesion.

6. In fracture dislocations of C6 on C7, the sixth cervical nerve innervating the elbow flexors and wrist extensors is usually not involved. The ability of the patient to control these functions is the key to potential self-sufficiency.

7. Horner's syndrome usually means a lesion at the level of C7–T1.

8. With involvement of the cord at C4–C5 there is complete quadriplegia, and respiratory paralysis is likely.

9. Paralysis from a fracture dislocation of C3 on C4 is usually fatal because of respiratory failure.

After initial evaluation of neurological status, the cervical spine injury should be further evaluated by means of x-ray taken in the emergency room without moving the patient.

Radiographic Evaluation

REMARKS

The ease with which severe cervical trauma may occur is surpassed only by the frequency with which it may be overlooked. Injuries to the uppermost and lowermost cervical vertebrae are especially notorious for going unrecognized.

The patient with neck pain after any motor vehicle collision, any diving accident, or injury of any kind should have thorough radiographic evaluation to rule out the possibility of fracture.

Do not be reluctant to order cervical spine radiographs, which are far more important than radiographic studies of the skull for most injured patients.

For the severely injured patient with suspected neck fracture, a lateral view should be obtained by means of a portable x-ray machine used under a physican's supervision and without moving the patient from the emergency litter.

Be sure to visualize the entire cervical spine from the occiput to C7 and to pull downward on the arms and upward on the neck to demonstrate the C7–T1 articulation. If the lateral view shows no fracture or dislocation, obtain anteroposterior, open-mouth, and oblique views as well as any special views that might be indicated by the mechanism of injury and the location of pain.

Special Views

1. A direct blow to the top of the head indicates a possibility of a C1 fracture, which may require tomography to visualize spread of the lateral masses.

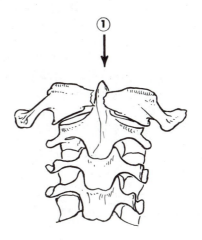

Special Views (Continued)

2. Odontoid fracture lines are frequently not seen on the initial x-ray, but any prevertebral soft tissue swelling greater than 5 mm anterior to body of C3 indicates bony injury.

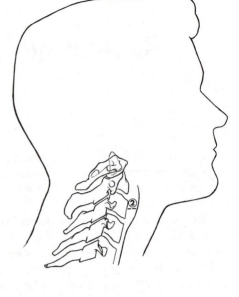

3. For hyperextension-rotation injury, as might be indicated by soft tissue injury to the side of the forehead, a pillar view may be necessary to visualize articular fractures.

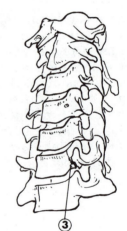

4. The x-ray is centered over the midcervical region with a 35-degree cephalocaudal tilt.

5. The patient's head is rotated 45 degrees to the side to visualize the articular pillars.

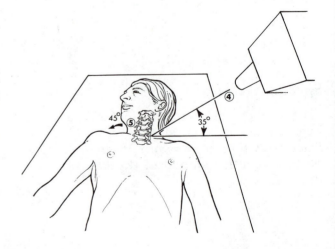

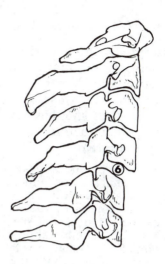

6. Anterior displacement of 25 per cent of the body width occurs with unilateral facet dislocation.

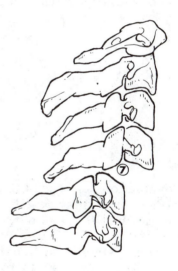

7. Displacement of 50 per cent indicates bilateral facet dislocation.

8. Flexion-extension views may be necessary to demonstrate instability, particularly at C1–C2.

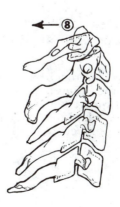
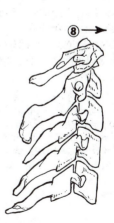

295

Special Views (Continued)

9. Fracture dislocations of C6–7 are frequently missed on inadequate x-rays obscured by shoulder structures. Cervical spine x-rays must visualize down to C7-T1. Pull shoulders down, out of the x-ray field in order to visualize this important area.

Note: Myelogram is not indicated for acute cervical spine injury, unless the cause of a neurologic deficit is not evident on standard x-ray studies or the level of the neurologic deficit does not correlate with the levels of the spinal column fracture. Occasionally, an air myelogram with tomography is useful if a partial cord lesion does not recover as anticipated or a displaced disc or bone fragment is suspected to be causing anterior cord syndrome.

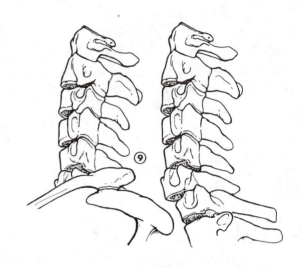

Cervical Spine X-Ray in Children

X-ray evaluation of the injured child's cervical spine may be difficult because of the child's lack of cooperation as well as:

1. Numerous epiphyseal centers that usually fuse after six to eight years of age.

2. Normal wedge-shaped vertebral bodies that square off only after seven years.

3. Pseudosubluxation permitted by the horizontal angle of the child's facets.

Note: Frequently, the best approach when in doubt is to protect the injured child's neck with a cervical support and repeat x-rays in one or two days when the child is sedated or is more willing to cooperate.

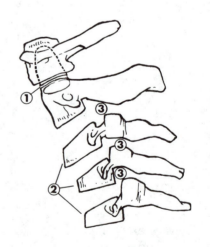

Radiographic Signs of Instability

In addition to obvious facet fracture comminution and disruption of both anterior and posterior support structures, suspect an unstable spine if there is

1. Greater than 3.5 mm horizontal shift of one vertebra on the other, evident on either a resting view or a flexion-extension lateral view.

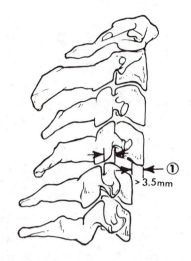

2. Greater than 11-degree fanning between two adjacent vertebral segments on lateral view, compared with segments above or below.

Note: Fanning is measured by horizontal lines from two discrete points on the vertebral body. The angle of intersection is compared with similar angles above and below the involved segment.

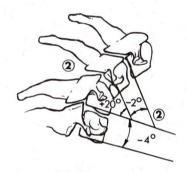

Other Immediate Considerations

1. Take necessary measures to prevent respiratory embarrassment. Administer oxygen, because in the early phase of spinal cord injury, particularly in spinal shock, the patient's vital capacity is severely reduced.

If necessary, perform a tracheostomy.

Observe the patient closely, preferably in an intensive care unit, until all vital signs are stable and normal respiratory exchange is established.

2. Meticulous skin care must be maintained in order to prevent pressure sores. Patient with complete paralysis should be turned every hour.

3. Insert an inlying Foley catheter to prevent bladder distension.

4. Ileus is a common complication of spinal cord injury. Give only intravenous fluid for the first few days until there is evidence of audible peristalsis, indicating return of normal bowel function.

5. Do not mistake hypotension from spinal shock for hypovolemic shock. Overhydration of the patient with spinal cord injury frequently precipitates pulmonary edema.

Skull Traction

REMARKS

Skull traction should be employed for most cervical spine fractures and dislocations with or without neurologic deficit.

Simple flexion fractures of the vertebral body may require only brace immobilization.

Injuries to the occiput–C1–C2 region (e.g., odontoid fractures) and extension fractures of the spine are treated using halo immobilization without traction.

For cervical spine injuries in the elderly, arteriosclerotic patient, the patient with central cord lesion, or the patient with ankylosing spondylitis, traction should be avoided, since postural reduction with halo immobilization is safer and more effective.

TECHNIQUE OF APPLYING SPRING-LOADED (GARDNER-WELLS) TRACTION*

This is the easiest skull traction to apply in the emergency room and may be used for temporary immobilization prior to halo application or during operative treatment of fracture.

The points of the device are tilted in the direction of pull, and one point is spring-loaded in order to indicate when force is applied sufficient to penetrate just the outer skull table.

The instrument is designed for emergency bedside application under antiseptic rather than aseptic conditions, and sterilization of the needle-sharp points in antiseptic solution is sufficient.

After sterilizing the patient's scalp with aerosol spray, inject local anesthesia into the points of application in line with the mastoid process.

---

*Gardner-Wells tongs are available from Codman Corporation, Randolph, Massachusetts, 02368

1. Tapered points are inserted 3 cm above the ear and in line with the mastoid.

2. When the spring-loaded pin barely protrudes beyond its flat surface, it is fully compressed, ensuring that only the outer table is penetrated.

3. Metal plate with instruction is fastened to the assembly.

Note: Pins may need to be retightened within 24 hours. The tongs may be exchanged for a halo ring if so desired at a later time.

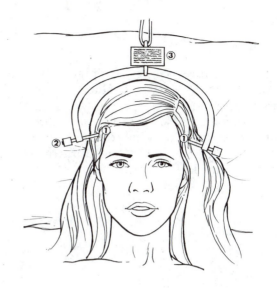

TECHNIQUE OF APPLYING HALO TRACTION

REMARKS

The halo ring is an ideal method of applying traction to acute spine injuries, since it allows reduction of the fracture or dislocation and permits subsequent immobilization by either operative or nonoperative means.

The operator should check that all necessary materials for application are immediately available including: 4 positioning pins, 2 torque wrenches, 4 skull pins, 1 extra skull pin, 5 various-sized halo rings.

1. While the patient's head is supported by the hands of an assistant or by a small wooden board, 10 cm wide, his hair is trimmed (not shaved), and the 4 pin sites are prepared with antiseptic spray.

2. Pin sites are 1 cm above the lateral third of the eyebrows and 1 cm above the ears in the mastoid region.

3. A sterilized halo ring is chosen that will allow 1.5-cm clearance around the skull. The number 2 halo fits most heads.

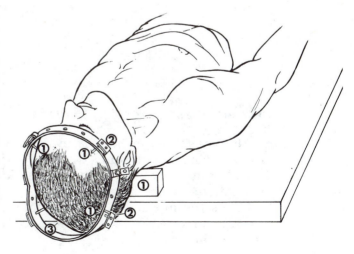

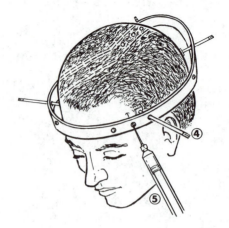

4. Positioning rings are placed in holes adjacent to those selected for the skull pins.

5. Inject local anesthetic into the entry site for the pins through the center of the 3-hole set, and infiltrate down to the skull. *Wait 3 minutes.*

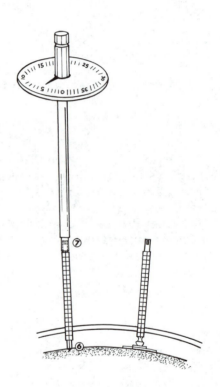

6. Without making a skin incision, screw the skull pins through the halo into the scalp and then into the outer table.

7. Exert equal pressure on all 4 pins by alternately tightening the diagonally opposite pins up to 6 lbs (2.7 kg) as measured by the torque wrenches. In children tighten only 4 lbs (1.7 kg).

Note: Lock the nuts over the pins to secure position.

Management After Application

Alignment of the halo is evaluated and the pins are treated with local antibiotic ointment.

Obtain a tangential x-ray of the skull to insure that the pins have not penetrated the inner table.

Check the torque on the pins daily for the first few days, but avoid excessive tightening. If the pins become loose or drainage is excessive, change the pin sites.

1. Traction may be applied to the ring for reduction, but if the patient develops nystagmus or unequal extraocular motion, excessive distraction is occurring.

If reduction of the fracture or dislocation is stable, attach the halo to a vest or cast and allow the patient to be mobilized.

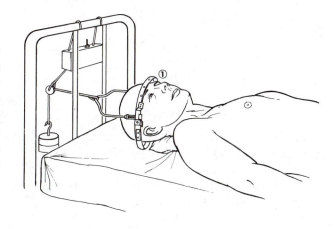

Technique of Applying Halo Vest

1. With halo traction applied, the back section of the vest is slid under the patient and is positioned to fit snugly on his shoulders.
2. The anterior portion of the vest is secured by sheepskin-lined straps.

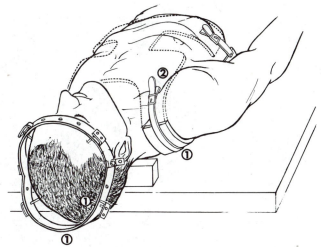

3. The metal framework is attached to shoulder bars, to the anterior vest, and to the halo ring.
4. With the patient sitting, the unit is tightened with the head and neck in the desired position.

Note: If a halo vest is not available, a halo cast may be applied. For patients with impaired protective sensation or susceptibility to pressure sores, a halo-pelvic hoop may be used.

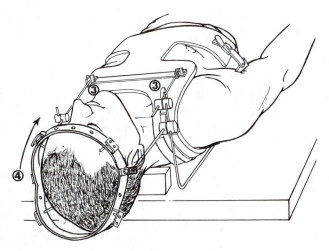

Technique of Applying
Halo-Pelvic Hoop for Cervical
Injuries with Sensory
Impairment (After Dewald and
Ray)

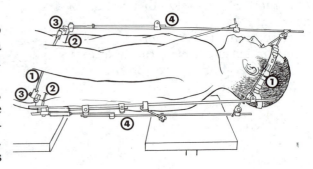

1. With neck controlled by halo traction, the patient is placed on a fracture table and the hoop is passed over his lower limbs and pelvis.

2. Threaded iliac rods are drilled, entering lateral and inferior to the anterior superior iliac spines and exiting by the posterior iliac spines. Rods should be level with the pelvis and parallel to the floor when the patient stands.

3. Hoop is attached to rod.

4. Halo and pelvic hoop are secured by four turnbuckles.

MANAGEMENT OF SUBLUXATIONS, DISLOCATIONS, AND FRACTURE-DISLOCATIONS

REMARKS

Management of cervical spine injury varies depending on the location and degree of spinal column instability, the presence or absence of neurologic deficit, and whether or not the deficit is complete.

The age of the patient and the presence of underlying conditions such as ankylosing spondylitis, osteoarthritis, and cerebrovascular insufficiency also modify the treatment.

For the first few days after injury, neurologic examination, which must be complete, detailed, and recorded, should be performed frequently.

Total neurologic deficit is not improved by laminectomy. Stability of the spinal column can usually be achieved using a halo vest or halo-pelvic rings (see page 301). If closed reduction and stabilization prove inadequate, open reduction and internal fixation are indicated to allow prompt rehabilitation.

The persistence of any sensory or motor function, such as perianal sensation or active toe flexion, indicates the lesion is incomplete with significant chance for recovery.

The most common incomplete injury, the central cord lesion (see page 275), is characterized by greater involvement of the upper limbs due to hemorrhage and edema in the central area of the cord. These lesions, which result from hyperextension of the osteoarthritic cervical spine, are not benefited by laminectomy because spontaneous recovery is frequent.

The anterior cord syndrome, which is characterized by motor paralysis associated with partial sensory preservation, results from compression-flexion injuries producing teardrop fracture and shattering of the vertebral body (see page 271). Anterior decompression and fusion may be indicated to relieve cord and spinal artery compression from the shattered fracture. Posterior stability should be present before anterior decompression and fusion are performed.

The Brown-Séquard syndrome results from a unilateral injury, usually a gunshot wound, causing ipsilateral motor loss and contralateral hypesthesia. Operative treatment is necessary to debride the open fracture, but neurologic recovery tends to occur in varying degrees unrelated to surgical treatment.

Spinal column injuries without neurologic deficit heal with stability if the bony fracture is reduced and supported by external means. If the injury has disrupted articular facets and is mainly ligamentous, as demonstrated by persistent widening of spinous processes, open reduction and posterior wiring with fusion are frequently necessary to restore stability.

Halo traction in extension is the usual method for reducing most cervical spine fractures and dislocations. The traction should be applied in 10-lb (5-kg) increments, and x-rays should be taken frequently to insure against overdistraction.

For some injuries, particularly to the rings of C1, C2, and the odontoid, traction in extension may be detrimental. Cervical traction in the elderly patient with cerebrovascular disease or cervical osteoarthritis or in any patient with ankylosing spondylitis is hazardous and should be minimized or avoided.

Management of cervical spine injuries is never routine and always demands an informed understanding of the varying types of injuries to the spinal structures and a mature appreciation of the risks and benefits of nonoperative and operative treatments.

GOALS OF MANAGEMENT

The objectives of treatment are to:

1. Protect the spinal cord from further damage.
2. Reduce fractures, dislocations, and fracture-dislocations completely to insure decompression of neural structures.
3. Stabilize the reduction by external or internal support, including fusion where indicated.
4. Begin the patient's rehabilitation promptly by anticipating the complications that follow spinal cord injuries and maximizing the use of the uninjured neuromuscular structures.

INDICATIONS FOR IMMEDIATE SURGICAL INTERFERENCE

Keep in mind that spinal shock after cord injury makes the patient extremely sensitive to anesthetic agents such as succinylcholine and very liable to cardiac arrest. Also, quite frequently the hypotension of spinal shock may have been treated with excessive fluid, overloading the circulatory system and causing pulmonary edema.

The occasional indications for immediate surgical treatment include:

1. Penetrating injuries from gunshot wounds or stab wounds requiring debridement and cleansing of the wound.

2. Injuries associated with conditions such as ankylosing spondylitis in which epidural bleeding worsens the neurologic deficit.

3. The rare incomplete injury that worsens despite or because of traction treatment.

4. Obvious evidence of displacement of bone fragments into the canal that are likely to produce cord or nerve root compression.

Note: Myelography and spinal fluid monometrics (Queckenstedt's test) are misleading indicators of the need for acute surgical interference, since edema from the injury is usually sufficient to block flow temporarily.

INDICATIONS FOR DELAYED SURGICAL INTERFERENCE

The majority of cervical spine fractures and fracture-dislocations can be readily reduced and adequately stabilized by halo brace techniques allowing prompt mobilization of the patient.

The rare occipito-atlantal dislocation and the more frequent atlanto-axial dislocation from trauma, with or without underlying congenital odontoid deficiencies or ligamentous destruction from rheumatoid arthritis, require internal fixation and fusion to insure stability.

The odontoid fracture that displaces and fails to heal sufficiently for flexion-extension stability following adequate closed treatment requires C1–C2 fusion to prevent myelopathy.

Dislocations of the spine with significant ligamentous disruption, as indicated by persistently wide separation of spinous processes or facet fractures and disruption, are likely to be unstable and to require operative reduction, internal fixation, and posterior fusion.

Unilateral facet dislocations sometimes lock and require open reduction and fusion to prevent pain and impingement on the nerve root.

Anterior decompression and fusion are applicable to flexion-compression (teardrop) fractures of the vertebral body, which produce anterior cord syndrome.

Surgical fusion may also be needed for the patient with progressive instability following laminectomy. This is especially likely to follow laminectomy in children and young adults.

Except for these instances, closed treatment has the most favorable risk-benefit ratio for the majority of cervical spine injuries.

OCCIPITO–ATLANTAL DISLOCATIONS

REMARKS

Survival of a patient with this injury is rare, since the medulla oblongata or the spinomedullary junction is usually severed.

Spontaneous, nontraumatic occipito-atlantal dislocation may occur secondary to inflammatory diseases such as rheumatoid arthritis, and severe instability can cause sudden death.

The patient who survives the acute injury may have brainstem and cord involvement with cranial nerve palsy and respiratory distress requiring respiratory assistance.

The lateral x-ray should be scrutinized carefully to identify the relation of the odontoid, atlas, and the base of the skull, because superficial review may fail to detect the injury.

Cranial displacement is accentuated by traction.

Use postural reduction with the halo apparatus for immobilization, and proceed with posterior craniocervical fusion when the patient's respiratory distress has subsided.

Preoperative X-Ray

1. Lateral cervical x-ray shows occipito-atlantal dislocation, which was associated with respiratory distress. The respiratory distress was relieved by tracheostomy, and the spine was stabilized by occipitocervical fusion.

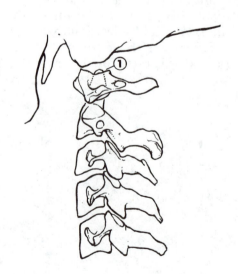

OCCIPITOCERVICAL FUSION (AFTER ROBINSON-SOUTHWICK)

Positioning Technique

Note: Endotracheal anesthesia is performed with the patient face up while the surgeons and team maintain the head, neck, and trunk positions.

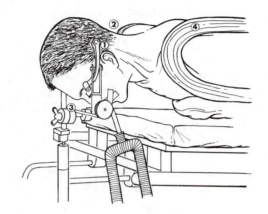

1. A Gardner pin vise head holder* is attached to the patient's head and the patient is carefully turned over onto the operating table. The position of the vertebra and occiput are then determined using lateral x-rays.

2. The head is in neutral position.

3. The head-holding device is attached to its base and is positioned so as to align the occiput to C1.

4. Adhesive straps are taped to the end of the operating table to depress the patient's shoulder, and the iliac crest is prepared for bone graft.

Operative Technique

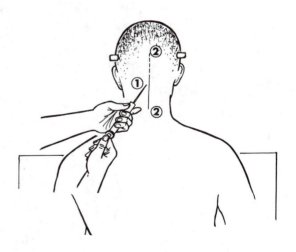

1. The incision site is infiltrated with epinephrine (1:100,000) and the incision is carefully centered over the ligamenta nuchae in the midline to minimize bleeding.

2. The incision runs from the external occipital protuberances to mid-cervical region.

---

*Obtainable from Codman & Shurtleff, Inc., Randolph, Mass. 02368

Operative Technique (Continued)

3. Three drill holes are made at least 1 cm from the foramen magnum and are large enough to allow

4. Separation of dura from the inner table of the skull with nerve hook.

5. The vertebral artery is deep to the atlanto-occipital membrane and must be avoided.

6. 20-gauge wires are passed through the occipital drill holes and under the ring of C1 as well as through holes drilled in the laminae of C2 and C3.

7. Two iliac grafts are drilled and fixed to the occiput and cervical vertebrae.

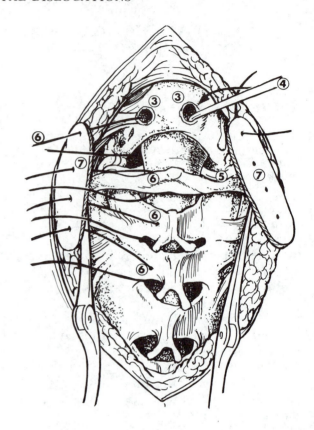

Postoperative X-Ray

Fusion extends from occiput to at least C3.

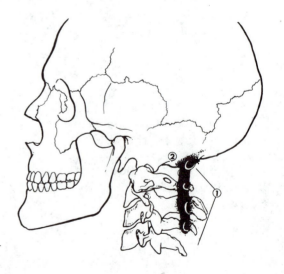

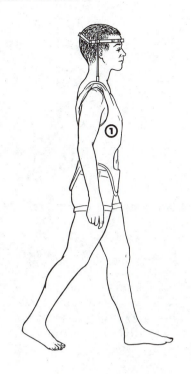

Postoperative Management

1. Halo cast immobilization is continued for twelve weeks until healing is evident radiographically.

2. Following removal of the halo cast, a Philadelphia collar is used for four months until flexion x-rays show stable occipitocervical fusion.

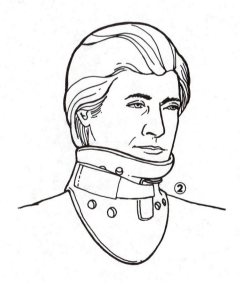

FRACTURE OF THE ATLAS (BURSTING OR JEFFERSON'S FRACTURE)

REMARKS

This lesion is the result of a force directed vertically downward through the skull while the spine is straight (see page 271).

The lateral masses of the atlas are forced outward.

Generally no neurologic deficit results, because the spinal canal is widened.

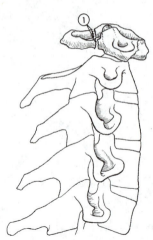

Prereduction X-Ray

1. Fracture through posterior neural arch.

Note: Fracture may not be as evident on lateral x-ray as it is on anteroposterior tomograms of C1, which show widening of lateral masses.

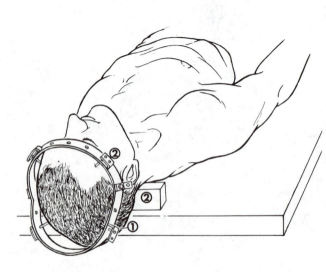

Immediate Management

1. Apply halo ring.
2. A support under the neck during application of halo cast or vest permits postural reduction.

Note: Traction is usually unnecessary to achieve fracture reduction.

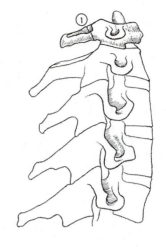

Postreduction X-Ray

1. Neural arches are reduced by the extension position.

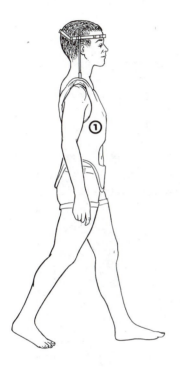

Postreduction Management

1. Halo cast or vest is used to maintain the head in neutral position for eight weeks.

2. This is followed by use of Philadelphia collar or similar orthosis for approximately six weeks.

Note: Be sure there is no injury to other regions such as the odontoid, particularly if there are any neurologic signs or symptoms.

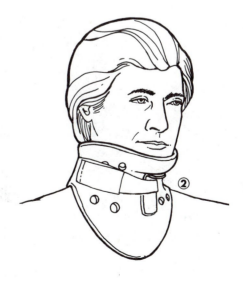

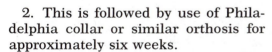

FRACTURE OF THE NEURAL ARCH OF C2 (HANGMAN'S FRACTURE)

REMARKS

This injury results from hyperextension forces compressing the posterior elements of the atlas (see page 277). The fracture may produce wide separation of the fragment and anterior displacement of the body of C2.

Any neurologic deficit, if present at all, is usually not severe because of the large capacity of the spinal canal at this level.

The body of C2 may or may not be displaced.

If a severe neurologic deficit is present, look for a fracture-dislocation at a lower cervical level. The following case is an example.

X-Ray

UPPER CERVICAL SPINE

1. Comminution of neural arches of C2.

2. Forward displacement of C2 on C3.

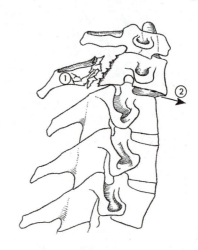

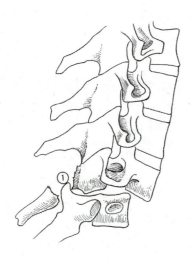

LOWER CERVICAL SPINE

1. Fracture-dislocation of C7 on T1.

Prereduction X-Ray of Common C2 Fracture

1. Marked comminution of the neural arch of C2.
2. Forward displacement of C2 on C3 (not marked).
3. Narrowing of the intervertebral disc.
4. Articular processes are in normal alignment.
5. Widening of interval between C1 and C2.

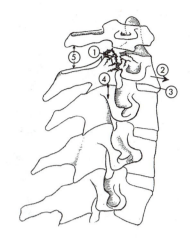

Immediate Management for Fracture of C2 Without Injury Elsewhere

1. Apply halo cast or vest.
2. Hold the neck in a straight position to achieve postural reduction. Avoid hyperextending the neck, since this was the initial mechanism of injury.

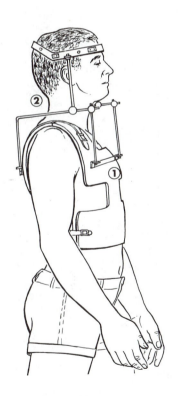

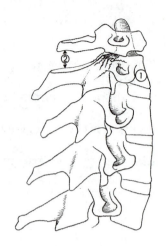

X-Ray After Application of Halo Cast or Vest

1. Anterior displacement of C2 is reduced.
2. Interval between C1 and C2 is normal.

Postreduction Management

Surgical stabilization of this comminuted fracture is usually unnecessary unless gross anterior displacement occurs.

Maintain halo immobilization for at least twelve weeks until stability is evident on flexion-extension x-rays.

Protect with a cervical orthosis for twelve weeks more.

314

UNILATERAL ATLANTO-AXIAL SUBLUXATION

REMARKS

This lesion may occur in adults as well as children after infections in the cervical region or after minor trauma that displaces the lateral mass of the atlas anteriorly over the articular facets of the axis (see page 286).

The lesion is not usually complicated by compression of neural elements unless there is anterior displacement as well as rotatory subluxation.

The usual wryneck or acute torticollis is short-lived and easily correctible with rest and immobilization. Occasionally, reduction may be obstructed by swollen capsular and synovial tissue so that rotatory subluxation becomes fixed.

Persistence or recurrence of the deformity for longer than three months sometimes requires skeletal traction and fusion of C1–C2 if torticollis is severe.

Possible diagnoses that should always be considered include cervical spine infection, congenital abnormality of the dens, syringomyelia, cerebellar tumors, and ocular problems.

Typical Deformity

1. Head is displaced forward.
2. "Cock robin" position. The patient may rotate head further to his left but rotation to right is extremely limited.

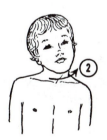
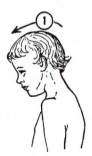

Prereduction X-Ray

OPEN MOUTH VIEW

1. Lateral mass of the atlas rotates forward and appears wider and closer to the dens.

2. Where the atlas has rotated backwards, the joint between the lateral mass of the atlas and the axis is obscured.

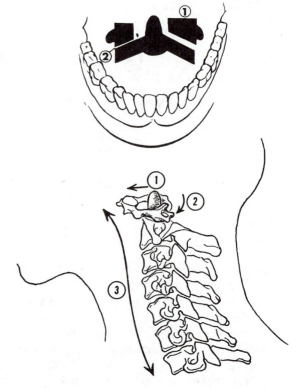

LATERAL VIEW

1. Occasionally there may be anterior displacement of the atlas.

2. Because of the tilt of the atlas, its spinous process is rotated toward the same side as the chin.

3. Normal anterior curve of the cervical spine is lost.

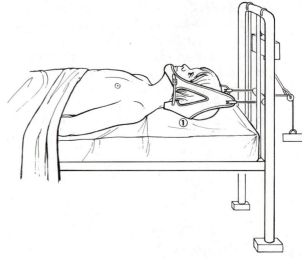

Treatment

1. Head halter traction for three days followed by cervical collar for three weeks relieves most of these problems.

If torticollis persists, manipulation may be of value.

REDUCTION BY MANUAL TRACTION

Reduction is performed with patient under thiopental sodium anesthesia.

1. Patient's head and neck extend beyond the end of the table.

2. Operator makes gentle steady traction backward in the line of the deformity of the head.

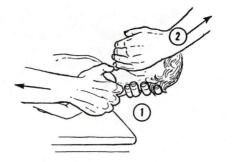

316

3. The chin is now rotated to the midline.

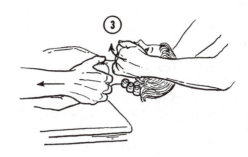

4. The neck is slowly hyperextended.

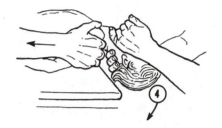

Postreduction X-Ray

OPEN MOUTH VIEW

1. The dens is centered between the lateral masses.

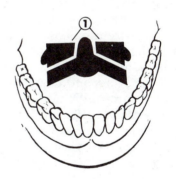

LATERAL VIEW

1. The atlas has returned to its normal position.

2. The normal cervical curve is restored.

The spinous process of the axis is in the midline and the chin is no longer tilted.

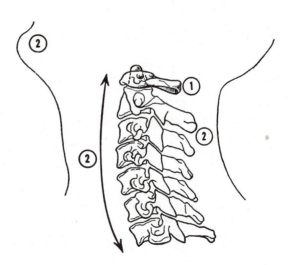

Cast

1. Extends from the forehead to the iliac crests.

2. Must fit snugly under the chin.

3. Mold the cast well under the chin and occiput, behind the neck, over the shoulder, and over the iliac crests.

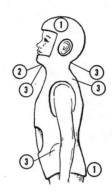

Postreduction Care

Plaster fixation is maintained for twelve weeks.
Recheck cast for:
    Excessive motion of the head.
    Recurrence of the deformity.
    Slipping of the chin inside the cast.
    Pressure areas over bony prominences.
For the first four weeks take x-rays at weekly intervals.
Check for:
    Loss of normal cervical curve.
    Forward migration of the atlas.
    Should a significant deformity recur or persist beyond three months, rotatory fixation may require skeletal traction and C1–C2 fusion.

Open mouth views with cervical rotation or cineroentgenograms should be taken to determine the presence of C1–C2 rotatory fixation.

Rotatory Fixation of Three Months' Duration

1. Open mouth view shows persistent asymmetric relation of the dens to the articular masses with the head rotated 15 degrees to the right or 15 degrees to the left.

Note: Symptomatic fixation of this type for more than three months should be treated by halo traction and fusion (see page 321).

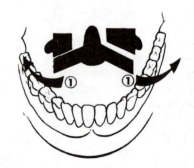

TRAUMATIC FORWARD DISLOCATION OF THE ATLAS

Without Fracture of the Odontoid Process

REMARKS

This lesion occurs most frequently when superimposed on chronic rheumatoid arthritis or congenital abnormalities that cause instability of the atlanto-axial articulations.

When acute injuries tear the transverse ligament (see page 283), the lesion may be very unstable, and death is common.

If patient survives the injury, he is likely to have acute respiratory distress, which must be corrected promptly, usually with tracheostomy.

Reduction is achieved by positioning in extension and is maintained by light halo traction (5 lb, 2.3 kg) until the patient's condition permits fusion of C1 to C2.

Dislocation of the atlas occurs in 20 to 25 per cent of patients with generalized rheumatoid arthritis, but only 5 to 10 per cent develop neurologic symptoms. Occasionally these patients also manifest vertical migration of the odontoid upward into the foramen magnum, which causes brainstem compression (see page 284).

The presence of brainstem symptoms such as dysphagia or cranial nerve palsies indicates the need for occipitocervical fusion with widening of the foramen magnum to relieve vertical compression.

Prereduction X-Ray

1. The atlas is displaced forward.
2. The position of the spinous process of the atlas indicates some rotatory displacement.

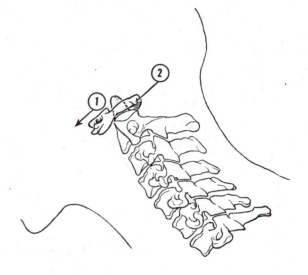

Reduction by Positioning and Halo Traction

1. Halo ring is applied and light traction is used to extend C1 or C2. Heavier traction is necessary only if there is vertical migration of the odontoid. Halo traction is continued until fusion (Brooks' technique) is performed.

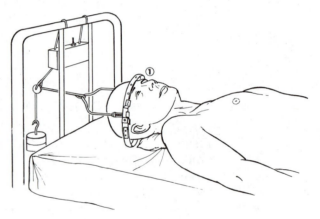

Postreduction X-Ray

1. Normal curve of the cervical spine is restored.
2. Atlas has receded to its normal position.

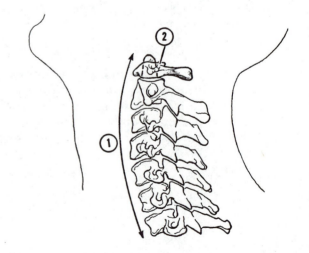

TECHNIQUE OF C1–C2 FUSION (AFTER BROOKS)

REMARKS

Usually C1–C2 fusion with wiring is sufficient to stabilize the dislocation.

If brainstem symptoms and cranial nerve palsies indicate upward migration of the dens, occipitocervical fusion with widening of the foramen magnum is necessary.

Positioning Technique

Note: Endotracheal anesthesia is performed with the patient face up while the surgeons and team maintain the head, neck, and trunk position.

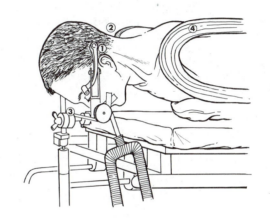

1. A Gardner pin vise head holder* is attached to the patient's head, and the patient is carefully turned over onto the operating table. The position of the vertebra is then determined using lateral x-ray.

2. The head is in neutral position.

3. The head-holding device is attached to its base and is positioned to reduce C1 on C2.

4. Adhesive straps are taped to the end of the operating table to depress the patient's shoulder.

Note: Prepare iliac crest for bone graft.

Operative Technique

1. Incision site is infiltrated with epinephrine solution (1:100,000), and incision is carefully centered over the ligamenta nuchae in the midline to minimize bleeding.

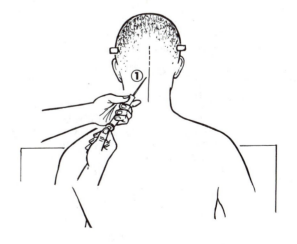

*Obtainable from Codman & Shurtleff, Inc., Randolph, Mass. 02368.

321

Operative Technique (Continued)

2. After C1 and C2 are carefully exposed, an aneurysm needle is used to pass a number 2 suture beneath the arch of the atlas and lamina of the axis.

3. The suture is then used to pull two double 18-gauge wire sutures beneath the arch of C1 and the lamina of C2.

4. Atlanto-axial membrane is left intact.

Note: If difficulty is encountered in passing the wire under the lamina of C2, the wire may instead be fixed around the spinous process of C2. The stability immediately achieved, however, is not as good.

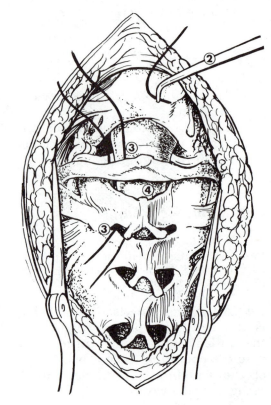

5. Four wires are teased laterally from the midline, with care taken to avoid injury to the vertebral artery.

6. Two cortical cancellous grafts are taken from the posterior iliac spine and fitted between lamina of axis and ring of atlas and notched slightly.

7. The four wires are twisted.

Note: The lateral position controls rotation as well as flexion-extension at C1–C2, but care should be taken to avoid the vertebral artery. Wires should not be allowed to angulate into the spinal canal.

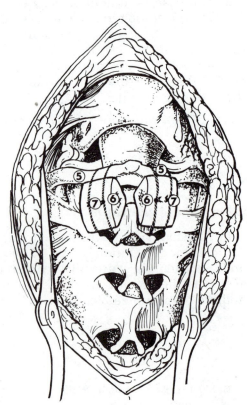

TRAUMATIC POSTERIOR DISLOCATION OF THE ATLAS WITHOUT FRACTURE OF THE ODONTOID PROCESS

REMARKS

This is an extremely rare lesion, or at least it is extremely rare for a patient to survive this lesion and so require treatment.

If ligaments and soft tissue attachments remain sufficiently intact to lock the atlas in its displaced position, survival without cord damge is possible.

Reduction is accomplished by traction and manipulation under anesthesia, and C1–C2 fusion is advisable.

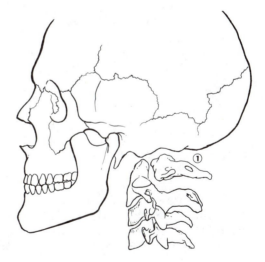

Preoperative X-Ray

1. The anterior arch of atlas is posterior to odontoid on lateral view.

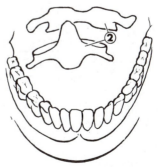

2. Anteroposterior view shows lateral shift of atlas.

Technique of Reduction (after Harralson and Boyd)

1. After tracheostomy, inhalation anesthesia is given. Respiration is carefully monitored so that if respiratory distress occurs, the operator is alerted to the possibility of neurologic damage.

2. Under fluoroscopic guidance, traction is applied to the halo apparatus in increments of 5 lb (2.3 kg) to pull the ring of the atlas back to the tip of the odontoid.

3. An assistant pulls caudally on the shoulder opposite to the atlas displacement.

4. The head is extended by manual traction on the chin, and the occiput and is gradually rotated to neutral. The dislocation should reduce with an audible "snap."

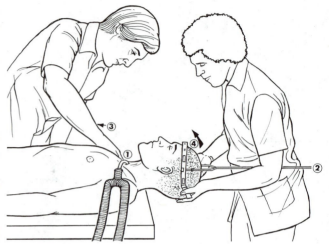

X-Ray During and After Reduction

5. With 20-lb (9-kg) traction, the ring of the atlas is nearly at the tip of the odontoid. Further traction causes no further change in position.

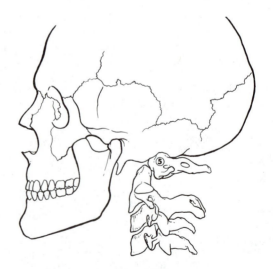

6. After manual reduction, normal relationship is restored.

Note: Following reduction the patient will experience difficulties in breathing and eating and will require continued tracheostomy and probably gastrostomy.

When the condition stabilizes, a C1–C2 fusion may be elected (see page 321).

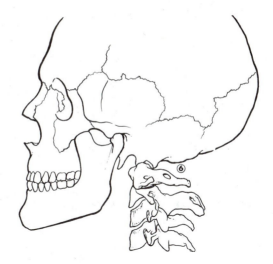

Postoperative X-Rays

A C1–C2 fusion has been performed.
1. Relationship of the atlas to the axis is corrected.
2. Bone graft is easily visualized to determine the status of the fusion.

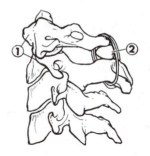

Postoperative Management

The patient need not be placed in a cast postoperatively, but the neck should be protected with a collar or brace until the patient is up and walking.

A Philadelphia collar is worn at all times as soon as the patient is ambulatory and is kept on until radiographic evidence of fusion is seen, usually 12 to 16 weeks after operation.

325

LESIONS OF THE ODONTOID PROCESS

CONGENITAL ABNORMALITIES

Three congenital lesions of the odontoid process may be encountered:

1. Complete absence of the odontoid process.

2. Partial absence of the odontoid process.

3. Nonfusion of the odontoid process (os odontoideum).

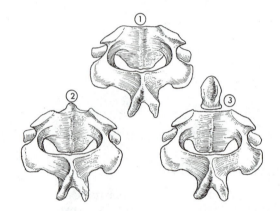

REMARKS

Generally, injury, even minor injury, initiates the symptoms. Occasionally, symptoms appear without trauma.

Quite often the patient will suffer "drop attacks," or transitory episodes of tetraparesis or hemiparesis, during which he suddenly flexes his neck. Typically these episodes are labeled "hysterical," since the neck region is usually pain-free.

These lesions are potentially lethal and require C1–C2 fusion when recognized.

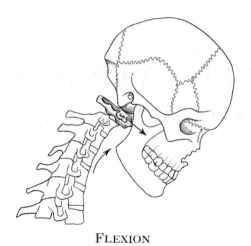

FLEXION

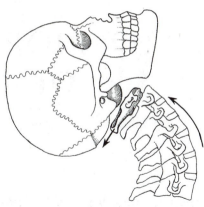

EXTENSION

MANAGEMENT

If the displacement occurs as the result of trauma, apply halo immobilization to position the head and neck in straight alignment. Traction is unnecessary, since it tends to distract C1 from C2.

When alignment is achieved, fuse C1–C2 using the Brooks technique (see page 321) and brace immobilization for postoperative care.

327

SUPERIOR SUBLUXATION
OF ODONTOID

In the rheumatoid patient, if neurologic symptoms persist despite adequate C1–C2 fusion or if there is any cranial nerve palsy, superior migration of the dens should be suspected.

1. The tip of the odontoid has slipped more than 5 mm above McGregor's line.

2. Erosion of the occipital–C1–C2 articulation allows upward migration.

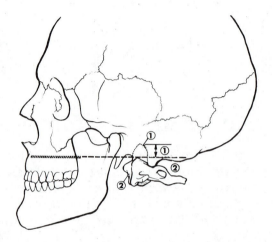

Surgical Management

1. Occipital–C1–C2–C3 fusion is performed, along with

2. Widening of the foramen magnum to decompress the brainstem.

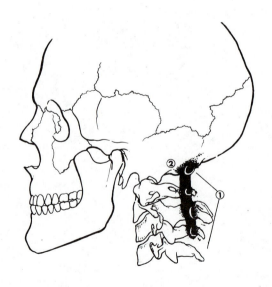

Fracture of the Odontoid Process
Without Displacement

REMARKS

These lesions may be easily missed and must be seriously considered in any patient with neck pain after injury.

No neurologic complications are associated with this lesion.

Healing occurs either with fibrous or bony union.

Surgical intervention is indicated only if there is evidence of displacement following conservative treatment.

Radiographic Findings
ANTEROPOSTERIOR VIEW

1. Fracture line is visible at the base of the odontoid in the anteroposterior (open mouth) view.

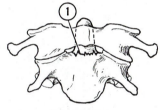

Anteroposterior

LATERAL VIEW

2. No displacement of the odontoid is noted.

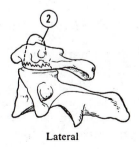

Lateral

Radiographic Findings
(*Continued*)

3. Since fracture line may not be evident on initial x-ray, always look for prevertebral soft tissue swelling of more than 5 mm in front of C3, which indicates hemorrhage from fracture.

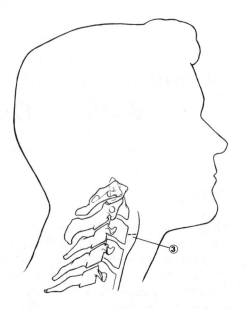

Management

A halo cast is preferable to a halo vest or Minerva jacket, since elimination of C1–C2 rotation is desirable to insure healing. Avoid traction, which distracts the fracture site.

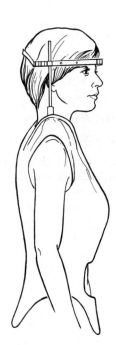

Postimmobilization Care

Maintain the patient in the halo cast for twelve weeks and evaluate the stability of the fracture by flexion and extension x-ray.

Change to a Philadelphia collar for two to three months and repeat the flexion-extension views before discarding the collar.

A fibrous union of the odontoid fracture does not require fusion provided the fracture is stable 5 months after injury.

Fracture of the Odontoid Process with Displacement (Atlanto-Odontoid Fracture-Dislocation)

REMARKS

Depending on the direction of the force, the odontoid process with the atlas may be displaced anteriorly or posteriorly. The former is more common.

Backward displacement of the odontoid is more likely to produce pressure on the cord.

Symptoms may vary from none or only minor neurologic deficits to tetraplegia and death. Odontoid fracture may produce a cruciate paralysis or involvement of motor fibers to the upper limb while sparing lower limb innervation. This is very similar to a central cord lesion.

These unstable lesions require prompt reduction usually by posture techniques and halo immobilization.

Healing by closed treatment is likely if the fracture is not distracted by traction treatment.

Fibrous union is fairly frequent, and if C1–C2 stability is not evident by 16 weeks, fusion is indicated.

Prereduction X-Ray

FORWARD DISPLACEMENT (MORE COMMON TYPE)

1. Atlas and odontoid process are displaced forward.

2. Atlas shows some rotatory displacement. This is the usual finding.

3. Spinous process of C2 is unusually prominent.

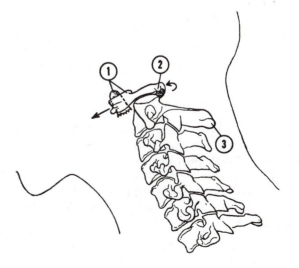

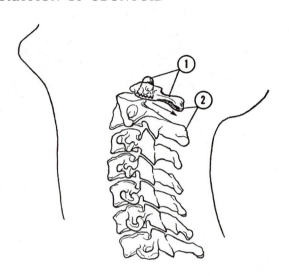

Prereduction X-Ray (Continued)

BACKWARD DISPLACEMENT (LESS COMMON)

1. Atlas and odontoid process are displaced backward.
2. Tips of spinous processes of C1 and C2 are almost in the same plane.

Immediate Management

FORWARD DISPLACEMENT

1. Apply a halo ring. Under fluoroscopic guidance, apply traction in a straight line, beginning with 10 lb (4.5 kg). When the displaced odontoid is pulled up superior to the level of the axis,
2. Extend the neck slightly by
3. Placing a pillow under the head and
4. Lowering the pulley.

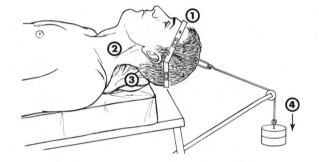

BACKWARD DISPLACEMENT

The treatment is similar: application of halo ring and traction beginning with 10 lb (4.5 kg).
1. Flex the neck slightly by
2. Raising the pulley and by
3. Increasing the height of the head pillow.

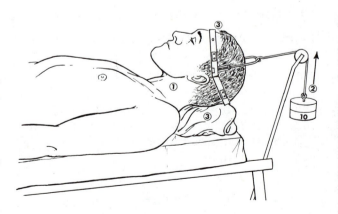

Postreduction X-Ray

1. Displacement of the odontoid process and atlas is corrected.
2. Rotatory displacement of the atlas is corrected.
3. Spinous process of C2 is in normal relation to that of the vertebra above and below.

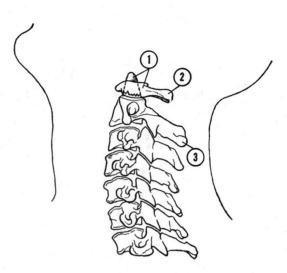

Postreduction Care

A halo cast gives slightly better rotatory immobilization, but a halo vest is better tolerated by elderly patients with this lesion who must be mobilized early and must not remain recumbent.

Evaluate the position of the odontoid fracture radiographically after the patient is ambulatory and avoid distracting the fracture line.

Maintain the halo support for four months and then evaluate stability on flexion-extension x-rays taken without the halo cast or vest.

If odontoid instability is evident, perform a C1–C2 posterior fusion (see page 321).

If the injury is stable protect against reinjury for two to three months longer by means of a Philadelphia collar.

UNILATERAL AND BILATERAL DISLOCATION OF A CERVICAL VERTEBRA

REMARKS

UNILATERAL DISLOCATION

This lesion is produced by lateral and rotatory forces. A unilateral dislocation without fracture can occur only if the interspinous ligaments and joint capsule on the dislocated side rupture completely.

As a rule the cord is not involved, but approximately 30 per cent of these injuries involve the nerve root and produce pain or nerve root paralysis.

Lateral x-rays of these injuries characteristically show anterior displacement of 25 per cent of the width of the vertebral body. Reduction should restore the posterior surfaces of the vertebral bodies to congruent alignment.

Attempted reduction of a unilateral dislocation by straight skeletal traction is fruitless because of the integrity of the disc and capsule on the undislocated side.

Reduction is facilitated by skeletal traction along with slight lateral flexion away from the side of the dislocation and then gentle rotation toward the side of the dislocation.

BILATERAL DISLOCATION

As uncomplicated lesions (without fracture) bilateral dislocation is indeed rare but does occur.

There is severe disruption of all posterior ligaments, including the posterior longitudinal ligament, the annulus, and the disc.

The vertebra may be displaced forward on the body below more than one half of its width. The lesion is very unstable.

These lesions reduce easily but also recur easily. Surgical stabilization is necessary.

In most instances the cord is severely damaged but occasionally the neurologic injury occurs from uncontrolled application of heavy traction.

Apply traction cautiously, following the effects closely by fluoroscopy.

TYPICAL DEFORMITIES:

In any suspected or diagnosed vertebral dislocation, check for:
Motor and sensory deficits along the nerve roots at the site of dislocation.

Evidence of cord compression.

Minor fractures: fractures of the spinous processes, chip fractures of the vertebral bodies.

Severe fractures: crushing of the inferior vertebral body, fractures of the articular processes, fracture of the pedicles.

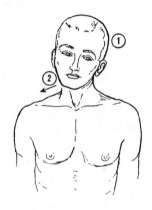

UNILATERAL DISLOCATION

1. Head is tilted toward the site of the lesion.
2. Chin is directed to the opposite shoulder.

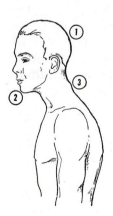

BILATERAL DISLOCATION

1. Head is displaced forward.
2. Chin is in the midline.
3. Prominence of the spinous process of the inferior vertebra at the level of the dislocation.

Note: This is an extremely unstable lesion. The patient who escapes paralysis is likely to be holding his neck with his hands.

335

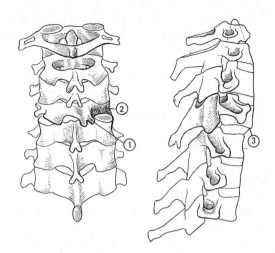

Prereduction X-Rays

UNILATERAL DISLOCATION
(BETWEEN C4 AND C5)

1. Spinous process of C4 is deviated from the midline.

2. Inferior facet of C4 is displaced in front of superior facet of C5.

3. Slight anterior displacement of C4 on C5.

BILATERAL DISLOCATION
(BETWEEN C4 AND C5)

1. Flattening of the anterior cervical curve.

2. Overriding of the articular processes.

3. Forward displacement of body of C4 on C5. (This may vary from half to total displacement of the body.)

4. Narrowing of the intervertebral disc. (The disc must be severely damaged. A chip of bone may be avulsed from the anterior margins of the vertebra above or below, indicating tearing of the anterior longitudinal ligament.)

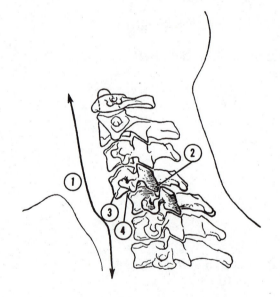

Attempted Closed Reduction by Longitudinal Traction

Note: Longitudinal traction is only effective if the facet has fractured or has been disrupted on the side opposite the injury. Usually closed reduction of a pure unilateral facet dislocation is possible only with cervical manipulation.

1. The patient is on a firm bed in a horizontal position.

2. The head of the bed is elevated on blocks.

3. Tongs or halo is applied as previously described (page 299).

4. Traction is directed upward and backward in line with the vertebra above the dislocation.

5. Begin with 15 lb (6.8 kg) of weight. Add 5 lb (2.3 kg) every 15 minutes, up to 35 lb (15.9 kg). Check constantly for any neurologic change. When traction has been at 20 lb (9 kg) for 30 minutes, check anatomy with radiography. If disengagement has not been effected, add 5 lb (2.3 kg) to traction every 15 minutes until 35 lb (15.9 kg) is reached. If disengagement is not complete, allow traction to remain at this weight for 12 to 24 hours, and take another radiograph to check anatomy.

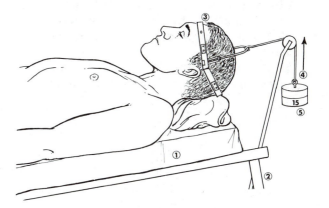

Appearance on X-Ray

Following application of 35 lb (15.9 kg) of traction, the facet remains locked because of the integrity of the opposite facet and disc.

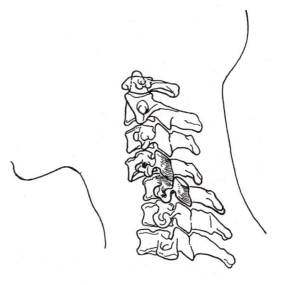

Technique of Manipulation

FOR UNILATERAL DISLOCATION

If the facets are not disengaged within 24 hours, give the patient general anesthetic with nasal intubation.

1. While longitudinal traction is acting,

2. Apply gentle lateral flexion away from the side of the lesion; then

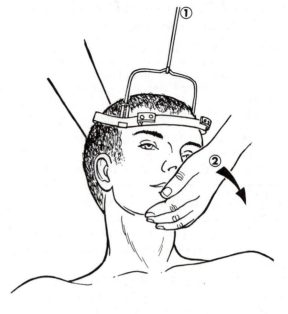

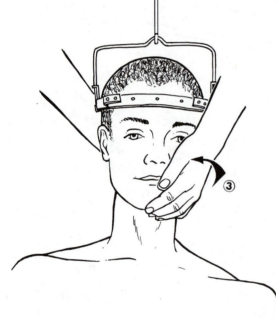

3. Rotate the head so the chin is in the midline and

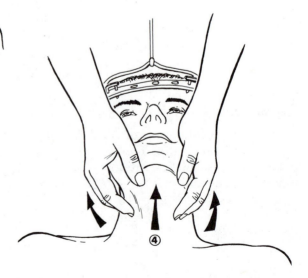

4. Hyperextend the neck.

POSTREDUCTION X-RAY

1. Normal anterior cervical curve is restored.

2. Posterior borders of the vertebral bodies are congruent.

3. The inferior articular processes are posterior to the superior processes of the lower vertebra.

Note: These maneuvers are usually successful in achieving reduction of unilateral facet dislocation. The cervical spine may then be immobilized in a halo device.

If they are unsuccessful, open reduction and posterior stabilization are necessary.

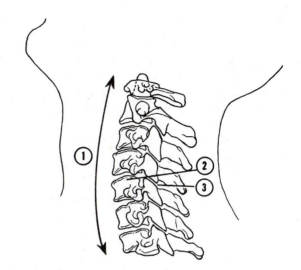

FOR BILATERAL DISLOCATIONS

Generally, reduction is readily achieved through minimal skeletal traction. Avoid overpulling these unstable injuries and producing or worsening neurologic deficit. Following reduction, stabilize the spine by posterior fusion. Surgery is performed as soon as the patient's general condition permits.

Open Reduction, Wiring, and Posterior Cervical Fusion

REMARKS

This method is applicable to:

1) Unreducible and unstable unilateral and bilateral facet dislocations and fracture-dislocations.

2) Injuries that have damaged the anterior vertebral body support structures and disrupted the posterior ligamentous structures and that have remained unstable after adequate closed treatment.

Laminectomy is not necessary with this method, except where it aids in facet reduction.

Wiring and posterior fusion may also be necessary for stabilization of a spine that has been made unstable by laminectomy.

Endotracheal anesthesia is performed with the patient face up while the surgeon and surgical team maintain head, neck, and trunk position.

Position of Patient

1. While the patient is supine, Gardner pin vise head holder* is attached. The patient is carefully turned over onto the operating table.

2. Head is kept in neutral position.

3. Head-holding device is attached to its base to maintain neutral position.

4. Adhesive straps are taped to the end of the operating table.

Note: The posterior iliac crest is prepared for bone graft.

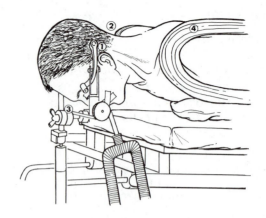

Operative Technique

1. Inject epinephrine solution (1:100,000) and then make a vertical midline incision through the skin and subcutaneous tissues.

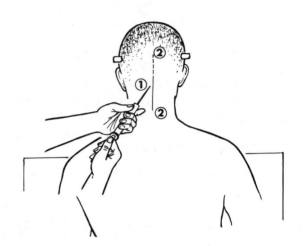

2. Incise the ligamentum nuchae in the line of the skin incision. Stay in midline and avoid cutting muscle fibers to reduce the amount of bleeding.

3. By sharp periosteal dissection expose the spinous processes and laminae of the involved vertebra and

4. Of one vertebra above and one below the involved vertebra.

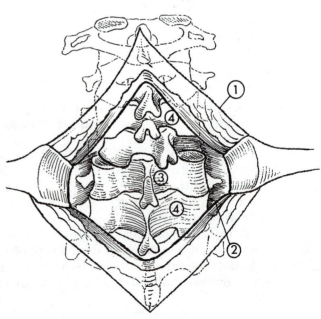

---

*Available from Codman & Shurtleff, Inc., Randolph, Mass. 02368

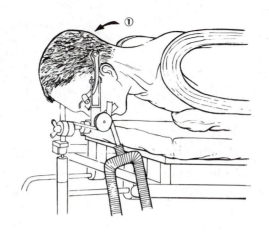

Surgical Management of a Dislocated Vertebra

STEP I

1. Lower the head holder until the head and neck are in a horizontal position.

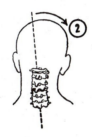

2. Tilt the neck toward the opposite side of the lesion.

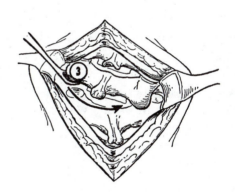

3. Hook a long stout curette under the dislocated articular processes and gently lever them into their normal position. Do not snap them back.

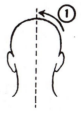

STEP II

1. Return head to the midline.

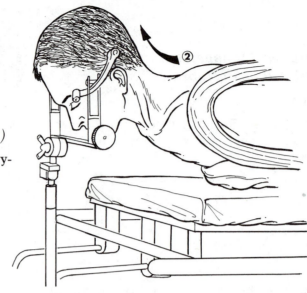

Surgical Management of a Dislocated Vertebra *(Continued)*

2. Raise the head holder to hyperextend the spine.

If the previous method of reduction fails,

1. Resect carefully the superior processes of the inferior vertebra with a rongeur.

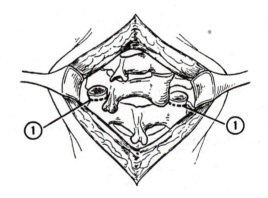

2. Bring head to the midline and hyperextend the neck by elevating the head holder.

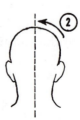

Wiring of Vertebrae

1. With a 2-mm drill make a drill hole on each side of the base of the spinous process of the vertebra above and below the dislocation.

Note: While making the drill holes, stabilize the spinous processes with a bone clamp. Direct the drill point at an angle of 45 degrees on each side of the spinous process so that the drill holes meet.

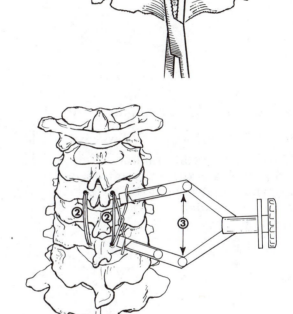

2. Pass a double 18-gauge wire through the drill holes in the spinous processes above and below the dislocation.

3. Tighten the wires snugly with a Kirschner wire bow to hold the facets reduced.

1. Take cortical and cancellous bone grafts from pelvis for fusion.

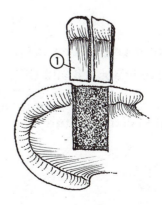

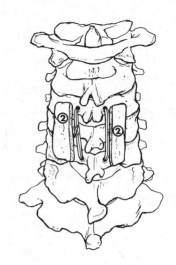

Wiring of Vertebrae (Continued)

2. Apply bone grafts to laminae and facets for fusion. For a unilateral dislocation a two-level fusion is adequate, but three-level fusion is necessary to stabilize bilateral dislocation.

Postoperative Management

UNSTABLE BILATERAL DISLOCATION

1. Maintain skull traction of 8 to 10 lb (3.6 to 4.5 kg) until soft tissues heal, which takes about three weeks.
2. Neck is slightly hyperextended in traction.

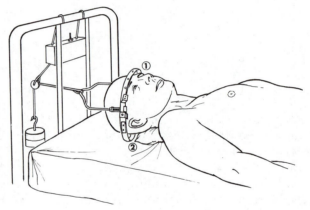

FOR STABLE UNILATERAL DISLOCATION

A Somi brace is applied and the patient is ambulatory. The neck is protected with the brace for four to six months, until fusion is mature.

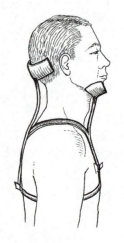

MANAGEMENT OF FLEXION INJURIES

Simple Compression Fractures

REMARKS

Compression of a vertebral body with disruption of the osseous elements may occur as the result of vertical loading with the neck in slight flexion.

Greater forces may produce marked disruption of the posterior osseous elements (see page 269).

Simple compression of a vertebral body is usually associated with injury to the intervertebral discs and articular plates. In these lesions the posterior ligamentous apparatus is intact, but if capsule ligaments tear, subluxation of the articular processes will occur.

Generally the posterior portion of the body is not compressed and there is no encroachment on the cord.

These may be unstable fractures if both the anterior and posterior elements of the spinal canal are injured.

Prereduction X-Ray

1. Normal cervical curve diminished or even reversed.

2. Compression of C5 (lesion is most common at C5–C6–C7).

3. Narrowing of the intervertebral disc.

4. Subluxation of articular processes.

Note: If the posterior ligaments rupture, there is wide separation of the spinous processes (in this case between C4 and C6).

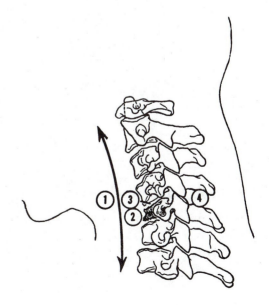

Immediate Management

1. Apply halo traction of 15 lb (6.8 kg).

2. Line of pull is straight.

Note: Add 5 lb (2.3 kg) of traction every 15 minutes, up to 35 lb (15.9 kg). Check constantly for any neurologic change. When traction has been at 20 lb (9 kg) for 30 minutes, check anatomy with radiography. If realignment is not effected, add 5 lb (2.3 kg) every 15 minutes until 35 lb (15.9 kg) is reached. If alignment is still not complete, allow traction to remain at this weight for 12 to 24 hours, and take another radiograph to check anatomy.

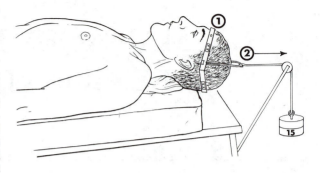

Postreduction X-Ray

1. Posterior processes are in alignment.

2. Height of vertebra is restored.

3. Height of disc space is restored.

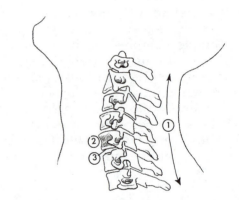

Postreduction Management

1. Lower pulley until neck is hyperextended.

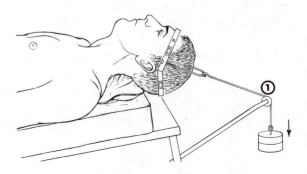

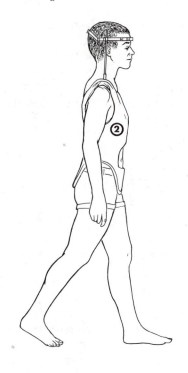

2. When patient's condition permits, apply halo cast with neck in neutral position.

Indications for Posterior Surgical Stabilization of Cervical Spine

Following closed reduction and halo traction, open reduction and wire fixation are necessary if there is

1. Greater than a 3.5-mm horizontal shift of one vertebra on the other, evident on either a resting view or a flexion-extension lateral view.

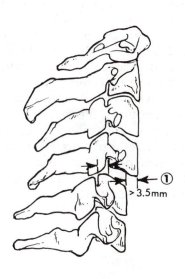

2. More than 11 degrees of fanning between two adjacent vertebral segments on the lateral view compared with the segments above and below.

Note: Fanning is measured by horizontal lines from two discrete points on the vertebral body. The angle of intersection is compared with similar angles above and below the involved segment.

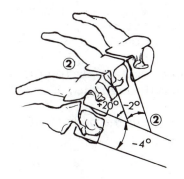

347

Postreduction Care

The patient is allowed to ambulate and may be discharged in the halo cast, which is worn for at least four months. The cervical spine is then protected with a Philadelphia collar for two months longer, until stability is evident on flexion and extension x-rays.

Fracture-Dislocations Produced by Hyperflexion Mechanism

REMARKS

Hyperflexion is the most common mechanism of fracture-dislocation in the cervical spine and is associated with neurologic complications, which can vary from transient paresis to complete tetraplegia and death (see page 292).

Associated features may be:
1. Crushing of one or more cervical bodies.
2. Fracture of the pedicles.
3. Fracture through the articular process.
4. Fracture of one or more spinous processes.
5. Fracture of the laminae.

Dislocation of the articular processes may be unilateral or bilateral.

Progressive paralysis may be the result of hemorrhage in the cord or of unrelieved pressure from displaced fragments or articular processes.

Perform neurologic examination at frequent intervals to determine evidence of increasing cord compression.

Lesions occur most commonly between C4 and C6.

Prereduction X-Ray

1. Flattening or reversal or distortion of anterior cervical curve.
2. Forward displacement of C4 on C5.
3. Associated fracture or fractures (here fracture is through the pedicle of C4).
4. Compression of the body of C5.

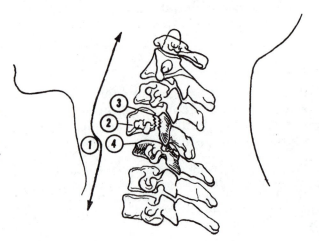

348

Reduction by Skeletal Traction

1. Patient is placed on a firm bed in the horizontal position.

2. The head of the bed is elevated on blocks.

3. Halo ring is applied for reduction by traction.

4. Traction is made in a straight line.

5. Pulley must be free to slide from side to side on the cross bar. Start with 15 lb (6.8 kg) of traction.

Note: Proceed cautiously and slowly until reduction is achieved. Add 5 lb (2.3 kg) every 15 minutes. Check constantly for signs of neurologic change. When traction has been at 20 lb (9 kg) for 30 minutes, check anatomy with radiography. If disengagement has not been effected, add 5 lb (2.3 kg) every 15 minutes until 35 lb (15.9 kg) is reached. If disengagement is not complete, allow traction to remain for 12 to 24 hours, and take another radiograph to check anatomy.

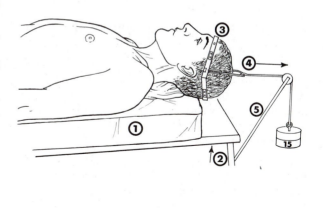

X-Rays During Reduction

WITH TRACTION AT 15 LB (6.8 KG)

If during the course of adding 5-lb (2.3-kg) weights the neurologic abnormalities become worse, remove the last 5 lb (2.3 kg) and prepare the patient for exploration of the cord (laminectomy).

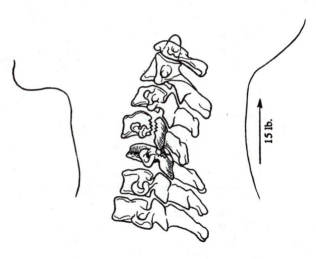

WITH TRACTION AT 20 LB (9.0 KG) AFTER 30 MINUTES

1. Beginning of disengagement of articular processes. Add 5 lb (2.3 kg), for a total of 25 lb (11.3 kg).

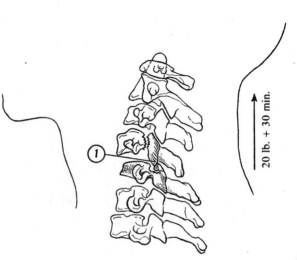

X-Rays During Reduction
(Continued)

WITH TRACTION AT 25 LB (11.3 KG)
AFTER 30 MINUTES

1. Articular processes show further disengagement, but it is not complete.

2. Fragments of the pedicle are coming closer together. Add 5 lb (2.3 kg) more, for a total of 30 lb (13.6 kg). Wait 15 minutes and add another 5 lb (2.3 kg).

Note: Take x-rays when traction has been at 35 lb (15.9 kg) for 30 minutes; if disengagement is not achieved, leave traction on for 12 to 24 hours, and take x-rays again.

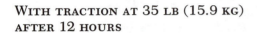

WITH TRACTION AT 35 LB (15.9 KG)
AFTER 12 HOURS

1. Articular processes are completely disengaged and overriding is corrected.

2. Distance between fragments of pedicles is markedly reduced. Spine is now ready to be hyperextended — slowly.

Note: If disengagement is not achieved within 24 to 48 hours after adequate traction, open reduction, posterior wiring, and fusion may be necessary (see page 342). However, operative intervention should be delayed until patient's general condition allows.

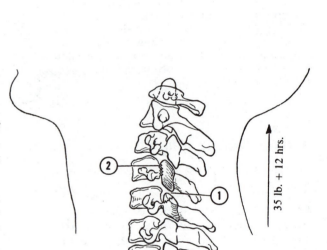

Hyperextension of the Spine

1. Lower pulley slowly until neck is hyperextended.

2. If x-rays show reduction, reduce weights to 10 lb (4.5 kg).

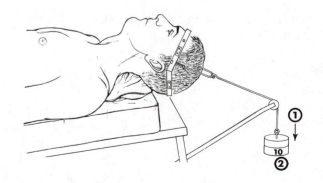

Postreduction X-Ray

1. Normal cervical curve is restored.

2. Forward displacement of C4 is corrected.

3. Fragments of the pedicles are approximated.

4. Height of the body of C5 is restored.

5. Joint surfaces of articular processes of C4 and C5 are now parallel.

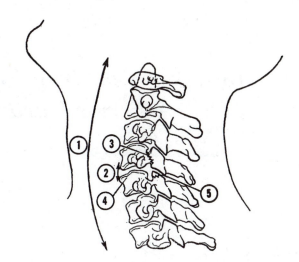

Postreduction Care

When the patient's condition permits, apply halo cast or halo pelvic cast if there is loss of protective sensation.

Continue halo immobilization for four months, and then protect neck with a brace for two months longer until stability is evident on flexion and extension x-rays.

Bursting Teardrop Fractures Causing Anterior Cord Syndrome

REMARKS

A bursting teardrop fracture is typically sustained from hyperflexion and compression. A posterior teardrop fracture is displaced into the spinal canal.

Anterior decompression and fusion may be necessary.

Note: The characteristic neurologic picture is that of anterior cord syndrome with motor paralysis but some preservation of sensation.

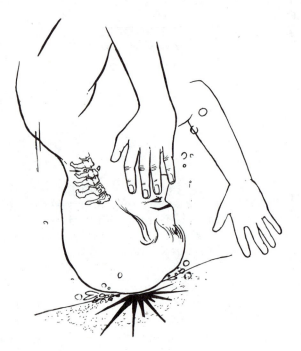

Immediate Management

1. Apply halo ring and traction.
2. Pull is in a straight line; start with 15 lbs (6.8 kg).

Note: Add 5 lb (2.3 kg) every 15 minutes. Check often for any change in the neurological pattern, if there is a neurologic pattern. When traction has been at 20 lb (9.0 kg) for 30 minutes, take an x-ray. If realignment of the bony elements has not been effected, add 5 lb (2.3 kg) every 15 minutes until 35 or 40 lb (15.8 or 18.0 kg) is reached. If reduction on x-ray taken at this time is not satisfactory, allow traction to remain for 12 to 24 hours, taking x-rays at 6-hour intervals.

If during the course of adding 5-lb (2.3-kg) weights the neurological deficits become worse, remove the last weight and evaluate the patient's condition in preparation for anterior decompression and fusion.

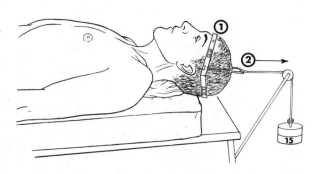

352

X-Rays During Reduction by Skeletal Traction

WITH TRACTION AT 15 LB (6.8 KG)

1. Fragmentation of body of C6.
2. Backward displacement of posterior fragment of C6. This teardrop fracture causes anterior cord compression.
3. Collapse of disc between C5 and C6.
4. Fracture of laminae of C6.

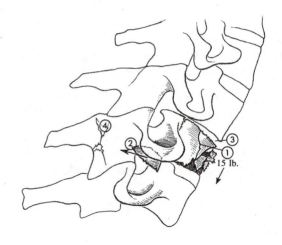

WITH TRACTION AT 20 LB (9.0 KG) AFTER 30 MINUTES

1. Beginning realignment of bone fragments. Add 5 lb (2.3 kg) to fracture.

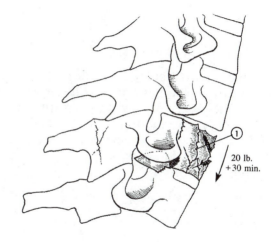

WITH TRACTION AT 25 LB (11.3 KG) AFTER 30 MINUTES

1. Further realignment of bone fragments out of the spinal canal.
2. Opening of disc space.

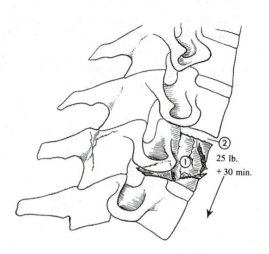

X-Rays During Reduction by
Skeletal Traction (Continued)

WITH TRACTION AT 35 LB (15.9 KG)
AFTER 12 HOURS

1. Realignment of anterior surface of spinal canal.
2. Some residual displacement of anterior fragments.
3. Restoration of disc space.

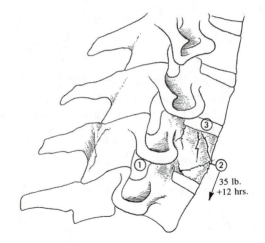

Postreduction Care

If a satisfactory reduction of the fragments is achieved with traction continue the patient in traction for a period of four to six weeks.

This is a very unstable injury and should be evaluated periodically for loss of reduction.

After four to six weeks a halo cast may be applied or a halo pelvic hoop used for the patient without protective sensation and rehabilitation started.

Indications for Surgical
Stabilization

1. The patient with persistent anterior cord syndrome and evidence of anterior compression from the teardrop fracture or disc material is a candidate for anterior decompression and fusion.
2. Before carrying out operative procedure, make sure posterior elements are not disrupted (see page 362).

Anterior Decompression and Cervical Spine Fusion for Anterior Cord Syndrome

REMARKS

This procedure is preferred when a teardrop fracture persistently compresses the cord or anterior spinal artery, producing anterior cord syndrome.

The objective is to decompress the anterior cord structures by removal of bone fragments and stabilize the anterior spine with a fibula strut.

The posterior ligamentous structures should be intact or an anterior operation will contribute to further instability.

ANESTHESIA

Use endotracheal anesthesia; in case of dislocations or fracture-dislocations of the cervical spine, the tube, if passed orally, must be passed without flexion or extension of the neck. If this is impossible, pass the tube through the nose.

Position of Patient

1. Skeletal traction of 10 to 15 lb (4.5 to 6.8 kg) is maintained throughout the procedure.

2. The cervical spine is in slight extension.

3. The head is rotated slightly to the right.

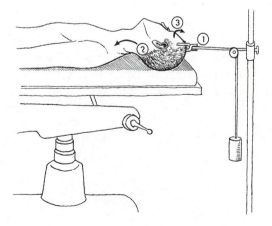

Incision

1. Locate the cricoid cartilage; this is opposite the sixth cervical vertebra.

2. Make an incision along the anterior border of the sternocleidomastoid muscle, 5 cm above and 5 cm below the affected level.

3. Cut the platysma in the same line as the skin incision.

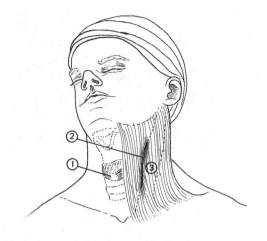

Exposure Down to the Pretracheal Fascia

1. Divide longitudinally the anterior layer of the cervical fascia along the anterior border of the sternocleidomastoid muscle.

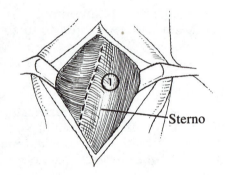

Sterno

2. By scissor dissection mobilize the anterior margin of the sternocleidomastoid muscle and gently retract it laterally.

3. Now the pulsating carotid sheath and the omohyoid muscle are visualized.

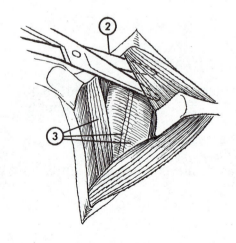

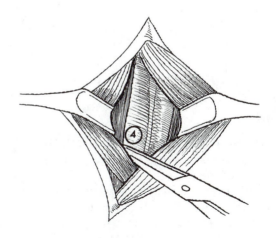

4. By blunt dissection develop the interval medial to the carotid sheath.

Exposure of the Anterior Aspect of the Vertebral Bodies

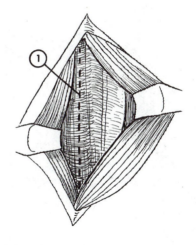

1. Make a small incision in the pretracheal fascia.

2. With the index finger develop the retropharyngeal space for the full length of the incision.

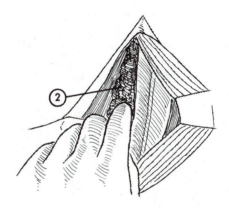

357

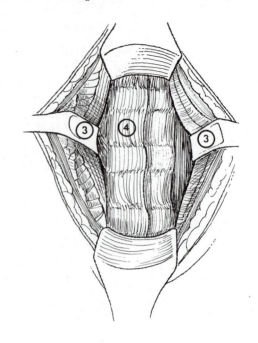

Exposure of the Anterior Aspect of the Vertebral Bodies (*Continued*)

3. Retract the thyroid gland, trachea, and esophagus medially and the carotid sheath laterally.

4. The prevertebral fascia is seen as a glistening sheath covering the vertebral bodies, longitudinal ligament, discs, and longus colli muscles.

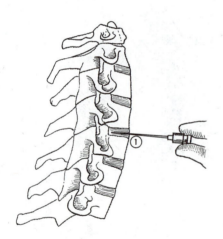

Orientation of Vertebra

1. Insert a fine straight needle in a disc space and take a lateral x-ray.

Note: The site of the lesion, such as in a dislocation, may be recognized at this stage of the procedure by characteristics of the disc, which may be mushy and bulging.

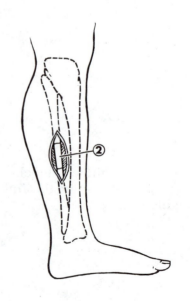

2. While x-ray film is being developed, take a full-thickness strut of bone from the mid third of the fibula.

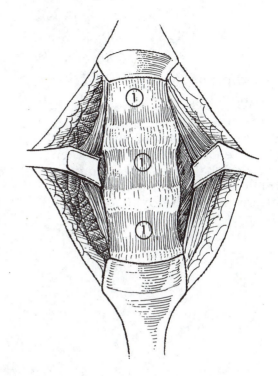

Preparation of the Graft Bed

1. Identify the area to be decompressed and the vertebrae to be fused.

2. Incise longitudinally and in the midline the prevertebral fascia, and with a sharp elevator reflect the fascia off the vertebral bodies.

3. Cut a trough in the anterior aspects of the vertebral bodies, 1 cm in width and 0.5 cm in depth.

Note: Use an air drill to cut the trough.

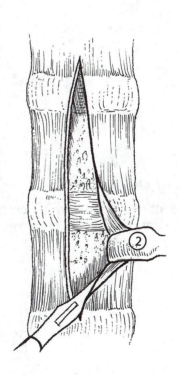

Preparation of the Graft Bed (*Continued*)

4. The trough in the end vertebrae spans three quarters of the vertical height of each vertebra and the entire vertical height of the comminuted fractured vertebra. A notch is cut superiorly and inferiorly to lock in the fibula strut.

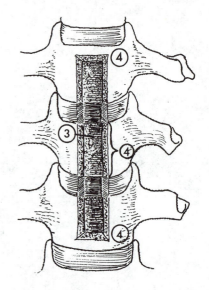

5. Remove the anterior portion of the comminuted body as well as the contiguous discs.

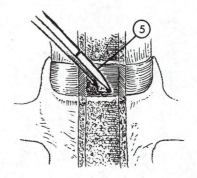

Placement of the Bone Graft

1. Fix the fibula strut into a notch cut into the superior and inferior vertebrae.

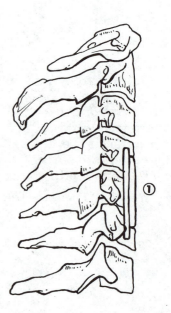

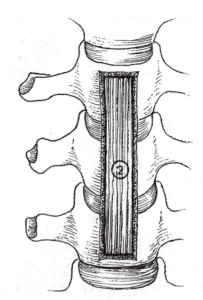

2. Cut the graft so that it fits snugly in the trough.

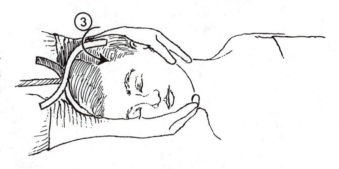

3. Now bring the neck to the neutral or slightly flexed position. This position firmly seats the graft in its bed.

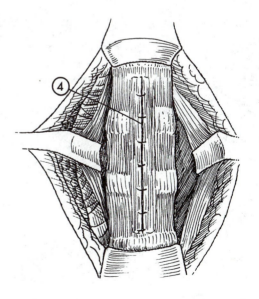

4. Approximate the edges of the prevertebral fascia over the graft.

361

Postoperative Care

Maintain skull traction until the patient has recovered from the operation. On the third to fifth postoperative day, apply a halo vest or halo-pelvic device to allow the patient to be mobilized and rehabilitation to be started.

CAUTION

Anterior decompression and fusion may increase the displacement if the posterior elements are disrupted.

Posterior instability is indicated by:

1. Greater than 3.5-mm horizontal shift of one vertebra on the other.

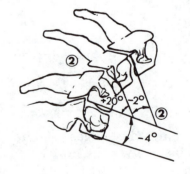

2. More than 11 degrees of fanning between two adjacent vertebral segments when compared with the segments above and below.

Note: Both anterior and posterior fusions may be necessary for anterior cord syndrome with posterior instability.

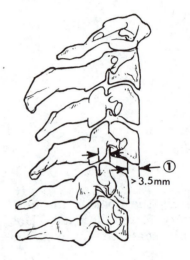

MANAGEMENT OF EXTENSION INJURIES

Backward Dislocation Without Disruption of Osseous Elements

REMARKS

This lesion is the result of a forceful hyperextension mechanism (see page 272).

The anterior longitudinal ligament is ruptured, occasionally causing avulsion of a chip of bone from the anterosuperior margin of the inferior vertebra.

The disc is detached from the articular plate.

The cord is pinched between the posterior aspect of the displaced vertebra and the lamina of the inferior vertebra.

Spontaneous relocation occurs.

The neurologic damage is usually severe, and the prognosis is poor.

There is no radiographic abnormality except occasionally for a chip of bone from the inferior vertebra if avulsion has occurred.

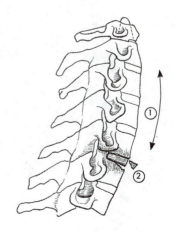

Appearance on X-Ray

1. Osseous elements are in normal alignment.
2. Chip of bone from anterior superior surface of lower vertebra (not always present).

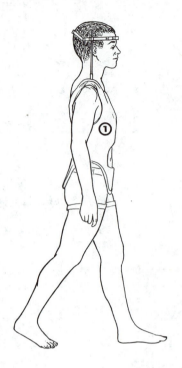

Immediate Management

1. Apply a halo cast immediately, but do not use traction, which would distract the vertebral bodies.

Allow the patient to begin ambulation or rehabilitation as needed.

Indications for Stabilization of the Spine

In paralyzed patient, if there is no evidence of the site of the cord injury on plain film, obtain a myelogram. If this shows signs that anterior cord syndrome is caused by a disc protrusion or fragment in the canal, anterior decompression and fusion should be performed (see page 355).

Hyperextension of the Cervical Spine With Osteoarthritis Causing Central Cord Syndrome

REMARKS

This lesion (see page 275) occurs in elderly victims.

The neck is forcefully hyperextended.

The cord is pinched between the posterior osteophytes and the ligamentum flavum.

The neurologic damage is usually severe, consistent with an acute central cord lesion.

The immediate prognosis is good, but usually some permanent neurologic deficit remains.

The only radiographic evidence of abnormality is the degenerative changes.

Avoid the use of skeletal traction, which is unnecessary and is poorly tolerated by the elderly patient.

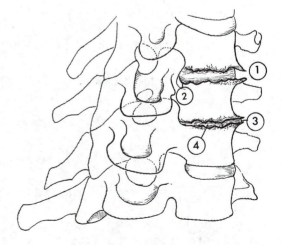

X-Ray

1. Normal alignment of osseous elements; no fracture.
2. Posterior osteophytes.
3. Anterior osteophytes.
4. Thin intervertebral discs.

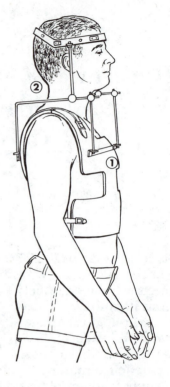

Immediate Management

1. Apply a halo vest.
2. Neck is in neutral position.

Note: If patient cannot tolerate a halo, use a Somi brace.

Postimmobilization Care

Mobilize these patients promptly and begin rehabilitation for any neurologic damage with the anticipation that some improvement is likely.

If injury is stable, external support may be discarded in approximately eight to ten weeks.

Cervical fusion is usually unnecessary and does not increase chance of neurologic recovery from central cord syndrome.

Fracture-Dislocation Produced by Hyperextension and Compression

REMARKS

These lesions are characterized by severe disruption of the posterior bony elements.

The anterior longitudinal ligament may rupture, avulsing a chip of bone from the anterior margins of the lower vertebra. The disc may be detached from the articular plates.

In some of these lesions the vertebral body may slip forward, simulating a hyperflexion lesion.

If a lateral flexion force is added, the bony elements may be involved on one side only (on the side opposite the side from which the force was delivered).

The neurologic deficit may vary from none to pain caused by root pressure to severe cord damage.

Be sure to establish the true mechanism of these lesions because traction in extension may reproduce or exaggerate a deformity or may cause further damage to neural elements.

Occasionally, special x-ray views of the vertebral pillars are necessary to define a fracture (see page 294).

Types of Hyperextension Compression Lesions— Appearance on X-Ray

BACKWARD DISPLACEMENT

1. Backward displacement of C3 on C4.
2. Fracture of laminae.
3. Fracture-dislocation of articular processes.
4. Fracture of base of spinous process of C4.

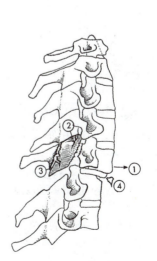

FORWARD DISPLACEMENT

1. Body of C5 is displaced forward on C6.
2. Fracture through the pedicles of C5.
3. Fracture of the articular processes of C5.

Note: The fractured processes have been displaced upward.

4. Chip off the anterior superior surface of C6 (indicating rupture of the anterior longitudinal ligament).

Note: If the compression force has a lateral flexion component, a unilateral lesion may result, with an asymmetrical neurologic deficit.

These lesions are frequently mistaken for flexion injuries.

Types of Hyperextension Compression Lesions — Appearance on X-Ray (*Continued*)

Avulsion

1. Triangular fragment off the anterior portion of C5 is a teardrop fracture from extension injury.

2. Body of C5 displaced slightly backward.

3. Thinning of disc (usually the disc and the articular plate are severely disrupted).

4. Fracture of base of spinous process of C5.

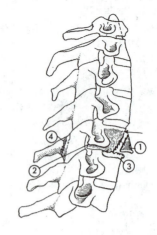

Immediate Management

1. Apply halo traction.

2. Pull must be in a straight line (no flexion, no extension); start with 5 lb (2.3 kg).

Note: Add 5 lb (2.3 kg) every 15 minutes. Take x-rays every 30 minutes. Generally, these fracture-dislocations are readily reduced. Do not overdistract the vertebra by using too much weight.

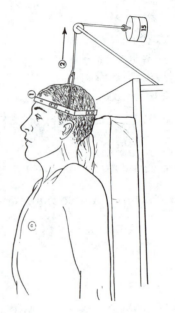

X-Ray During Reduction

With traction at 20 lb (9.0 kg) after 30 minutes

1. Posterior displacement of C5 is realigned with the body above and below.

2. Slight distraction of disc.

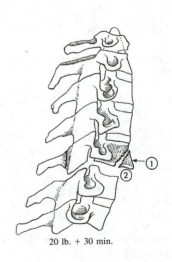

20 lb. + 30 min.

Postreduction X-Ray

1. Reduce weight to 10 lb (4.5 kg).
2. Normal alignment is retained.
3. Distraction is reduced.

If reduction is not achieved in a patient with no implication of the neural elements, reduce weight to 10 lb (2.3 kg) and perform open reduction and spine fusion in one to three weeks.

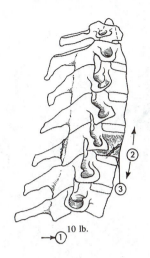

Postreduction Care

Most can be reduced and stabilized with a halo cast or a halo-pelvic hoop.

Apply the halo cast as soon as the patient's general condition allows.

Allow the patient to begin ambulation and rehabilitation promptly.

Continue with halo immobilization for six to twelve weeks, and then use a Somi brace for two months longer.

POSTERIOR FUSION FOR INSTABILITY FOLLOWING LAMINECTOMIES (ROBINSON AND SOUTHWICK)

REMARKS

Although indications should be relatively few, cervical laminectomy is still used to decompress the spinal cord and nerve roots following encroachment from such conditions as dislocation, tumor, and osteoarthritis.

Removing the spinous processes and lamina may not cause immediate instability, but progressive angulation and deformity are frequent. This results in increasing pain, weakness, and progressive neurologic deficit. The delayed progressive deformity is attributable to the viscoelastic stretching of ligaments produced by muscle forces and the weight of the head.

Fusion should be performed lateral to the area of laminectomy by denuding the articular processes, passing wires through drill holes in the inferior articular processes, and then binding two longitudinal struts of cortical cancellous bone to the posterior columns of the articular processes at each segment.

This type of fusion does not interfere with any decompression that has been accomplished, and it allows early mobilization of the patient with external support.

Preoperative X-Ray

1. Extensive laminectomies at C4–C6 produce
2. Swanlike deformity of the cervical spine,
3. Anterior displacement of the lower vertebrae and progressive neurologic symptoms, and
4. Thinning of the discs.

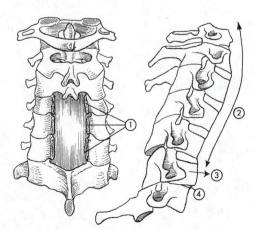

370

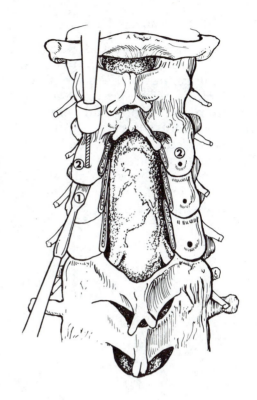

Wiring of Vertebrae

1. After the articular cartilage is removed from each joint surface with a small curette, the articular processes are pried open with a small angled elevator.

2. Drill holes are made in each inferior articular process, at a 90 degree angle to the plane of the surface.

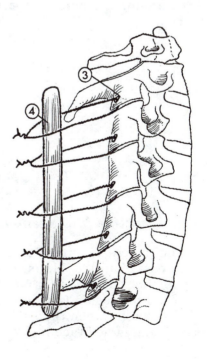

3. A wire of two strands of 24-gauge wire twisted together with a hand drill, is inserted into each hole and is advanced through the joint with a fine-angle clamp.

4. The wires are passed around cortical cancellous grafts taken from the posterior iliac crest.

371

Wiring of Vertebrae (Continued)

5. Bone grafts from the posterior iliac crest are concave in two surfaces, conforming to the normal cervical lordosis and preventing the graft from impinging on exposed dura and cord. Each graft strut should be at least 1.5 cm wide.

The grafts extend from the top of the laminae of the most proximal vertebra to the bottom of the lamina of the most distal vertebra.

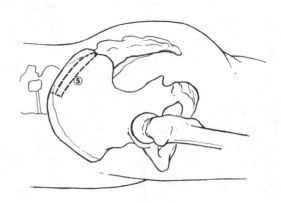

6. To secure graft to the spinous process at the bottom of the laminectomy a hole is drilled at the base of the spinous process at its junction with the lamina and 2 separate wires are twisted around the lateral aspects of each graft.

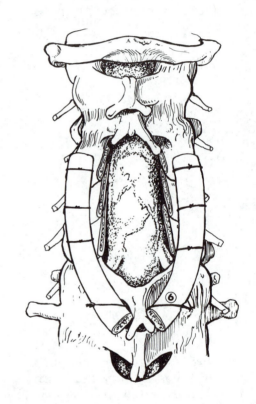

Postoperative Management

The patient is nursed on a bed for several days until pain and muscle spasm subside. He is then mobilized with a cervicothoracic brace protecting the fusion for 6 to 12 months.

When the fusion is seen radiographically to be maturing and there is no motion between the fused segments on flexion-extension views, the cervicothoracic brace may be discarded.

MANAGEMENT OF INJURIES OF THE CERVICAL DISCS AND SOFT TISSUES

REMARKS

The cervical disc structure is subject to a variety of injuries, the most common being the hyperextension-hyperflexion trauma of rear-end auto collisions.

A displaced disc may compress ligaments, nerve roots, dura, the anterior spinal artery, or the cord itself, resulting in symptoms ranging from a chronic headache and neckache to quadriplegia and sudden death.

Persistent disc bulging produces a traction effect on the posterior longitudinal ligament, resulting in periosteal overgrowth and osteophyte formation. Prompt treatment of the displaced disc fragment will relieve neck and scapular pain and will prevent persistent cervical disc syndrome and osteophyte formation.

The nerve roots commonly involved are C6 or C7, causing scapular pain or pain radiating down the back of the arm and outer forearm to the long, ring, and middle fingers.

Thorough history and physical examination are more reliable diagnotic tools than x-ray studies. The cervical spine motion should always be evaluated for any limitation of flexion, extension, lateral bending, or rotation. Although cervical disc protrusion frequently causes pain and limitation of neck movements without nerve root involvement, testing for abnormal nerve root function should always be performed.

Clinical Pattern from Dural Compression Without Nerve Root Compression

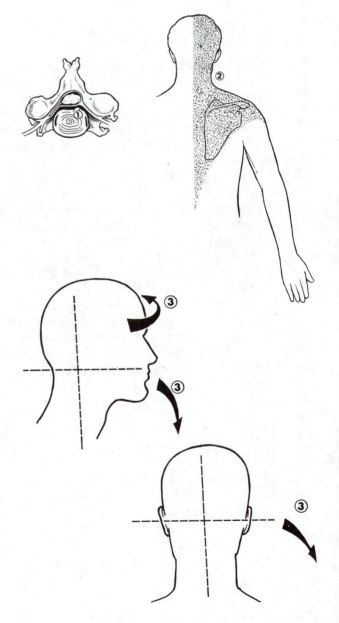

1. Disc impingement on the dura or dural sleeve produces

2. Pain radiating to neck, trapezius region, and occipital and intrascapular areas without radiation down the arm.

3. Flexion, extension, rotation, or lateral bending of the neck will worsen the pain as the sensitive dura is pulled over the protruded disc.

Note: This is the best time to begin effective treatment to reduce the disc before root symptoms make the diagnosis obvious.

Clinical Patterns of Specific Root Compression

Sixth Nerve Root (Between C5 and C6)

1. Distribution of pain — root of neck, trapezius muscle, vertebral borders of scapula, anterior aspect of chest wall, outer aspect of arm into thumb.

2. Paresthesias — thumb.

3. Diminished muscle power — biceps.

4. Reflexes — decreased or absent biceps reflex.

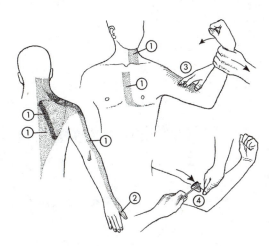

Seventh Nerve Root (Between C6 and C7)

1. Distribution of pain — root of neck, trapezius muscle, vertebral border of scapula, anterior chest wall, outer aspect of arm into index and middle fingers.

2. Paresthesias — index and middle fingers.

3. Diminished muscle power — triceps.

4. Reflexes — decreased or absent triceps reflex.

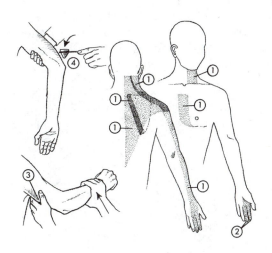

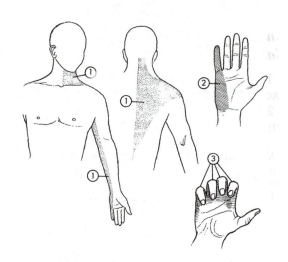

Eighth Nerve Root (Between C7 and T1)

1. Distribution of pain — neck, trapezius, inner border of arm into little finger.

2. Paresthesias — ulnar aspect of hand and little finger.

3. Diminished muscle power — all fingers (occasionally).

Reflexes — none.

Radiographic Features of Cervical Disc Injuries

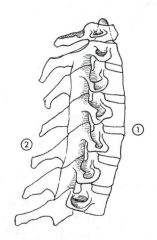

Normal X-Ray Features

1. No change — x-ray appears normal in every respect.

2. Loss of cervical lordosis may result from voluntary positioning of the chin and is not necessarily indicative of cervical disc syndrome.

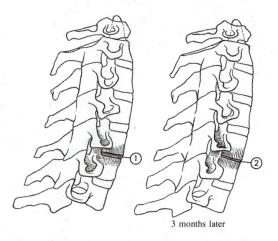

3 months later

Collapsing Disc (Best Seen in X-Rays Taken Every Four to Six Weeks)

1. Thin disc space at C5–C6.

2. Further thinning three months later.

Note: This may lead to chronic myelopathy from osteophyte formation, one of the most common causes of chronic cord injury in middle-aged and older patients.

376

Chip of Bone off Anterior Rim of Caudal Vertebra

1. X-ray of cervical spine is normal except for
2. Small chip of bone from anterior superior rim of caudal vertebra.

Note: This indicates a rupture of the anterior longitudinal ligament and a possible subluxation or dislocation of the cervical spine that has reduced spontaneously.

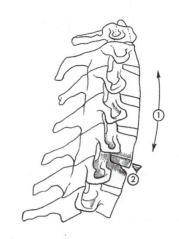

Degenerative Changes Localized at One Level

1. Thin disc.
2. Anterior osteophytes.
3. Posterior osteophytes.
4. Narrowing of intervertebral foramen.

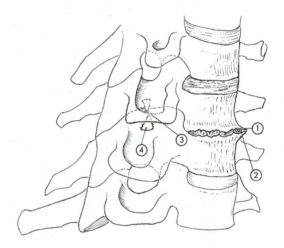

5. After heavy traction, of 150 lb (70 kg), the disc space from C2 to C7 will open a total of 1 cm.

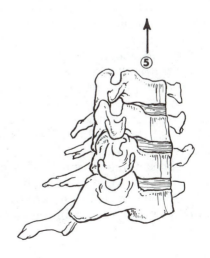

Hypermobile Cervical Vertebra

Note: Usually seen in late cases in which the disc was severely crushed or detached.

1. Forward displacement of C4 on C5.
2. Backward displacement of C4 on C5.

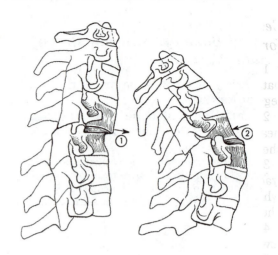

Management of Acute Disc Protrusion by Traction and Manipulation

REMARKS

The acutely displaced cervical disc protrusion may be reduced by heavy cervical traction and carefully applied manipulation in the direction of rotation and lateral flexion.

Traction is essential and must be sufficient to open the disc spaces at least 1 cm. Depending on the size of the patient, this may require a force of 150 lbs (70 kg) or more (see page 377).

The traction and manipulation are carried out with the patient fully awake and cooperating. After each maneuver the patient sits up and evaluates neck motion.

The manipulation is first directed at restoring full rotation in the direction that is pain free. When the patient's confidence is gained, rotation manipulation is carried out in the direction that had been painful. After each manipulation, the patient informs the physician of any neurologic symptoms.

The occasional patient with long-tract neurologic signs (hyperactive reflexes, et cetera) and the elderly patient with symptoms of cerebral or vertebral artery ischemia are the only patients in whom this treatment of acute cervical disc problems is contraindicated.

Cervical Traction – Manipulation for Disc Protrusion (After Cyriax)

1. Fully conscious and cooperative patient lies supine on the table with legs held by an assistant.

2. Physician stands at the patient's head with his foot supported against the table leg.

3. Hand under mandible applies traction and extends patient's neck while avoiding pressure on the trachea.

4. Hand supports occiput, using towel while applying heavy traction.

5. Most of traction is effected by physician's body weight rather than muscle force.

6. Rotate neck first toward the pain-free side and then in a direction that is painful.

Note: After each brief manipulation, patient sits up and evaluates the range of neck motion and pain. The physician then resumes traction manipulation and adds side flexion if indicated by patient's limitation of motion. One or two 15-minute sessions usually relieve patient's symptoms. If disc symptoms recur, the patient uses home traction unit with suspension bar.

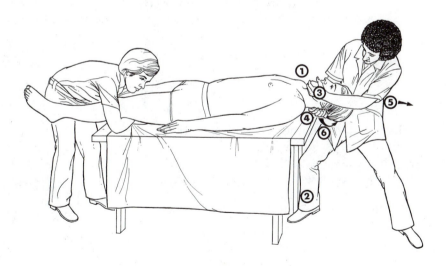

Overhead Traction

1. Patient sits on a stool with feet on ground.

2. Collar is adjusted to clear patient's trachea while supporting mandible.

3. Patient's head is in neutral position.

4. Spreader bar prevents squeezing of patient's ears.

5. Patient or therapist pulls suspension rope sufficiently to lift buttocks from stool. Suspension is maintained for one to five minutes.

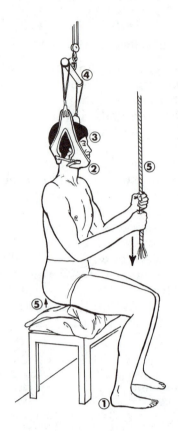

Cervical Supports

REMARKS

Occasionally the disc symptoms recur, and cervical supports may help prevent further symptoms.

The support is applied immediately after traction or manipulation and is used in conjunction with the treatment program until disc symptoms stabilize, which may take several weeks or months.

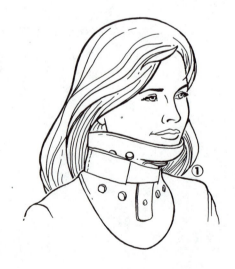

Soft collars do not immobilize the neck of the patient in an upright position but may be useful to wear while sleeping. For adequate support of recurrent disc symptoms use:

1. Philadelphia collar or

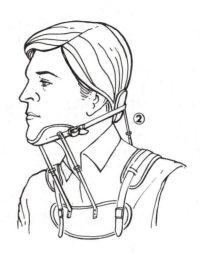

2. Two-piece chin and occiput support or a four-poster.

SLEEPING POSITION

1. Patient should sleep without a pillow and should avoid sleeping on the stomach with the head forced to one side.

2. A soft cervical collar or a heavy bath towel is a simple, useful cervical support during sleeping.

Note: Hot shower before bed and ice massage can relieve localized neck pain.

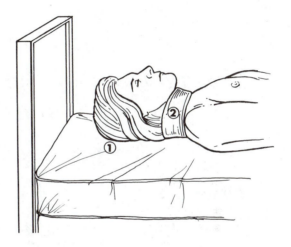

Injection of Arthritic Facet Joints

REMARKS

If a specific point of facet tenderness can be elicited by direct joint palpation, injection with triamcinolone and bupivacaine may effectively relieve pain. The joint to be injected is selected by palpation for tenderness.

1. The patient lies prone with the neck fully flexed toward painless side to open up the involved facet joint. In this position the articular facets are readily palpated.

2. One-ml syringe with 22-gauge needle at least 3 cm long is inserted 2 cm from midline.

3. If tip strikes bone directly, withdraw it and insert it obliquely and laterally. The needle then passes into the facet joint, which is infiltrated with mixture of triamcinolone and bupivacaine.

Note: Injection of "trigger points" in region of trapezius or rhomboids is illogical, because the pain in these regions is referred from a pathologic condition of the cervical disc and facet joints.

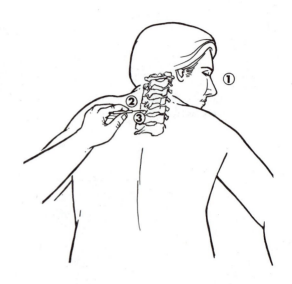

Management of the Chronic Cervical Syndrome

REMARKS

In this category are patients with dural and nerve root pain caused by chronic disc degeneration and osteophyte formation as well as patients with myelopathy from chronic cord compression. Chronic disc disease represents the most common cause for cervical myelopathy seen today, and the diagnosis should always be considered in any middle-aged patient with progressive neurologic deficit.

Osteophytes are not always pathologic and may actually be beneficial in limiting facet joint motion and preventing dural impingement that causes pain.

When disc narrowing and osteophytes cause pain that is unrelieved by or recurs after traction and disc reduction, surgical stabilization is necessary.

Selection of the effective level is based on:

1. Clinical evaluation of neck motion and nerve root impingement.

2. Radiographic findings, particularly osteophyte formations consistent with physical findings.

3. Disc distension test.

4. Myelography including evaluation of spinal fluid protein for possibility of spinal cord disease and tumors.

DISC DISTENSION TEST

REMARKS

The purpose of this test is to identify the intervertebral disc responsible for the cervical syndrome.

It is performed under image-intensified fluoroscopic guidance.

A strict aseptic technique must be employed.

Sudden distension of the pathologic disc will reproduce the patient's pain.

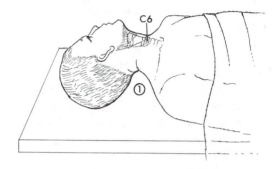

1. The patient is in the supine position with the head turned slightly to the left.

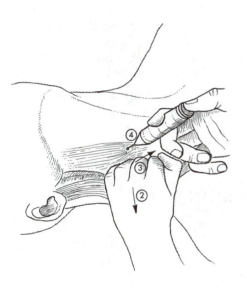

2. With the fingers of the left hand, displace laterally the medial border of the sternocleidomastoid muscle and the carotid sheath.

3. With downward pressure, the anterior surfaces of the cervical vertebrae are felt.

4. Using a number 20 hypodermic needle tilted outward 15 to 20 degrees, inject 3 to 5 ml of procaine in the skin and underlying soft tissues down to the bodies of the vertebrae.

5. With the fingers of the left hand still in position, insert a number 20 needle at the end of a 5-ml syringe containing normal saline and tilted outward 15 to 20 degrees into the same area previously injected with procaine. The needle is pushed inward until the point makes contact with a vertebra.

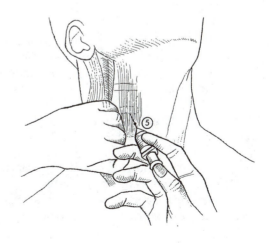

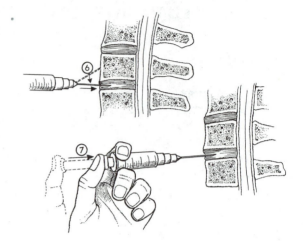

6. Move the needle up or down until a "soft spot" is felt, then push the needle in one cm. (Check the position of the needle with the fluoroscope and identify the disc penetrated.)

7. With the needle in position, thrust downward the plunger of the syringe quickly and firmly.

Note: If the site injected is the responsible disc, the patient will experience a reproduction or an aggravation of his pattern of pain.

A normal disc may take 0.5 ml of fluid without symptoms, and in some instances it will take more.

A pathologic disc producing no symptoms may take up to 3 ml of fluid.

Sudden distension of a responsible disc with even minimal fluid reproduces the pain pattern.

When the responsible level is identified, also test the disc above and below, because in some instances multiple levels are involved.

Note: Discography to show leakage on injection of radiopaque dye into the disc is not as reliable diagnostically as pain reproduced by disc injection.

ANTERIOR CERVICAL SPINE FUSION USING INTERBODY BONE PLUGS

REMARKS

Either the right or left approach can be used; a left approach is less likely to damage the recurrent laryngeal nerve.

Either a vertical or a transverse incision can be made; this depends on the number of levels to be fused. Employ the transverse incision if one or two levels are to be fused and the vertical incision if three or more levels are to be fused.

The region from C3 to T1 can be readily approached through these incisions.

For orientation of the incisions use the cricoid cartilage that is opposite C6 and is readily palpable.

Use endotracheal anesthesia through the oral route; the tube in the trachea helps identify the trachea during the operation.

Position of the Patient

1. Place a folded towel beneath the interscapular region to hold the head in slight hyperextension.

2. Turn the head slightly to the right (15 to 20 degrees).

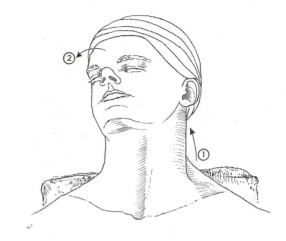

Incision

TRANSVERSE INCISION

1. Locate by palpation the cricoid cartilage opposite C6 for orientation.

2. Make the incision in a skin crease opposite the desired level beginning at the midline and extending laterally for 7.5 to 9.0 cm across the belly of the sternocleidomastoid muscle.

3. Cut the platysma in the same line as the skin incision.

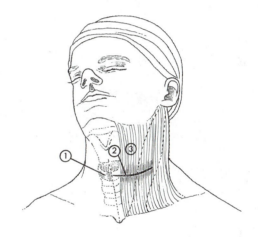

Incision

VERTICAL INCISION

1. Locate by palpation the cricoid cartilage opposite C6 for orientation.

2. Make the incision along the anterior border of the sternocleidomastoid muscle, 5 cm above and 5 cm below the desired level.

3. Cut the platysma in the same line as the skin incision.

Note: For both the transverse and the longitudinal incisions the following steps are the same:

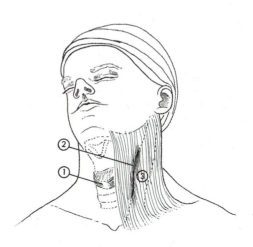

Incision (Continued)

EXPOSURE DOWN TO THE PRETRACHEAL FASCIA

1. Divide longitudinally the anterior layer of the cervical fascia along the anterior border of the sternocleido-mastoid muscle.

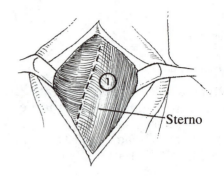

Sterno

2. By scissor dissection mobilize the anterior margin of the sternoclei-domastoid muscle and gently retract the muscle laterally.

3. Now the carotid sheath and the omohyoid muscle are visualized.

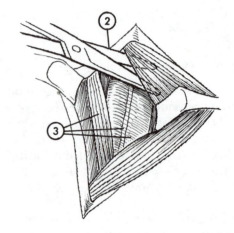

4. By blunt dissection develop the interval medial to the carotid sheath and retract the omohyoid muscle me-dially.

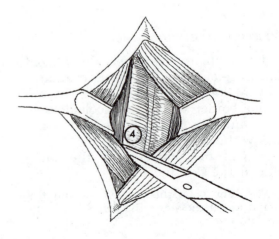

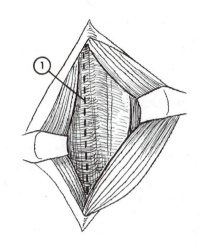

EXPOSURE OF THE INTERVERTEBRAL DISC

1. Make a small longitudinal incision in the pretracheal fascia.

2. With the index finger develop the retropharyngeal space for the full length of the incision. This is easily accomplished because the space comprises loose areolar tissue that is readily displaced in all directions.

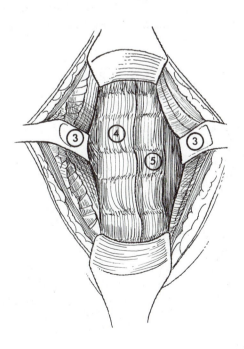

3. Gently retract the thyroid gland, trachea, and esophagus medially and the carotid sheath laterally.

4. Now the prevertebral fascia is seen as a glistening sheath covering the vertebral bodies, the anterior longitudinal ligament, and the longus colli muscles.

5. The intervertebral discs are clearly visualized through the prevertebral fascia.

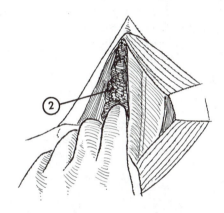

Incision (Continued)

CAUTION

1. When dividing the pretracheal fascia look for the middle thyroid vein; divide and ligate it.

2. In high incisions (C2 and C3), the superior thyroid artery and vein and the superior laryngeal nerve are encountered; displace them proximally. Occasionally it may be necessary to divide the vessels.

3. In low incisions (C6 to T1) it may be necessary to divide the inferior thyroid artery and vein.

4. In low incisions, do not injure the recurrent laryngeal nerve. Remember, it descends along the carotid sheath and ascends between the esophagus and trachea.

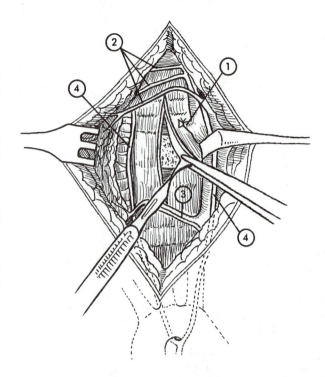

Localization of the Intervertebral Disc

1. Insert a fine straight needle in the disc and take a lateral x-ray.

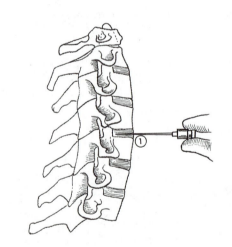

2. While the x-ray film is being developed, remove a block of bone from the anterior iliac crest. The piece of bone should comprise the full thickness of the crest of the ilium.

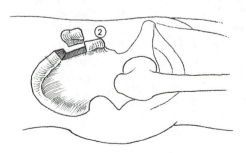

Excision of the Affected Intervertebral Disc

1. By blunt dissection, without traumatizing the sympathetic chains, mobilize and displace the longus colli muscles laterally, directly opposite the disc to be removed.

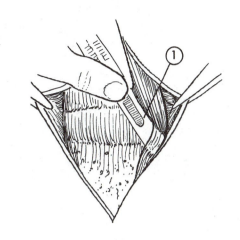

2. Hook flat blade retractor (1 to 1.5 cm wide) under the muscles.

3. With the electrocautery, coagulate and divide transversely the tissues directly over the intervertebral disc.

Note: Using the electrocautery renders the field bloodless. There is no need to preserve the edges of the divided prevertebral fascia. If the bone block to be inserted fits snugly between the vertebrae, the chances of extrusion or displacement of the graft are practically nil.

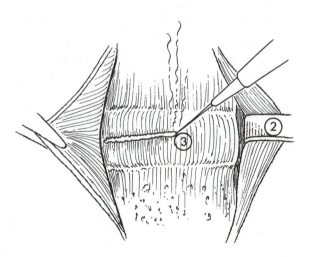

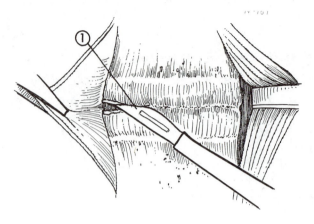

Removal of the Disc

1. With a scalpel cut the annulus fibrosus across the entire width of the disc.

2. Have an assistant make strong manual traction on the head to open up the disc space.

Note: Traction is made with the neck only slightly hyperextended. Manual traction is preferred to continuous traction with a head halter because it can be applied and released as desired. If the fusion is performed to stabilize dislocations and fracture-dislocations, skeletal traction of 15 lbs (6.8 kg) is maintained at all times during the operation. The weights can be increased if widening of the disc space is desired.

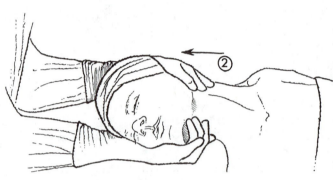

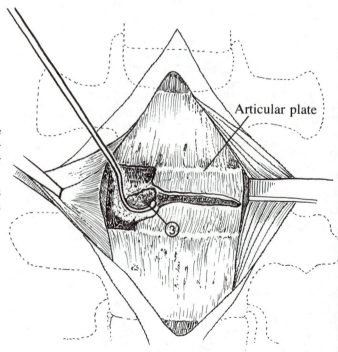

Articular plate

3. With a curette remove the entire disc piece by piece. Also remove the articular plate above and below down to subchondral bone.

Note: Curved curettes of varying sizes facilitate removal of disc material from the uncovertebral joints.

Insertion of Bone Graft

1. Cut out a bone block from the iliac bone previously removed.

Note: The width of the graft should be same as the width of the intervertebral space exposed between the longus colli muscles; the height of the graft should be such that it fits snugly between the two vertebral bodies; the graft should have cortical bone on both sides.

2. While manual traction is applied to open the disc space, gently tap the graft into position.

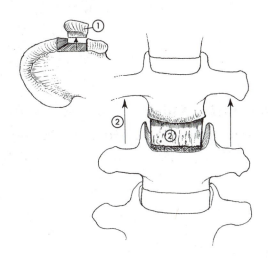

3. The anterior surface of the graft should be behind the anterior margins of the vertebrae.

4. Bring the head to a slightly flexed position and close the wound in layers. There should be no need to place a drain in the wound.

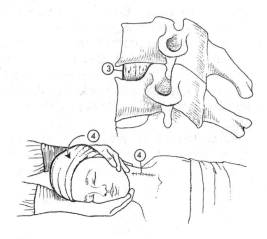

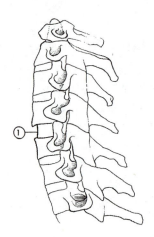

Postoperative X-Ray

1. Graft in position between C4 and C5.

Postoperative Care

Immediately after operation apply a felt collar holding the head in a position of slight flexion. (If operation was done with tongs in place, remove the tongs at this time.)

Ambulate the patient on the second day.

Before discharging the patient from the hospital (five to seven days after surgery), replace felt collar with a cervical brace.

After eight to ten weeks, fusion is solid enough that the brace may be discarded and replaced with a felt collar. Now start daily isometric exercises.

After two more weeks remove the collar for longer periods of time each day; it should be discarded within two more weeks.

Take x-rays every four weeks to note the status of healing at the fusion site.

REHABILITATIVE MANAGEMENT OF THE PATIENT WITH SPINAL CORD INJURY

REMARKS

Rehabilitation of patients with this lesion should be of primary concern from the start of treatment.

Ideally these patients are cared for at centers staffed to meet their complex medical, musculoskeletal, social, family, and vocational needs in a way that maximizes the use of their uninjured neuromusculoskeletal function.

Rehabilitation can be considerably aided by attention to complications likely to occur during immediate treatment. These include a number of problems, but the most common are pulmonary edema from fluid overload during spinal shock, respiratory failure, gastric distension and bleeding, urinary retention, and pressure sores. All of these potential and real complications should be kept in mind in treating the spinal column injury itself.

1. The patient is positioned in traction in a regular bed and is turned every two hours. Turning frames, especially beds, are poorly tolerated and are hazardous to the paralyzed patient.

2. Use intermittent positive pressure breathing and observe the patient carefully for respiratory insufficiency and pulmonary edema.

3. Gastric dilatation and gastric bleeding require intubation and lavage with iced water.

4. Indwelling urethral catheter should be used for the first 48 hours, but when diuresis occurs intermittent catheterization may be employed.

5. Start bowel control program with Dulcolax or other suppository every two to three days.

6. Splints should hold limbs in functional positions but should be as light as possible.

Note: Attention to these basic needs of the paralyzed patient from the start of immediate care will mitigate the complexity of rehabilitation problems considerably.

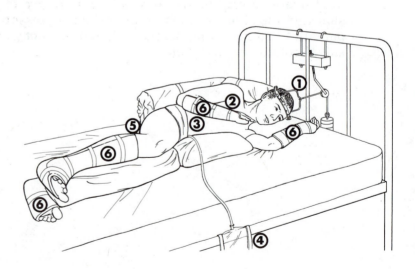

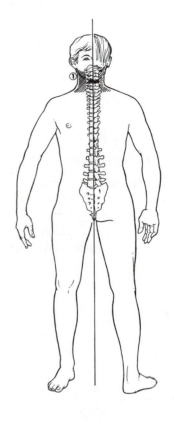

Functional Levels in Spinal Cord Injury

The level of nerve root involvement or nerve root sparing makes significant difference in key muscle control and functional potential, in the cervical spine.

1. Involvement from C5 down leaves only neck muscle control. This requires the patient to use electrically powered wheelchair and externally powered hand splints for limited self-care.

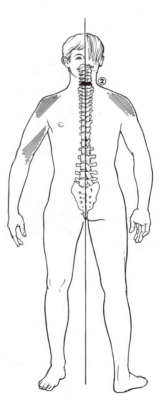

2. Involvement from C6 level down leaves the patient with control of shoulder muscles and elbow flexors. These permit self-transfer with an overhead sling and allow the patient to propel a wheelchair and have limited self-care using externally powered assistive devices.

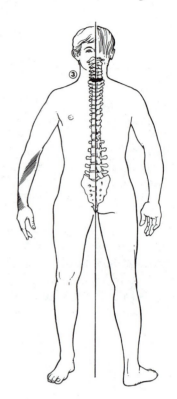

Functional Levels in
Spinal Cord Injury (Continued)

3. Involvement from C7 level down leaves the patient with wrist extensors and supinator muscles. These permit more independence for transfer, self-care and driving an auto with hand controls.

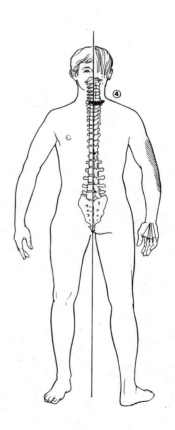

4. Involvement of C8 level down leaves the patient with elbow extension and a weak hand grip for most self-care activities without the need for hand splints.

SUMMARY: THE PITFALLS OF CERVICAL SPINE FRACTURES AND DISLOCATIONS

The pitfalls of these injuries as outlined in this chapter are both diagnostic and management problems.

Diagnostic assessment must include thorough neurologic evaluation as well as radiographic examination. Be particularly alert to intermittent symptoms of motor paralysis or "drop attacks," which should prompt investigation for cervical spine instability, particularly at C1–C2.

The ease with which the cervical spine is fractured is exceeded only by the ease with which the injury is undetected. Injuries to the upper and lower regions of the cervical spine in particular are missed by inadequate x-rays. X-rays should completely visualize the odontoid regions as well as the cervical spine down to C7–T1.

Careful assessment of the x-ray should help in analyzing the mechanism of the fracture. Most cervical spine fractures result from flexion mechanisms, but the physician should be alert to signs of extension injuries, including avulsions of the anterior vertebral body (see page 367).

Management of these injuries should be biomechanically rational and should avoid common pitfalls such as excessively heavy traction for odontoid fractures or the C2 "hangman's fracture".

Heavy traction should also be avoided for unilateral facet dislocation, which requires lateral flexion for reduction (see page 338).

Heavy traction is also inappropriate and even dangerous for bilateral facet dislocations and is likely to inflict further neurologic damage.

Management should be individualized for each patient rather than for each fracture. The elderly patient with a cervical spine fracture and central cord syndrome from hyperextension injury to an osteoarthritic neck is in danger of being overtreated. This injury is best managed by prompt halo or brace application, which eliminates the need for traction in recumbency.

One of the most common management pitfalls is the overuse of laminectomy, which is performed in hopes of improving the neurologic deficit. Acute laminectomy most often increases only the chances of the patient's rapid demise. The ultimate pitfall to avoid in managing these injuries is overextensive laminectomy, which produces spinal instability. The surgical management all too frequently becomes part of the patient's disease and then requires surgical refusion (see page 370).

The final pitfall to avoid is failure to recognize that managing any of these fractures and dislocations is but a small part in caring for patient with serious injury, particularly nerve deficits. The physician who undertakes management of cervical spine fractures and dislocations must be oriented toward rehabilitation needs and complications as well as the acute problem of the injury itself.

REFERENCES

Boshch, A., Stauffer, E. S., and Nickel, V. L.: The risk of neurologic damage with fractures of the vertebrae. J. Trauma, 17:126, 1977.

Braakman, R., and Penning, L.: Injuries of the cervical spine. *In* Injuries of the Spine and Spinal Cord, 26:227. New York, American Elsevier Publishing Co., Inc., 1976.

Brooks, A. L., and Jenkins, E. B.: Atlanto-axial arthrodesis by the wedge compression method. J. Bone and Joint Surg., 60-A:279, 1978.

Callahan, R. A., Johnson, R. M., Margolis, R. N., et al.: Cervical facet fusion for control of instability following laminectomy. J. Bone and Joint Surg., 59-A:991, 1977.

Cyriax, J.: Textbook of Orthopaedic Medicine. Baltimore, The Williams & Wilkins Company, 1975, pp. 129–165.

Davidson, R. C., Horn, J. R., Herndon, J. H., et al.: Brain-stem compression in rheumatoid arthritis. JAMA, 238:2633, 1977.

Dewald, R., and Ray, R.: Skeletal traction for the treatment of severe scoliosis. J. Bone and Joint Surg., 52-A:233, 1970.

Fielding, J. W., and Hawkins, R. J.: Atlanto-axial rotatory fixation. J. Bone and Joint Surg., 59-A:37, 1977.

Fried, L. C.: Cervical spinal cord injury during skeletal traction. JAMA, 229:181, 1974.

Funk, F. J., and Wells, R. E.: Injuries of the cervical spine in football. Clin. Orthop., 109:50, 1975.

Gardner, W. J.: The principle of spring-loaded points for cervical traction. Technical note. J. Neurosurg., 39:543, 1973.

Griswold, D. M., Albright, J. A., Schiffman, E., et al.: Atlanto-axial fusion for instability. J. Bone and Joint Surg., 60-A:285, 1978.

Haralson, R. H., Boyd, H. B.: Posterior dislocation of the atlas on the axis without fracture. J. Bone and Joint Surg., 51-A:561, 1969.

Nickel, V., Perry, J., Garrett, A., et al: The halo: a spinal skeletal traction fixation device. J. Bone and Joint Surg., 50-A:1400, 1968.

Prolo, D. J., Runnels, J. B., and Jameson, R. M.: The injured cervical spine. Immediate and long-term immobilization with the halo. JAMA, 224:591, 1973.

Riggins, R. S., and Kraus, J. F.: The risk of neurologic damage with fractures of the vertebrae. J. Trauma, 17:126, 1977.

Robinson, R. A., and Southwick, W. O.: Surgical approaches to the cervical spine. *In* Instructional Course Lectures, American Academy of Orthopaedic Surgeons, 9:299, Mosby, St. Louis, 1960.

Schneider, R. C., and Kahn, E. A.: Chronic neurological sequelae of acute trauma to the spine and spinal cord. I. The significance of the acute-flexion or "tear-drop" fracture-dislocation of the cervical spine. J. Bone and Joint Surg., 38-A:985, 1956.

Schneider, R. C., Livingston, K. E., Cave, A. J. E., et al: "Hangman's fracture" of the cervical spine. J. Neurosurg., 22:141, 1965.

Weir, D. C.: Roentgenographic signs of cervical injury. Clin. Orthop., 109:9, 1975.

White, A. A., Johnson, R. M., Panjab, M. M., et al.: Biomechanical analysis of clinical stability in the cervical spine. Clin. Orthop., 109:85, 1975.

DISLOCATIONS, FRACTURES, AND FRACTURE-DISLOCATIONS OF THE THORACIC AND LUMBAR SPINE

ANATOMIC FEATURES AND MECHANISMS OF INJURIES

REMARKS

The goal of managing injuries to the thoracic and lumbar spine is to achieve a painless, strong, flexible back without neurologic deficit.

In spite of the implications that a "broken back" has for the lay person, only 15 per cent of patients with thoracolumbar fractures suffer neurologic injury. This minority, however, demands considerable knowledge and critical judgment on the part of the physician for maximum recovery.

Prognosis and treatment of thoracolumbar spinal cord injuries vary considerably depending on the level and degree of injury.

Paraplegia following thoracic spine injury carries the poorest prognosis for return of neurologic function.

Thoracolumbar or lumbar spine injuries, which usually spare important nerve roots, are essentially lesions of peripheral nerves rather than the cord. They have the best prognosis for neurologic recovery provided that the bony injury is reduced.

A review of the anatomic differences in the thoracic and lumbar spine and nerve structures and a correlation of this anatomy with clinical findings are critical for effective evaluation of these injuries.

Understanding the various mechanisms that disrupt these structures is also basic to rational treatment.

Anatomic Features

REMARKS

The thoracic spine, because of the shape and size of its articular processes and the reinforcement provided by the ribcage, is more stable than the cervical or lumbar segments.

In addition to the ribcage and articular facets, support structures include the interspinous and interlaminal ligaments, facet joint capsules, anterior and posterior longitudinal ligaments, and disc structures.

NORMAL ANATOMY

1. The superior articular facets face backward in the thoracic spine, permitting rotation and limiting flexion and extension.

2. This is contrasted with the articular facets in the cervical region, which face upward, and

3. The articular facets in lumbar region, which turn abruptly inward, permitting flexion and extension but restricting rotation.

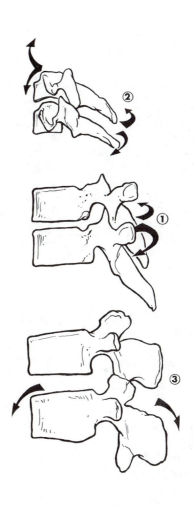

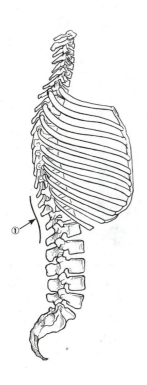

1. Abrupt transition from thoracic kyphosis to lumbar lordosis along with the loss of the ribcage support and the changes in axes of motion combine to make T12 through L2 the most common site for fracture-dislocations.

401

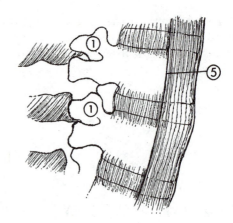

The major anterior and posterior support structures of the spine include:

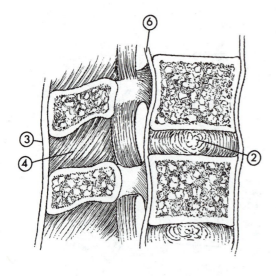

1. Articular facets.
2. Disc and annulus.
3. Supraspinous ligament.
4. Interspinous ligament.
5. Anterior longitudinal ligament.
6. Posterior longitudinal ligament.

ANATOMY RELATED TO NEUROLOGIC SIGNS

1. Cord segments end at L1; this level varies considerably from person to person.

2. Cord occupies one half of thoracic spinal canal. Neural damage here is usually permanent.

3. Neural structures take up only one third of lumbar canal, and are less likely to be permanently damaged than neural structures in the thoracic spine.

4. The most common fracture-dislocation at T12–L1 produces a combination of nerve root and conus injury. The injured peripheral nerves can recover, but the central nerve or conus damage is permanent.

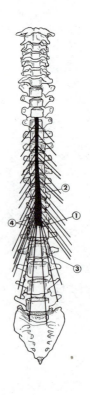

Motor and Sensory Innervation in the Lower Body

Note: To separate peripheral from central lesions, the physician should identify the specific muscle groups and sensory levels involved.

1. Abdominal muscles innervated by T7 through T12.
2. Hip flexors, adductors and internal rotators, L2–L3.
3. Knee extensors, L3–L4.
4. Hip extensors, abductors, and external rotators, L5–S1.

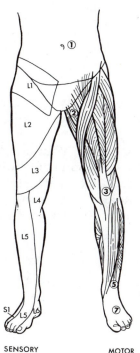

SENSORY   MOTOR

5. Ankle dorsiflexors, L4–5.
6. Knee flexors, L4–5, L5–S1.
7. Toe extensors, L5–S1.
8. Calf muscles, L5–S1.
9. Perineal and foot muscles, S1–S2.

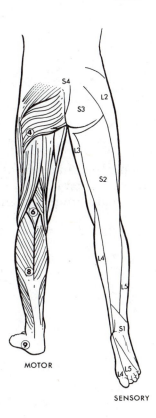

MOTOR

SENSORY

403

GOOD PROGNOSTIC SIGNS

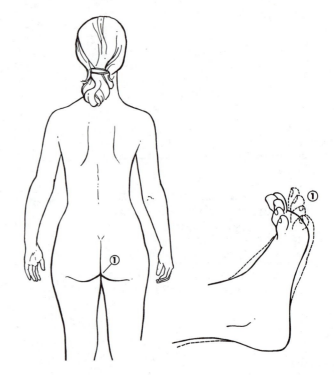

Always test completely for any residual sensory or motor function whatsoever.

1. Preservation of any voluntary motion including toe motion or voluntary anal sphincter contraction after lumbosacral injury indicates an incomplete lesion with the possibility of significant recovery.

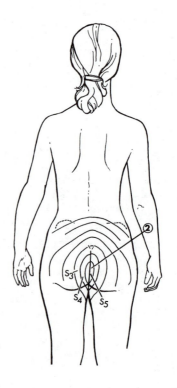

2. Preservation of perianal sensation indicates that the sacral roots are spared and neurologic improvement is possible.

POOR PROGNOSTIC SIGNS

Flaccidity of initial injury ("spinal shock") lasts no more than 24 hours. The return of any superficial reflexes in the total absence of motor and sensory function indicates a complete cord injury and a poor prognosis. These include:

1. Bulbocavernous reflex — pulling on catheter causes bulbous urethra and rectal sphincter to contract, as felt on rectal examination.

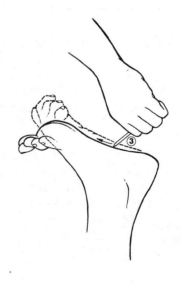

2. Superficial anal reflex — pricking perineum causes contraction of rectal sphincter.

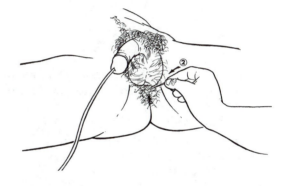

3. Slow toe flexion and extension on plantar stimulation.

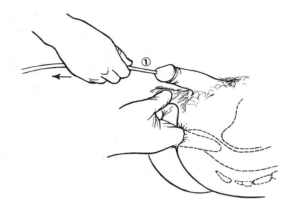

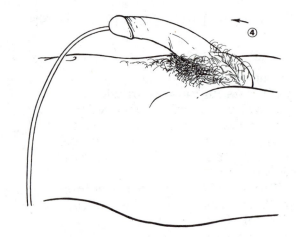

4. Priapism.

Mechanisms of Injury

Injuries to the thoracolumbar spinal column are produced most often by any of the following mechanisms:
1. Hyperflexion.
2. Compression.
3. Flexion-rotation.
4. Hyperextension-shear.
5. Distraction.
6. Lateral bending.
7. Lateral shear.
8. Gunshot fracture.

For the injury to be unstable, both anterior and posterior support structures of the spinal column must be disrupted.

HYPERFLEXION MECHANISM

REMARKS

A fall in which the victim lands on his heels or sits down hard on his buttocks causes a hyperflexion injury to the spine.

Pure hyperflexion produces a wedge-shaped compression fracture of the vertebral body of the thoracic or lumbar spine.

These injuries usually are stable and cause no nerve deficit, because the ribs and posterior support structures are intact.

If the ribs and posterior elements are fractured, the vertebral body is compressed more than 50 per cent of its height, or multiple vertebral bodies are fractured, the injury can be quite unstable and can cause progressive neurologic deficit or kyphosis.

Stable Hyperflexion Injury

1. Posterior ligaments are intact.

2. Anterior portion of body has absorbed most of compression load.

3. Posterior portion of body shows minimal loss of height, indicating posterior stability.

4. Intervertebral discs and vertebrae above and below may be implicated, but wedging of the body may be seen on x-ray only several months later.

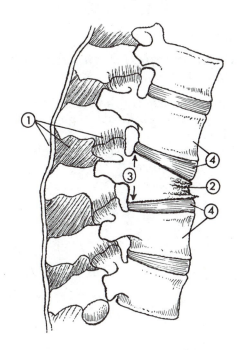

Unstable Hyperflexion Injuries

1. Wedge fracture of T8 in a patient who at first was neurologically intact.

2. Fractures of the ribs and posterior elements were not recognized.

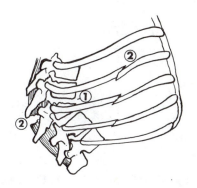

3. Horizontal displacement occurred, producing neurologic damage.

Note: The rib fractures indicate that this injury resulted not from a hyperflexion mechanism but from a direct blow to the back that produced a shearing mechanism (see page 414).

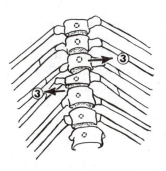

Unstable Hyperflexion Injuries (Continued)

1. Multiple vertebral body compression fractures indicate potential instability.

2. Progressive kyphosis can develop, which would require

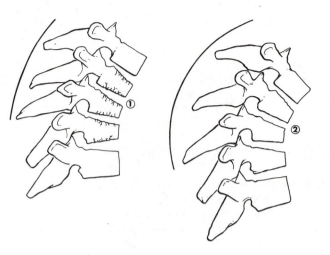

3. Surgical stabilization.

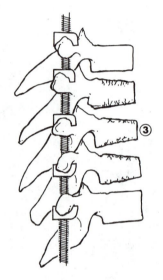

COMPRESSION MECHANISM (BURSTING FRACTURE)

REMARKS

The disrupting force is transmitted vertically downward along the line of the vertebral bodies when the spine is in a neutral position. Characteristically, this occurs in the patient with an osteoporotic spine who "sits down hard" and drives the intervertebral disc through the articular endplates into the weak vertebral bodies. This low-violence injury does not usually cause neurologic deficit.

If the vertical loading is sufficient to shatter the vertebral body, neurologic structures will be damaged from protrusion of the posterior vertebral body fragments into the cord or cauda equina.

Anterior decompression and interbody fusion may occasionally be necessary for partial neurologic lesions, but surgical treatment does not benefit the patient with total neurologic loss.

Low-Violence Mechanism

The typical compression fracture in an osteoporotic spine produces:

1. Increased dorsal curve.

2. Collapsed, codfish-shaped vertebral bodies.

3. Other vertebral bodies may show cupping.

4. Intervertebral discs may become biconvex.

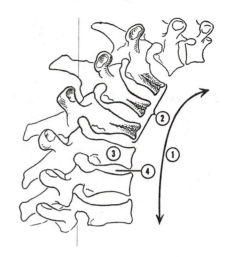

High-Violence Mechanism

If vertical compression loading is severe,

1. The verterbal body may shatter, and

2. Disc material is displaced into the body.

3. The body disintegrates.

4. The posterior portion of the body is displaced backward, producing cord damage. Removal of this fragment and interbody fusion may benefit the patient with incomplete paralysis.

5. Anterior and posterior ligaments are usually intact.

Note: Compression fractures of the spine are stable and are the only vertebral body fractures likely to fuse spontaneously. Operative treatment is usually not necessary except to decompress partial nerve injuries.

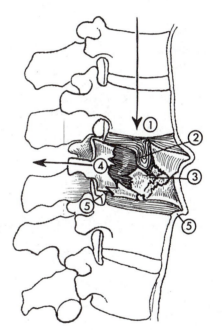

FLEXION-ROTATION MECHANISM

REMARKS

The most common mechanism of fracture-dislocation in the thoracolumbar spine is a combination of flexion and rotation.

Formerly, the typical victim was a coal miner who, while working in the flexed position, had a load fall on his back. Today, the injury is most commonly seen in the motor vehicle occupant thrown about in his car.

Severe flexion disrupts the anterior support structures, but rotation is necessary to tear the posterior ligaments and fracture the posterior spinal elements.

The result is a slice fracture of the superior aspect of the vertebral body and horizontal displacement of the entire vertebra.

The injury most commonly occurs at the thoracolumbar junction and produces paraplegia resulting from both conus and nerve root damage.

This lesion is quite unstable, and open reduction with internal fixation (not laminectomy) is the most effective method to insure decompression of the injured neural structures.

1. Fracture of the articular process with displacement.

2. Rupture of posterior ligaments.

3. Spinous process of T12 is to the right of that of L1. This indicates significant instability.

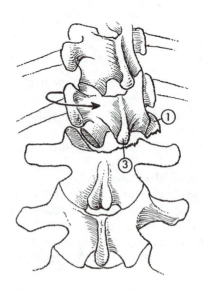

4. Slice fracture of superior portion of L1.

5. Disc is intact.

6. Separation of spinous processes of T12 and L1.

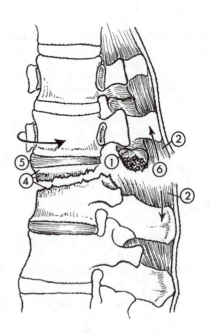

410

Rarely, the flexion-rotation mechanism may rupture the posterior ligaments and capsule along with the anterior disc structures without fracturing the articular facets or the vertebral body.

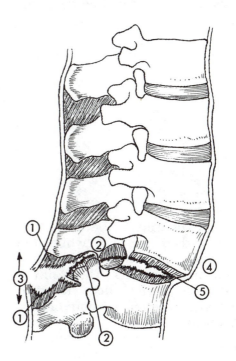

1. Rupture of posterior ligaments.
2. Articular process of L4 in front of that of L5.
3. Separation of the spinous processes of L4 and L5.
4. Forward displacement of body of L4 on L5.
5. Disruption of disc.

Note: This infrequent dislocation without fracture is unstable because of anterior and posterior disruption.

HYPEREXTENSION-SHEAR MECHANISM

REMARKS

Hyperextension-shear mechanism occurs most typically when the victim is hit from behind by a motor vehicle. The force pushes the lower lumbar vertebra suddenly forward while the upper part of the spine hyperextends because of inertia.

Rupture of the articular capsules allows the superior articular processes to disengage from the inferior articular processes of the upper vertebra, causing the whole upper vertebra to slip backward (retrolisthesis).

Should the shearing force continue, the pedicle of the lower vertebra will fracture, and significant damage will result from stretching of neural structures.

The separation of the neural arch from the body produced by such a mechanism is extremely unstable and difficult to reduce.

411

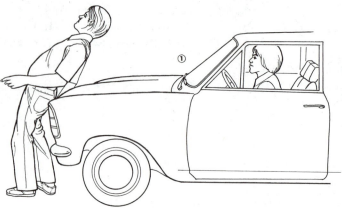

1. Typically, injury occurs when victim is struck from behind by motor vehicle.

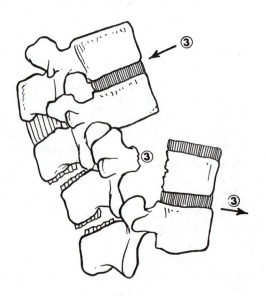

2. Under the impact the lower vertebra is forced forward while the upper spine and trunk are hyperextended owing to inertia. The result is retrolisthesis with slice fracture through the inferior portion of the superior body.

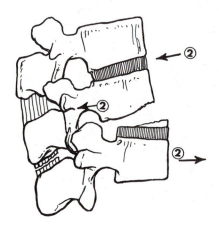

3. With more violent force, further displacement of the slipped vertebra will fracture and separate the posterior elements of the vertebra from the vertebral body, causing neurologic damage.

Note: This mechanism differs from flexion-rotation fracture-dislocations, in which the superior body slips forward and the slice fracture occurs through the superior aspect of the inferior body (see page 410).

DISTRACTION MECHANISM (SEAT BELT FRACTURE)

REMARKS

Distraction loading of the spine produced by the lap seat belt of an auto occupant has become a recent addition to the mechanism of thoracolumbar injuries.

The fulcrum for spinal flexion becomes the point of impact of the lap belt against the anterior abdominal wall, resulting in a tensile or distraction loading of the spinal structures.

The bony structures may fail first, leaving the ligaments to stabilize the spinal articulations.

It is important with this type of injury to determine the degree of blunt abdominal injury, which may include rupture of a viscus or infarction of the bowel.

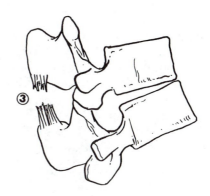

1. Hyperflexion over the seat belt causes compression loading of the abdominal wall.

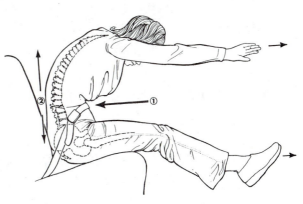

2. Spine is distracted, producing either complete bony injury, or

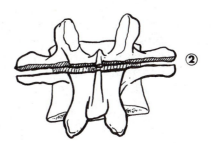

3. Disruption of ligaments.

Note: The possibility of serious intra-abdominal injury must always be carefully ruled out before embarking on treatment of the spinal injury.

LATERAL BENDING MECHANISM

1. Loading by lateral bending may rarely cause a unilateral compression fracture.

2. More commonly, this mechanism results in avulsion fractures of the transverse processes caused by violent contraction of the quadratus lumborum on the convex side during a fall.

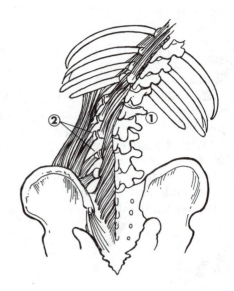

LATERAL SHEARING MECHANISMS

REMARKS

This results from a direct blow to the prominent thoracic region, as for example when someone jumps and lands on a swimmer's back or when a vehicle rolls over a prone victim.

This violent mechanism usually causes a complete fracture-dislocation and a total cord injury. Occasionally the victim may escape neurologic involvement (see page 450).

1. A direct blow to the prominent thoracic spine fractures the posterior elements.

2. This shearing mechanism displaces the superior vertebra laterally on the inferior vertebra (see pages 423 and 449).

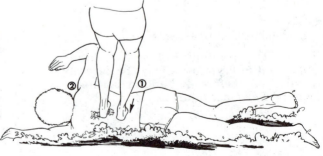

414

GUNSHOT MECHANISMS

REMARKS

Gunshot wounds are second only to automobiles as a cause of spinal cord injury in many treatment centers. They are usually produced by low-velocity, low-energy wounds from .22-caliber or .38-caliber hand guns.

Prognosis for recovery is almost entirely dependent on the degree of initial neurologic deficit. The majority of gunshot wounds cause complete lesions in the lumbar spine.

The fracture produced by a gunshot wound is usually stable. Laminectomy for these injuries does nothing but add to the complication rate, particularly causing spinal instability, wound infection, and draining fistulae.

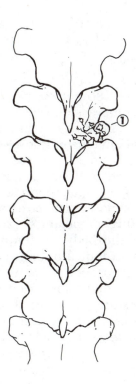

1. The typical gunshot mechanism results from a low-velocity missile that produces a stable fracture of either the thoracic or the thoracolumbar spine.

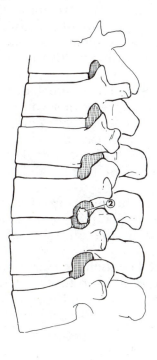

2. Rarely, the bullet will remain lodged within the spinal canal.

EVALUATION AND MANAGEMENT OF INJURIES TO THE THORACIC AND LUMBAR SPINE

REMARKS

Between 80 and 85 per cent of injuries in this region are stable flexion or compression types without neurologic impairment.

Take nothing for granted. Progressive instability and neurologic damage have been known to occur after injury is presumed stable.

These lesions must be carefully evaluated to ensure that they are stable and will not cause delayed neurologic injury. Even minimal neurologic impairment such as loss of sphincter control should alert the physician to the possibility of an unstable injury.

Fracture of posterior elements, compression of more than 50 per cent of the body, widening of interspinous spaces, or horizontal displacement indicates an injury in which further displacement is possible.

In the absence of signs of instability or neurologic deficit, the usual flexion-compression fracture is best managed symptomatically with early restoration of functional activity.

Injuries from flexion-rotation or hyperextension-shear mechanisms carry at least a 70 per cent risk of neurologic damage, either complete or incomplete. The degree of persistent neurologic deficit relates more to the injury than to the type of surgical or nonsurgical treatment.

The objectives in treating fracture-dislocations with neurologic impairment should be to achieve adequate reduction, ensure stability of the spine, and allow injured nerve roots to recover.

Routine laminectomy, which is still practiced in many areas of the United States, is ineffective in achieving these objectives or in relieving neural compression, which is most often in the anterior spinal canal.

Reduction and stabilization of the fracture-dislocation by Harrington distraction instrumentation and fusion can relieve anterior neural compression and at the same time prevent progressive and painful deformities that follow wide laminectomies.

416

For the occasional unstable fracture-dislocation resulting from hyperextension-shear mechanism and for progressive kyphotic deformities following unstable hyperflexion (wedge) fractures, Harrington compression-rod fixation meets the biomechanical demands for stability.

Management of these hazardous, unstable injuries by operative or nonoperative means is not without complications and should only be undertaken by physicians thoroughly familiar with these techniques and their limitations.

INITIAL EVALUATION

REMARKS

Always keep the patient with an injured spine supported by a spine board during transportation.

Obtain history if possible to establish a mechanism of injury, such as flexion-rotation, hyperextension-shear, or seat belt fracture.

Inspect the patient's back for gibbus, hemorrhage, or deformity of the spine when he is positioned on the litter for clinical and radiographic examination.

Clearly establish and record any sensory, motor, or reflex findings, no matter how subtle or gross. Check carefully for perianal sensation, toe motion, and anal sphincter contraction, which would indicate incomplete neurologic injury.

Evaluate for commonly associated problems of intestinal ileus, bladder distension, and signs of blunt abdominal injury as well as for any other injuries.

On x-rays, look for the site of the lesion and for any signs of instability including anteroposterior, mediolateral, or horizontal displacement, disruption of both anterior and posterior support structures, and superior or inferior slice fractures of vertebral bodies.

Perform neurologic evaluation repeatedly during the first 24 hours and daily thereafter.

Manage the spinal injury by postural reduction for the first few days while the need for surgical stabilization is considered.

Internal fixation and fusion may be done, but only under ideal conditions and by experienced personnel.

Nonoperative and Operative Methods

Fracture management should be based on the degree of the spinal column instability as well as the neurologic damage.

The usual fracture produced by a hyperflexion or compression mechanism does not cause neurologic damage and may be treated symptomatically with bed rest and early mobilization.

Cast or external orthosis to support the fracture adds nothing but a longer disability time. The radiographic appearance of a wedged vertebral body may be improved initially by a hyperextension cast, but this fracture of the cancellous bone will return to its collapsed position quite promptly after the cast is removed.

For the less common but still significant injury in which spinal instability or neurologic damage has occurred or is likely to occur, the physician must selectively employ management techniques of both nonoperative and operative types.

The indications for both nonoperative and operative management of spinal cord injuries have been widely studied and compared. Any physician caring for the patient with this serious problem should be thoroughly familiar with the advantages and disadvantages of both methods.

NONOPERATIVE POSTURAL REDUCTION METHOD

REMARKS

A patient with complete paraplegia and minimal translational displacement, i.e., less than 20 per cent of the body, can be treated by this method.

A perfectly satisfactory result can follow nonoperative management, but keep in mind that some of the most chronically deformed spines in paraplegic patients after fracture showed very little primary fracture displacement.

Try conservative treatment of "stable" injuries, but follow the status of the fracture closely by radiographic scrutiny. Any tendency of the spine to deform indicates the need for internal fixation.

The major complications from conservative treatment on long-term follow-up have been residual spinal deformity and serious back pain.

Spinal deformity is virtually certain to follow paraplegia occurring in childhood injuries and after wide "decompression" laminectomy.

Back pain is more likely to afflict the paraplegic patient treated by nonoperative methods than the patient treated by operative stabilization. Pain occurs particularly frequently with multiple wedge fractures of the vertebral body causing thoracic kyphosis.

Postural Reduction Method

1. When the patient is in the supine position, pillows support the head, lumbar region, ankles, and feet.

2. The patient is turned by an experienced lifting team or is log-rolled every two hours.

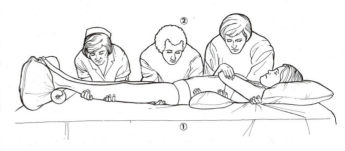

3. In the lateral position, pillows support the patient's head, lumbar spine, legs, and feet.

Note: The postural reduction method may improve the position of the vertebra, but the technique requires a trained nursing team, and its effect on vertebral alignment is unpredictable. The spinal alignment must be scrutinized closely by x-ray for several weeks to ascertain that the injury is truly stable.

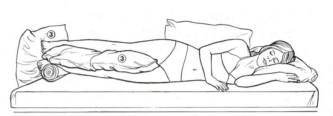

OPERATIVE REDUCTION AND INTERNAL FIXATION METHODS

REMARKS

Most spinal injuries with or without neural damage are sufficiently stable to be managed by postural or nonoperative methods.

The return of neurologic function is almost completely dependent on the degree and completeness of the original injury. Operative treatment has never been shown to increase chances for neurologic recovery. Indeed, wide laminectomy has been repeatedly shown to increase the patient's problem by producing iatrogenic spinal instability.

The prime indication for operative treatment is to stabilize an unstable spine and at the same time decompress the neural structures by adequate reduction of the fracture.

The technology of spinal instrumentation has advanced to the point that spinal stability can be accomplished effectively to permit early mobilization and rehabilitation of the paraplegic or paraparetic patient.

Internal fixation of the spine is especially indicated for incomplete neurologic deficit from unstable injuries.

Operative fixation is of moderate benefit for the patient with complete paralysis in allowing early rehabilitation.

Surgical reduction is probably not indicated, at least acutely, for the patient with a dislocated spine but no, or minimal neurological impairment.

419

Methods of spinal stabilization include:

Distraction Harrington Rods

1. These rods are applicable to unstable flexion-rotation injuries with an intact anterior longitudinal ligament.

2. The distraction rod reduces the spinal fracture by elongating the column.

3. The anterior longitudinal ligament limits elongation.

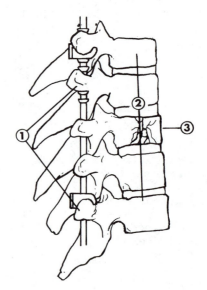

Contraction Harrington Rods

1. Contracting type of Harrington rods are effective in reducing and stabilizing progressive thoracic kyphosis by compressing on the convex side of the kyphosis.

2. Contracting rods are applicable to multiple compression fractures or

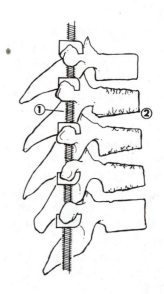

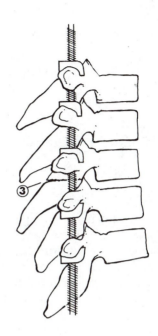

3. Hyperextension (seat belt) fractures.

Circumferential Wiring

1. Circumferential wiring can be used to stabilize dislocated vertebra, or
2. Wire may effectively supplement spinal rods, particularly to allow fixation and segmental fusions.

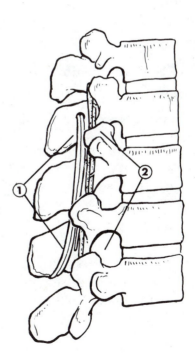

Hyperflexion (Wedge) Fractures of the Vertebral Bodies

REMARKS

This lesion is the result of a pure flexion mechanism.

The posterior ligaments and discs are intact.

This group accounts for over 60 per cent of all spinal injuries.

Vertebrae in the spinal segment between T10 and L3 are most frequently involved. More than one body may be compressed.

Look for associated fractures, such as fractures of one or both calcanei and fractures of bones of the lower legs.

These are stable fractures and require no reduction or immobilization.

If there is any suspicion of neurologic impairment or disruption of posterior support structures, be alert to possible displacement.

Appearance on X-Ray

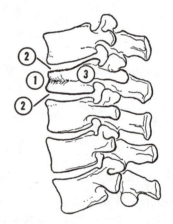

STABLE WEDGE FRACTURE

1. Vertebral body is compressed less than 50 per cent of its height into a wedge shape.

2. Intervertebral discs above and below are intact.

3. Posterior elements are intact and alignment is normal.

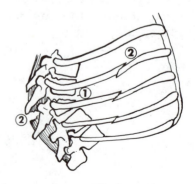

UNSTABLE WEDGE FRACTURE

1. Vertebral body is compressed more than 50 per cent of its height.

2. Adjacent ribs are fractured, and posterior support is lost.

3. Posterior element disruption permits horizontal shift of vertebrae.

Note: These unstable injuries combine hyperflexion and shear mechanisms (see page 414).

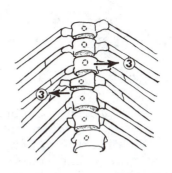

MANAGEMENT OF STABLE HYPERFLEXION (WEDGE) FRACTURE WITHOUT NEUROLOGIC DEFICIT

Immobilization through bed rest for three to five days relieves acute pain.

Ileus may require intravenous fluids.

Begin crutch walking at five to seven days and add hyperextension exercises. Increase these as patient's muscle soreness diminishes.

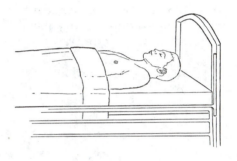

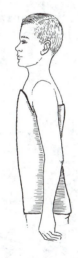

An external extension orthosis or cast usually only adds to the patient's disability and should generally be avoided.

Healing should be complete at four to six months.

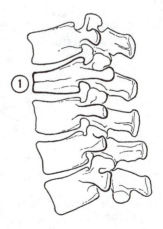

X-Ray After Healing

1. Consolidation of the vertebra is complete without an increase in deformity. This deformity does not preclude excellent function.

Note: Occasionally, compression fractures of adjacent vertebrae may become evident only after several months.

MANAGEMENT OF HYPERFLEXION (WEDGE) FRACTURE WITH NEUROLOGIC DEFICIT

REMARKS

These apparently benign lesions may occasionally produce paraplegia, particularly when instability is not recognized.

In addition, the injured spine may develop progressive kyphotic angulation, causing pain and pressure sores. This frequently follows decompression laminectomy or injury to a child's spine.

Harrington compression instrumentation and fusion are useful for these complications.

1. Wedge compression fracture of T10 with 35-degree deformity prior to decompressive laminectomy.

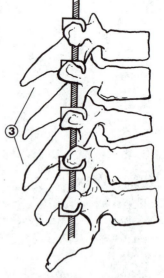

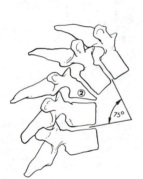

2. Following laminectomy the kyphotic angulation increased to 75 degrees.

3. Stabilization by compression rods and posterior fusion were necessary.

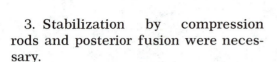

Note: Laminectomy of a fractured spine in a child will inevitably lead to structural deformity.

Flexion-Rotation Fracture-Dislocation of the Thoracolumbar Spine

REMARKS

This mechanism is the most common cause of fracture-dislocation in the spinal segment from T12 to L2.

The momentum of injury ruptures the posterior ligaments or fractures the posterior processes and produces a wedge-shaped slice fracture off the superior portion of the lower vertebra.

The lesion is unstable and is often associated with significant neurologic injury, but in 50 to 60 per cent of cases the nerve roots are spared, and in incomplete lesions there is a good chance for return of neurologic function.

Because of the unstable nature of this injury, open reduction and Harrington distraction-rod fixation offer the best method of decompressing and stabilizing the spinal canal, provided that the anterior longitudinal ligament is intact.

Prereduction X-Ray

ANTEROPOSTERIOR VIEW

1. Lateral displacement of the body of T12.

2. Fracture of the articular processes.

3. Horizontal fracture through the superior portion of the body of L1.

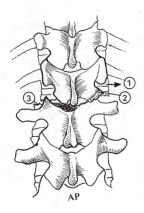

AP

Prereduction X-Ray (Continued)

LATERAL VIEW

    1. Forward displacement of T12.

    2. Fracture of the articular facets.

    3. Slice fracture through the superior portion of the body of L1.

    4. Anterior longitudinal ligament is intact. This is critical for the use of distraction rods.

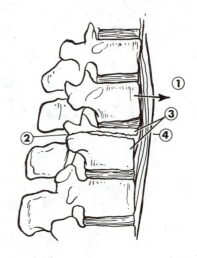

Stabilization by Harrington Distraction Rods and Fusion

STEP I

    1. The patient is in a prone position on the operating table.

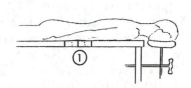

    2. Expose by sharp periosteal dissection two levels above and two levels below the fracture-dislocation.

    3. Carry the subperiosteal dissection laterally to expose the articular facets and the transverse processes.

Note: Don't make any move that might make pressure on the cord. If the spinous processes are freely movable, steady them with a bone forceps while performing the subperiosteal dissection. Remove all loose fragments of bone.

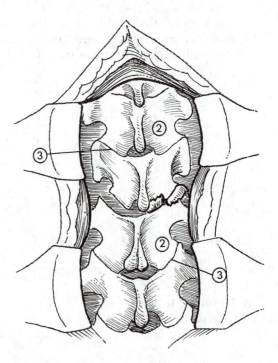

    At this time, inspect the spinal canal and the dura through the tear in the ligamentum flavum. Remove any bone or disc fragment that may be making pressure on the cord.

STEP II

1. Notch the articular facets of the vertebrae two interspaces above and two below the fracture site to seat the superior and inferior hooks.

2. The outrigger is attached to hooks on one side, and distraction is applied slowly while the injured area is carefully observed.

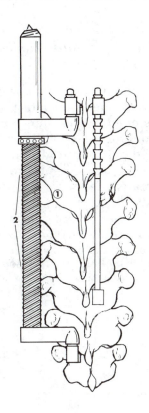

3. During elongation a resistance is encountered as the anterior longitudinal ligament tightens. (If resistance is not felt or the vertebrae are seen to separate, the anterior ligament is torn and a compression rod is needed.)

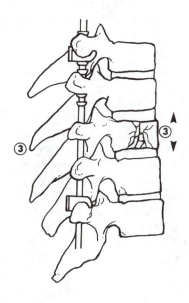

427

Stabilization by Harrington Distraction Rods and Fusion (Continued)

4. A distraction rod of appropriate length is positioned opposite the outrigger. The outrigger is then removed to make room for the second rod.

5. Proceed with lateral gutter fusion two levels above and two below the fracture-dislocation.

Note: Obtain x-rays to evaluate reduction prior to closure. Occasionally, dye left in place after myelogram will demonstrate relief of interspinal obstruction. The fusion should include all the segments fixed by the rods.

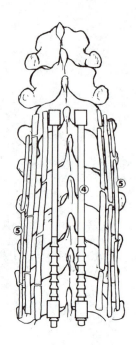

Postoperative Management

For the first 10 days, treatment includes complete bed rest, careful positioning, and regular turning by log-rolling.

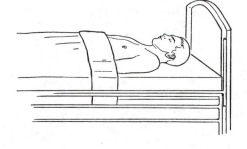

A bivalved body cast or customized polypropylene body jacket is then applied to allow the patient out of bed while protecting any insensitive areas from pressure breakdown.

External support must be continued for at least 20 weeks or until stability is evident.

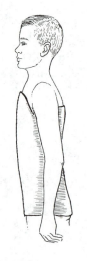

Dislocations of the Lumbar Spine Without Fracture

REMARKS

Lumbar dislocations, which are infrequent, result from either a flexion-rotation mechanism in which flexion predominates or hyperextension-shear mechanism that does not fracture the pedicle (see pages 411–412).

The result of these injuries is rupture of the posterior ligaments with disruption of the disc support structures and either forward or backward dislocation.

Since ligament and disc supports are lost, these lesions are usually unstable.

If postural reduction methods are inadequate, open reduction and posterior stabilization should be employed.

Prereduction X-Rays

FLEXION-ROTATION MECHANISM

1. Forward displacement of L2 on L3.

2. The inferior articular process of L2 is in front of the superior articular process of L3.

3. Wide separation between spinous processes of L2 and L3.

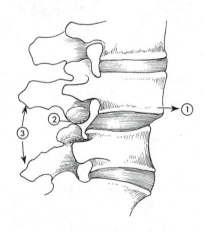

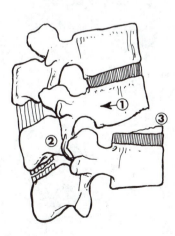

HYPEREXTENSION-SHEAR MECHANISM

1 Posterior displacement (retrolisthesis) of L2 on L3.

2. Inferior articular process of L2 is in back of the superior articular process of L3.

3. Slice fracture off inferior aspect of body of L2 may or may not be evident.

429

Management

This injury frequently can be reduced by simply turning the patient to the prone position. However, redislocation is likely, and open reduction with internal fixation and fusion is needed to prevent further displacement or nerve damage.

Surgical Treatment

POSITION OF PATIENT

1. Patient is in the prone position on an operating table that can be broken in the middle.

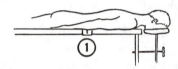

EXPOSURE OF VERTEBRAE

2. Expose by sharp subperiosteal dissection the spinous processes of the dislocated vertebra and of the vertebrae above and below.

3. Carry the subperiosteal dissection laterally as far as the apophyseal joints. Laminectomy is unnecessary, since the dislocation has already opened the canal for inspection.

Note: At this time, if a neurologic deficit exists inspect the dura and the spinal canal through the tear in the ligamentum flavum.

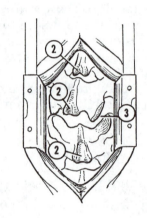

REDUCTION OF DISLOCATION

1. Break the table; this flexes the spine and may disengage the facets.
2. Place a curette under the inferior process of the dislocated vertebra and correct the rotatory displacement.
3. Straighten the table to engage the two articular processes.

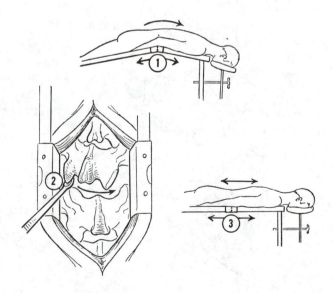

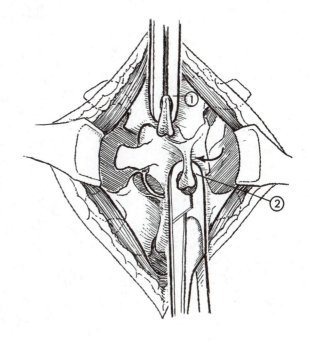

Or:

1. Grasp the spinous processes immediately above and below the dislocation by strong bone forceps, and

2. Reduce the displacement by manipulation under direct vision.

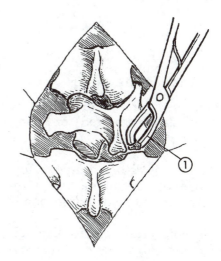

Or:

If the previously described methods of reducing the dislocation fail, a third method may be used.

1. With a small rongeur, nibble away the superior processes of the lower vertebra.

Surgical Treatment *(Continued)*

2. Grasp the spinous processes immediately above and below with strong bone forceps, and

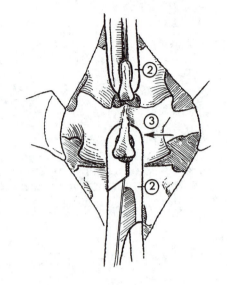

3. Reduce the dislocation by manipulation under direct vision.
4. Extend the table.

STABILIZATION OF THE SPINE

Fixation may be accomplished by Harrington distraction-rod or compression-rod technique (see page 427).

Wire fixation is also a simple, effective method of stabilizing these injuries if Harrington instrumentation is not applicable.

1. Drill hole transversely through spinous process above level of dislocation.

2. Pass two 18-gauge soft wires* through the hole and loop them around the spinous process below the level of dislocation.

3. Use wire tightener to draw neural arches of the dislocated segments together.

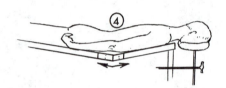

---

*Available from Zimmer Corp, Warsaw, Indiana.

432

4. Laminae and spinous processes above and below dislocation are prepared and are fused with autogenous iliac crest graft.

Note: Obtain interoperative x-ray prior to closure to ascertain completeness of reduction.

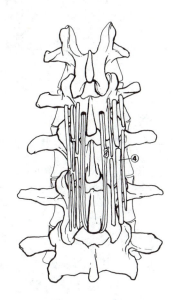

Postoperative X-Ray

LATERAL VIEW

1. L2 is in normal relationship to L3.

2. Articular facets of L2 and L3 are in their normal anatomical positions.

3. Wire is fixed to the spinous processes of L1 through L3.

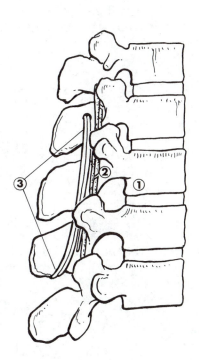

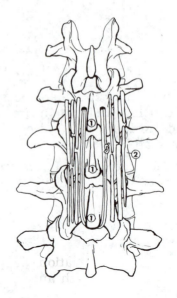

Postoperative X-Ray (Continued)

ANTEROPOSTERIOR VIEW

1. Spinous processes are in normal alignment.
2. Lateral displacement of dislocated facets has been corrected.

Postoperative Management

For the first seven to ten days, treatment includes complete bed rest, careful positioning, and regular turning by log-rolling.

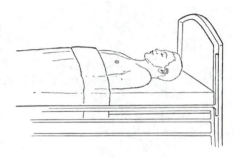

A bivalved body cast or customized polypropylene body jacket is then applied to allow the patient out of bed while protecting any insensitive areas from pressure breakdown.

External support must be continued for at least 20 weeks, or until stability is evident.

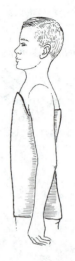

COMPRESSION FRACTURES ASSOCIATED WITH OSTEOPOROSIS

REMARKS

These fractures are usually encountered in elderly patients.

More than one vertebra at different levels may be involved.

Generally, only minimal flexion trauma is sufficient to cause compression of the bodies.

Reduction of fractures is not necessary.

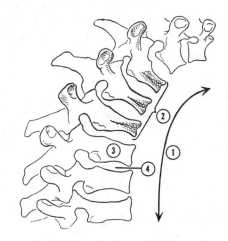

Appearance on X-Ray

1. Dorsal curve is usually increased, and the vertebral column exhibits diffuse osteoporosis.

2. Compression of affected vertebrae may vary in degree.

3. Other vertebral bodies may show cupping.

4. Intervertebral discs may become biconvex.

Management

1. A thoracic extension brace may be used. Frequently, however, this is more uncomfortable than the injury itself, and the patient soon discards it.

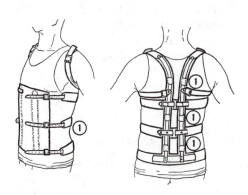

General Therapy

Bed rest should be kept to the minimum needed to relieve symptoms, since any immobilization adds to the primary problem of osteoporosis.

Calcium carbonate, 1 tablet 3 times a day, helps prevent further demineralization, as does a high-protein diet with vitamin D supplement.

Estrogens are of slight value for symptomatic relief.

After acute symptoms subside the patient should begin hyperextension exercises (see page 135).

COMPRESSION FRACTURE — BURSTING TYPE

REMARKS

These are stable injuries because the posterior support elements remain intact. This fracture frequently results in spontaneous interbody fusion, in contrast with other spinal fractures that infrequently fuse spontaneously.

In the lumbar spine, where neural structures occupy only 30 per cent of the canal, neurologic involvement may be minimal and spontaneous recovery is likely without surgical intervention.

Since posterior displacement of the fragmented body into the canal produces the neural injury, decompression, if necessary, should be done anteriorly.

CLOSED TREATMENT WITH SPONTANEOUS FUSION

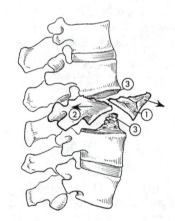

Appearance on X-Ray

1. Disrupted body of L3.
2. Posterior displacement of posterior fragment, which did not produce neurologic injury.
3. Collapsed and disrupted intervertebral disc.

Nonoperative Treatment

Use postural reduction technique for one to two weeks and evaluate neurologic status (see page 419). Then, if nerve function remains unimpaired, apply body cast or polypropylene brace.

1. Enough head traction is applied to force the patient on his toes.
2. The spine is in neutral position.
3. The cast extends from below the clavicles to the symphysis pubis.
4. All bony prominences are well padded.

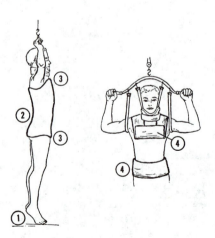

436

Aftercare

The patient begins hyperextension exercises and is then allowed to ambulate with crutches.

Cast is maintained for at least four months. An x-ray taken at four months without the cast often shows that the affected vertebra is fusing spontaneously to the superior vertebral body.

POSTEROLATERAL DECOMPRESSION FOR NEURAL DEFICIT (UNIVERSITY OF MINNESOTA TECHNIQUE)

REMARKS

Compression-burst fractures of the thoracic spine associated with incomplete paralysis from anterior compression of neural elements may be managed first by anterior transthoracic decompression and fusion similar to the procedure for cervical spine injuries (page 355).

Posterior Harrington rod instrumentation should be done first and should be followed in two to three weeks by anterior decompression if the vertebral body fragments remain displaced.

For compression-burst fractures in the thoracolumbar and lumbar regions, a combined posterolateral decompression, Harrington instrumentation, and posterior fusion is most effective. This should only be attempted by individuals thoroughly familiar with anterior and posterior spinal surgery.

Preoperative X-Ray

1. Compression burst fracture of L1 with posterior protrusion of vertebral body fragment has caused incomplete neurologic damage.

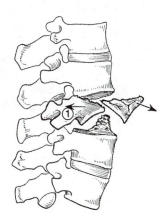

Operative Technique

POSITION OF PATIENT

1. The patient is in the prone position on an operating table.

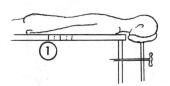

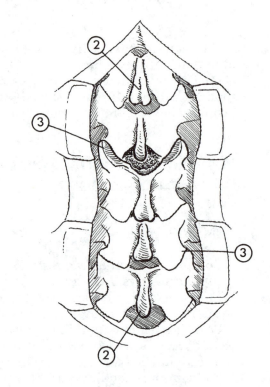

Operative Technique (Continued)

EXPOSURE OF AFFECTED VERTEBRA

2. Expose by sharp subperiosteal dissection the spinous process of the fractured vertebra as well as two vertebrae above and two below.

3. Carry the subperiostel dissection laterally out through the facet joints and transverse processes.

APPLICATION OF HARRINGTON DISTRACTION INSTRUMENTATION

(See also page 427.)

1. After Harrington outrigger is applied, the lateral portion of L1 lamina, the articular processes, and the pedicles are removed with a burr to expose the lateral part of the spinal canal.

2. Nerve root is identified and is followed to the lateral aspect of the dural sac. Loose fragments are removed.

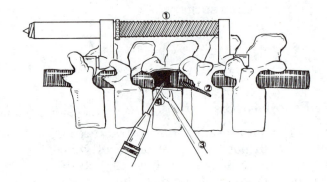

3. The posterior cortex of the vertebral body is undermined with a curette, leaving a thin shell of cortex to protect the dura.

4. The cortical shell of the body is fractured anteriorly away from the dura to complete decompression.

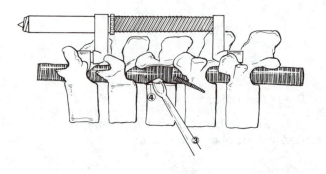

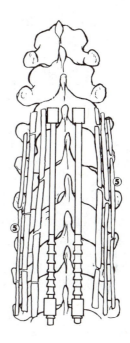

5. Harrington distraction instrumentation and posterior fusion are completed.

Postoperative Management

For the first 10 to 14 days, treatment includes complete bed rest, careful positioning, and regular turning by log-rolling.

A bivalved body cast or customized polypropylene body jacket is then applied to allow the patient out of bed while protecting any insensitive areas from pressure breakdown.

External support must be continued for at least 20 weeks, until stability is evident.

For rehabilitation considerations for patients recovering from paraplegia, see page 453).

Hyperextension-Shear Fracture-Dislocations

REMARKS

The mechanism of this relatively infrequent injury may be recognized clinically by posterior hematoma or abrasions produced when the victim's spine is struck from the rear by a vehicle (see page 412).

Radiographically the mechanism is recognized by a retrolisthesis and by a slice fracture of the inferior aspect of the vertebral body with or without separation of the posterior portion of the vertebra from the anterior portion.

Should both anterior and posterior support structures be disrupted, the spine becomes very unstable and requires internal fixation.

Occasionally hyperextension forces applied to the lower lumbar spine cause a traumatic spondylolisthesis (football lineman's back), which is not unstable but may benefit from a flexion-cast immobilization.

Appearance on X-Ray

1. Dislocation of L2 on L3 with retrolisthesis of L2.

2. If anterior border of L3 strikes the posterior border of L2, a slice fracture of L2 will result.

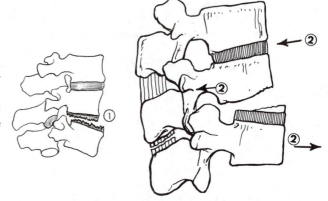

3. With more violent forces the posterior portion of L3 will fracture through the pedicle, producing a very unstable injury.

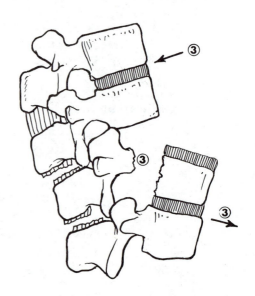

4. Occasionally, pure hyperextension loading of the lower lumbosacral spine will produce a traumatic spondylolisthesis.

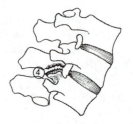

TREATMENT

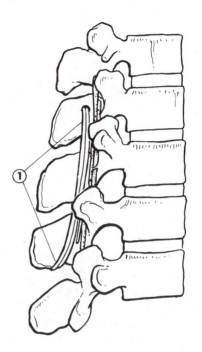

Operative Fixation of Unstable Shear Fracture

The technique chosen for operative fixation depends on the degree of instability.

1. For the unstable dislocation with ligamentous rupture, wire fixation and posterior fusion are sufficient (see page 432).

2. For unstable separation of the anterior and posterior elements, apply Harrington compression rods to the transverse processes and perform posterolateral fusions.

3. Additional stability by means of wiring of the posterior elements may be necessary.

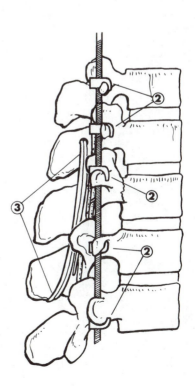

POSTOPERATIVE MANAGEMENT

For the first 10 to 14 days, treatment includes complete bed rest, careful positioning, and regular turning by log-rolling.

A bivalved cast or customized polypropylene body jacket is then applied, and the patient is allowed out of bed. The cast or jacket should remain for at least 20 weeks, or until bony stability is evident on x-ray.

If the patient is paraplegic, a rehabilitation program should be planned and begun as soon as the injuries stabilize.

Application of Cast for Stable Traumatic Spondylolisthesis

1. Body cast is applied with patient flexed 40 degrees at the lumbrosacral spine.

2. The cast extends from the symphysis pubis to the sternum.

3. All bony prominences are well padded.

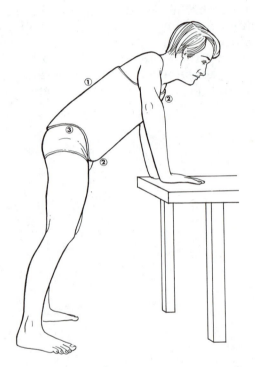

MANAGEMENT

The patient may be allowed to ambulate after the cast has been applied.

Cast immobilization should be continued for six weeks. Then for 6 to 10 weeks longer, flexion exercises should be performed and a lumbosacral flexion orthosis should be worn.

Distraction (Seat Belt Fracture)

REMARKS

This is usually a stable injury, but if both anterior and posterior support structures of the spine are disrupted, internal fixation with Harrington compression rods or wires may be necessary.

Remember that the abdominal contents absorb a good deal of the blunt trauma and may be injured seriously (see page 413).

1. Typical "all-bone" fracture through vertebral body and posterior elements resulting from seat belt injury.

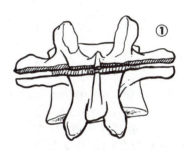

2. Bone and ligament injury from seat belt injury.

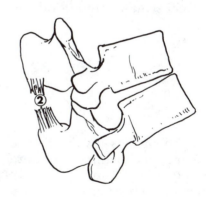

3. Bruising from impact against the seat belt indicates possible damage to abdominal viscus.

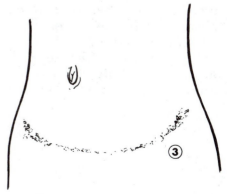

443

Management

Use postural management in bed for seven to ten days and observe closely for any indication of neurologic or abdominal injuries.

Extension body jacket for twelve weeks is sufficient immobilization for healing of "all-bone" injury.

If damage is mainly ligamentous, internal fixation with wire or Harrington compression instrumentation and fusion may be necessary for stability and healing (see page 426).

Lateral Bending Injuries

REMARKS

These are unusual lesions but can produce significant damage to nerve roots or the kidneys.

The usual injury from lateral flexion is an avulsion of the transverse processes on the convex side.

Occasionally, unilateral compression fractures may result.

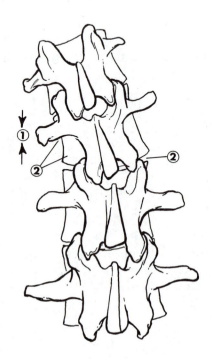

1. This patient was involved in an auto accident and sustained a lateral flexion fracture of L2 and kidney injury requiring nephrectomy.

2. Three months after injury she complained of left knee weakness when climbing stairs. X-rays showed unilateral compression fracture with subluxation of contralateral facets. Myelogram showed compression of L3 root.

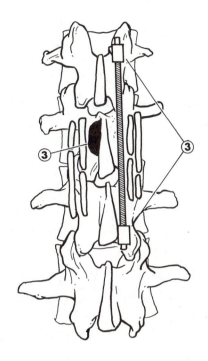

3. Decompression of nerve root, Harrington compression instrumentation, and fusion relieved nerve symptoms.

Isolated Fractures of Lumbar Transverse Processes

REMARKS

These fractures most often involve L2, L3, and L4 and cause little difficulty despite displacement.

It is important not to overtreat the injury. Most require no more than three to five days of bed rest followed by wearing of a lumbosacral corset, if necessary, to allow the patient to return to light work.

The patient should not confuse these isolated avulsion injuries with more serious fractures of the spine.

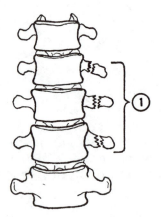

Appearance on X-Ray

1. Fracture of the transverse processes of L2, L3, L4.

Immediate Care

If pain symptoms require, bed rest for three to five days is usually adequate.

Heat and ice massage are helpful, as are flexion and extension exercises.

Lumbosacral corset may allow the patient to walk without rotating the transverse process fractures, but this is purely symptomatic treatment. The corset should be discarded when the patient is free of pain.

Isolated Fractures of Spinous Processes

FRACTURE OF CERVICAL AND FIRST DORSAL SPINOUS PROCESSES

REMARKS

These are usually insignificant fractures and occur as the result of sharp forward flexion of the neck or by a direct blow.

Do not overtreat the lesion.

Consider the associated soft tissue trauma.

Prognosis is good.

Bony union is the rule.

Fibrous union occurs rarely; it may or may not be painful.

In case of fibrous union with pain, excise the fragment.

This fracture does not involve the laminae or the pedicles or bases of the spinous processes, and it differs from an extension injury in this respect.

Appearance on X-ray

CERVICAL FRACTURE

1. Fracture of the spinous process of C7.
2. Displacement is minimal.

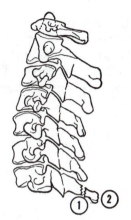

DORSAL FRACTURE

1. Fracture of spinous process of T1.
2. Displacement is minimal.

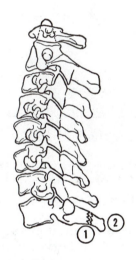

Immobilization

1. Felt collar is applied.
2. Collar is fixed by elastic bandage.
3. Head is in a neutral position.

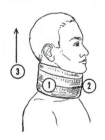

Management

Maintain immobilization for three to four weeks.
Follow with heat and gentle massage.
Avoid strenuous activity for two to four more weeks.

Note: If pain is persistent excise the fragment.

447

FRACTURE OF LUMBAR SPINOUS PROCESSES

REMARKS

This fracture may be produced by sharp hyperflexion or a direct blow; usually the tip of the process is avulsed.

Do not confuse this lesion with fractures of the posterior elements, including fractures of the bases of the spinous processes in hyperextension injuries of the cervical spine (see pages 278–279).

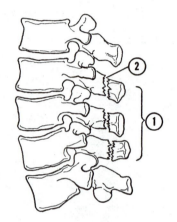

Appearance on X-ray

1. Fracture of spinous processes of L2, L3, and L4.
2. Displacement of fragments is minimal.

Nonsurgical Management

In cases of multiple fractures, bed rest on a firm mattress for seven to ten days relieves pain symptoms.

Follow by crutch walking and wearing of a corset-brace for two to four weeks.

Heat and gentle massage are beneficial.

Normal activity should be resumed.

Flexion and extension back exercises should begin after the third week.

Note: If pain is persistent, excise the fragment.

X-Ray of Fibrous Union

1. Fracture line is still clearly visible. No evidence of bony union is demonstrable.

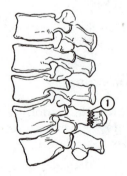

Excision of Loose Fragments

1. The fragment is exposed by subperiosteal dissection.

2. Pick up fragment with forceps and cut it loose from its fibrous tissue bed.

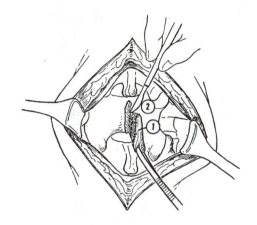

Postoperative Management

In the cervical region, apply a felt collar for two weeks.

In the lumbar region, apply a corset-brace for two to three weeks.

Allow the patient to ambulate on the first or second day.

After removal of sutures, apply heat and allow the patient to begin range-of-motion exercises for the spine.

Shearing Mechanism Producing Complete Lateral Dislocation– With and Without Cord Injury

REMARKS

A violent direct blow to the prominent thoracic spine frequently shears the vertebrae laterally off one another by fracturing the posterior elements and disrupting the anterior support structures.

This commonly results from another person's jumping on or being thrown violently against the victim's back. Most often this occurs with swimming accidents or during plane crashes (see page 414).

Shearing fracture-dislocations may also be produced from the wheel of a vehicle rolling directly over the victim's thoracic spine.

The lateral dislocation usually causes total destruction of the cord structures and complete paraplegia. Rarely the victim will escape neurologic injury.

Open reduction and fixation may prove difficult even for surgeons experienced in Harrington instrumentation.

For the fortunate patient who sustains a lateral shearing fracture-dislocation without neurologic involvement, postural management in bed for two to three months and protective brace support permit spontaneous healing of the displaced bodies. The lateral dislocation of this type is frequently surprisingly stable and does not cause long-term pain symptoms as it fuses spontaneously.

Appearance on X-Ray

1. A direct blow to the back of the thoracic spine during a plane crash has sheared T6 laterally off T5.

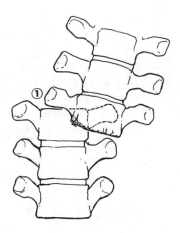

2. The overlap of T5 on T6 is seen on lateral x-ray.

This patient completely escaped neurologic damage! Management was nonoperative with postural turning in bed for two months followed by external brace support for an additional four months.

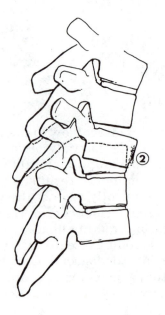

450

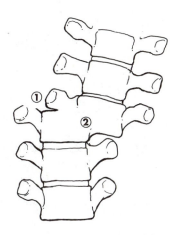

X-Ray After Three Months of Postural Management

1. The dislocation remains unreduced.

2. The fractures are healing and the vertebral bodies are fusing spontaneously.

Gunshot Fractures of the Spine

REMARKS

These unfortunately common civilian injuries are the yields of the production of low-caliber hand guns in this country.

Most often, the victim is an adult man less than 30 years old, and the gunshot fracture produces total paralysis from thoracic or sometimes cervical cord involvement.

Should the bullet fracture the lumbar region, the neurologic deficit is usually incomplete.

These low-velocity gunshot fractures do not cause spinal instability, and there is no real indication for a laminectomy. A laminectomy only increases the chance of spinal instability or leads to problems of spinal infection or draining fistulae.

Occasionally, when the bullet remains lodged in the canal, it may be removed surgically. This should only be done after 3 to 4 days of observation during which the patient's clinical condition can stabilize.

1. A .22-caliber gunshot injury has fractured the thoracic spine and produced total paraplegia.

Note: Laminectomy or fusion is not indicated since this is a stable injury.

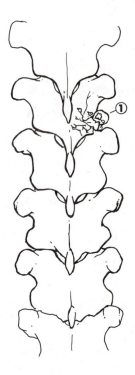

2. A gunshot fracture to the lumbar spine produces an incomplete neurologic deficit. Laminectomy to remove the bullet, which is retained in the canal, should be carried out only after three to four days of observation to permit the patient to stabilize neurologically.

Note: Frequently these patients have gunshot wounds to other structures besides the spine.

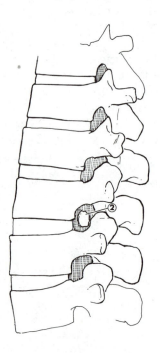

REHABILITATION OF THE PATIENT WITH TRAUMATIC PARAPLEGIA

REMARKS

The physician caring for the patient with a spinal cord injury should not make a commitment solely for the immediate care. Rehabilitation should begin with initial treatment in order to maximize useful recovery of neuromuscular structures.

Pay particular attention to common complications such as pressure sores, urinary retention, and loss of bowel control.

1. Begin a turning regimen as part of the initial care, turning patient from back to side every two hours and using a conventional hospital bed with pillow supports. Avoid special turning frames, especially the circle-electrical types, which add to potential complications.

2. Use an indwelling Foley catheter for the first three to five days until postinjury diuresis occurs. Then institute a program of intermittent catheterization.

3. A bowel program using rectal suppositories regularly each morning will permit bowel control and prevent rectal impaction.

4. Splint limbs in functional position until braces are applied.

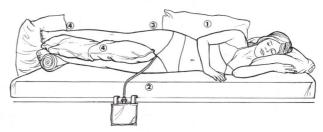

The psychological response to a sudden loss of neuromuscular function varies tremendously but rehabilitation will succeed only if the patient learns to make the most of remaining function rather than bemoan what is lost.

The ideal setting for primary and continuing rehabilitation care of these severely injured patients is a spinal cord center.

Functional Levels in
Spinal Cord Injury

REMARKS

The level of the nerve root involvement or nerve root sparing makes significant differences in key muscle control and functional potentials, either in the cervical or thoracolumbar spine.

1. Involvement from T-1 down to T-8 level leaves the patient with normal hand muscles, permitting independent hygiene and some limited therapeutic standing with posterior leg splints.

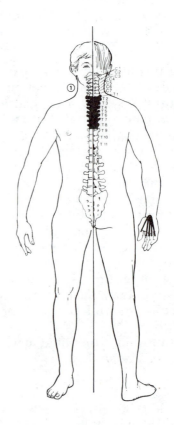

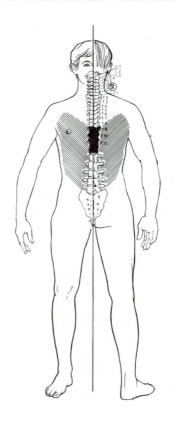

2. Involvement from T-9 down to T-12 level provides trunk stabilizing muscles, which allow some physiologic ambulation with the use of bilateral long leg braces.

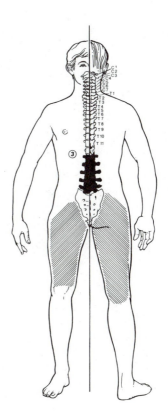

3. Involvement from L-1 down to L-5 level allows pelvic stability, which permits the patient to ambulate with bilateral long leg braces and crutches.

4. Involvement of S-1 to S-2 level leaves the patient with knee extension and hip flexion and permits effective ambulation with short leg braces, crutches, or canes.

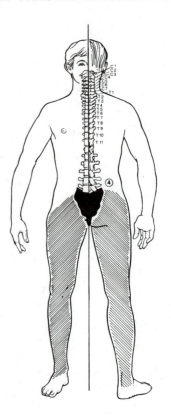

PITFALLS OF MANAGING THORACIC AND LUMBAR SPINE FRACTURES AND DISLOCATIONS

The outcome of spinal fracture or dislocation is generally determined by the mechanism of the original injury and the location and degree of initial damage to the spinal contents. Nevertheless, the opportunities to mitigate or worsen the problem by treatment are truly impressive.

Thoracic and lumbar spine fractures should not be assumed to be stable because the patient has no neurologic deficit. The physician should carefully evaluate for signs of potential instability such as contusion of the spine from direct blows, associated multiple rib fractures, and translational displacement or disruption of both anterior and posterior spinal support structures.

Should the patient complain of even minimal numbness or demonstrate motor or sphincter weakness, the injury must be approached cautiously and judiciously. The degree of spinal injury and instability may not be apparent on the initial x-ray.

Any residual sparing of even slight sensory or motor function indicates an incomplete neurologic lesion. Check the patient carefully for voluntary toe motion, sphincter control, and perianal sensation.

Other injuries that may be life-threatening must be considered. For example, seat belt fractures may cause significant trauma to the patient's liver or diaphragm or may produce bowel infarction. Look for other injuries.

Stable hyperflexion injuries without neurologic damage do not require elaborate closed reduction methods or prolonged immobilization in casts or braces, which would only magnify the patient's problem and add to his disability.

Unstable injuries with neurologic deficit do not require extensive laminectomy to make them more stable. Rather, the neural structures can be decompressed by adequate fracture reduction and fixation using either closed or open methods.

Not every displaced spinal fracture with neurologic damage requires operative fixation. However, ignoring the potential long-term benefits of effective methods of internal fixation because of conservative management is as great an error as inappropriately extensive laminectomy has been. The patient who requires spinal fixation should have the benefit of the best technology available utilized by a surgeon thoroughly familiar with the advantages and disadvantages of current management techniques.

Hasty operative management of the spinal injury does not improve the chances for neurologic recovery, but frequently it can make them worse.

Surgical management of the fractures and dislocations of the spine depends on careful assessment of the skeletal and neurologic problems. It should only be carried out under ideal conditions and after thorough planning.

References

Bedbrook, G. M.: Spinal injuries with tetraplegia and paraplegia. J. Bone and Joint Surg., 61-B:267, 1979.

Bedbrook, G. M.: Treatment of thoracolumbar dislocation and fractures with paraplegia. Clin. Orthop., 112:27, 1975.

Bergqvist, D., Dahlgren, S., and Hedelin, H.: Rupture of the diaphragm in patients wearing seatbelts. J. Trauma, 18:781, 1978.

Bradford, D. S., Akbarnia, B. A., Winter, R. B., et al.: Surgical stabilization of fracture and fracture dislocations of the thoracic spine. Spine, 2:185, 1977.

De Oliveira, J. C.: A new type of fracture-dislocation of the thoracolumbar spine. J. Bone and Joint Surg., 60-A:481, 1978.

Flesch, J. R., Leider, L. L., Erickson, D. L., et al.: Harrington instrumentation and spine fusion for unstable fractures and fracture-dislocations of the thoracic and lumbar spine. J. Bone and Joint Surg., 59-A:143, 1977.

Gertzbein, S. D., and Offierski, C.: Complete fracture-dislocation of the thoracic spine without spinal cord injury. J. Bone and Joint Surg., 61-A:449, 1979.

Holdsworth, F. W.: Fractures, dislocations, and fracture-dislocations of the spine. J. Bone and Joint Surg., 52-A:1534, 1970.

Kaufer, H., and Hayes, J. T.: Lumbar fracture-dislocation. A study of twenty-one cases. J. Bone and Joint Surg., 48-A:712, 1966.

Lewis, J., and McKibbin, B.: The treatment of unstable fracture-dislocations of the thoraco-lumbar spine accompanied by paraplegia. J. Bone and Joint Surg., 56-B:603, 1974.

Roberts, J. B., and Curtiss, P. H.: Stability of the thoracic and lumbar spine in traumatic paraplegia following fracture or fracture-dislocation. J. Bone and Joint Surg., 52-A:1115, 1970.

Skold, G., and Voigt, G. E.: Spinal injuries in belt-wearing car occupants killed by head-on collisions. Injury, 9:151, 1978.

Smith, W. S., and Kaufer, H.: Patterns and mechanisms of lumbar injuries associated with lap seat belts. J. Bone and Joint Surg., 51-A:239, 1969.

Stauffer, E. S., Wood, R. W., and Kelly, E. G.: Gunshot wounds of the spine: The effects of laminectomy. J. Bone and Joint Surg. 61-A:389, 1979.

FRACTURES AND DISLOCATIONS OF THE PELVIS

PERTINENT ANATOMIC
FEATURES AND
MECHANISMS OF INJURY

REMARKS

One of the by-products of the current frequency of motor vehicle accidents is a high incidence of pelvic fractures and disruptions.

Although pelvic fractures should never be taken lightly, approximately 40 per cent may be classified as minor fractures because they are infrequently associated with injury to adjacent structures.

Between 60 and 65 per cent of all pelvic fractures are complicated by other injuries involving the central or peripheral nervous system, the viscera of the thorax, abdomen, or pelvis, or other bones. These are classified as major fractures.

Open pelvic fractures have a 50 per cent death rate from hemorrhage or sepsis, whereas the death rate for all pelvic fractures exceeds 10 per cent.

The most severe pelvic fracture is a crushing injury sustained by a pedestrian or motorcyclist. Victims of this type of injury have as high as 30 per cent chance of dying. Crushing fractures of the pelvis are almost as lethal as injuries to the central nervous system or the chest.

Knowledge of the pertinent anatomic features of the pelvis and of the important adjacent structures as well as recognition of the signs of major and minor pelvic fractures and of their mechanisms of injury are essential for rational and effective treatment.

Anatomic Features

Arch of the Pelvis

1. Summit of the arch (sacrum).
2. Sides of the arch (ilia).
3. Interpubic ligaments.

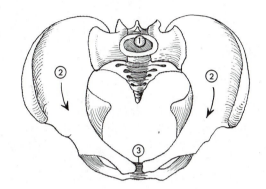

The body weight is transmitted as a vertical force through the sacrum; it then traverses the sacroiliac joints, the bodies of the ilia to the acetabula, and finally the femora.

In the erect position the anterior portion of the pelvic arch bears no weight. The direction of transmission of the body load is discernible in the trabecular pattern of the pelvic arch.

1. Vertical load (body weight).
2. Transmission of thrust through the ilia to
3. The acetabula to
4. The femora.
5. Trabecular pattern of pelvic arch and upper end of the femora.

Note: Pubic and ischial rami are not weight-bearing structures.

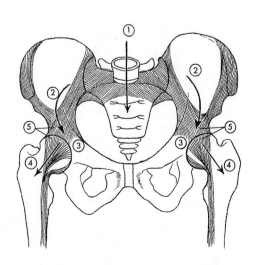

461

Adjacent Structures

Arterial injury is the major cause of death after pelvic fracture.

The vessels within the rich blood supply to the pelvic region that are frequently injured include:

1. External iliac.
2. Internal iliac (hypogastric).
3. Iliolumbar.
4. Lateral sacral.
5. Internal pudendal.
6. Obturator.
7. Common femoral.

In pelvic fractures, peripheral nerves are injured less frequently than arteries, but any adjacent nerve is exposed to damage.

8. Lumbosacral trunk (L4, L5).
9. Femoral nerve (L2, L3, L4).
10. Sciatic nerve (L4, L5, S1, S2, S3).
11. Obturator nerve (L2, L3, L4).
12. Pudendal nerve (S2, S3, S4).

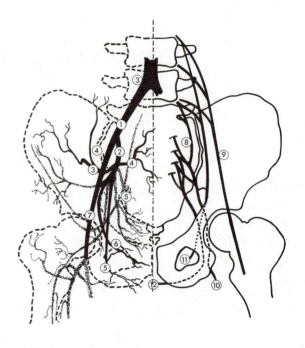

Intrapelvic Structures

Structures commonly injured (in 15 per cent of cases) in pelvic fracture and palpable on rectal or abdominal examination are:

1. Urethra.
2. Urogenital diaphragm.
3. Prostatic urethra.
4. Rectum (any blood on examining finger indicates significant rectal injury).
5. Bladder (if bladder is palpable it is usually not injured).

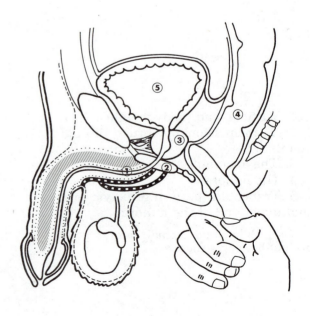

CLASSIFICATION OF PELVIC FRACTURES

Major Fractures

Because of the nature and location of these fractures, injury of adjacent vascular or visceral structures is likely.

1. Fractures of the acetabulum.

2. Bilateral fractures of the pubic or ischial rami.

3. Fracture-separation of the hemipelvis (Malgaigne fracture) combines separation of symphysis pubis or fractures of pubic rami with fractures through the ilium or sacrum or dislocation of the sacroiliac joint.

4. Separation of the symphysis pubis.

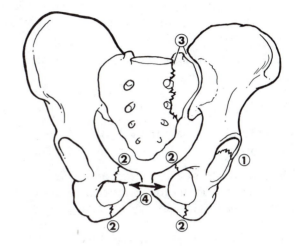

Minor Fractures

These fractures *infrequently* injure the adjacent structures.

1. Fracture of a single pubic ramus.

2. Fracture of a wing of the ilium.

3. Fracture of the ischium.

4. Avulsion fracture from muscle attachments.

5. Undisplaced fracture of the sacrum or coccyx.

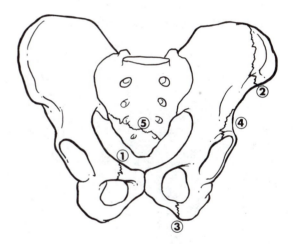

Mechanisms of Injury

Four basic mechanisms are responsible for pelvic fractures:
1. Transmitted force.
2. Direct compression.
3. Avulsion forces.
4. Fatigue forces.

Note: Usually, several mechanisms are working simultaneously.

FORCE TRANSMITTED TO THE PELVIS

The force is transmitted to the pelvis along the shaft of the femur. The type of the resultant injury depends upon the degree of flexion, the position of abduction or adduction of the femur, and the intensity of the force.

Note: This is the basic mechanism acting on victims in automobile accidents.

With Femur Flexion in Neutral Position

When the femur is flexed less than 90 degrees and is in a neutral position, the following injury may be produced:

1. Rupture of the interpubic ligaments and diastasis of the symphysis pubis.
2. Dislocation of the sacroiliac joint.

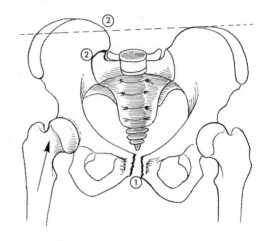

1. Fracture of both pubic rami.
2. Dislocation of the sacroiliac joint.

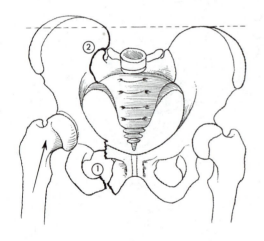

1. Fracture of the superior ramus of the pubis.
2. Fracture of the ischium.
3. Dislocation of the sacroiliac joint.

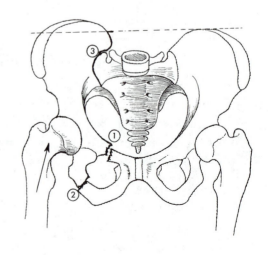

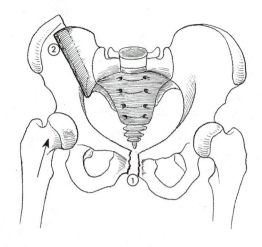

1. Diastasis of the pubic symphysis.
2. Fracture of the ilium adjacent to the sacroiliac joint.

With Femur Flexion and Adduction

When the femur is severely flexed and adducted,
1. Posterior dislocation of the hip may occur.

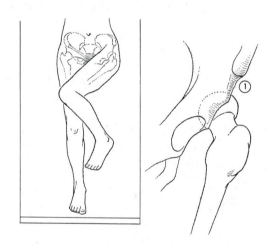

Moderate adduction and flexion of the femur may produce:
1. Posterior dislocation of the hip.
2. Fracture of the posterior rim of the acetabulum.

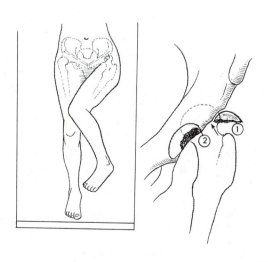

465

With Femur Flexion and Abduction:

1. Fracture of the acetabulum.
2. Central dislocation of the hip.

Note: Fractures and dislocations of the hip are considered separately.

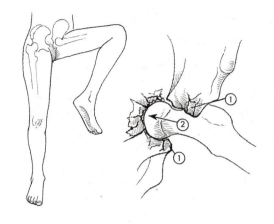

DIRECT COMPRESSION OF THE PELVIS

REMARKS

The fractures produced by direct compression of the pelvis appear similar to those from transmitted force, but the direct compression force disrupts adjacent vessels and pelvic and abdominal viscera much more frequently than transmitted force.

The usual victim of this mechanism is a pedestrian run over by a car, the motorcyclist thrown from his bike, or the farmer dragged by his tractor.

The injury compresses the pelvis from side to side, from back to front, or from inferior to superior (as in a straddle injury).

The prognosis with this type of injury is most serious because of the frequent disruption of adjacent structures.

Side-to-Side Compression

1. Disruption of the interpubic ligaments.
2. Dislocation of the sacroiliac joint.
3. Medial displacement of one half of the pelvic arch.

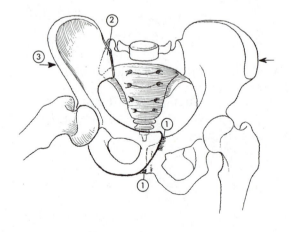

Anterior-Posterior (Front-to-Back) Compression

1. Disruption of the interpubic ligaments and wide diastasis of the symphysis pubis.
2. Dislocation of the sacroiliac joint.

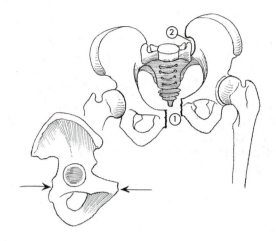

Inferior-Superior Compression (Straddle Injury)

1. Fractures of both superior pubic rami.
2. Fractures of both inferior pubic rami.

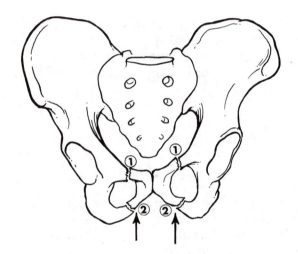

AVULSION FORCES

REMARKS

Minor pelvic fractures are produced by excessive muscle contraction, especially in adolescents engaged in strenuous activity.

They are not complicated by injuries to abdominal or pelvic viscera.

467

1. Avulsion of the anterior superior iliac spine (by action of the sartorius).

2. Avulsion of the anterior inferior iliac spine (by action of the rectus femoris).

3. Avulsion of the tuberosity of the ischium (by action of the hamstring muscles).

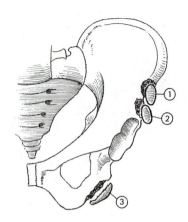

FATIGUE FORCES

Fatigue fractures, or stress fractures, although rare, may occur in the pubic rami.

These lesions may occur in women during the last months of pregnancy or in army recruits after forced marches.

1. Stress fracture of superior ramus in a pregnant woman.

2. Stress fracture of the inferior ramus in a young adult male.

Note: Fractures of this type should not be confused with more serious fatigue fractures of the femoral neck.

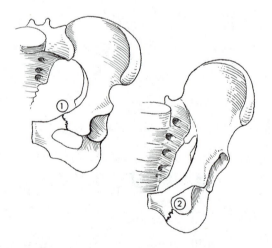

GENERAL PRINCIPLES OF TREATMENT FOR PELVIC INJURIES

Differentiate promptly between the relatively uncomplicated minor pelvic fracture and the major fracture with complications that may kill the patient.

While obtaining the patient's history, determine and note the cause of injury. Motorcycle accident and injury to pedestrian by motor vehicle are the most lethal, as they are most likely to cause disruption of adjacent vessels and viscera by direct violence.

Determine the time the patient last voided. If the patient has not voided recently, do not try to make him void, because urine extravasation might occur. Also, note the time the patient last ate or drank; a bladder that was empty when the pelvis was fractured is not likely to be ruptured.

Note any associated injuries to the head, chest, abdomen, and limbs.

On initial physical examination, check the vital signs and the status of the airway. Then remove all the patient's clothes to permit complete anterior and posterior examination of the head, chest, spine, abdomen, pelvis, and limbs.

Be sure to inspect the perineum for evidence of open pelvic fracture as well as for ecchymosis, swelling, or urine extravasation.

Bleeding from the rectum or vagina may indicate lacerations and direct communication with the pelvic fracture.

Evaluate pelvic stability by palpating the symphysis pubis and pubic rami and by gently compressing and distracting the iliac wings.

In a male patient, always check by rectal examination for displacement of the prostate gland, which would indicate rupture of the urethra. In females, check for vaginal lacerations and perineal injury.

Before and during physical examination, if the patient shows any signs of shock, treat by administering oxygen, promptly replacing blood volume, and monitoring with a central venous pressure line. Avoid turning the patient with an unstable pelvis; instead, for signs of shock, apply external compression or military antishock trousers (MAST, or "G" suit).

Obtain x-rays of the chest, pelvis, and other regions of suspected injury. A plain film of the abdomen and a simultaneous "one-shot" intravenous pyelogram should also be obtained, but treatment of the severely injured patient should never be delayed for a complete IVP series.

Urologic investigation should include one attempt at clean catheterization, which if successful virtually excludes the possibility of complete rupture of the urethra. If the perineum shows sign of direct or straddle injury, a urethrogram should be obtained before catheretization is attempted. If catheretization is unsuccessful, a cystostomy should be performed.

If catheterization is successful, two x-rays should be taken, one of the bladder with 200 ml of radiopaque dye and one after the bladder is drained of the dye. These will demonstrate intraperitoneal or retroperitoneal rupture.

Peritoneal aspiration or lavage to look for signs of blood in the cavity is the next step in detecting intra-abdominal injury associated with pelvic fracture, especially in a patient who is unconscious or in severe shock. Lavage the peritoneum in the midline above the umbilicus—a lavage catheter inserted below the umbilicus may penetrate into the retroperitoneal hematoma.

If shock persists despite adequate replacement of blood volume (5 to 6 units are usually sufficient) and examination of peritoneal aspirate is unrevealing, arteriographic studies should be performed in order to locate the site of bleeding. Selective arterial embolization of bleeding vessels is particularly useful for treatment of retroperitoneal hemorrhage. Before moving a patient whose status is precarious, apply military antishock trousers (MAST) and arrange for blood volume replacement to be continued during arteriographic study.

Operative treatment is indicated for a nonretroperitoneal source of bleeding and for rupture of a viscus. Prompt surgical treatment is also necessary for the life-threatening open pelvic fracture that communicates with the rectum. A diverting colostomy with disimpaction and antibiotic irrigation of the rectum, primary urethral repair, and perineal drainage are essential to avoid the lethal septic complications of open pelvic fracture.

One major intraabdominal injury associated with pelvic fractures but frequently overlooked is rupture of the diaphragm. Keep this possibility in mind on initial evaluation and during follow-up care.

Intraperitoneal rupture of the bladder should be repaired surgically.

Retroperitoneal urethral disruption is treated by primary repositioning of the prostatic urethra with repair of any resultant short stricture of the urethra. This procedure should be delayed, however, until hemorrhage from the fracture has ceased because retroperitoneal dissection would accelerate hemorrhage and cause exsanguination.

The major orthopedic problem in management of pelvic injuries relates to the sacroiliac joint, for which closed reduction methods usually give satisfactory results.

MANAGEMENT OF MINOR PELVIC FRACTURES

REMARKS

In minor pelvic fractures, the continuity of the pelvic ring remains intact, and adjacent structures are rarely injured. Examples of such fractures are:

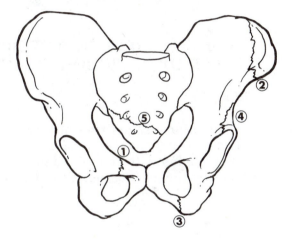

1. Fracture of a single pubic ramus.
2. Fracture of a wing of the ilium.
3. Fracture of the ischium.
4. Avulsion fracture.
5. Undisplaced fracture of the sacrum or coccyx.

   Note: A displaced sacral fracture frequently causes neurologic injury.

   This group of lesions exhibits no or only minimal displacement of the fragments.
   Isolated fractures of the wing of the ilium may cause rigidity of the abdominal muscles and tenderness in the lower quadrant of the same side. (The abdominal muscles arise from the iliac crest.)
   Blood loss in fractures of the wing of the ilium may be substantial.
   Isolated fractures of the sacrum may be difficult to demonstrate on x-rays; a rectal examination may be helpful in establishing the diagnosis.
   Fractures of the sacrum are frequently associated with bilateral fractures of the pubic rami and may well be considered major fractures (see page 475).
   Isolated pelvic fractures require no external fixation, suspension, or operative intervention.
   Perfect anatomic alignment of the fracture is not essential for complete recovery of function.
   Adjacent vessels and viscera are infrequently injured.

GENERAL MANAGEMENT

The patient should be recumbent on a firm bed until pain symptoms remit.

Protected crutch walking is begun usually by the third to fifth day.

Crutches may be discarded when the patient is free of pain, usually three to five weeks after injury.

This general management is applicable to fracture of a single pubic ramus, fracture of a wing of the ilium, and fracture of the ischium.

Avulsion Fractures

AVULSION OF THE ANTERIOR SUPERIOR OR ANTERIOR INFERIOR ILIAC SPINE

REMARKS

This injury results from powerful contracture of muscles, especially in adolescents engaged in strenous activity.

Bony union with complete restoration of function is the rule.

Restoration of fragments to their anatomic position is not essential.

Appearance on X-Ray

1. Avulsion fracture of anterior superior iliac spine (by action of sartorius).

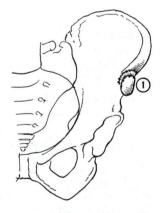

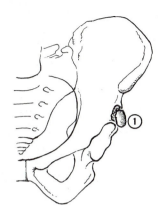

1. Avulsion fracture of anterior inferior iliac spine (by action of rectus femoris).

Management

The patient should rest in bed with the hip and knee slightly flexed for two to three days, until acute pain subsides.

Hip muscles should be protected by crutch walking for four to six weeks.

Complete restoration to normal function should occur.

AVULSION OF TUBEROSITY OF ISCHIUM

REMARKS

This injury results from powerful contractions of the hamstring muscles and is common in athletes who run track or hurdle.

The amount of separation of fragments varies.

Bony union is the rule. Occasionally, fibrous union occurs (especially if fragments are widely separated).

Repositioning of fragments is not necessary for a good result.

Normal function is the rule in all cases of bony union and in most cases of fibrous union.

Excision of the fragments is indicated only in patients in whom fibrous union has occurred and who still have pain.

Appearance on X-Ray

1. Avulsion of the tuberosity of the ischium with minimal displacement.

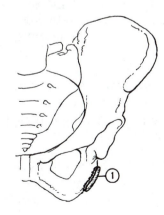

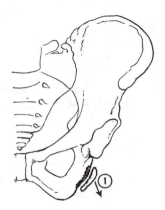

Appearance on X-Ray (*Continued*)

1. Avulsion of the tuberosity of the ischium with excessive displacement.

Management

In acute cases, rest in bed for one or two weeks should be sufficient. Activity should be restricted for ten to twelve weeks.

Note: In cases of fibrous union, if pain persists, excise the avulsed fragments.

Transverse Fracture of the Sacrum with Displacement

A direct, violent blow to the low back as the patient stands with the hips flexed and the knees extended produces a fracture at the junction of S1 and S2. This is, in essence, a traumatic spondylolisthesis of the sacrum.

Owing to the superimposed bony structures, this injury may be difficult to detect on a standard anteroposterior x-ray. A true lateral view of the sacrum will demonstrate forward displacement of the upper portion of the sacrum on the lower.

Frequently, the sacral fracture is associated with multiple transverse process fractures produced by a violent contraction of the quadratus lumborum.

The significance of the transverse fracture of the sacrum depends on the degree of displacement but, quite commonly, the injury causes a significant neurologic impairment.

A displaced sacral fracture is unstable and may displace further with flexion.

Consistently, the patient sustains damage to the sacral nerve roots that may not be recognized for several days after injury. The major problem is the loss of bowel and bladder control as well as loss of sensation in the perineum and upper thigh.

If displacement is minimal, the injury may be treated by closed methods with anticipation that the neurologic function will return.

When displacement is pronounced, operative treatment is indicated in order to decompress the sacral nerves and reduce and fuse the fracture.

Patients with displaced and unreduced transverse sacral fractures frequently suffer from chronic pain problems and inability to stand for very long.

Transverse Fracture with Minimal Displacement

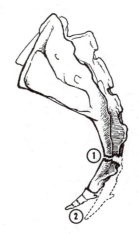

1. The fracture line was not evident on the anteroposterior view but is demonstrable on the lateral view.

2. There is minimal forward displacement of the sacrum, which was associated with urinary retention and some numbness in the perineum.

Note: Displacement of this minimal degree requires no reduction, and with time, the neurologic deficit will clear.

Transverse Fracture with Marked Displacement (Traumatic Spondylolisthesis of the Sacrum)

PREOPERATIVE X-RAY

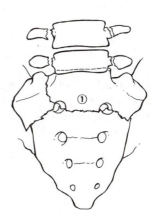

1. Anteroposterior x-ray of the lumbosacral region, occurring in a man who was injured by a heavy weight falling on his back while he was leaning forward, shows multiple transverse process fractures and a suspicion of a sacral fracture.

Transverse Fracture with Marked Displacement (Traumatic Spondylolisthesis of the Sacrum) (Continued)

2. The lateral view shows pronounced forward displacement of the upper sacrum. This patient had loss of bowel and bladder control as well as severe back pain.

Note: Transverse fractures of this degree of displacement should be treated by laminectomy and fusion to provide the patient with a relatively pain-free back.

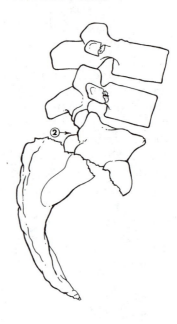

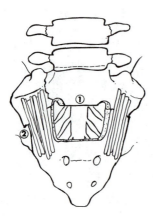

Postoperative X-Ray

1. The sacral laminectomy was done to decompress the sacral nerve roots.

2. The sacrum was fused laterally across the fracture site.

3. The position of the fracture was improved by hyperextending the hips at the time of laminectomy.

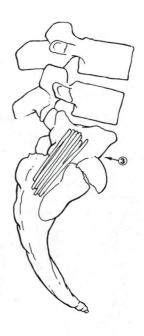

Fracture of the Coccyx with Displacement

REMARKS

This lesion is usually the result of direct violence.
It may occur in women during a difficult delivery.

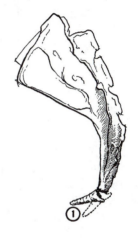

Appearance on X-Ray

1. Forward dislocation of the distal segments of the coccyx.

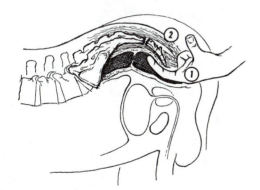

Reduction by Digital Manipulation

1. A finger is inserted into the patient's rectum.
2. The coccygeal fragment is manipulated backward into its normal position.

Postreduction Management

If pain is severe, bed rest for seven to ten days is indicated.
Apply an adhesive strapping around the buttocks for two to four weeks.
Hot tub baths once or twice a day aid healing.

Note: If pain persists after several months of conservative treatment, surgical excision of the coccyx is indicated.

477

MANAGEMENT OF MAJOR PELVIC FRACTURES AND DISLOCATIONS

Single Breaks in the Continuity of the Pelvic Ring

REMARKS

Unilateral fractures of the pubic and ischial rami are the most common fractures of the pelvis, accounting for 35 to 50 per cent of all pelvic fractures.

They are infrequently associated with arterial, urinary, or abdominal injuries, in contrast to bilateral fractures of the pubic rami.

However, fractures of the sacrum and ilium may be associated with severe local hemorrhage.

In all degrees of separation of the symphysis pubis, check the sacro-iliac joints for possible subluxation.

All the lesions described here are treated in the same manner.

Appearance on X-Ray

1. Separation of the symphysis pubis.

2. Fracture of the pubic rami; this is the most common fracture.

3. Fracture of the ilium.

4. Vertical fracture of the sacrum. Unlike transverse sacral fracture, this injury does not usually cause neurologic deficit (see page 475).

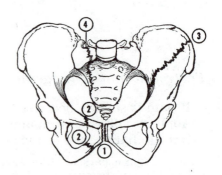

Management

The patient should be recumbent on a firm bed for one to two weeks.

He should walk with crutches after a few days and should discard them by six to eight weeks.

Active exercises of lower extremities and trunk, first assisted and within the patient's tolerance of pain, then against resistance, are started after seven to ten days. This stimulates soft tissues to return rapidly to normal and prevents cicatrix formation and fixation of joints.

Complete recovery should occur in eight to ten weeks.

Subluxation of the Sacroiliac Joint

REMARKS

This rare injury can usually be treated by application of a mini-spica cast.

Prereduction X-Ray

1. The ilium is displaced upward and backward in relation to the sacrum.

2. The ilium is closer to the midline than the opposite ilium.

Note: As an isolated lesion, subluxation of the sacroiliac joint is rare.

It may be difficult to establish the diagnosis by x-ray.

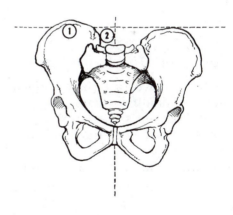

Reduction

Anesthesia is rarely indicated.

1. Patient is placed on a fracture table on his uninjured side; the ilium and trochanter of the sound side rest on the pelvic support.

2. An assistant supports the legs, one above the other.

3. The surgeon stands behind the patient and makes firm pressure on the iliac crest, pushing downward and forward and rotating the displaced ilium toward the unaffected side of the pelvis.

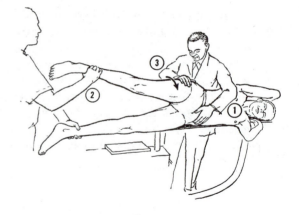

Application of Mini-Spica Cast

1. Apply cast over a lightly padded stockinette, molding firmly downward on the patient's iliac crest.

2. Use a hinged knee-joint for ease of ambulation.

3. The other hip is left out of plaster.

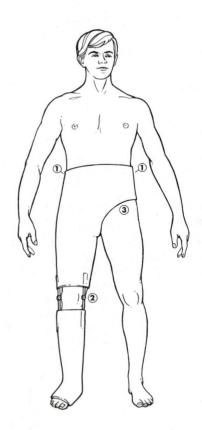

480

X-Ray After Cast Application

1. The displacement of the ilium is reduced.

2. Articular surfaces of the ilium and sacrum on the affected side are in anatomic position when compared with the normal side.

Note: For severe disruption of the sacroiliac joint with fracture, skeletal traction in conjunction with application of mini-spica cast may be necessary (see p. 492).

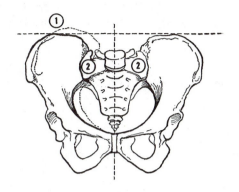

Postreduction Management

Plaster immobilization is continued for eight to ten weeks. The patient is encouraged to walk in the cast using crutches.

If pain persists and is severe for some time after removal of the cast, surgical arthrodesis of the sacroiliac joint may be necessary. A decision regarding arthrodesis should not be made for at least a year after injury.

High-Risk Major Pelvic Fractures

REMARKS

Certain types of pelvic fractures carry a high risk of associated injury, particularly when they result from a severe, direct crushing accident. Most commonly they are produced by automobile-pedestrian or motorcycle accidents.

Death from exsanguination or infection of the pelvic hematoma is frequently a sequela of:

Open pelvic fractures.

Malgaigne's fracture-dislocation of the hemipelvis.

Double breaks in the anterior segment of the pelvic ring.

To abort the lethal complications from these injuries, the physician should systematically consider the following protocol while resuscitating the patient:

Potential Problem	*Evaluation and Treatment*
Hypovolemic shock from intra-abdominal injury.	Upper midline peritoneal lavage (watch for diaphragmatic rupture.)
Shock requiring less than 2000 ml in 8 hours.	Continue standard replacement therapy.
Shock requiring blood replacement of more than 2000 ml in 8 hours.	Apply military antishock trousers. (Caution: If MAST is applied, it can be released only when the patient is normotensive and the blood pressure is being carefully monitored.
Continued bleeding after application of MAST	Angiography and venography to detect site of bleeding.
Bleeding from major iliac or femoral vessels.	Direct (surgical) repair.
Bleeding from retroperitoneal vessels. Genitourinary injury.	Selective embolization. Urethrogram and cystogram to determine site of injury. Intraperitoneal bladder rupture should be repaired. Retroperitoneal rupture may be treated by repositioning of the prostate, if necessary.
Open pelvic fracture with rectal laceration.	This is evident on rectal examination and requires bypass colostomy with irrigation from above and below.
Open pelvic fracture with vaginal laceration.	Close mucosa and drain retrovaginal space.

HYPOVOLEMIC SHOCK FROM PELVIC FRACTURES

REMARKS

Hypovolemic shock is indicated when the patient remains hypotensive despite adequate blood volume replacement (2000 ml given over 8 hours should be adequate).

1. Evaluate for intraperitoneal bleeding by peritoneal lavage using a supraumbilical midline approach to avoid retroperitoneal hematoma.

2. Apply military anti-shock trousers (MAST) to compress the pelvis externally and immobilize the fracture. This also provides an autotransfusion by shunting blood from the legs.

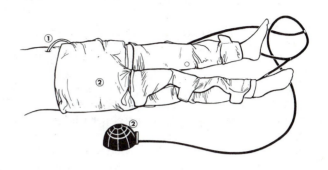

Note: If there are associated fractures of the femur or tibia, MAST application for longer than two to three hours can produce ischemic muscle necrosis from compartment syndromes. Apply a spica cast promptly for an unstable pelvic fracture combined with lower limb fractures.

For a complete description of MAST application see Appendix (page 2146).

3. If the hypovolemic shock continues despite application of MAST or pelvic spica, perform arteriograms and venograms, if necessary, to locate the bleeding site.

4. If internal iliac (hypogastric) artery or its branches are the source of extraperitoneal bleeding, selective arterial embolization with Gelfoam strips is most effective for controlling hemorrhage. (Apply mini-spica after embolization.)

5. If external iliac artery or its branches are the source of bleeding surgical repair is necessary.

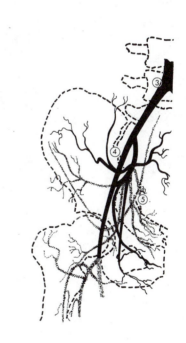

UROLOGIC INJURY

Any major pelvic fracture is likely to injure the urinary tract, especially in males.

Suspect urologic injury if there is:

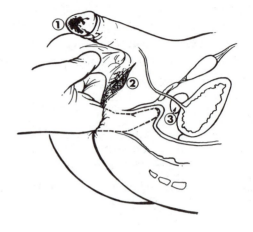

1. Blood at the external meatus.
2. Contusion, laceration, or ecchymosis in the perineum from straddle injuries.
3. Upward and backward displacement of the prostate (as revealed by rectal examination).

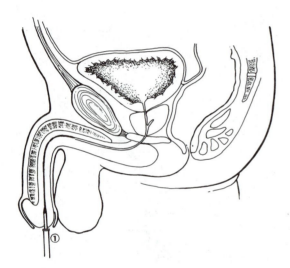

If any of these findings are present:
1. Perform urethrography by injecting 20 ml water-soluble radiopaque solution into the urethral meatus to demonstrate urethral tear on x-ray.

2. If the urethrogram is normal, insert catheter and fill bladder with 200 ml of radiopaque solution to show intraperitoneal rupture by cystography.

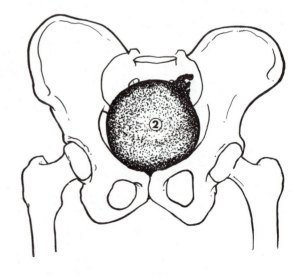

3. Take another x-ray after bladder is empty to show retroperitoneal rupture.

Note: An intraperitoneal bladder rupture should be repaired promptly. Attempted primary repair of retroperitoneal rupture, however, is fraught with technical difficulty and accelerates hemorrhage. If the membranous urethra is completely ruptured and the prostate is dislocated, primary repositioning of the prostate is indicated when patient is no longer in danger of exsangination.

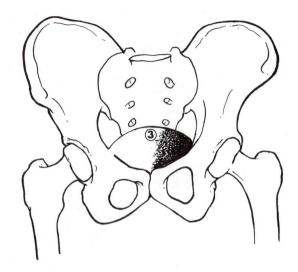

Repositioning of Fracture-Dislocated Prostate (After Turner-Warwick)

1. Retropubic hematoma is evacuated and drained.
2. Plastic Foley catheter is passed through penile urethra and is used for aligment of urethral end.
3. Suprapubic catheter is inserted for bladder drainage.
4. A single nylon sling suture passes through the perineum and through the prostate in front of the urethra.
5. The suture is tied over perineal packs.

Note: Management of the disrupted urethra permits drainage without aggravating hemorrhage. Secondary repair of any short urethral stricture may be necessary later.

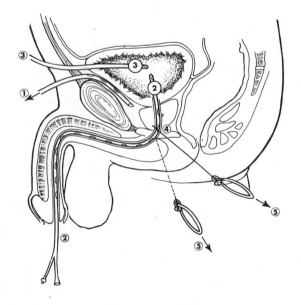

Occasionally, stabilization of the symphysis pubis fracture-dislocation may be necessary in conjunction with the repair of the urethral injury.

A mini-spica cast is most helpful when applied promptly to aid pelvic stability and diminish hemorrhage.

STABILIZATION OF PELVIC FRACTURE-DISLOCATION WITH URETHRAL INJURY

Open reduction of a pelvic fracture or symphysis pubis disruption is rarely necessary except in conjunction with a urethral repair.

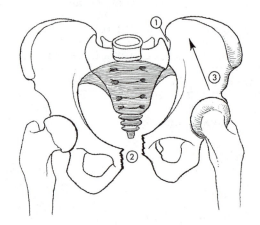

Appearance on X-Ray

1. Subluxation of sacroiliac joint.
2. Wide diastasis of symphysis pubis.
3. Upward and backward displacement of the hemipelvis.

Operative Reduction

1. In conjunction with the urethra repair the pubic bones are exposed extraperitoneally.
2. Make pressure on the sides of the pelvis to reduce the diastasis.
3. Insert heavy screws through each pelvic bone.
4. Bind the screws together with 18-gauge wire.

Note: Add additional stability by immediate application of a mini-spica cast.

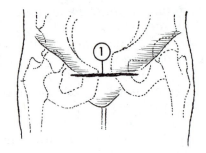

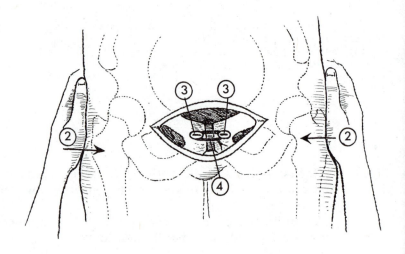

Postoperative Management

Institute a daily program of arm and leg strengthening exercises.

The patient may begin walking in the mini-spica cast if the urologic problem allows.

At ten to twelve weeks the cast is removed and progressive weight bearing is permitted.

Lethal Injuries from Open Pelvic Fractures

REMARKS

Because of the frequency of massive hemorrhage or sepsis, mortality from open pelvic fractures exceeds 50 per cent.

Blood volume replacement must be prompt in conjunction with surgical repair of major vascular injuries and selective arteriographic embolization for retroperitoneal hemorrhage.

Rectal and vaginal examination should be done in all pelvic fractures so as to detect any direct communication with the fracture. Any blood on the finger indicates significant associated damage.

Communicating rectal injuries are best treated aggressively with diverting colostomy and disimpaction and irrigation of the rectum to avoid otherwise inevitable sepsis.

Repair of urethral injuries and perineal (not peritoneal) drainage must also be done promptly to avoid sepsis.

Tetanus and intravenous antibiotics are begun preoperatively and adjusted postoperatively according to results of wound cultures.

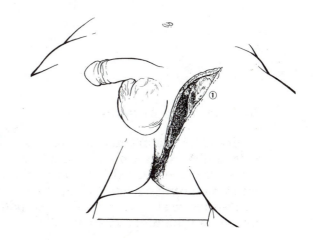

1. Open pelvic fracture may be grossly obvious, as in this farmer who was dragged by his tractor or

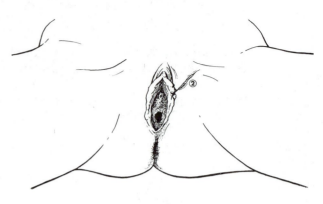

2. May be subtle, as in this woman with a straddle injury.

3. Diverting colostomy is performed promptly.

4. A second surgical team disimpacts and irrigates the distal rectal segment with an antibiotic solution.

5. Transperineal drains or packs are essential.

Note: If the vagina has been lacerated by the pelvic fracture, the vaginal mucosa should be sutured and the retrovaginal space should be drained transperineally.

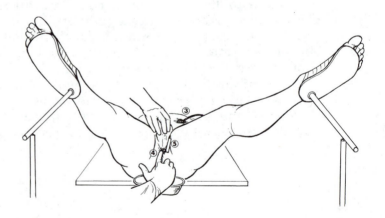

Postoperative Management

Additional wound debridement and drain adjustment are essential, as is antibiotic administration according to results of wound culture.

A mini-spica cast should be applied to immobilize the pelvis while accommodating colostomy apparatus and perineal wounds.

Intensive systemic care of these patients' multiple problems will increase their chances of survival.

488

Upward Dislocation of the Hemipelvis (Malgaigne Fracture-Dislocation)

REMARKS

Dislocation of the hemipelvis carries all the risk of associated injuries described above but, unlike most pelvic fractures, frequently requires reduction.

Except for an occasional case of separation of the symphysis pubis that requires internal fixation after urethral repair, the major problems of orthopedic management of pelvic injury are related to disruption of the sacroiliac joint.

Upward dislocation of the hemipelvis (Malgaigne fracture-dislocation), in which there are breaks in both the anterior and posterior segments of the pelvic ring, can be reduced by distal femoral traction combined with use of a double sling that rotates the pelvic arches internally and forward.

Once accomplished, the reduction can be maintained with a femoral traction pin incorporated in a mini-spica cast.

Reduction of the sacroiliac joint will not ensure the patient freedom from occasional sacroiliac pain during healing. Significant sacroiliac pain that persists for longer than one year after injury can be relieved by sacroiliac fusion.

MALGAIGNE FRACTURE-DISLOCATIONS NOT REQUIRING REDUCTION

REMARKS

Reduction is indicated primarily for the sacroiliac joint. Persistent dislocation of the symphysis pubis is surprisingly asymptomatic.

Appearance on X-Ray

1. Fractures of both pubic rami.
2. Separation of the sacroiliac joint without dislocation.

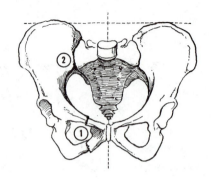

1. Fracture of the superior ramus of the pubis.
2. Fracture of the ischium.
3. Separation of the sacroiliac joint without dislocation.

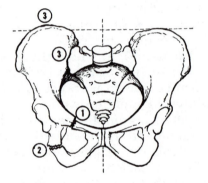

1. Dislocation of the symphysis pubis.
2. Fracture through the ilium.

Note: These fractures may be treated primarily by a mini-spica cast without preliminary skeletal traction.

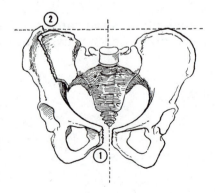

MALGAIGNE FRACTURE-DISLOCATION REQUIRING REDUCTION

Appearance on X-Ray

1. Wide separation of the symphysis pubis.

2. Wide upward displacement of sacroiliac joint.

Note: Preliminary skeletal traction is necessary to reduce the upward displacement of the hemipelvis prior to spica cast application.

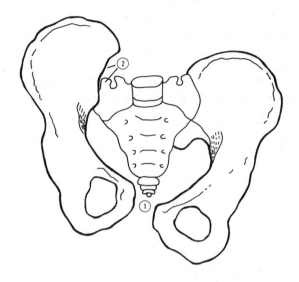

Reduction by Traction and Double Pelvis Sling

1. A threaded 6-mm or 8-mm Steinmann pin is inserted in the distal femur and 25 lb (11.3 kg) of traction is applied to reduce upward displacement.

2. Crossover pelvic slings rotate the pelvic arch internally and forward.

Note: The displacement usually reduces promptly so that a mini-spica cast may be applied when the patient is comfortable, usually within the first three to five days.

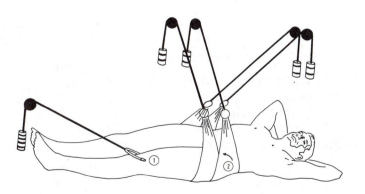

491

Application of Mini-Spica Cast

Light sedation should be used, but anesthesia is rarely necessary.

1. The patient is placed on a fracture table while femoral traction is maintained by an assistant.

2. Mini-spica cast is applied over a lightly padded stockinette.

3. Molding well over the iliac crest helps maintain reduction of the pelvic arch.

4. The other hip is left out of the plaster.

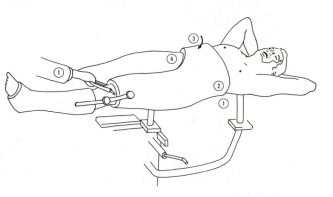

5. Femoral pin is incorporated in plaster.

6. Knee hinge allows easier crutch walking.

Note: Prompt application of mini-spica cast diminishes blood loss and decreases the risk of pulmonary embolism that is associated with prolonged immobilization.

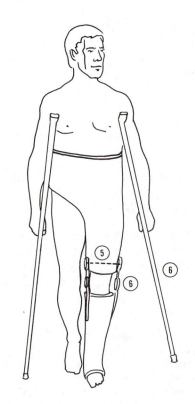

Postreduction X-Ray

1. Widening of symphysis pubis has diminished.

2. Limb length has been restored.

3. Sacroiliac joint has been approximated. Slight widening is accepted.

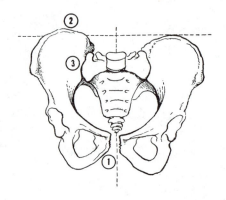

Postreduction Management

The patient is taught crutch walking and is allowed to ambulate in the mini-spica cast as tolerated.

The femoral pin is removed from the plaster 4 to 6 weeks after injury.

The mini-spica cast is removed at 12 to 14 weeks, following which sacroiliac stability is evaluated using x-rays of the joint in a weight-bearing position.

Note: If sacroiliac pain persists for more than a year after injury, sacroiliac fusion may be required.

Double Breaks in the Anterior Segment of the Pelvic Ring

REMARKS

Displacement of the fragments in all these lesions is, as a rule, minimal.

The posterior segment of the pelvic ring is intact; therefore, the weight-bearing portion of the pelvis is not impaired and no leg length inequality occurs.

Often, these fractures are sustained when the victim falls while straddling a solid object like a fence, which strikes directly against the anterior pelvic arch. The disruption of perineal structures may be considerable.

Of this group, bilateral fractures of the pubic rami are most important because of a high incidence of associated injuries to vessels, and genitourinary and rectal structures. For these, the associated injuries have urgent priority, as described previously (see page 482).

For fractures without associated injuries, management is mainly symptomatic.

Appearance on X-Ray

1. Fractures of both pubic rami.
2. Separation of symphysis pubis.

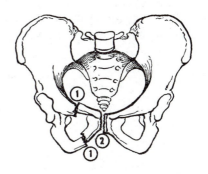

493

Appearance on X-Ray (Continued)

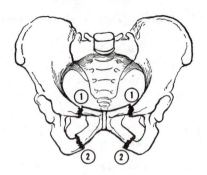

1. Fractures of both superior pubic rami.

2. Fractures of both inferior pubic rami.

Note: This straddle fracture frequently has associated urethral damage.

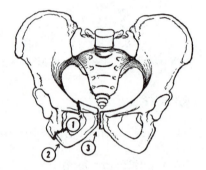

1. Fracture of superior pubic rami.
2. Fracture of ischium.
3. Separation of symphysis.

Management

If careful examination has demonstrated that there are no associated injuries, the patient with this type of fracture should be kept recumbent on a firm bed for three to five days.

Crutch walking is allowed at five to seven days and is continued for six to eight weeks, depending on pain symptoms.

Usually, recovery is complete by eight to twelve weeks.

If the patient has excessive discomfort when out of bed, a mini-spica cast will support the pelvis while permitting continued ambulation.

A Potentially Lethal Complication of Pelvic Fractures—Retroperitoneal Abscess

REMARKS

O'Keefe has shown that retroperitoneal infection may occur after a closed pelvic fracture.

Clinical manifestations of the infection most consistently are pain in the abdomen and flank or pain referred to the groin and thigh region.

Characteristically, the patient is a victim of multiple injuries in whom septic embolization produces contamination of the retroperitoneum.

The signs of sepsis may begin anywhere from three weeks to three months after the original injury.

The retroperitoneal abscess may not be detected until a mass develops in the groin from distal dissection. Characteristically, the delay in diagnosis allows extension of a massive abscess and is likely to result in death from sepsis or hypovolemic shock.

The retroperitoneum is a potential space bounded by
1. The peritoneum anteriorly,
2. The transversalis fascia posteriorly,
3. The diaphragm superiorly, and
4. The pelvis inferiorly.
5. Hemorrhage from the pelvis may breech the transversalis fascia and frequently may extend proximally into the retroperitoneum. As much as 4000 ml of blood may extravasate into this potential space.

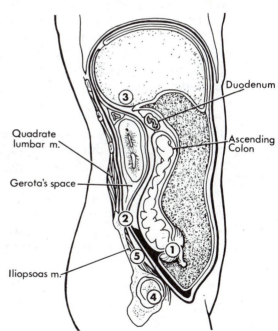

Keep this potential, but fortunately rare, complication in mind in caring for any patient with signs of sepsis after a closed pelvic fracture.

SUMMARY:
PITFALLS IN MANAGING
PELVIC FRACTURES
AND DISLOCATIONS

The major problems of pelvic fractures and dislocations stem from management of injuries to adjacent vascular and visceral structures.

Although some prove to be relatively minor, pelvic fractures remain extremely lethal injuries, particularly when they result from a crushing type of mechanism.

Caring for the patient who steadily exsanguinates from a severe pelvic fracture can be one of the most frustrating experiences of a trauma surgeon's career. A plan to locate and treat the source of hemorrhage and other major visceral injuries is essential. One such protocol has been proposed in this chapter; it utilizes a sequential approach to consider and care for the numerous associated injuries common to pelvic fractures.

The initial orthopedic management should be concerned with stabilization of the pelvis to diminish blood loss. In the acute stage this can be done by application of military antishock trousers; later a spica cast is most effective.

The major area of concern regarding the pelvis itself is the sacroiliac joint. This can be reduced by applying a well-molded spica cast with or without preliminary skeletal traction to correct the upward displacement of the hemipelvis.

Displacement of the symphysis pubis is asymptomatic on long-term follow-up of most patients. Overmanagement of this injury, particularly by operative means, may result if the physician relies too heavily on radiographic evidence of injury rather than on symptoms when choosing treatment.

References

Bucknill, T. M., Blackburne, J. S.: Fracture-dislocations of the sacrum. J. Bone and Joint Surg., 58-B:467, 1976.

Conolly, W. B., and Hedberg, E. A.: Observations on fractures of the pelvis. J. Trauma, 9:104, 1969.

Flint, L. M., Brown, A., Richardson, J. D., et al.: Definitive control of bleeding from severe pelvic fractures. Am. Surg., 189:709, 1979.

Fountain, S. S., Hamilton, R. D., and Jameson, R. M.: Transverse fractures of the sacrum. J. Bone and Joint Surg., 59-A:486, 1977.

Heckman, J. D., and Keats, P. K.: Fracture of the sacrum in a child. J. Bone and Joint Surg., 60-A:404, 1978.

Holm, C. L.: Treatment of pelvic fractures and dislocations. Clin. Orthop., 97:97, 1973.

Kaplan, B. H.: Pneumatic trousers save accident victims' lives. J.A.M.A., 225:686, 1973.

Langloh, N. D., Johnson, E. W., and Jackson, C. B.: Traumatic sacroiliac disruptions. J. Trauma, 12:931, 1972.

Maull, K. I., Sachatello, C. R., and Ernst, C. B.: The deep perineal laceration-aggressive surgical management. J. Trauma, 17:685, 1977.

O'Keefe, T. J.: Retroperitoneal abscess. A potentially fatal complication of closed fracture of the pelvis. J. Bone and Joint Surg. 60-A:1117, 1978.

Patterson, F. P., and Morton, K. S.: Neurological complications of fractures and dislocations of the pelvis. J. Trauma, 12:103, 1973.

Peltier, L. F.: Complications associated with fractures of the pelvis. J. Bone and Joint Surg., 47-A:1060, 1965.

Rothenberger, D. A., Fischer, R. P., Strate, R. G., et al: The mortality associated with pelvic fractures. Surgery, 84:356, 1978.

Rothenberger, D. A., Fischer, R. P., and Perry, J. F.: Major vascular injuries secondary to pelvic fractures: An unsolved clinical problem. Am. J. Surg. 136:660, 1978.

Turner-Warwick, R. T.: Three approaches to the management of acute disruption of the membranous urethra. In Current Controversies in Urologic Management,. edited by Russell Scott, Jr., Philadelphia, W. B. Saunders Company, 1972, pp. 144–151.

Van Urk, H., Perlberger, R. R., and Muller, H.: Selective arterial embolization for control of traumatic hemorrhage. Surgery, 83:133, 1978.

INJURIES TO THE THORACIC CAGE

GENERAL
CONSIDERATIONS

Rib fractures are among the most common fractures and can result from minor injury such as a fall or from major injury such as that sustained in motor vehicle accidents.

The majority of isolated rib fractures are uncomplicated by damage to underlying thoracic structures and are best treated symptomatically for pain relief.

The patient with multiple rib fractures may suffer complications including pulmonary contusion, hemothorax, tension pneumothorax, flail chest with respiratory failure, lacerations of major vessels, cardiac contusions, pericardial tamponade, heart valve ruptures, diaphragmatic rupture, or tears of abdominal viscus, among others.

The patient with multiple rib fractures must be suspected of having associated injuries to cardiorespiratory structures until they are ruled out by examination.

Injuries to the flexible ribcage of the young child, e.g., as from being thrown forward in the restraint seat of a car, are very likely to damage heart or lungs with little external evidence of damage to the ribcage itself. When a child's chest is significantly bruised or contused, severe trauma to thoracic or abdominal viscera must be considered.

Thoracic injuries in children are even more prone to complications than in adults. The child has limited reserves and must have blood replaced promptly. The child's air passages are readily obstructed by edema, mucus, and bronchospasm.

Gastric dilatation frequently follows chest injuries in adults but especially follows such injuries in children. Stomach contents should be decompressed, and the status of the diaphragm and abdominal contents should be thoroughly evaluated.

Steering wheel injuries in which fracture of the sternum or multiple rib fractures have occurred and in which mediastinal widening is found on x-ray also produce injury to the great vessels in about one third of cases. Any mediastinal widening seen on x-ray after blunt chest trauma is indication for angiographic study to determine the status of the aorta. Prompt diagnosis and surgical repair of a partial aortic tear are the only ways to avoid catastrophic rupture.

CARDINAL POINTS IN THE MANAGEMENT OF PATIENTS WITH MAJOR CHEST INJURIES

1. Treat shock while simultaneously relieving hypoxia and hypotension. The goal in correcting the hypoxic state is to maintain arterial Po_2 over 100 mm Hg. Nasal administration of oxygen may be sufficient for the contused lung, but any significant pulmonary compromise or collapse requires pleural cavity catheter drainage and endotracheal intubation for adequate oxygenation.

2. Find the source of bleeding and control it. As a rule, bleeding from pulmonary vessels stops spontaneously. Occasionally, bleeding into the pleural cavity from a systemic vein may be difficult to control. Rarely, thoracotomy may be necessary to control bleeding.

3. If paradoxical respiration occurs from a flail chest, control the ribcage movement and the patient's breathing by positive pressure respirator via endotracheal intubation. Insert chest tubes for drainage prior to beginning mechanical ventilation to avoid creating a tension pneumothorax.

4. Clear the airway of all secretions and obstructions, especially if the patient is a child. Quite frequently this requires endotracheal intubation. Emergency tracheostomy can be avoided by intubation, but if respiratory control is necessary for more than five to seven days, elective tracheostomy can be done with endotracheal tube in place.

5. Always aspirate any blood from the pleural cavity so as to avoid early as well as late pulmonary compromise.

6. Evaluate the patient carefully for any evidence of cardiovascular or intra-abdominal injuries. Employ arteriography promptly after any sudden deceleration injury or direct blow to the chest that can readily rupture the aorta.

7. Replace lost blood promptly, especially in children.

8. Control pain but avoid drugs that depress respiratory and cough reflexes. Pain is effectively relieved by intracostal nerve block, which may be repeated if necessary.

9. External, open chest wounds must be thoroughly debrided, cleansed, and covered with a dressing that allows egress but not ingress of air to the chest.

FRACTURES AND DISLOCATIONS OF THE RIBS

REMARKS

Fractures may be single, double, or multiple and may be associated with minimal to massive complications as previously reviewed.

Fractures of the ribs are rare in child, but severe cardiac contusion may be produced by blunt trauma to the child's flexible chest.

Overriding and angulation do not preclude prompt and satisfactory healing of fractured ribs, which usually occurs within three weeks after injury.

Recognition and prompt management of numerous complications from rib fracture are of far more significance than treatment of the fracture itself.

Dislocations of the ribs may cause more persistent and recurrent pain than do fractures.

Upper Ribs

REMARKS

Pain associated with rib fractures is the result of local tissue damage, and motion at the fracture site caused by excursion of the thorax accentuates the pain.

In the absence of complications, pain can be relieved by injection of a local anesthetic around the intercostal nerves, provided that the physician and patient understand the possibility of pneumothorax.

Following injection, recurrence of the pain can be relieved by supporting the thoracic cage.

With involvement of the upper ribs, the pain is accentuated by movements of the neck and shoulders rather than of the thoracic cage.

If test expansion of the chest causes little pain there is no need to bind the thoracic cage.

Appearance on X-Ray

1. Fracture of the first rib with no displacement.

Note: Evaluate the patient carefully for injury to the great vessels associated with this unusual fracture.

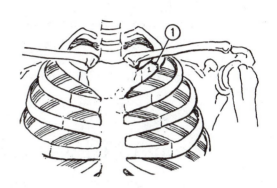

1. Fracture of the second, third, and fourth ribs.
2. Dislocation of the fourth rib at the vertebra.

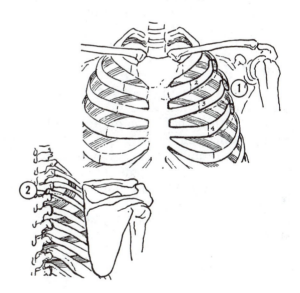

INJECTION OF INTERCOSTAL NERVES

Injection of one rib may be effective but, as a rule it may be necessary to inject two to four ribs to obtain the required relief of pain. Pneumothorax may occur, and the physician and patient should be aware of this possibility and willing to accept it for relief of the pain.

This method is especially helpful for the elderly patient who is likely to breathe inadequately and develop pneumonia after rib fracture.

1. Insert the needle a hand's-breadth proximal to the fracture site, toward the spine and under the margin of the rib.

2. Withdraw the plunger to ascertain that no blood or air is withdrawn.

3. Inject at least 5 ml of a long-acting anesthetic such as bupivacaine with epinephrine, 1:200,000.

Note: This may be repeated several times during the first three to five days after fracture.

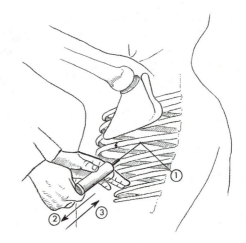

METHODS OF IMMOBILIZATION

Immobilization may be accomplished by strapping or by application of a binder.

Avoid immobilizing any elderly patient's chest, because this can lead to atelectasis and pneumonia.

Strapping

Cleanse the skin and paint with tincture of benzoin.

Have patient hold his breadth following expiration.

Apply two long strips of adhesive 7 cm wide across the shoulder.

1. In front, the strips extend well down on the abdomen.

2. In back, they extend to the lower back.

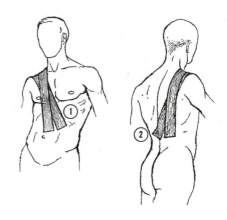

Application of Binder

Apply a tight muslin binder from below the costal cage to below the level of the axilla. Total immobilization of the thorax must be avoided.

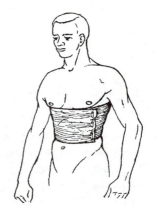

POSTIMMOBILIZATION MANAGEMENT

Whichever method is used, seven to ten days of immobilization is usually sufficient to relieve the pain.

Reinforcement of strapping or reapplication of binder may be necessary if the patient's pain is severe. However, the treatment is mainly symptomatic, and most patients are more comfortable without a binder or strapping after the first week.

Lower Ribs

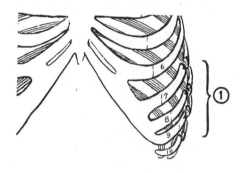

Appearance on X-Ray

1. Fracture of the seventh, eighth, ninth, and tenth ribs with displacement.

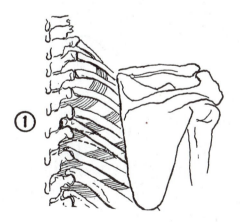

1. Dislocation of the sixth rib at the vertebra.

Management

Treatment for these injuries is symptomatic and may include analgesics, local injection, and strapping as described on pages 504–507.

FRACTURES AND DISLOCATIONS OF COSTAL CARTILAGES

REMARKS

Unless cartilages are calcified, these lesions are not demonstrable by x-ray.

The diagnosis is essentially a clinical one, especially in the presence of a deformity.

Reduction should be attempted in the face of a deformity.

Generally, healing and functional results are excellent, with or without displacement.

Types of Injuries

1. Fracture of the sixth chondral element.
2. Dislocation of the seventh costochondral joint.
3. Dislocation of the sixth costosternal joint.
4. Separation of the eighth and ninth costal cartilages.

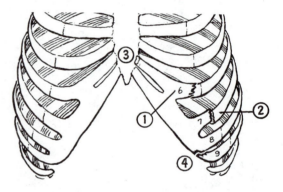

Reduction

Note: Use intercostal nerve block anesthesia.

1. An assistant draws the shoulders backward while the patient holds his breath with the chest in position of full inspiration.

2. Surgeon makes firm pressure on the displaced chondral element, forcing it into normal position.

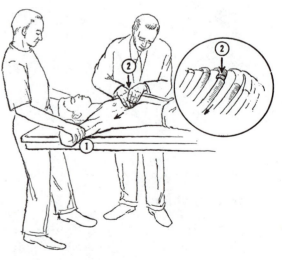

Immobilization

1. If reduction has been attempted, place a piece of felt measuring 4 cm by 5 cm by 2 cm thick over the displaced cartilage.

2. While pressure is maintained, 7-cm adhesive strips are applied, extending anteriorly and posteriorly across the midline.

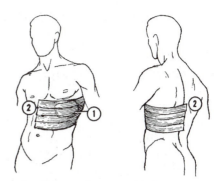

Note: The same type of strapping without the felt pad is applied in cases with no displacement or in cases in which reduction fails. If adhesive tape cannot be tolerated, apply an elastic bandage or a muslin binder firmly around the lower half of the rib cage. This prevents wide excursion of the ribs and reduces the intensity of the pain.

Postimmobilization Management

Reinforce strapping at the end of five days.

Since this treatment is symptomatic, most patients are more comfortable without the strapping by the end of seven to ten days.

Recurrent Subluxation or Dislocation of Costochondral Joint

REMARKS

Click associated with pain often is demonstrable on certain movements of trunk or arm.

Displaced rib or cartilage may be demonstrated clinically.

Some lesions respond to Marcaine and steroid injections and strapping, as in fresh lesions. If not, surgery is indicated.

Lesion

Displaced sixth costochondral joint associated with pain and clicking.

(These lesions are not seen on x-rays unless cartilages are calcified.)

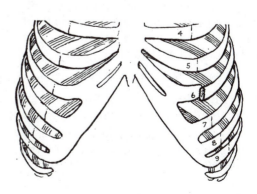

METHODS OF IMMOBILIZATION

Strapping

Prepare chest wall and paint with tincture of benzoin.

1. Apply felt pad measuring 4 cm by 5 cm by 2 cm over the rib; do not overlap the cartilage.

2. Encircle chest with strips of 7-cm adhesive, extending across the midline in front and back.

Note: If pain is severe, inject Marcaine and a steroid into the joint before applying strapping. If adhesive strapping is not tolerated, apply an elastic bandage or a muslin binder around the lower thoracic cage.

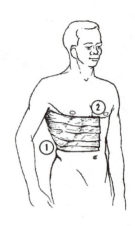

POSTIMMOBILIZATION MANAGEMENT

Reinforce strapping at the end of 5 days.

Reapply strapping at the end of 12 to 14 days.

Remove strapping at the end of four weeks; healing is slow — it may require 6 to 8 weeks.

Surgical Repair

1. Make a 7.6-cm skin incision over the prominence parallel to the affected rib.

2. Continue incision down to rib and cartilage, and by subperiosteal dissection free the end of the rib and cartilage of all soft tissue.

Note: Do not puncture the chest wall.

3. With a bone-cutting forceps, cut out the displaced end of the cartilage.

Note: Cut out enough cartilage (1 to 2 cm) to prevent any impingement of the ends during excursion of the chest wall.

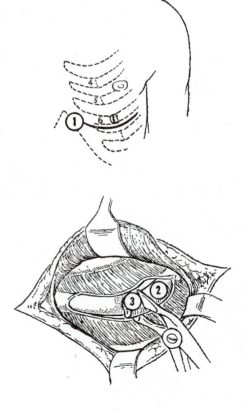

508

EMERGENCY MANAGEMENT OF COMPLICATIONS FROM RIB FRACTURES

Tension Pneumothorax

REMARKS

This condition may result from a valvular wound of the chest wall or lung.

The air enters the pleural cavity during inspiration but cannot be expelled on expiration.

If positive pressure is great, respiratory embarrassment results (dyspnea, cyanosis).

This is an emergency.

In some cases of pneumothorax, air is forced through a tear in the parietal pleura into the tissues of the chest wall, producing interstitial emphysema. Generally no treatment is indicated. Air is rapidly absorbed in tissues.

Appearance on X-Ray

This patient has tension pneumothorax after sustaining fractures of the fifth and sixth ribs.

1. Lung is collapsed and trachea has shifted to the right.

2. Mediastinum is displaced to the opposite side and apical heart sounds are in midline.

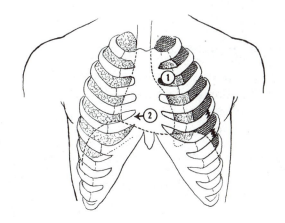

Emergency Management

INSERTION OF INTRAPLEURAL DRAINAGE TUBE

1. Insert an intrapleural drainage tube into the pleural cavity through the second intercostal space, 5 cm from the edge of the sternum.

2. Fix tube in place with a suture.

3. Submerge connecting tube in sterile water.

4. Place bottle below level of the bed.

Note: Suction may be required if lung does not subsequently expand (see also page 516).

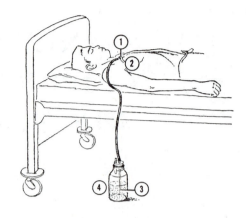

Emergency Use of Flutter Valve

If intrapleural drainage tube is not immediately available, use a flutter valve, which consists of an

1. 18-gauge needle with

2. Rubber valve, which permits egress but not ingress of air.

Note: Flutter valves are most useful for well-trained rescue squad personnel who can insert the simple emergency device prior to transporting patient.

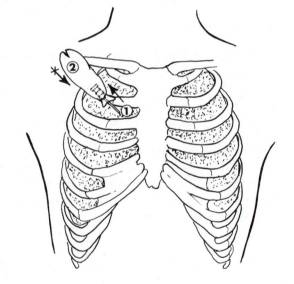

X-Ray Following Aspiration

1. Lung is partially expanded.

2. Mediastinum has returned to its normal position.

Note: Catheter drainage is continued until valvular defect in lung closes, as indicated by the fact that air no longer bubbles through the water. As a rule, 48 hours of closed drainage is sufficient.

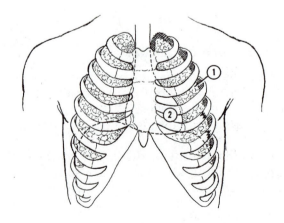

Hemothorax

REMARKS

Intrathoracic bleeding or hemothorax results usually from a rent in the lung, injury to an intercostal artery or vein, or rupture of mammary vessels.

Usually, hemorrhage is not progressive, and no immediate intervention is needed unless the hemorrhage is massive and causes respiratory impairment.

Occasionally hemothorax results from high pressure in systemic vessels, which continue to bleed.

Any hemothorax that is clinically detectable or that causes 25 per cent of the underlying lung to collapse should be aspirated and drained by intrapleural catheter (see page 516).

Appearance on X-Ray

1. Fractures of the sixth and seventh ribs with
2. Hemothorax.

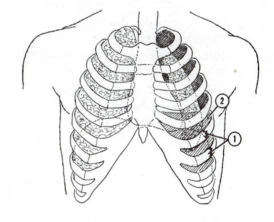

Aspiration

1. The blood is withdrawn slowly using an 18-gauge needle.

Note: Insert intrapleural catheter for suction drainage after aspiration. If bleeding continues at a rate greater than 150 ml/hour, thoracotomy should be done promptly.

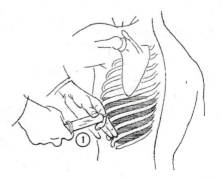

Open Chest Wounds

Large open wounds to the chest wall result in collapse of the lung and pendulum motion in the mediastinum.

The patient cannot tolerate this situation. The pendulum action must be stopped immediately by endotracheal intubation to gain respiratory control and by direct pressure dressing over the sucking wound to the chest wall.

Emergency Management

1. Apply and strap a large voluminous dressing over the wound so that the dressing allows the escape of air and does not give airtight coverage to the chest cavity.

Note: Prompt endotracheal intubation and intrapleural drainage are necessary to allow adequate ventilation of the lung.

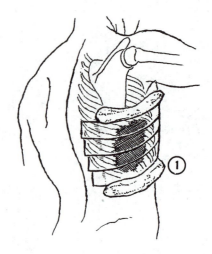

Definitive Care

When the airway has been insured, the chest wound should be excised and cleaned.

Associated injuries to lung and thoracic contents must be treated, and the chest cavity should be thoroughly irrigated.

Following this, the wound of the chest wall should be closed and the pleural cavity should be drained by suction drainage.

DOUBLE FRACTURES OF THE RIBS (STEERING WHEEL INJURY, FLAIL CHEST, STOVE-IN CHEST)

REMARKS

This lesion in its severe form is not compatible with life. The efficiency of a rigid chest wall is lost and paradoxical respiration occurs; that is, during inspiration the detached segment of the chest wall retracts and during expiration it bulges outward.

Under these conditions the diaphragm loses its effectiveness and the underlying lung is not ventilated and may become the air space from which the other lung is ventilated. The underlying lung collapses, secretions accumulate, cough is ineffective, and a state of hypoxia ensues.

Direct impact on the sternum causing bilateral anterior fractures (the steering wheel injury) is the most common cause of this problem. Correction of this emergency condition demands stabilization of the chest wall, expansion and ventilation of the lung, and reestablishment of a normal cough reflex.

The thoracic wall is best stabilized by intermittent positive pressure breathing, which also improves alveolar ventilation, decreases the patient's work in breathing, and relieves his pain and anxiety.

In order for the respirator to be effective the following requirements must be met:

1. Endotracheal intubation is performed using a cuffed endotracheal tube.

2. Intercostal drainage for pneumothorax or hemopneumothorax is accomplished.

3. Humidified oxygen is administered to maintain the arterial Po_2 over 100 mm Hg.

4. The upper respiratory tract is carefully suctioned to remove any secretions or foreign material that might have been aspirated.

5. If control of respiration is necessary for more than seven days, a tracheostomy is performed with the endotracheal tube in place.

6. When the airway has been established, careful evaluation is made for associated injuries to the heart as indicated by electrocardiographic changes or murmurs and x-ray films of the chest are reviewed for signs of mediastinal widening, which is indicative of vascular damage.

7. Arteriograms should be done promptly after this type of injury to detect frequent damage to great vessels.

Appearance on X-Ray

INSPIRATION

1. The detached segment of the chest wall retracts.

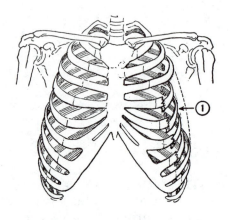

EXPIRATION

1. The floating segment bulges outward. The lung may be partially or totally collapsed.

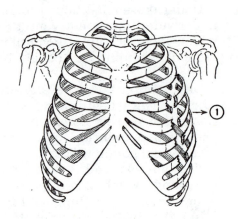

Steering Wheel Injury

LATERAL VIEW

Anterior bilateral rib fractures of second, third, and fourth ribs and fracture of the sternum.

1. The detached sternum and ribs retract.

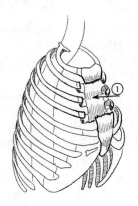

514

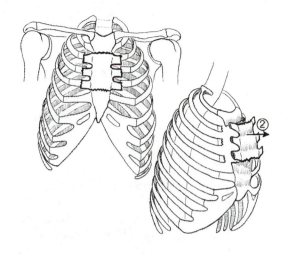

2. During expiration the detached sternum and ribs bulge anteriorly.

ANTEROPOSTERIOR VIEW

1. Widening of the mediastinum indicates strong possibility that there may be a tear of the aorta and arteriographic investigation is imperative.

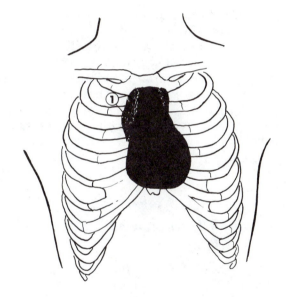

ARTERIOGRAM

1. Traumatic pseudoaneurysm is demonstrated in descending aorta, the most common location for this lesion.

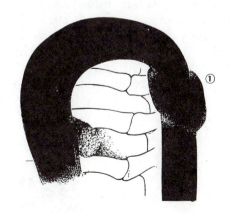

515

Management of the Flail Chest

REMARKS

These injuries may be dangerously deceptive. The patient initially may not appear to be in respiratory distress, and the paradoxical respiration may not be recognized because of soft tissue swelling.

Death may be directly related to the failure to recognize the degree of injury and to begin prompt treatment.

Any patient with a direct injury to the chest should be carefully evaluated for paradoxical respiration, particularly if there are multiple fractures of the anterior chest wall.

The simplest, quickest way of temporarily stabilizing the flail chest is by turning the patient on the affected side and placing a sandbag against the involved segment.

Obtain arterial blood gases promptly, even in the absence of dyspnea. If arterial Po_2 is less than 60 mm Hg, begin mechanical ventilation.

Any pneumothorax should be drained prior to mechanical ventilation so as to avoid a tension pneumothorax.

Insertion of Intrapleural Drainage Tube

1. For hemothorax, insert plastic intrapleural drainage tube in the mid-axillary region, in the fifth interspace.

2. For pneumothorax, insert tube in the second anterior interspace.

3. Pass a forceps through the stab wound made for the tube.

4. Push drainage tube into the pleural cavity and attach it to a suction system. Suture drainage tube in place.

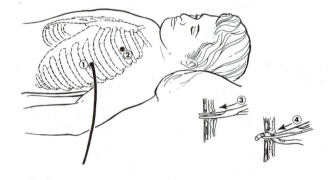

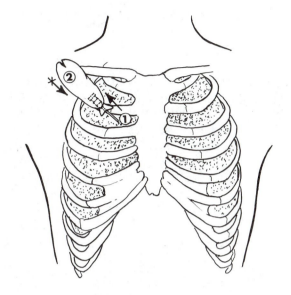

Use of Flutter Valve

If there is no time for the insertion of a drainage tube,

1. A flutter valve needle allows egress of air but

2. The rubber valve prevents ingress of air.

Management

1. Intrapleural drainage tube is attached to a suction system.

2. Endotracheal tube is in place. Perform tracheostomy if respiratory control will be used for more than seven days.

3. A mechanical respirator allows positive pressure breathing, expands the collapsed lung, and maintains arterial Po_2 over 100 mm Hg. This also provides internal pneumatic stabilization of flail chest.

Note: Respiratory control may have to be used for ten days or longer.

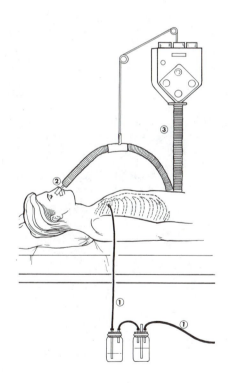

INTERNAL FIXATION OF A FLAIL CHEST

REMARKS

If the patient requires thoracotomy to correct major intrathoracic injuries, the unstable fracture should be stabilized.

Operative fixation of the rib fractures, however, is not usually indicated, because mechanical ventilation can give effective internal pneumatic stabilization.

1. The multiple rib fractures are stabilized by intramedullary Kirschner wires bent to prevent migration or

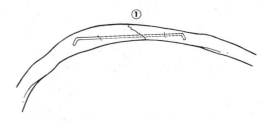

2. Cerclage 18-gauge stainless steel wire wrapped around the oblique rib fracture.

Note: The Kirschner wire should be removed at three weeks.

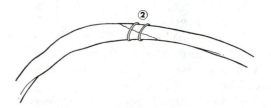

FRACTURES OF THE STERNUM

REMARKS

Although rare, fracture of the sternum is frequently associated with fractures of other bones—ribs, scapula, clavicle, and especially the dorsal vertebrae.

The most common site is at the junction of the manubrium and the body of the sternum.

Displacement of the lower fragment may be forward or backward.

Open reduction is rarely indicated.

Always make sure there are no injuries to underlying structures between the lungs. Check for cardiac murmur, which might indicate valve damage, and for electrocardiographic signs of cardiac contusion.

Widening of the mediastinum on x-ray is caused in one third of cases by tears of the aorta and should be investigated thoroughly by means of arteriography.

Obtain arteriograms promptly after this injury because of the strong possibility of major vascular damage.

Check for signs of hemothorax, pneumothorax, and subcutaneous emphysema.

Appearance on X-Ray

1. Fracture of the sternum with no displacement.

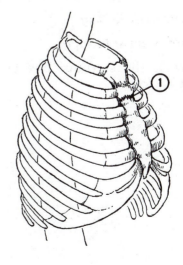

Strapping

Prepare the chest wall and paint with tincture of benzoin.

1. Apply a piece of felt 2 cm thick over the site of the lesion.

2. Apply cross strappings of Elastoplast over the felt.

3. Apply a plaster posterior figure-of-eight bandage on the shoulders.

Note: Have patient lie on a sandbag placed between the scapulae until the plaster has set firmly.

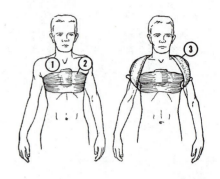

With Displacement

REMARKS

Displacement may be forward or backward.

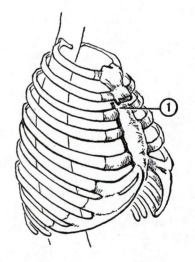

Appearance on X-Ray

BACKWARD DISPLACEMENT

1. Body of the sternum has been displaced backward.

Forward displacement

1. Body of the sternum has been displaced forward.

Reduction

Note: Attempt reduction only after an arteriogram shows that no injury of cardiovascular structures has occurred.

1. Patient assumes the supine position with the spine hyperextended, shoulders back, and arms over the head. The table is tilted.
2. After injection of procaine into the affected area, the surgeon makes firm downward pressure over the fragment displaced anteriorly.

Note: Anatomic reduction is not essential to healing. Do not manipulate forcefully because of potential damage to underlying cardiovascular structures.

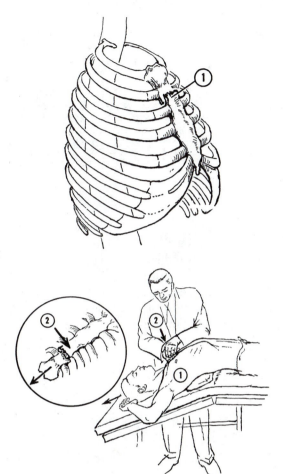

Strapping

Prepare the chest wall with tincture of benzoin.

1. Apply a piece of felt that measures 3.8 by 5.4 by 1.8 cm over the site of the lesion.
2. Apply cross strappings of Elastoplast over the felt.
3. Apply a plaster posterior figure-of-eight bandage on the shoulders.

Note: Have patient lie on a sandbag placed between scapulae until the plaster posterior figure-of-eight bandage has set firmly.

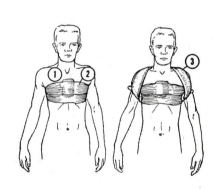

If closed reduction fails, healing will occur and the functional result is usually good in spite of a deformity.

Open reduction of a grossly displaced sternal fracture is best referred to the cardiovascular surgeon, who is prepared to deal with potential damage to underlying major vessels.

SUMMARY: PITFALLS OF MANAGING INJURIES TO THE THORACIC CAGE

This section has been written to emphasize for the trauma surgeon that the major problems of fractures and dislocations of the ribcage result from the significant injuries to underlying cardiovascular and pulmonary structures.

For a complete review of these problems, the reader is referred to the text by Kirsh and Sloan.

REFERENCE

Kirsh, M. M., and Sloan, H.: *Blunt Chest Trauma, General Principles of Management.* Boston: Little, Brown and Company, 1977.

FRACTURES AND DISLOCATIONS OF THE SHOULDER GIRDLE

FRACTURES OF THE CLAVICLE

REMARKS

The clavicle is one of the most frequently fractured bones, especially in young children. Management of the usual childhood fracture is by simple reduction and immobilization for three weeks in a figure-of-eight harness. Healing usually occurs without complications.

Management of an adult's fractured clavicle is a good deal more difficult, requiring more complete and prolonged immobilization than does the child's fracture. Even in the adult clavicular fracture, unless there is severe disruption of soft tissues and wide separation of the fragments, union usually occurs with adequate closed treatment.

Displaced fragments may unite with some deformity, but this does not preclude good function. However, a large callus mass may produce neurovascular impingement 20 or more years after the injury. Marked posterior displacement of clavicular fragments should be corrected to prevent thoracic outlet syndrome.

Nonunion is rare but does occur, most commonly after open reduction of clavicular fractures in adults. Surgical intervention should result in adequate fixation, which is best provided by a compression plate or Knowles pins, and should be strictly limited to specific indications such as:

1. Widely separated fragments that cannot be reduced by closed method and that are liable to produce thoracic outlet impingement.

2. Occasional fractures involving the acromioclavicular joint associated with disruption of the coracoclavicular ligament, which would prevent adequate reduction.

In all fractures of the clavicle, check for injuries to the brachial plexus, the subclavian vessels, and the lungs and pleura.

Fractures of other bones, especially in the upper limb, and dislocations of the inner and outer ends of the clavicle are frequently associated with clavicular fractures.

Mechanisms and Classification of Fractures of the Clavicle

REMARKS

Fractures of the clavicle may be the result of either a direct or an indirect force acting on the bone. The type, direction, and concentration of the force determines the type of fracture produced.

Fractures of the clavicle can be grouped into three categories: fractures of the middle third, fractures of the outer third, and fractures of the inner third.

FRACTURES OF THE MIDDLE THIRD OF THE CLAVICLE

This is by far the most frequently encountered fracture of the clavicle.

It may be produced by a direct impact; the fracture is usually segmental at the juncture of the outer and middle thirds of the clavicle.

It may be produced by an indirect force acting along the humerus such as occurs when one falls on the upper extremity with the arm flexed and abducted at least 45 degrees. The counter points in this mechanism are the glenohumeral and sternoclavicular joints. Usually a spiral fracture occurs.

It may be produced by direct violence applied to the top of the shoulder forcing the clavicle against the first rib. The result is a spiral fracture of the middle third of the clavicle.

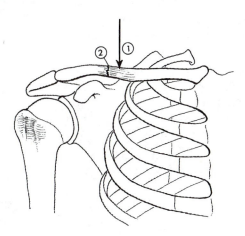

1. Direct force applied to middle third of the clavicle.

2. Fracture at the juncture of the middle and outer thirds.

1. Indirect force travels along the shaft of the humerus.

2. Counter points are the glenohumeral joint and the sternoclavicular joint; the result is

3. An oblique fracture of the middle third of the clavicle.

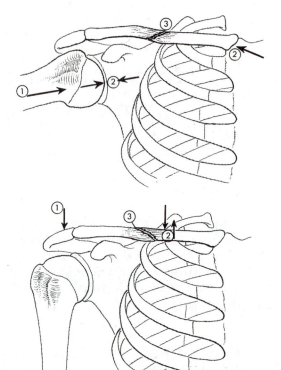

1. Direct force is applied to the top of the shoulder.

2. Clavicle is forced against the first rib. The result is

3. A spiral fracture of the middle third of the clavicle.

FRACTURES OF THE OUTER THIRD OF THE CLAVICLE

These lesions are the result of a direct force applied to the top of the shoulder. The result may be a comminuted fracture of the distal third.

The fracture may extend into the acromioclavicular joint.

The fracture may be distal to the coracoclavicular joint.

The fracture may be associated with rupture of the capsular ligaments and the coracoclavicular ligaments.

Note: Fractures distal to the coracoclavicular ligaments frequently fail to unite if the major fragment is displaced superiorly.

1. Direct force on the distal third of the clavicle.

2. Communication of the distal third of the clavicle.

Note: All ligaments are intact, and acromioclavicular joint is not involved.

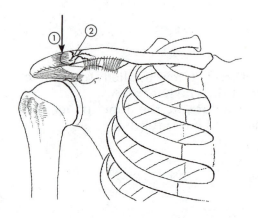

1. Direct force on the distal third of the clavicle.

2. Comminution of the distal third of the clavicle.

3. Fracture extends into the acromioclavicular joint.

4. All ligaments are intact.

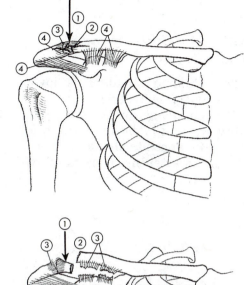

1. Direct force on the distal third of the clavicle.

2. Fracture is distal to coracoclavicular ligaments.

3. All ligaments are disrupted, and reduction of the displaced fragment may be incomplete, so that nonunion results.

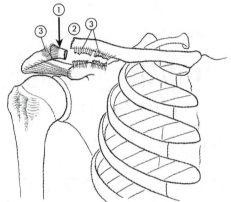

FRACTURES OF THE INNER THIRD OF THE CLAVICLE

These fractures are the result of a direct impact applied at an angle from the lateral side.

Displacement is usually minimal, unless there is disruption of the costoclavicular ligament.

1. Direct force is applied from the side.

2. Fracture of the inner third of the clavicle occurs.

3. All ligaments are intact.

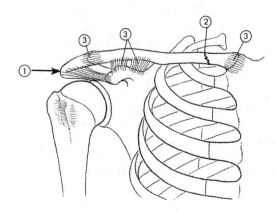

TYPICAL DEFORMITY

Complete Fracture of the Clavicle

1. The affected shoulder is lower than the opposite shoulder.
2. The shoulder drops downward and forward and is closer to the midline than the opposite shoulder.
3. There is swelling over the clavicle.

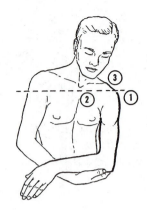

Management of Specific Fractures of the Clavicle: Closed Reduction

IN INFANTS AND CHILDREN

Application of Posterior Figure-of-Eight Harness

This method is useful for all fractures encountered in infants and children.

If displacement is pronounced, injection of 5 ml of bupivacaine into the hematoma will relieve the pain.

1. The patient sits on a stool.
2. The operator stands behind the patient and places one knee between the scapulae while applying the harness.
3. A commercially available figure-of-eight harness or a stockinette filled with cast padding is applied and is tightened so as to elevate the shoulder and reduce the fracture fragments.

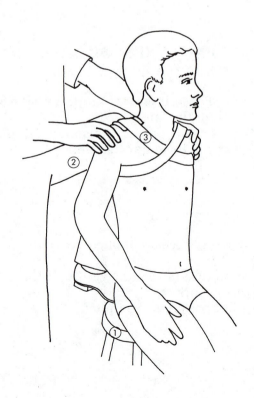

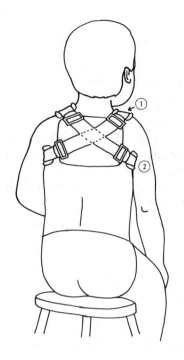

Back View of Figure-of-Eight Harness

1. Harness pulls shoulders up and back.
2. If circulation or neurologic function in the upper limb is affected, the harness should be loosened.

IN ADOLESCENTS AND ADULTS

REMARKS

The following treatment applies to all fractures of the clavicle except those likely to produce thoracic outlet impingement and those distal to the coracoclavicular ligament with gross upward displacement.

Application of Clavicular Spica Cast

1. The patient sits on a stool.
2. Using a body stockinette and light pads over the fracture, the operator applies the shoulder spica while pushing the shoulder superiorly and posteriorly.
3. The arm on the fracture side is incorporated in the plaster.

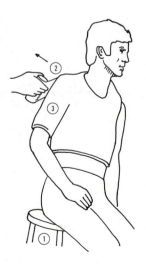

Application of Clavicular Spica Cast *(Continued)*

Before plaster sets:

1. Have the patient lie supine with a sandbag between the scapulae and the arms at the sides.

2. Hold shoulders back by molding upward in the deltoid region.

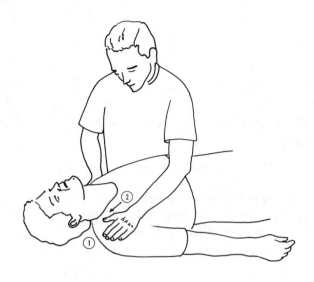

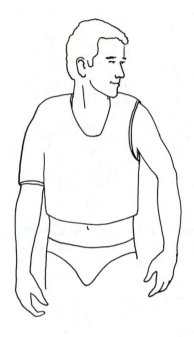

Front View of Clavicular Spica Cast

Note: Support arm on fractured side with sling until pain subsides.

Back View of Clavicular Spica Cast

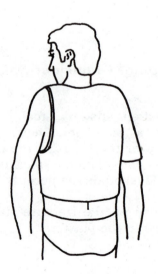

Postreduction Care

A child is immobilized in a figure-of-eight harness for three weeks.

An adult must be immobilized for six to eight weeks in the clavicular spica cast, and then the shoulder is generally supported in a sling while motion is regained.

Healing is best determined clinically by fracture stability and absence of pain. Radiographic signs lag far behind clinical evidence of union, particularly in children.

Encourage free use of the arm and hand on the affected side, especially in adults and elderly patients.

Frozen shoulder and stiffness of the fingers must be avoided.

Exercises must be carried out on a regulated program at least five to ten minutes every waking hour.

ALTERNATIVE METHOD OF IMMOBILIZATION: LATERAL TRACTION

This may be necessary for the occasional patient who must be confined to bed temporarily because of other injuries or for the fracture that cannot be reduced by the usual closed method.

1. Patient assumes the prone position.

2. Place a board under the mattress.

3. Elevate the side of the bed 10 cm.

4. Apply adhesive traction apparatus to upper arm and add 6 to 10 lb (2.7 to 4.5 kg).

5. Apply traction apparatus to forearm and 3 to 6 lb (1.4 to 2.7 kg) — just enough to counterbalance the weight of the forearm.

Note: Traction is made with arm abducted 90 degrees and externally rotated 90 degrees. Forearm is flexed 90 degrees.

Maintain traction for two weeks.

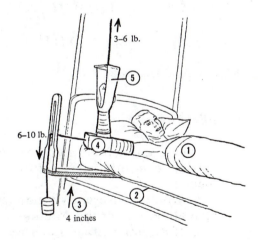

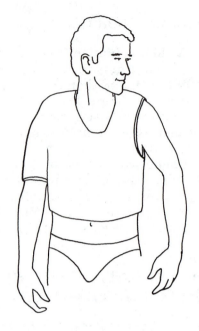

Postreduction Care

Apply shoulder spica, which should be worn for three to five weeks. Free use of arm and hand on the affected side, especially in elderly patients, should be encouraged.

Frozen shoulder and stiffness of the fingers must be avoided.

Exercises must be carried out on a regular program of at least five to ten minutes every waking hour.

Open Reduction of Fractures of the Adult's Clavicle

REMARKS

Open reduction is rarely indicated except:

1. In comminuted fractures with wide displacement of the fragments.

2. Where conservative management has failed to restore an acceptable alignment of the fragments.

3. If evidence of compression of the neurovascular structures in the thoracic outlet is present and it has not been relieved by closed reduction of the fractured clavicle.

4. Fractures distal to the coracoclavicular ligaments with disruption of these ligaments.

Do minimal stripping of soft tissues around the clavicle; otherwise, delayed union or nonunion results.

Avoid intramedullary Steinmann pin or Kirschner wire fixation for clavicular fractures and dislocations. Complications from pin migration are too frequent and too serious to warrant their use. If pin fixation is chosen, use a Knowles pin, which is designed to exert a compressive force and has a hub that prevents medial migration.

Tubular compression plating works well for the rare clavicular fracture that requires internal fixation.

Operative Procedure

POSITION OF THE PATIENT

1. Patient is in the supine position.
2. A sandbag is placed under the shoulder.

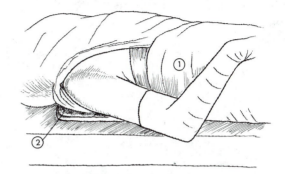

INCISION

1. Make a curved incision overlying the second rib — centered over the fracture site.

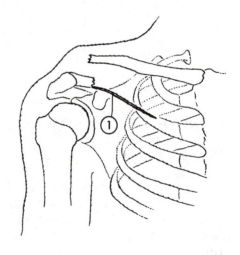

2. Divide the platysma and, with the overlying tissues, reflect it upward.

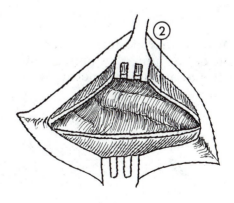

Operative Procedure (Continued)

EXPOSURE AND REDUCTION

1. Expose the fracture site and deliver the lateral fragment into the wound.

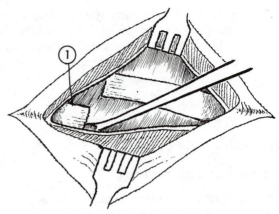

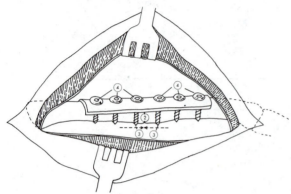

2. Reduce the fracture anatomically and apply a six-hole semitubular tension-band plate.

3. Inserting the first two screws nearest to the fracture promotes compression.

4. At least two and preferably three screws should fix each fragment.

Alternative Fixation Technique (After Neviaser)

REMARKS

The curved configuration of the clavicle makes it quite easy to drill an "intramedullary pin" into the thoracic cavity. The natural rotatory motion of the clavicle also promotes and encourages erosion of the intramedullary pin through the fracture and into major thoracic structures.

1. On an anteroposterior x-ray the position of the pin may appear adequate despite posterior penetration.

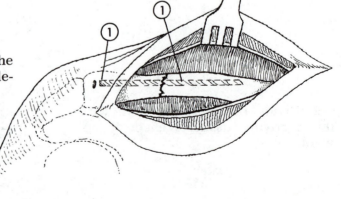

2. Curved clavicle encourages drilling the pin into the mediastinum.

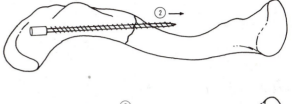

1. If an intramedullary pin is necessary, use a Knowles pin inserted from the posterior cortex.

2. The hub design of the Knowles pin promotes compression of the fracture and prevents medial migration.

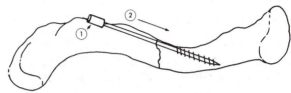

Postoperative Management

The arm is supported in a sling for one to two weeks. The patient is encouraged to use the arm for activities of daily living. Full functional activity and active range of motion is encouraged by the third to fourth week, depending on the degree of stability achieved by surgery.

Fixation is not removed until at least one year after operation, if at all.

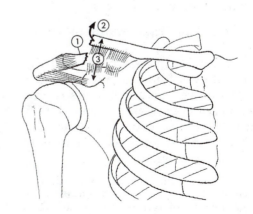

OPEN REDUCTION FOR FRACTURES DISTAL TO AND WITH DISRUPTION OF THE CORACOCLAVICULAR LIGAMENTS

Prereduction X-Ray

1. Fracture of the clavicle distal to the coracoclavicular ligaments.

2. Upward and backward displacement of the medial fragment.

3. Widening of the interval between the medial fragment and the coracoid process. (The coracoclavicular ligaments are ruptured.)

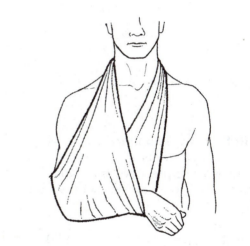

Note: Most injuries in this location are not this widely displaced and may be treated by sling immobilization.

Operative repair is necessary only if superior displacement of the clavicular fragment precludes healing.

535

Operative Procedure

INCISION AND EXPOSURE

1. Make a slightly curved 7.5-cm incision over the clavicle terminating at the tip of the acromion process.

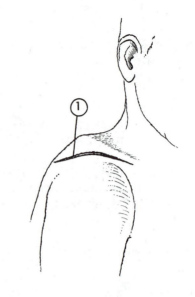

2. Reflect by subperiosteal dissection the attachments of the trapezius and the deltoid; preserve the capsular ligaments of the acromioclavicular joint.

Note: Do not perform any more subperiosteal stripping of the fragments than is absolutely necessary.

3. Expose the ends of the fragments.

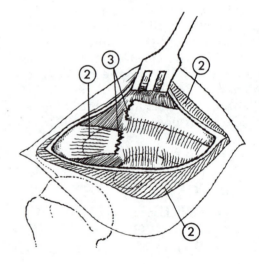

EXCISION AND REDUCTION

1. Excise the fragment distal to the coracoid.
2. Reattach the coracoacromial ligament into the fracture end.
3. Reinforce this newly constructed coracoclavicular ligament with heavy 5-mm Mersilene suture. Repair torn trapezius and deltoid muscle attachments to the clavicle.

Note: This method is an adaptation of the Weaver-Dunn procedure for acute acromioclavicular separation. (See page 552.)

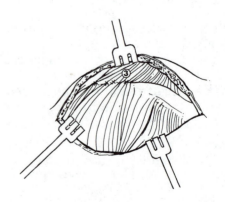

Postoperative Management

Arm is supported in a sling for four weeks and circumduction exercises are encouraged from the first day.

At the end of four weeks the patient is allowed full active use of the shoulder.

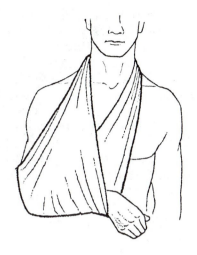

Complications of Fractures of the Clavicle

REMARKS

Although rare, complications associated with fractures of the clavicle do occur. These are most likely to follow clavicular fractures in adults.

The most common complications include: nonunion, excessive callus formation at the fracture site producing thoracic outlet syndrome, and direct injuries to neurovascular structures in the thoracic outlet.

Surgical misadventures may occur, primarily from the use of "intramedullary pin" fixation that migrates into mediastinum (see page 534).

NONUNION OF FRACTURES OF THE CLAVICLE

REMARKS

The most important factors predisposing to nonunion are:

The interval of immobilization may be too short. Although most fractures in adults unite in four to eight weeks, some fractures, particularly severely comminuted ones, require a longer period of immobilization.

Widely separated and comminuted fragments are also more likely to result in nonunion.

A figure-of-eight harness is inadequate to immobilize a clavicular fracture in an adult. Use a clavicular spica cast instead.

Open reduction as the primary treatment increases the incidence of nonunion. This is particularly true if open reduction is combined with inadequate internal fixation.

Most cases of nonunion cause sufficient pain to justify surgical repair, but occasionally the lesion produces no significant disability. Pseudoarthrosis of the clavicle in children is almost always congenital but still may require surgical repair.

Success of the surgical procedure depends on proper selection for the type of nonunion.

Nonunion of the clavicle may occur without shortening, and this allows tension-band plating without bone grafting. Nonunion of the clavicle with shortening or with a defect requires autogenous cortico-cancellous graft, taken usually from the iliac crest, so as to permit stable tension-band plating.

Preoperative X-Ray

1. Nonunion of clavicle with shortening and overriding may be plated without graft.

2. Nonunion with defect requires corticocancellous graft from the iliac crest along with plating.

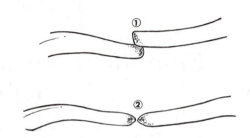

Operative Procedure (After Weber and Cech)

INCISION AND EXPOSURE

With the patient in the supine position and a sandbag under the involved shoulder:

1. Make a 10-cm incision along the inferior border of the clavicle centered over the fracture site.

2. Divide the platysma muscle and, with the overlying soft tissues, reflect it upward.

3. Expose the ends of the fragments by subperiosteal dissection.

Note: Do not strip off any more periosteum than is necessary.

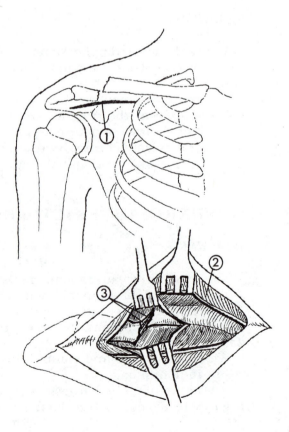

EXCISION AND FIXATION

1. Excise sufficient fibrocartilage to allow end-to-end contact of bone and application of the plate. The two screws closest to the fracture should be applied first so as to compress the fracture.

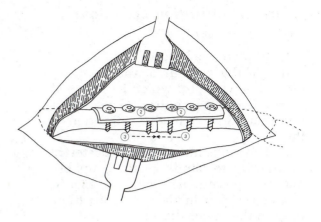

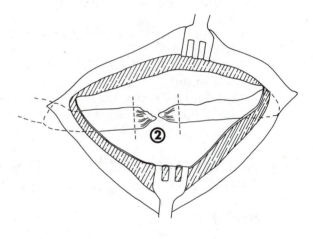

2. If nonunion has created a defect, remove the fibrous tissue and insert an interpositional bone graft. Use semi-tubular plate to hold bone graft in place.

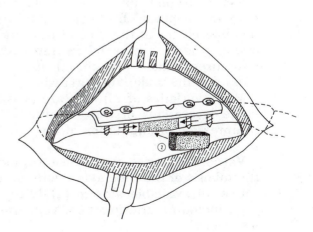

Alternative Fixation Technique (After Neviaser)

1. If plate cannot be applied because of the contour of the fracture, use a Knowles pin, which is designed to compress the fracture and also has a hub that prevents medial migration of the pin.

2. The pin is inserted from posterior to anterior to eliminate the palpable anterior prominence and to insure proper position in the clavicle rather than in the mediastinum.

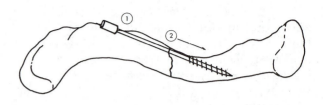

Postoperative Management

Fixation should be adequate to dispense with significant external immobilization.

Use a sling for three to five days and then begin circumduction exercises promptly.

Full activity is usually allowed by six weeks.

Plates should not be removed until at least one year after the procedure.

NEUROVASCULAR INJURIES FROM FRACTURES OR FROM EXCESS CALLUS AT THE FRACTURE SITE

REMARKS

Neurovascular injury from clavicular fracture may be acute or chronic. Displaced fragments may injure subclavian vessels and the brachial plexus at the time of fracture. Chronic obstruction or thoracic outlet syndrome may follow repetitive trauma to the neurovascular structures, which are chronically caught between the large callus mass and the underlying first rib.

Many varieties of injuries are possible, from simple compression to acute lacerations of the structures. The most common injuries are compression or angulation of the subclavian vessels and brachial plexus.

Vascular injuries may cause an aneurysm of the subclavian artery, thrombosis of the subclavian vein, or an arteriovenous fistula.

Use all available aids to establish the pathologic nature of the injury, including arteriograms, venograms, and electromyographic studies.

After severe fractures of the clavicle, check the vascular and neurologic function of the limb repeatedly.

Neurovascular injuries associated with fresh fractures should be recognized immediately. As a rule they respond to simple closed reduction and adequate immobilization of the fractures.

If the symptoms of neurovascular compression are not relieved in fresh fractures by closed reduction, open reduction and internal fixation should be carried out (see page 538).

In cases of long-standing compression caused by excessive callus formation, nonunited fractures, or malunited fractures of great deformity, excision of the fractured area is occasionally recommended. However, this usually does not solve the problem, because impingement on neurovascular structures by the remaining mobile portion of the clavicle, which frequently regenerates and forms spurs, is still possible.

Rather than excising the area of callus entirely, "debulk" or rongeur the fracture callus down into small fragments and then lay them back into the periosteal bed. External immobilization may be used until the defect heals.

This method of clavicular fragmentation has also been useful to heal defects created during surgical approaches to subclavicular vascular structures and the brachial plexus.

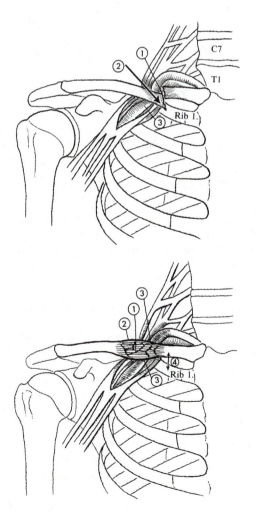

Acute Neurovascular Impingement from Displaced Fractures

1. Fracture of the clavicle.
2. Lateral fragment displaces downward, especially on forward flexion of the arm.
3. Neurovascular structures are compressed against the first rib.

Note: If closed reduction does not relieve neurovascular impingement, open reduction and internal fixation are indicated (see page 538).

Chronic Neurovascular Impingement from Excess Callus

1. Comminuted fracture of the middle third of the clavicle.
2. Massive callus formation.
3. Compression of the neurovascular structures.
4. The interval between the clavicle and the first rib is severely reduced.

Note: Avoid resection of the entire callus mass, which still would not prevent neurovascular impingement by the lateral fragment.

1. If the middle portion of the clavicle is completely resected to decompress the underlying neurovascular structures,

2. The lateral portion of the clavicle frequently regenerates or forms a bone spike that impinges on the vessels and brachial plexus whenever the patient flexes and adducts the shoulder.

Note: In preference to complete resection, use clavicular fragmentation (see page 543).

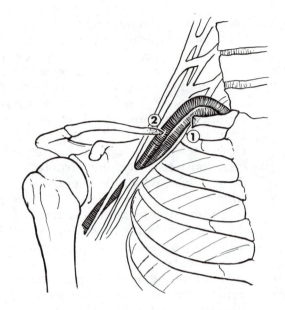

Excision of a Portion of the Clavicle

REMARKS

Certain segments of the clavicle can be excised with little or no dysfunction of the shoulder.
These include:

1. Excision of the clavicle distal to the coracoclavicular ligament.
2. Excision of the sternal end of the clavicle.
3. Excision of the entire clavicle.

Note: This is usually necessary only for tumors.

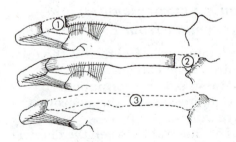

Caution: If the middle third or half of the clavicle is excised, the lateral portion tends to reform bone and scar, which impinge on neurovascular structures.

TECHNIQUE OF CLAVICULAR FRAGMENTATION (AFTER SHUMACKER)

Preoperative X-ray

1. Segmental fracture of the middle third of the clavicle.

2. Wide separation and malalignment of the fragments.

3. Massive callus formation impinging on the thoracic outlet.

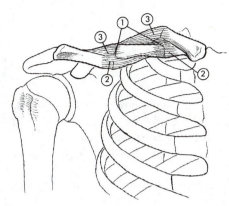

Position of Patient

The patient is placed in the supine position with a small sandbag between the shoulders.

Operative Procedure

INCISION AND EXPOSURE

1. Make a 10-cm incision along the inferior border of the clavicle.

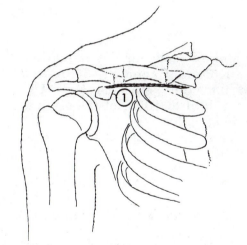

2. By superiosteal dissection, carefully free the clavicle.

3. Mark off the segment of the clavicle to be excised.

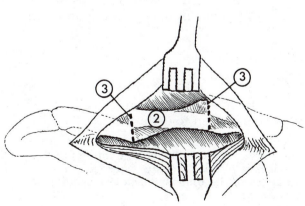

543

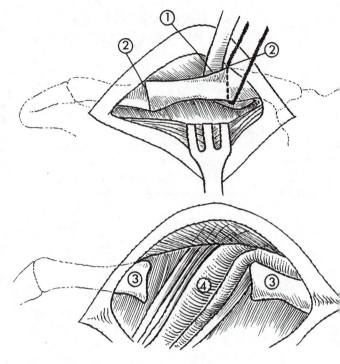

Operative Procedure (Continued)

EXCISION

1. Place a reverse retractor between the clavicle and the underlying soft tissues at the site of severance.

2. With a Gigli saw divide the bone at both sites.

3. The middle third of the clavicle has been excised.

4. The underlying structures are free.

FRAGMENTATION

1. Mill and rongeur the callus into 2-mm to 3-mm fragments and repack them into the periosteal bed. Use about a third to a half of the original amount of callus.

2. Close the periosteal sleeve over the chips.

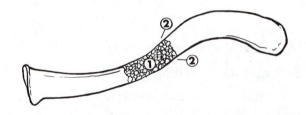

Postoperative Management

Immobilize the area postoperatively in a shoulder spica cast or a Velpeau sling, depending on the mobility at the fracture site.

Postoperative X-Ray

1. Osseous regeneration is well advanced by seven to eight weeks.

Note: This method is also useful to deal with large defects in the middle third of the clavicle created during surgical approaches to the underlying neurovascular structures.

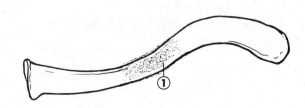

LIGAMENTOUS INJURIES OF THE ARTICULATIONS OF THE CLAVICLE

Lesions of the Ligaments of the Acromioclavicular Joint

REMARKS

Although injuries to the ligaments of the acromioclavicular joint may occur in any age group, they most frequently are seen in young athletic adults.

The typical mechanism of injury is a direct blow to the tip of the shoulder, e.g., when the football quarterback lands on his throwing shoulder after being tackled from the "blind side."

Involvement of the ligaments vary from a minor sprain, in which only a few fibers tear, to complete disruption of all fibers.

Complete disruption of the acromioclavicular joint is still compatible with normal shoulder function, but pronounced displacement may be painful or may cause an unsightly prominence.

An incompletely reduced acromioclavicular dislocation is likely to produce traumatic arthritis and painful shoulder function.

Management of these injuries requires an intelligent assessment of the patient's need rather than rote use of a set approach.

Muscular individuals who are most anxious to return to work or competitive sports may be treated symptomatically with sling support, ice applications, and exercises to strengthen the injured trapezius and deltoid muscles.

Corrective surgery may be done electively should the patient decide it is necessary for his functional needs.

Thin individuals who are likely to be bothered by the prominently displaced lateral end of the clavicle may be offered early surgical correction.

Attempts at closed reduction of a complete acromioclavicular dislocation with prolonged immobilization using shoulder supports are generally ineffective, since the basic problem is a poorly healing ligamentous injury. If the shoulder support or harness works, one tends to question its necessity in the first place. When the harness does not work, the patient is still faced with the alternative of surgical correction after six to eight weeks of ineffective treatment.

MECHANISMS OF INJURY

Most injuries result from a direct fall on the shoulder.
Occasionally, an indirectly applied force will injure the acromioclavicular joint.

Direct Mechanism

This is usually the result of a fall on the point of the shoulder, with the arm at the side or adducted slightly.

1. Direct force is applied to the point of the shoulder.

2. The scapula and the attached clavicle are forced downward and medially. The clavicle approaches the first rib. If the force continues,

3. The first rib abuts against the clavicle, producing a counter force that may cause

4. Rupture of the acromioclavicular ligaments and the coracoclavicular ligaments and

5. Tearing of the insertions of the deltoid and trapezius muscles.

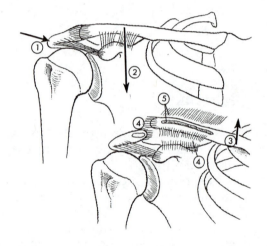

Depending upon the intensity of the forces acting, one of three lesions may result:

SPRAIN

1. Few fibers of the acromioclavicular ligaments stretch or even tear.

2. The acromioclavicular joint is stable; there is no laxity.

3. The coracoclavicular ligaments are intact.

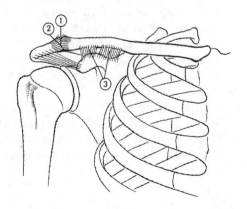

SUBLUXATION

1. Rupture of the capsule and acromioclavicular ligaments.

2. The acromioclavicular joint is unstable; there is obvious laxity.

3. The end of the clavicle is displaced upward, usually by less than half the width of the end of the clavicle.

4. The coracoclavicular ligaments are intact.

5. The attachments of the trapezius and deltoid muscles to the clavicle are intact.

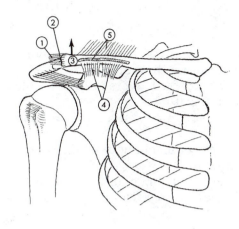

DISLOCATION

1. Rupture of the capsule and acromioclavicular ligaments.

2. Rupture of the coracoclavicular ligaments.

3. Avulsion of the attachments of the trapezius and deltoid muscles.

4. Upward displacement of the clavicle.

5. Wide separation between the clavicle and the coracoid process.

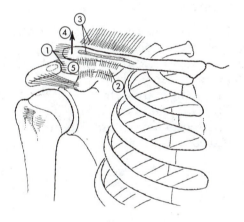

Indirect Mechanism

In an indirect mechanism the arm is usually slightly flexed and abducted.

From its point of application the force is transmitted along the shaft of the humerus, traverses the stable glenohumeral joint, and is expended on the acromion, forcing the scapula upward and medially.

In this mechanism the coracoclavicular ligaments are not injured but instead are forced into a relaxed position.

Depending on the intensity of the force, a sprain, a subluxation, or a dislocation is produced.

Indirect Mechanism (Continued)

SPRAIN

1. The force is transmitted along the shaft of the humerus.
2. The force traverses the stable glenohumeral joint.
3. The scapula is forced upward and medially.
4. The coracoclavicular ligaments are relaxed.
5. Few of the fibers of the capsule or of the acromioclavicular ligaments stretch or tear.

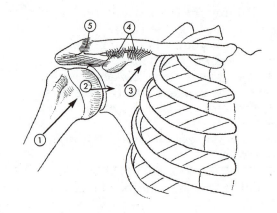

SUBLUXATION

If the force described above continues, subluxation occurs.

1. The capsule and acromioclavicular ligaments tear.
2. The joint is unstable.
3. The clavicle is freely movable.
4. The coracoclavicular ligaments are relaxed and intact.

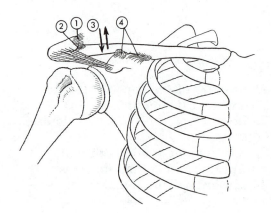

MANAGEMENT OF INJURIES OF THE ACROMIOCLAVICULAR LIGAMENTS

Sprain

1. There is minor stretching and tearing of the capsule and ligaments of the acromioclavicular joint.
2. Coracoclavicular ligaments are intact.

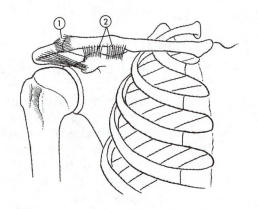

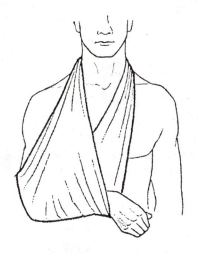

TREATMENT

Initially apply ice.

After three days, wet heat may be applied.

Rest the limb in a sling for three to five days.

Begin active exercises to strengthen deltoid and trapezius muscles when initial pain subsides.

Recovery should be complete in seven to ten days.

Subluxation

REMARKS

This lesion responds adequately to nonoperative methods.

Depending on the needs of the patient, the subluxation may be treated symptomatically, as described for sprain above, or by attempted closed reduction with acromioclavicular strapping.

Avoid the use of adhesive straps.

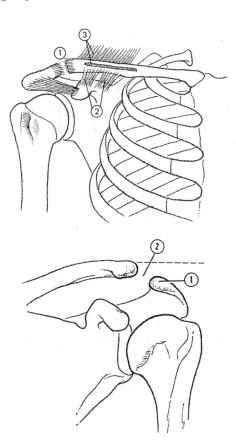

1. The capsule and the acromioclavicular ligaments are ruptured.

2. The coracoclavicular ligaments are intact.

3. The attachments of the trapezius and deltoid to the clavicle are intact.

PREREDUCTION X-RAY

1. The acromion is slightly below the level of the clavicle.

2. The acromioclavicular joint space is widened.

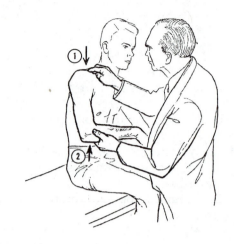

Subluxation *(Continued)*

MANIPULATIVE REDUCTION

1. Downward pressure on the clavicle and
2. Upward pressure on the forearm readily corrects the displacement.

Attempted reduction must be tailored to the needs of the patient.

If the patient must return to work or athletic competition promptly, symptomatic treatment for a few days with sling support is probably the wisest choice.

Otherwise, use a commercially available acromioclavicular (A-C) support.

USE OF A COMMERCIALLY AVAILABLE ACROMIOCLAVICULAR SUPPORT

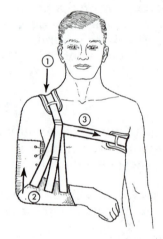

1. The shoulder strap applied over a piece of felt holds the clavicle down.
2. The sling supports the forearm and keeps the acromion in an elevated position.
3. The halter pulls both the shoulder strap and the sling inward.

After three weeks, allow free use of the arm.

Dislocation

REMARKS

Numerous methods, both closed and open, have been designed to treat this lesion.

The treatment for acromioclavicular dislocation should be tailored to the needs of the patient, since normal shoulder function is possible despite a chronically dislocated acromioclavicular joint.

The injury is not a surgical emergency but one that can well be treated promptly by simple shoulder support and early active range-of-motion exercises depending on the needs of the patient. This allows most individuals to return to work or to participation in sports within one to two weeks, much earlier than with surgical treatment.

Should surgical treatment be decided upon, the procedure should avoid:

1. Use of fixation pins across the acromioclavicular joint, which migrate all too frequently.

2. Use of fixation devices likely to erode bone or to fail.

3. Incomplete reduction of the acromioclavicular joint, which leads to arthritis.

4. A secondary operation necessary to remove fixation.

For an excessively prominent acromioclavicular dislocation that produces discomfort, the disrupted coracoclavicular ligament should be repaired and the outer 2 cm of the clavicle should be resected so as to avoid later development of acromioclavicular arthritis.

TYPICAL DEFORMITY

1. In a well-muscled man a complete acromioclavicular dislocation is barely perceptible.

2. The injury was treated symptomatically with early active exercise, and at two weeks the patient had returned to full activities.

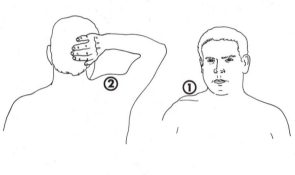

1. In this thin person the acromioclavicular dislocation completely disrupted muscles and became very prominent under the skin.

2. The shoulder drooped downward and forward.

3. There was a sulcus present between the outer end of the clavicle and the acromion.

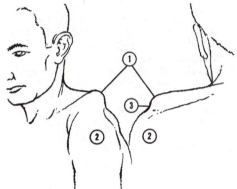

PATHOLOGIC PICTURE

1. Rupture of the acromioclavicular ligaments.

2. Rupture of the coracoclavicular ligaments.

3. Avulsion from the clavicle of attachments of the trapezius and deltoid muscles.

4. Acromion process is below and is widely separated from the clavicle.

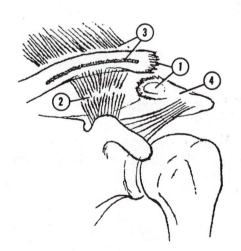

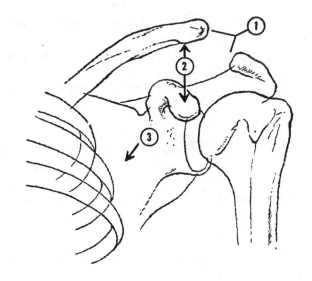

Dislocation *(Continued)*

PREREDUCTION X-RAY

1. There is complete displacement of the articular surfaces of the clavicle and the acromion process.

2. The interval between the clavicle and the coracoid is greatly increased.

3. The scapula is displaced downward and forward.

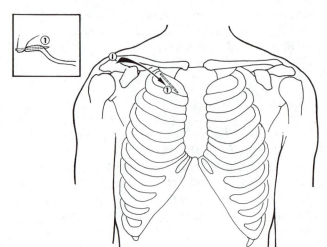

Caution: Avoid transarticular fixation of the acromioclavicular joint with pins. Too often this leads to symptomatic degenerative arthritis of the joint or

1. Migration of the pin into the mediastinum from the A-C joint "fixation."

OPERATIVE REPAIR (AFTER WEAVER AND DUNN)

1. Make a slightly curved 6-cm incision over the clavicle to the tip of the acromion.

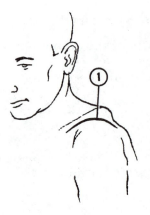

2. Reflect the deltoid and the trapezius to expose the coracoacromial ligament.

3. By subperiosteal dissection expose 5 cm. of the outer end of the clavicle.

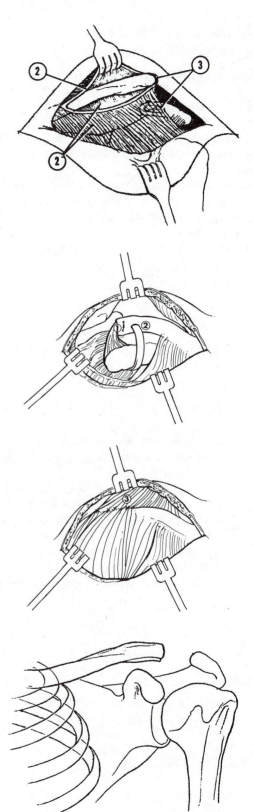

1. Suture the freed coracoacromial ligament into the distal end of the resected clavicle.

2. Use a heavy 5 mm. Mersilene suture passed around the coracoid process and into a hole drilled in the clavicle.

3. Repair the deltoid and trapezius muscles.

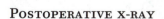

POSTOPERATIVE X-RAY

The distal clavicle has been resected and the coracoclavicular relationship has been restored.

553

Dislocation *(Continued)*

POSTOPERATIVE MANAGEMENT

Use a Velpeau sling for two to three days.

1. Pad the axilla.
2. Apply bias-cut bandage.
3. Support the arm with a sling until the initial postoperative pain subsides.

Start circumduction exercises by the third postoperative day, and discard the Velpeau sling when the patient is comfortable.

By the end of the fourth week, the patient is allowed full active use of the shoulder.

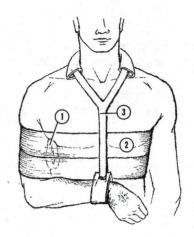

MANAGEMENT OF OLD ACROMIOCLAVICULAR DISLOCATIONS

REMARKS

Many chronically dislocated acromioclavicular joints are not painful and cause no dysfunction. These lesions generally do not require surgical repair.

Occasionally in a thin patient, a chronic dislocation becomes painful and interferes with complete elevation and abduction of the arm.

For some patients with subluxation or incompletely reduced dislocations, subsequent acromioclavicular arthritis becomes sufficiently painful to warrant treatment.

In both of these categories, resection of the outer 2 cm of the clavicle with or without repair of the coracoclavicular ligamentous supports is the procedure of choice.

Typical Deformity

1. Clavicle is unduly prominent.
2. Shoulder droops forward and downward.
3. Wide sulcus is apparent between acromion process and clavicle.

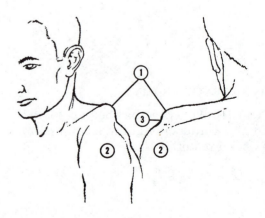

554

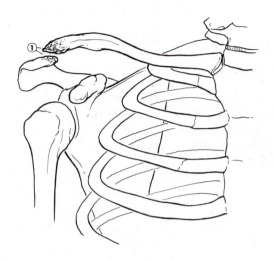

X-Ray of Acromioclavicular Arthritis

1. Partially reduced clavicle has developed symptomatic traumatic arthritis.

Operative Procedure

INCISION AND EXPOSURE

1. Make a slightly curved 7.6-cm incision terminating at the tip of the acromion process.

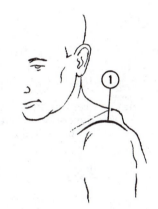

2. Deepen incision to bone.
3. By subperiosteal dissection, expose 5 cm of the outer of end of the clavicle.

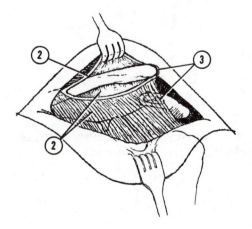

Operative Procedure (Continued)

EXCISION

1. With a Gigli saw remove 2 cm of the outer end of the clavicle.

2. Remove debris and remnants of meniscus from the acromioclavicular joint.

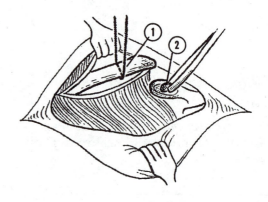

3. Approximate accurately by mattress sutures the detached margins of the trapezius and deltoid muscles.

Note: If the clavicle remains prominent after resection, repair the coracoclavicular ligament as described on page 553.

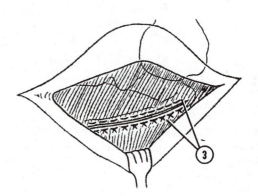

Postoperative X-ray

Approximately 2 cm of outer end of the clavicle has been resected.

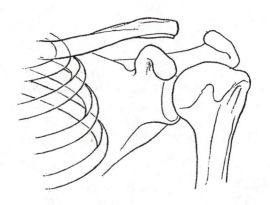

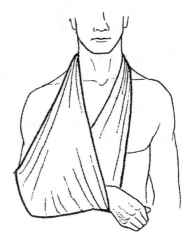

Postoperative Management

Apply triangular sling for one week.

Then allow free use of arm.

Institute physical therapy and progressive muscular exercises.

Injuries of the Sternoclavicular Joint

REMARKS

Injuries to the capsule and ligaments of the sternoclavicular joint are uncommon and consequently are frequently overlooked.

Typically, the patient complains of severe pain, and the medial end of the clavicle is as swollen and tender as in a fracture. No bone injury is evident unless specific x-ray views are taken to visualize the sternoclavicular joint.

The sternoclavicular joint has poor bony stability because only about half of the clavicle articulates with the manubrium, but the sternoclavicular ligaments offer strong compensatory support.

The medial end of the clavicle includes an epiphysis that does not appear on x-ray until the patient is about 18 years of age and is the last epiphysis in the body to close, usually at 26 years. Most sternoclavicular "dislocations" may actually be type I or type II epiphyseal fractures, which heal uneventfully.

Most lesions are the result of an indirect mechanism caused by laterally applied forces sustained when the individual falls on his shoulder. Most typically, this occurs in football when the patient lands on one shoulder as his tackler lands on the other shoulder. The sternoclavicular joint closest to the ground then absorbs the force of injury, and this usually causes an anterior dislocation or rarely a posterior dislocation of the joint.

557

A posterior or retrosternal dislocation may also occasionally be produced by a direct forceful blow to the front of the clavicle, e.g., with a baseball bat.

Posterior dislocation is much less common than anterior dislocation, but because of the threat to underlying cardiovascular and respiratory structures, posterior dislocation of the sternoclavicular joint can be life-threatening.

Depending on the degree of violence, the injury to the joint may be a sprain, a subluxation, or a complete dislocation.

MECHANISMS OF STERNOCLAVICULAR DISLOCATION

1. Most commonly the victim lands on one shoulder.

2. Someone else falls on the other shoulder, and the force is absorbed by the sternoclavicular joint closer to the ground. Depending on the position of the shoulder and the force vectors at time of injury, the clavicle may be displaced in one of three ways, anterosuperiorly, anteroinferiorly, or posteriorly.

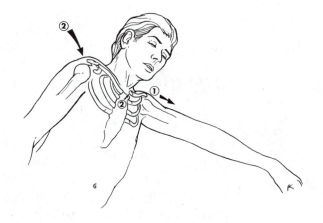

Anterosuperior Dislocation

1. The shoulder is depressed and extended during the fall.

2. The impact is applied to the anterolateral aspect of the shoulder.

3. The force is transmitted medially along the clavicle and posteriorly along the scapula.

4. The product of these forces is expended at the sternoclavicular joint, producing an anterosuperior dislocation.

5. If the force continues, the clavicle abuts against the first rib, which acts as a fulcrum to lever the clavicle anteriorly and superiorly.

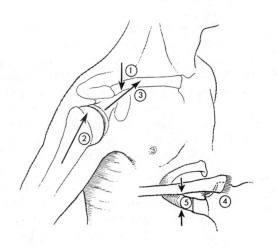

Anteroinferior Dislocation

1. The arm is abducted and the shoulder is extended during the fall.

2. Force travels along the humerus and medially along the clavicle.

3. The force is expended at the sternoclavicular joint, producing an anteroinferior dislocation.

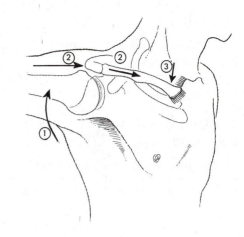

Posterior (Retrosternal) Dislocation

1. The shoulder is elevated and flexed forward during the fall.

2. The force travels along the humerus and medially along the clavicle.

3. The force is expended on the posterior aspect of the sternoclavicular articulation, producing a retrosternal dislocation.

Note: This same lesion may be caused by a direct blow to the anterior aspect of the sternal end of the clavicle.

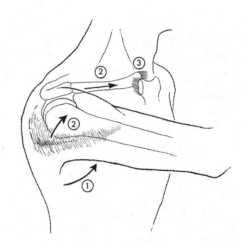

PATHOLOGIC PICTURE OF STERNOCLAVICULAR JOINT INJURY

Sprain

1. Some stretching and tearing of the sternoclavicular ligament.

2. No disalignment of the articular surfaces of the clavicle and the sternum.

3. The costocalvicular ligaments are intact.

4. Medial clavicular epiphysis is only partially separated.

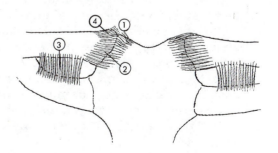

Subluxation

1. The capsule and the sternoclavicular ligaments rupture.

2. Some tearing and stretching of the costoclavicular ligament, but it is intact.

3. Partial separation of the medial clavicular epiphysis.

Note: The displacement of the clavicle may be anterosuperior, anteroinferior, or posterior, depending on the direction of the force.

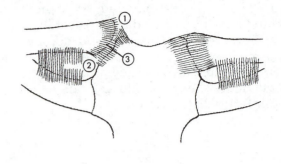

Dislocation or Epiphyseal Separation

1. Complete rupture of the capsule and sternoclavicular ligaments.

2. Complete rupture of the costoclavicular ligament.

3. Complete separation of the medial clavicular epiphysis.

4. Sternoclavicular ligaments are torn completely.

Note: The displacement of the clavicle may be anterior or posterior, depending on the direction of the force.

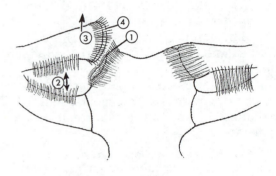

DIAGNOSIS OF STERNOCLAVICULAR JOINT INJURY

Diagnosis is primarily clinical and is based on swelling, tenderness, and instability of the medial end of the clavicle after injury.

The displacement of the clavicle is usually palpable, but the injured area may be too swollen and tender to permit adequate examination.

With a posterior dislocation, the medial end of the clavicle is not palpable, and the patient may be experiencing shortness of breath, choking, or circulatory damage, or may be in complete shock.

X-rays of the sternoclavicular joint are frequently difficult to interpret owing to superimposition of other structures. Special views are necessary.

X-Ray Technique for the Sternoclavicular Joint (Rockwood Technique)

1. X-ray is tilted 40 degrees toward the manubrium.
2. Tube distance is 100 cm in a child, 140 cm in an adult with a thick chest.
3. The cassette should allow visualization of both clavicles.

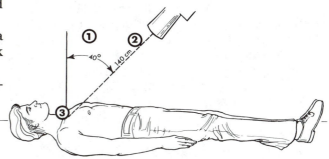

Appearance on X-ray

1. Normally, the clavicles appear in the same horizontal plane.
2. Anterior dislocation projects a clavicle above the horizontal plane.
3. Posterior dislocation projects a clavicle below the horizontal plane.

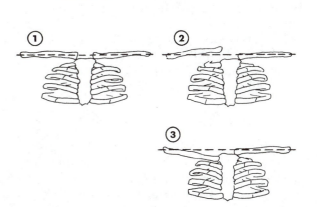

MANAGEMENT OF STERNOCLAVICULAR JOINT INJURY

Sprain

Sprains of the sternoclavicular joint require symptomatic treatment with a sling, ice application for 3 to 4 days, and gradual return to normal activities.

Recovery should be complete in 10 to 14 days.

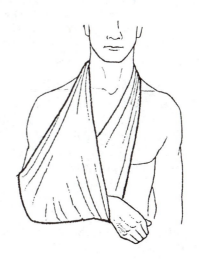

561

Subluxation or Anterior Dislocation

REDUCTION

1. Subluxations and anterior dislocations of this joint are reduced with the patient sitting on a stool.

2. A stockinette stuffed with cast padding is applied in a figure-of-eight manner around the shoulder.

3. The surgeon stands behind the patient and places his knee between the scapulae.

4. The surgeon applies 12 to 15 turns of 10-cm plaster in a figure-of-eight manner.

5. While the plaster is being applied, the shoulder is elevated and the surgeon pushes forward with a knee between the scapulae.

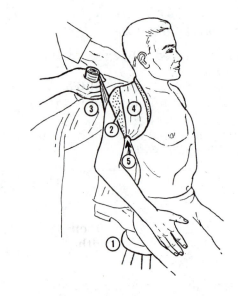

IMMOBILIZATION

1. Place patient in supine position with a sandbag between the shoulder blades and arms to the sides.

2. To reduce the anterior dislocation, apply firm pressure to the shoulder and the anteriorly displaced clavicle.

Note: Internal fixation of the sternoclavicular joint is too hazardous to warrant its use. If closed reduction is incomplete, open reduction is usually unnecessary. Should the sternoclavicular prominence produce chronic symptoms, delayed resection of the medial clavicle is an effective method of relieving symptoms (see page 565).

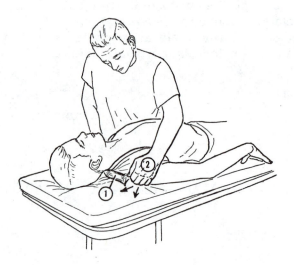

POSTREDUCTION MANAGEMENT

Watch for embarrassment of the circulation in the upper extremities.

Instruct the patient to pull the shoulders back voluntarily and to abduct the arms from the sides in case extremities become cyanotic.

Allow the patient free use of the arms, especially in the abducted position.

Plaster-of-Paris dressing is removed at the end of six weeks.

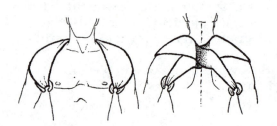

562

POSTERIOR DISLOCATION OF THE STERNOCLAVICULAR JOINT

REMARKS

This lesion is given special consideration because it may be associated with serious complications.

Posterior displacement of the sternal end of the clavicle may compress or may lacerate the contents of the thoracic outlet, the trachea, the esophagus, and the great vessels.

Reduction of the posterior dislocation can usually be readily accomplished by closed methods, but be sure to evaluate the patient carefully for hoarseness or any signs of respiratory or vascular impairment.

The patient usually does not require general anesthetic, although local anesthesia with sedation is helpful.

Manipulative Reduction

1. Place a sandbag between the scapulae of the patient.

2. The arm on the affected side hangs over the side of the table. An assistant makes steady traction downward.

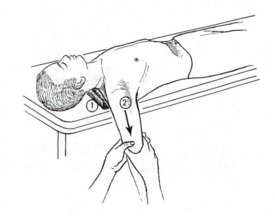

1. The operator grasps the clavicle; the fingers of both hands are placed on the posterior-superior surface of the clavicle and the thumbs on the inferior surface.

Pull the sternal end of the clavicle

2. Upward
3. Forward
4. Laterally.

Note: Reduction occurs with a click, and the medial end of the clavicle should then be palpable.

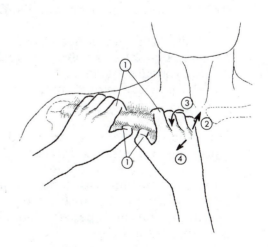

563

Manipulative Reduction (*Continued*)

Alternatively, if reduction is not achieved, prepare the area for surgery and with the patient under local anesthetic

1. Use a sterile towel clip to lift the clavicle upward and laterally.

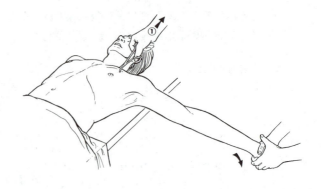

Immobilization

1. Apply a plaster-of-Paris posterior figure-of-eight bandage.

Note: These injuries, which are really epiphyseal fractures, are stable once they are reduced.

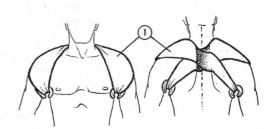

Postreduction Management

Posterior figure-of-eight bandage is removed at the end of three weeks.

MANAGEMENT OF UNREDUCED CHRONIC DISLOCATIONS OF THE STERNOCLAVICULAR JOINT

REMARKS

Many patients with unreduced or chronic anterior dislocations of the sternoclavicular joint have insufficient symptoms to warrant treatment.

Patients with unreduced posterior dislocation face too many potential complications and are best treated by resection of the inner end of the dislocated clavicle.

Patients with symptomatic, unreduced anterior dislocation of the joint are also best managed by resection of the medial clavicular prominence.

Reconstructive procedures and methods of open reduction for this injury do not offer sufficient advantages over simpler resection to discount their disadvantages.

Internal fixation with pins crossing the sternoclavicular joint is especially hazardous because of the high risk of vascular damage from pin migration and penetration. Several deaths have been reported from this catastrophe.

Resection of Chronic Dislocation

1. Expose the joint through a hockey stick incision 10 cm long.

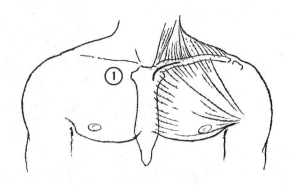

2. By subperiosteal dissection, reflect the clavicular head of the sternocleidomastoid upward and the insertion of the pectoralis major downward.

3. Resect obliquely 5 cm of the medial end of the clavicle.

4. Remove all remnants of the disc.

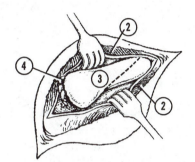

5. Approximate carefully the clavicular head of the sternocleidomatoid muscle to the pectoralis major muscle.

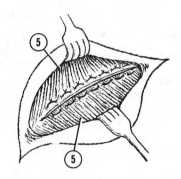

Postoperative Management

Apply a plaster-of-Paris posterior figure-of-eight dressing.

Remove dressing at the end of three weeks.

Encourage full use of the extremity.

Institute a regulated program of exercises (five to ten minutes every waking hour) to restore full motion of the shoulder girdle.

FRACTURES OF THE SCAPULA

Fractures of the Body, Spine, and Coracoid Process of the Scapula

REMARKS

Fractures of the body of the scapula are usually the result of a violent direct force.

On rare occasions muscle contractions may cause a fracture of the body and may also produce an avulsion fracture of the spine of the scapula.

Fractures of the scapula are frequently associated with fractures of the ribs and the spine.

In severe crushing injuries, fractures of the scapula may be overlooked.

Fractures of the body need no reduction; because the scapula is invested in muscle masses, separation of the fragments is never very great.

Complete anatomic alignment in fractures of the body of the scapula is not essential to attain an excellent functional result.

1. Fracture of the body.
2. Fracture of the spine.
3. Fracture of the acromion.
4. Fracture of the base of the coracoid process.

Note: Fractures of the acromion are frequently associated with underlying injuries to the rotator cuff. If shoulder weakness persists for six weeks or longer after these fractures, evaluate the rotator cuff mechanism by means of a shoulder arthrogram.

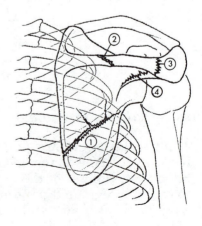

Management

All these fractures are treated as follows:

Apply ice to the part for the first 24 to 36 hours; then apply heat.

For the first 24 to 48 hours apply a compression bandage to hold the scapula firmly against the chest wall; then suspend the arm in a sling.

1. Firm compression bandage using moleskin to fix the scapula against the chest wall.
2. Suspend the arm in a sling.

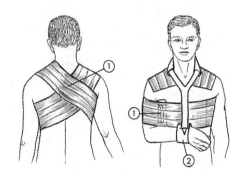

After Care

After 10 to 14 days, remove the supportive sling and encourage the use of the shoulder girdle within the tolerance of pain.

Institute a regimen of pendulum exercises progressively increasing in range and frequency.

Note: Inform the patient that although motion in the shoulder girdle will be promptly restored, some discomfort will be felt for many weeks, especially when forceful movements are attempted.

Fractures of the Neck of the Scapula

REMARKS

Fractures of the neck of the scapula are usually the result of direct violence applied to the anterior or posterior aspect of the shoulder.

The articular surface of the glenoid is not disturbed, and the capsular apparatus of the glenohumeral joint is intact.

Anatomic reduction is not essential to attain a good functional result.

Open reduction of this fracture is rarely indicated.

The type of management depends upon the degree of displacement of the distal fragment.

WITH MINIMAL DISPLACEMENT

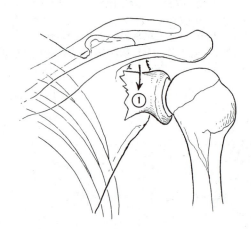

Appearance on X-Ray

1. The glenoid fragment is displaced downward and inward.

Management

Apply ice for the first 24 to 36 hours; then apply heat.

Apply a triangular sling.

After 10 to 14 days, begin graduated active exercises of the shoulder within the tolerance of pain.

Institute daily heat application and gentle massage to all the soft tissues of the shoulder girdle.

Discard the sling after three or four weeks and increase gradually the range and frequency of the pendulum exercises.

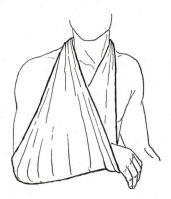

WITH MARKED DISPLACEMENT

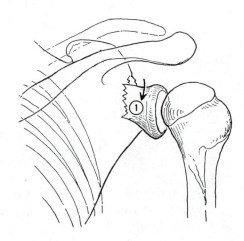

Appearance on X-ray

1. Glenoid fragment is markedly displaced downward and inward.

Reduction by Lateral Traction

1. Patient assumes the supine position.

2. Place a board under the mattress.

3. Elevate the side of the bed 10 cm.

4. Apply skeletal traction through the base of the olecranon and add 6 to 12 lb (2.7 to 5.4 kg).

5. Apply traction to forearm and add 3 to 6 lb (1.4 to 2.7 kg).

6. Traction is made with the arm abducted 90 degrees and the forearm flexed 90 degrees.

Note: Maintain traction for two weeks.

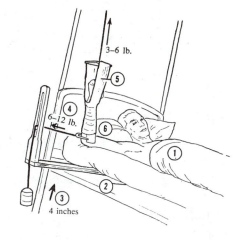

Postreduction X-Ray

Normal relation of glenoid fragment to the scapula is restored.

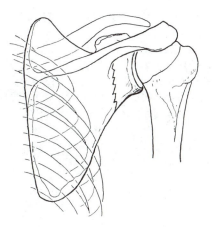

Postreduction Care

Apply a triangular sling for two weeks.

Institute progressive shoulder exercises on a regulated program (five to ten minutes every waking hour).

Institute daily heat and massage to the entire affected extremity.

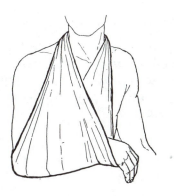

FRACTURES OF THE GLENOID

Mechanisms of Injury

REMARKS

Fractures of the glenoid are produced by either a direct or an indirect mechanism.

DIRECT MECHANISM: STELLATE FRACTURE

A direct force applied to the lateral side of the shoulder produces a stellate type of fracture; the degree of displacement of the fragments depends upon the intensity of the force.

Most stellate fractures require no reduction because the glenoid articular surface can tolerate much incongruity and still function normally; the glenohumeral joint is not a weight-bearing joint.

In severely displaced stellate fractures, an attempt should be made to reduce the deformity.

Minimal Displacement

1. A direct force is applied to the lateral side of the shoulder, and

2. Stellate fracture of the glenoid with minimal displacement of the fragments occurs.

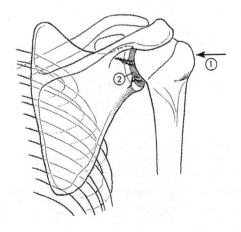

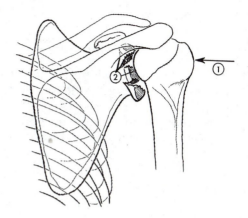

Marked Displacement

1. A direct force applied to the lateral side of the shoulder produces
2. Stellate fracture of the glenoid with severe comminution and separation of the fragments.

INDIRECT MECHANISM

This mechanism acts when the victim falls on the flexed elbow.

The force travels along the shaft and the head of the humerus and is expended on the glenoid, shearing off a portion of bone.

The site at which a fragment of bone is sheared off the glenoid depends upon the direction in which the humeral head is driven; if it is driven forward, a segment of the anterior aspect of the glenoid is sheared off; if it is driven backward a portion of the posterior region of the glenoid is displaced.

Management of the lesions is governed by the degree of the displacement of the detached fragment.

Fragments with greater displacements than 1 cm should be reattached surgically, because if not reattached they lead to recurrent dislocation of the glenohumeral joint.

Anterior Glenoid Fracture

1. The force travels along the shaft of the humerus, which is extended and abducted.
2. The head of the humerus abuts against the anterior portion of the glenoid.
3. A segment of the glenoid is driven forward.

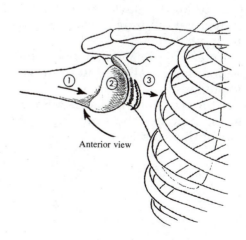

Anterior view

571

Posterior Glenoid Fracture

1. The force travels along the shaft of the humerus, which is flexed and abducted.

2. The head of the humerus abuts against the posterior portion of the glenoid.

3. A segment of the glenoid is driven backward.

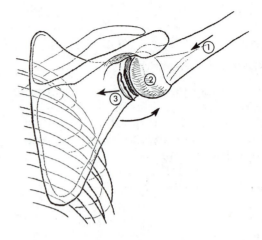

Management of Fractures of the Glenoid

STELLATE FRACTURES

With Minimal Displacement

Apply ice for the first 24 or 36 hours; then apply heat.

Apply a triangular sling.

After 10 to 14 days begin active, graduated pendulum exercises within the tolerance of pain.

Institute daily heat application and gentle massage to all the soft tissues of the shoulder girdle.

After three or four weeks discard the sling and increase the range and frequency of the exercises.

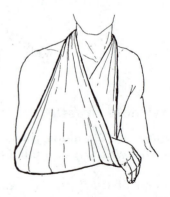

With Marked Displacement

REDUCTION BY LATERAL TRACTION

1. Patient assumes the supine position.

2. Place a board under the mattress.

3. Elevate the side of the bed 10 cm.

4. Apply skeletal traction through the base of the olecranon and add 6 to 12 lb (2.7 to 5.4 kg).

5. Apply traction to forearm and add 3 to 6 lb (1.3 to 2.7 kg).

6. Traction is made with the arm abducted 90 degrees and the forearm flexed 90 degrees.

Note: Maintain traction for two weeks.

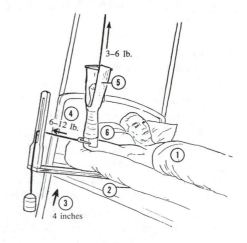

POSTREDUCTION X-RAY

Normal configuration of the glenoid fossa is restored.

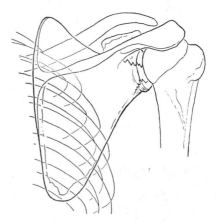

POSTREDUCTION CARE

Apply a triangular sling for two weeks.

Institute progressive shoulder exercises on a regulated program (five or ten minutes every hour).

Institute daily heat and massage to the entire affected extremity.

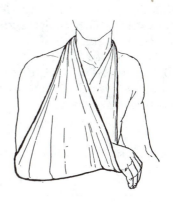

OPERATIVE MANAGEMENT OF SPECIFIC GLENOID RIM FRACTURES

Fractures of the glenoid rim commonly lead to shoulder instability, which requires operative repair. This is true even for minimally displaced fractures.

Fractures of the anterior or posterior portion of the glenoid result from dislocations of the shoulder and are frequently associated with recurrent instability and pain in the shoulder.

Even "minor," barely perceptible fractures of the inferior glenoid may produce symptoms of recurrent pain and subluxation, particularly in young, active individuals.

The larger fracture results most often from the humeral head impacting violently against the anterior glenoid rim at the time of the dislocation. The same mechanism produces the Hills-Sachs lesion, or a compression fracture of the posterolateral aspect of the humeral head.

A small inferior glenoid fracture may result from an avulsion mechanism that occurs when the shoulder is forcefully externally rotated and abducted, stretching the capsular attachment to the glenoid labrum.

Symptoms of shoulder pain and clicking or subluxation following such an avulsion injury can be confusing, because the shoulder may never completely dislocate. The physician should search carefully on x-ray for inferior glenoid rim fractures that would indicate the nature of the patient's problem.

Examples of Fractures

1. Fractures of the anterior portion of the glenoid with minimal displacement.

2. Fractures of the posterior portion of the glenoid with minimal displacement.

3. Avulsion fractures of the glenoid brim (associated with dislocations of the glenohumeral joint).

4. Avulsion fractures of the inferior glenoid brim caused by severe contracture of the triceps. This occurs most often in throwing athletes.

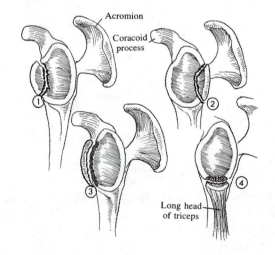

Appearance On X-Ray

1. An anterior subluxation of the humeral head produces
2. A subtle small avulsion fracture of the inferior glenoid.

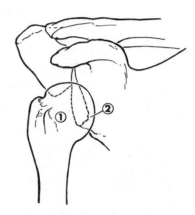

GLENOID FRACTURE ASSOCIATED WITH RECURRENT DISLOCATION

1. Fracture of the anterior portion of the glenoid.
2. The fragment is displaced forward more than 1 cm.

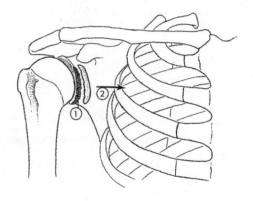

AVULSION FRACTURE ASSOCIATED WITH RECURRENT SHOULDER SUBLUXATION

1. An oblique axillary view is necessary to see the anterior inferior glenoid fracture.
2. A subtle fracture indicates the location of the avulsion injury which is producing symptoms of pain and instability on external rotation and abduction of the shoulder.

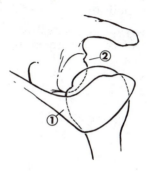

Position of Patient

Elevate shoulder with sandbag between scapulae and place patient on table so that arm is near the edge of the table.

Drape the arm separately to permit manipulation of the limb.

Tilt the whole table slightly away from the surgeon.

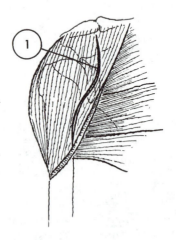

Operative Procedure

1. Make a curved incision on the anterior aspect of the shoulder, beginning at the inferior margin of the acromioclavicular joint and continuing through the deltopectoral interval.

2. Develop the interval between the deltoid and the pectoralis major and retract the cephalic vein with the pectoralis major medially.

Note: If more exposure is desired cut the proximal half of the tendon of the pectoralis major.

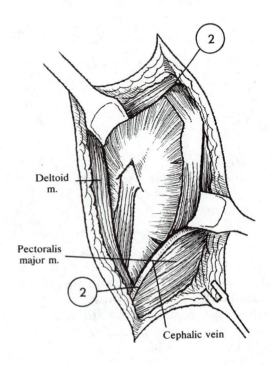

Deltoid m.

Pectoralis major m.

Cephalic vein

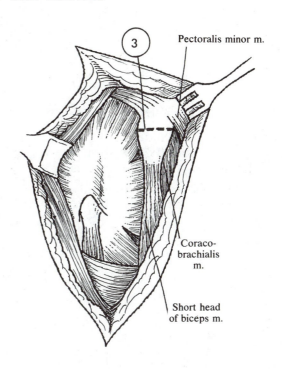

3. Isolate and divide the conjoined tendons of the muscles inserting into the coracoid process (the short head of the biceps, the coracobrachialis, and the pectoralis minor).

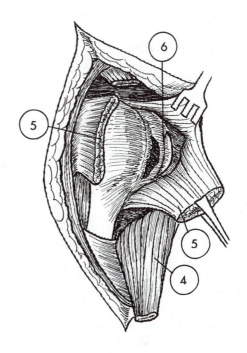

4. Retract the detached portion of the muscular attachments medially.

5. Divide the subscapularis tendon down to the capsule 1 cm medial to the lesser tuberosity, and by sharp dissection reflect the tendon from the capsule to beyond the anterior rim of the glenoid.

6. Isolate the site of the fracture—the displaced fragment will be found still attached to the capsule.

Operative Procedure (Continued)

7. Restore the fragment to its anatomic position and fix it with a screw.

8. Repair any rents in the capsule.

Note: For small avulsion fractures of the inferior glenoid, suture the capsule back into the glenoid.

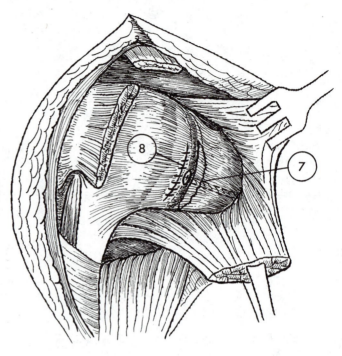

Postoperative X-Ray

1. Fragment is in its anatomic position

2. Screw is transfixing the fragment.

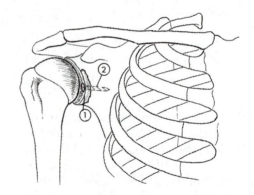

Postoperative Immobilization

1. Place a pad of cotton in the axilla.

2. Encircle the arm and trunk with a 10-cm bias-cut stockinette.

3. Apply a triangular sling or

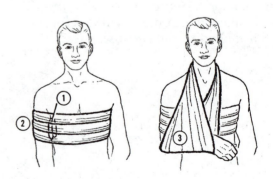

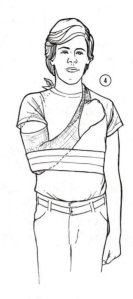

4. Apply a stockinette cut to immobilize the shoulder.

Postoperative Management

Fix the arm to the side in a position of internal rotation for four weeks.

During this time allow limited motion at the elbow and encourage motion at the wrist and in the fingers.

After four weeks discard all external immobilization and begin pendulum exercises in increasing arcs on a regulated regimen (five to ten minutes every waking hour).

After five weeks encourage active external rotation of the arm within the patient's tolerance.

Also, add abduction and external rotation exercises. Increase exercises progressively in range and frequency until movements are back to normal (see page 139).

FRACTURE OF THE POSTERIOR PORTION OF THE GLENOID

Preoperative X-Ray

1. Fracture of the posterior portion of the glenoid.

2. Fragment is separated more than 1 cm.

Note: Frequently this injury is associated with recurrent posterior instability and should be repaired.

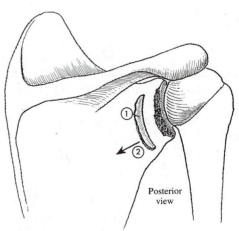

Posterior view

Position of Patient and Incision

1. Place the patient in the prone position.

2. Place a large sandbag under the shoulder.

3. Drape the arm free to aid exposure and place it on an arm board in the abducted position.

4. Begin the incision at the acromioclavicular joint and continue it posteriorly over the top of the acromion to the spine of the scapula; then curve it downward and outward to a point 4 cm above the posterior fold of the axilla.

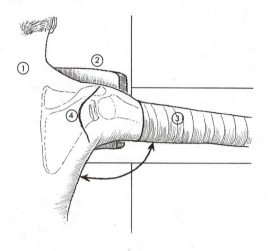

Operative Procedure

1. Identify and develop by blunt dissection the interval between the deltoid and the deeper muscles.

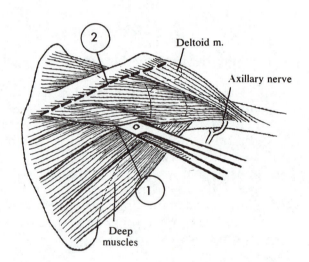

2. Divide the deltoid 1 cm from its bony attachment and then detach it subperiosteally as far as the acromioclavicular joint; retract the muscle laterally.

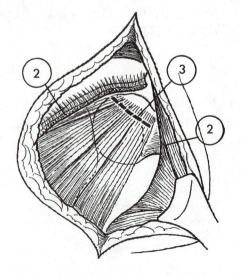

3. Divide the conjoined tendon, including the infraspinatus and teres minor and a portion of the supraspinatus (*Caution*: Do not sever the axillary nerve in the quadrilateral space), 1 cm from its insertion, and reflect the muscles medially as far as the posterior aspect of the glenoid.

4. Isolate the posterior detached fragment of the glenoid.

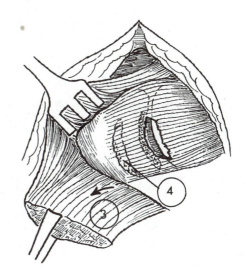

5. Restore the fragment to its anatomic position and fix it with a screw.

6. Repair any rents in the capsule by interrupted sutures.

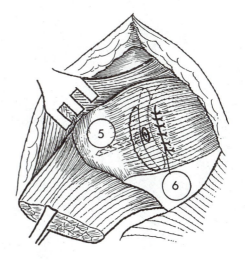

Postoperative X-Ray

1. Fragment in its anatomic position.

2. Screw is transfixing the fragment.

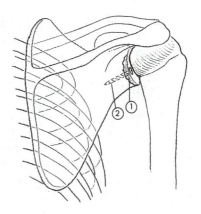

581

Postoperative Immobilization

1. Place a pad in the axilla.
2. Encircle the trunk with a 10-cm bias-cut stockinette.
3. Apply a triangular sling or

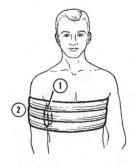
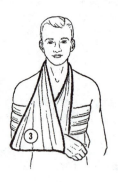

4. Apply a stockinette cut to immobilize the shoulder.

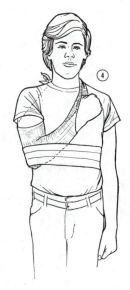

Postoperative Management

Fix the arm to the side in a position of internal rotation for four weeks.

During this time allow motion at the elbow and encourage motion at the wrist and in the fingers.

After four weeks discard all external immobilization and begin pendulum exercises in ever-increasing arcs on a regulated regimen (five to ten minutes every waking hour).

After five weeks encourage active external rotation and abduction exercises. Increase in frequency and range until normal range of motion is restored (see page 139).

DISLOCATION OF THE SCAPULA

REMARKS

Although rare, this lesion occasionally is encountered. Manipulative maneuvers will reduce the displaced scapula. Open reduction is usually not necessary.

Prereduction X-Ray

1. Entire body of scapula is displaced outward and rotated outward.
2. Lower angle is wedged between the ribs.

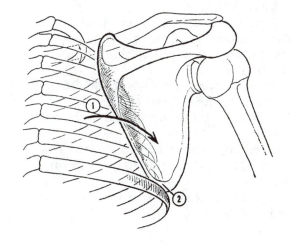

Manipulative Reduction

1. Assistant makes steady traction on the hyperabducted arm.
2. Surgeon grasps axillary border of scapula and by the same movement rotates bone forward and
3. Pushes scapula directly backward.

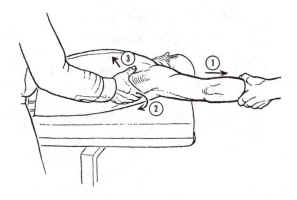

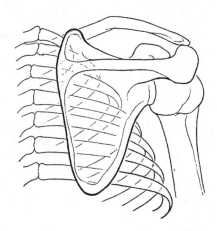

Postreduction X-Ray

Scapula has returned to its normal anatomic position.

Strapping and Immobilization

Use eight or ten long strips of 7.5-cm adhesive.

1. Beginning in front of chest, pass strips under arm, over the scapula, and around the chest to the top of the opposite shoulder.

2. Apply three strips over the affected shoulder from front to back.

3. Place a large cotton pad in the axilla.

4. Bind the arm to the side with a 10-cm bias-cut stockinette encircling the body.

5. Support the forearm with a collar and cuff sling.

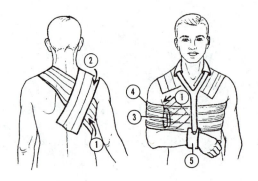

Postreduction Care

Reinforce dressing after seven to ten days.

Discard dressing after two weeks.

Encourage active free use of shoulder within tolerance of pain.

Institute regulated program of active exercises for the shoulder, hand, and fingers.

Normal function is achieved in four to five weeks.

SUMMARY: THE PITFALLS OF FRACTURES AND DISLOCATIONS OF THE SHOULDER GIRDLE

Fractures of the clavicle may lead to surprising pitfalls, particularly in the adult. Adequate reduction and immobilization require a shoulder cast for the adult's fracture rather than the simple figure-of-eight harness that works effectively in children.

Intramedullary pin fixation of the clavicular, sternoclavicular, or acromioclavicular injury is associated with an inordinate number of major complications due to pin migration out of the posterior clavicle. If pins are used at all for fixation of clavicular injuries, posterior migration should be anticipated and should be prevented by the use of Knowles pins inserted in a posterior-to-anterior direction.

Acromioclavicular dislocations may frequently be asymptomatic, particularly in well-muscled individuals. The treatment of this common injury must be particularly oriented toward the clinical needs of the patient rather than the radiographic appearance of the injury. Some types of surgical repair of this condition, particularly transarticular pin fixation, cause a more symptomatic problem than chronic dislocation.

Sternoclavicular dislocations lead to numerous pitfalls, the first one of which is an incorrect diagnosis. These fairly common injuries may not be recognized if the clinician depends more on the radiographic appearance than on the physical examination. Closed reduction of either the common anterior or the less common posterior sternoclavicular dislocation is usually quite simple and effective. Operative reduction with attempted internal fixation of these injuries is quite hazardous and is more likely to injure the underlying major vascular structures than is the dislocation itself.

Fractures of the scapula usually heal without complication except when the injury involves the glenoid labrum. Even subtle avulsion fractures of the labrum can cause symptoms of shoulder instability or subluxation out of proportion to the radiographic appearance. Once again, the physician's alertness to the patient's symptoms and physical findings rather than to the radiographic appearance is the most effective guide to avoid the pitfalls of treatment.

REFERENCES

Imatoni, R. J., Hanlon, J. J., and Cady, G. W.: Acute, complete acromioclavicular separation. J. Bone and Joint Surg. 57-A:328, 1975.

Neviaser, R. J., Neviaser, J. S., Neviaser, T. J., et al.: A simple technique for internal fixation of the clavicle. A long term evaluation. Clin. Orthop. 109:103, 1975.

Penn, I.: The vascular complications of fractures of the clavicle. J. Trauma 4:819, 1964.

Rockwood, C.: Dislocation of sternoclavicular joint. *In* Fractures, edited by C. Rockwood and D. Green, Philadelphia, Lippincott, 1975, pp. 756–786.

Shumacker, H. B.: Resection of the clavicle. With particular reference to the use of bone chips in the periosteal bed. Surg. Gyn. Obst. 84:245, 1947.

Weaver, J. K., and Dunn, H. K.: Treatment of the acromioclavicular injuries. J. Bone and Joint Surg. 54-A: 1187, 1972.

Weber, B. G., and Cech, O.: Pseudarthrosis. New York, Grune & Stratton, 1976, pp. 104–107.

INJURIES OF THE LIGAMENTS AND CAPSULE OF THE GLENOHUMERAL JOINT (SUBLUXATIONS AND DISLOCATIONS)

ANATOMIC FEATURES AND MECHANISMS OF INJURY

REMARKS

Knowledge of the anatomic features of the glenohumeral joint allows us to better understand the many injuries to which this joint is subject.

Comprehension of the mechanisms of these injuries is basic to prompt diagnosis and appropriate treatment.

The bony configuration of the glenohumeral joint provides minimal stability. The major stability of this articulation depends on the capsular structures and muscles, particularly the rotator cuff system and the deltoid and pectoralis major muscles.

The location of the glenohumeral joint and its wide range of motion makes this joint the most vulnerable in the body to dislocation.

Developmental differences in the shoulder support structures, particularly in the glenohumeral joints and the subscapularis muscles, also play a role in the susceptibility to recurrent dislocation.

The wide range of motion required in the shoulder joint causes surrounding soft tissue wear and degeneration, particularly in the supraspinatus tendon after the third decade. This common wear phenomenon results in frequent disruption of the rotator cuff support structures, sometimes with minor injury.

The close proximity of major neurovascular structures to the shoulder joint puts these structures in jeopardy from glenohumeral injury.

Muscles

REMARKS

Essentially, the important muscles enveloping the glenohumeral joint consist of two muscular sleeves, an inner sleeve made up of the rotator cuff muscles and an outer sleeve consisting of the deltoid, the teres major, and the pectoralis major muscles.

These two groups of muscles operate one within the other and are separated by an efficient gliding mechanism consisting of the sub-acromial bursa and fine, filmy areolar tissue.

Muscular Sleeves

1. The deltoid muscle makes up most of the outer sleeve, which also includes the teres major and pectoralis major muscles.

2. Subscapularis and supraspinatus components of the inner sleeve.

3. Subacromial bursa — the gliding mechanism between the two muscle strata.

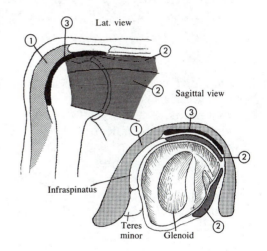

Arrangement of the Rotator Muscles Under the Coracoacromial Arch

1. Coracoacromial ligament.
2. Coracoid.
3. Acromion.
4. Subscapularis.
5. Supraspinatus.
6. Infraspinatus.
7. Teres minor.
8. Coracohumeral ligament.
9. Biceps tendon.

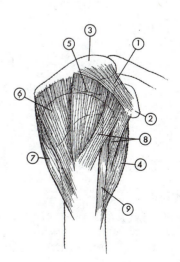

FUNCTIONAL MECHANISM OF MUSCLES OF THE GLENOHUMERAL JOINT

REMARKS

Abduction and flexion of the humerus is achieved by the synchronous action of two groups of muscles: (1) the deltoid, supraspinatus, and pectoralis major muscles and (2) the infraspinatus, teres minor, and subscapularis muscles.

The latter group constitutes a functional unit that depresses the humeral head and fixes it firmly against the glenoid so that the former group can abduct and flex the arm. Without the stabilizing effect of the rotator muscles, the deltoid would pull the humerus vertically under the acromion.

The rotator muscles pass from the scapula posteriorly, superiorly, and anteriorly and blend with one another and the fibrous capsule to form a tough musculotendinous cuff around the head of the humerus before inserting into the humerus. Together they hold the head of the humerus snugly against the glenoid.

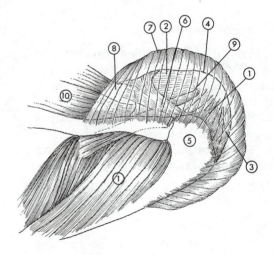

1. Supraspinatus.
2. Subscapularis.
3. Infraspinatus.
4. Musculotendinous cuff.
5. Acromion.
6. Coracoacromial ligament.
7. Deltoid.
8. Coracoid process.
9. Coracohumeral ligament.
10. Pectoralis minor.

Ligaments and Capsule

REMARKS

Ligaments, which are in essence areas of reinforced capsule, provide major support and stability to the shoulder joint. Numerous variations in the anterior ligament complex or the glenohumeral ligament, however, may be encountered in association with dislocation.

590

In its inferior portion, in order to permit the global range of motion in the glenohumeral joint, the capsule is redundant and folded on itself.

Anteriorly, the synovial portion of the capsule extends toward the coracoid process, forming the subscapularis recess and also the synovial covering of the bicipital tendon.

No communication ordinarily exists between the glenohumeral space and the subacromial or subdeltoid bursa. In later years the natural asymptomatic degeneration of the rotator cuff tendon allows communication between these spaces, but in most individuals communication between the glenohumeral joint and the subacromial bursa indicates disruption of the rotator cuff tendon.

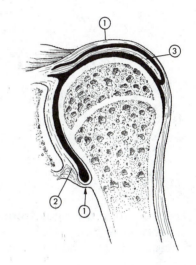

Capsule of the Glenohumeral Joint

1. Inferiorly the capsule is redundant and folds on itself like an accordion to allow full range of shoulder motion to the overhead position.
2. Glenoid labrum.
3. Biceps tendon.

Extension of the Synovial Capsule

1. Synovial capsule distended.
2. Prolongation under the coracoid process (subscapularis recess).
3. Prolongation along the bicipital groove and then onto the biceps tendon.
4. Transverse humeral ligament.

Note: The glenohumeral joint does not communicate with the subacromial space.

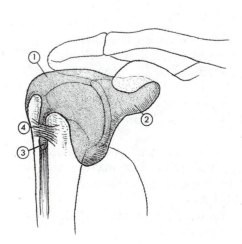

Glenohumeral Ligaments (From Behind)

1. Glenoid fossa
2. Glenoid labrum.
3. Biceps (long head).
4. Superior glenohumeral ligament.
5. Middle glenohumeral ligament.
6. Inferior glenohumeral ligament.
7. Subscapularis recess.

Note: Observe that all three ligaments are directed toward the superior aspect of the glenoid fossa.

The subscapularis recess communicates with the inside of the joint cavity.

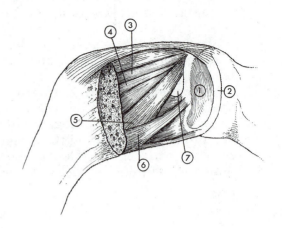

Degenerative Alterations of the Glenohumeral Joint

REMARKS

Degenerative changes from normal use of the arm occur early in the glenohumeral joint — as early as the second decade — and increase progressively in subsequent decades.

Representative models of the alterations in various decades are illustrated here.

Second Decade

1. The labrum in the lower half of the glenoid fossa is continuous with the capsule, and its upper portion is free.
2. The synovial membrane is smooth and adherent to all structures.
3. The capsule in the anterior aspect of the joint extends toward the base of the coracoid, forming a large synovial pouch.
4. The hyaline cartilage of the glenoid is normal.

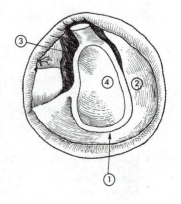

592

Fourth Decade

1. The labrum is detached from the anterior aspect of the glenoid.
2. The synovial membrane shows the formation of fringes and tabs.
3. In this specimen there is no synovial pouch extending under the coracoid.
4. The hyaline cartilage shows thinning and irregularity.

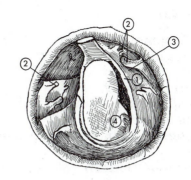

Sixth Decade

1. The labrum is frayed and detached from the glenoid in several areas.
2. The synovial membrane shows numerous fringes and tabs.
3. A small synovial pouch is present above the middle ligament.
4. Deterioration of the hyaline cartilage is advanced.
5. There is fraying and lamination of the musculotendinous cuff in the region of the supraspinatus and infraspinatus portions of the cuff.

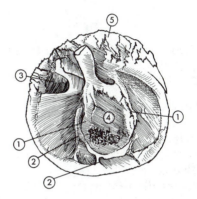

Neurovascular Structures in Close Proximity to the Joint

REMARKS

These structures may be injured during a dislocation or the reduction of a dislocation of the glenohumeral joint.

Axillary Nerve

1. Infraspinatus muscle.
2. Teres minor muscle.
3. Teres major muscle.
4. Triceps muscle.
5. Quadrangular space.
6. Axillary nerve.
7. Anterior branch of axillary nerve.
8. Posterior branch of axillary nerve.
9. Cutaneous branch of posterior branch of axillary nerve.
10. Nerve to teres minor.

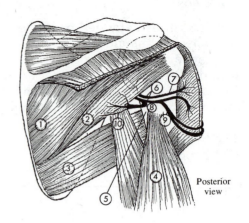

Posterior view

Large Neurovascular Structures

1. Axillary artery and brachial plexus.
2. Musculocutaneous nerve.
3. Clavicle.
4. Deltoid.
5. Pectoralis minor.
6. Biceps.
7. Pectoralis major.
8. Subscapularis.
9. Teres major.
10. Coracobrachialis.

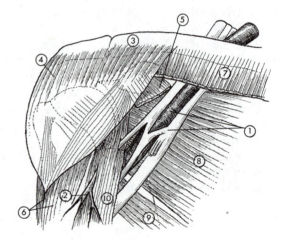

Normal Motions of the Glenohumeral Joint

REMARKS

The upper arm possesses a global range of motion (almost 360 degrees); this comprises the summation of the ranges of motion possible in four articulations — (1) the glenohumeral joint, (2) the sternoclavicular joint, (3) the acromioclavicular joint, and (4) the thoracoscapular joint.

594

Impairment of motion in any of these four components is reflected in the total performance of the shoulder girdle. They function as a single unit, yet they are capable of independent motion.

A special constant, delicate, intrinsic relationship (scapulohumeral rhythm) exists between the humerus and the scapula during elevation and abduction of the arm. After the first 30 degrees of abduction and 60 degrees of flexion, ranges in which the scapula finds a stable position in relation to the humerus, the ratio of motion in the two joints is constant, being 2 humeral and 1 scapular. For every 15 degrees of motion 10 degrees occurs at the glenohumeral joint and 5 degrees at the scapulothoracic joint.

Total motion is 120 degrees at the glenohumeral joint and 60 degrees at the scapulothoracic joint. The glenohumeral joint is capable of 90 degrees of independent motion.

Normal scapular motion on the chest wall is dependent upon normal motion at either end of the clavicle. Any interference at the sternoclavicular or acromioclavicular joint is reflected in the total range of elevation of the arm.

The sternoclavicular joint contributes 40 degrees and the acromioclavicular joint 20 degrees to the total range of elevation.

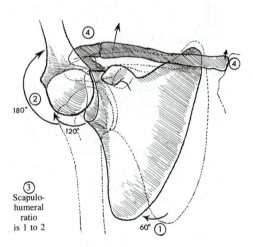

1. The scapula has moved upward and forward on the chest wall 60 degrees.

2. The humerus has reached 180 degrees elevation, having moved 120 degrees in relation to the glenoid.

3. Scapulohumeral ratio is 1 to 2.

4. Elevation of the clavicle at the sternoclavicular joint and at the acromioclavicular joint permits 60 degrees of scapular motion (40 degrees at the sternoclavicular joint and 20 degrees at the acromioclavicular joint).

Mechanisms of Injury

REMARKS

The mechanics of motion in the glenohumeral joint have been lucidly described by Codman and accurately measured by Inman, Saunders, and Abbott. Sudden alteration in these mechanics results in a sprain, dislocation, or fracture of the head of the humerus.

Normally, to reach the overhead position in the sagittal plane, the arm must be rotated internally, and in the coronal plane it must be rotated externally.

During elevation, if rotation of the humerus is in the correct plane, the greater tuberosity slips under the acromion and motion is smooth and rhythmical from beginning to end.

If rotation of the humerus is obstructed, the greater tuberosity impinges against the acromion and becomes locked in this position. Forcing the humerus beyond the locked position results in either a dislocation or a fracture of the humerus. A typical mechanism is football tackling in which the runner does not stop but drives the tackler's arm backward in forceful abduction and external rotation.

Most individuals sustain an anterior dislocation from vigorous activities, particularly participation in sports. Consequently, the majority of patients with an anterior dislocation are young adults.

Forceful abduction and external shoulder rotation may also be produced by a fall on the outstretched arm in which the humerus is in a fixed position but the glenoid moves away from it. Dislocations in older individuals are usually sustained by this mechanism.

Five per cent of glenohumeral dislocations are posterior and are produced by forceful internal rotation and adduction. The most common cause of this is a seizure from epilepsy or alcohol withdrawal.

Direct impact on the anterior aspect of the humerus during a fall may also produce posterior glenohumeral dislocation or fracture-dislocation.

Direct impact to the posterior aspect of the shoulder, e.g., in a fall from a horse, may cause anterior dislocation, but more often a fracture-dislocation results from direct violence to the shoulder.

In order for the humerus to be displaced out of the glenoid, the soft tissue support structures must be torn and stretched. The structures most often injured anteriorly are the glenoid labrum, the glenohumeral ligaments of the capsule, and the subscapularis muscle. The structures most often injured posteriorly are the glenoid labrum, the capsule, and the infraspinatus muscle.

INJURIES FROM ABDUCTION AND EXTERNAL ROTATION: SPRAIN, SUBLUXATION, AND ANTERIOR DISLOCATION

The severity of the injury is determined by the magnitude of the applied forces. Subluxation is produced by forces greater than those causing a sprain and less than those producing anterior dislocation.

Sprain

1. The humeral head is in the locked position.

2. The arm is abducted and externally rotated.

3. The acromion impinges against the greater tuberosity.

4. The anterior ligaments and capsule are severely stretched — some fibers tear, but the continuity of the structures remains intact.

Note: The defect in the anterior capsule may lead to recurrent anterior subluxation.

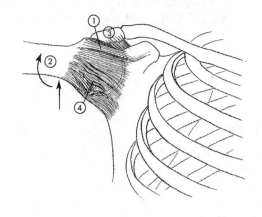

Subluxation

1. The acromion impinges against the greater tuberosity and levers it partially out of the glenoid cavity.

2. The anterior ligaments and capsule are stretched and the glenoid labrum may be avulsed or fractured. Recurrent subluxation may occur through this weakened area.

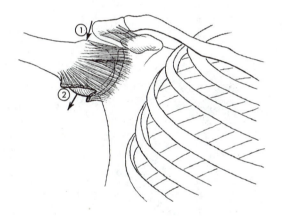

Anterior Dislocation

1. The acromion impinges against the greater tuberosity and levers it out of the joint anteriorly.

2. The anterior ligaments and capsule are severely stretched and torn, thus permitting a dislocation.

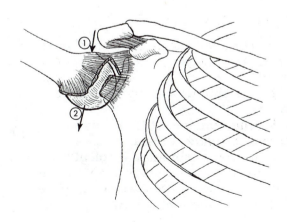

INJURIES FROM HYPERABDUCTION: SPRAIN, SUBLUXATION, AND INFERIOR DISLOCATION

The severity of the injury is determined by the magnitude of the acting forces. Subluxation is produced by acting forces greater than those causing a sprain and less than those producing inferior dislocation.

Sprain

1. The arm is in the locked (pivotal) position.

2. The scapula is rotated completely.

3. The acromion, acting as a fulcrum, impinges against the greater tuberosity and stretches the inferior portion of the capsule, thus producing a sprain.

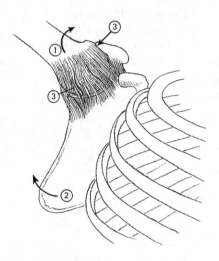

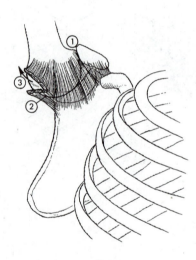

Subluxation

1. The acromion acts as a fulcrum, displacing the greater tuberosity downward and outward.

2. The inferior capsule is stretched and partially torn.

3. The head subluxates.

Inferior Dislocation

1. The head leaves the glenoid cavity and is displaced directly downward.

2. The inferior capsule is completely torn.

3. The rotator cuff is stretched across the glenoid fossa.

If this force continues a typical luxatio erecta results; this is a serious injury because of the severe damage inflicted on the rotator cuff.

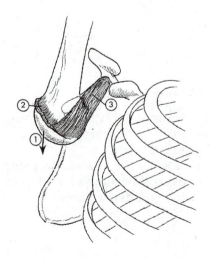

Inferior Dislocation *(Continued)*

1. The arm drops to the side.
2. The head is in the subglenoid position.

Note: From this position it may assume a subcoracoid position.

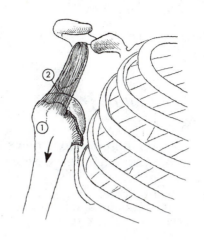

Superior Subluxation

1. Hyperabduction also results when the body weight is caught by one shoulder in a fall from a height.
2. The rotator cuff insertion is avulsed from the greater tuberosity.
3. The capsule is avulsed superiorly from the glenoid.
4. Superior subluxation results from deltoid pull.

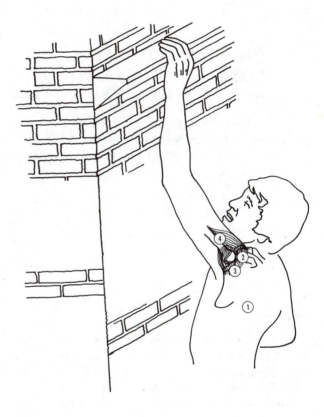

Inferior Subluxation from Hemiplegia

1. Inferior subluxation from disuse atrophy or hemiplegia after cerebrovascular accident.

Note: Early institution of range-of-motion exercises for the shoulder and use of sling support prevent this subluxation.

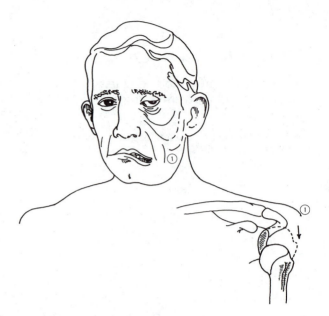

INJURIES FROM ADDUCTION AND INTERNAL ROTATION (POSTERIOR LESIONS): SPRAIN, SUBLUXATION, AND POSTERIOR DISLOCATION

The severity of the injury is determined by the magnitude of the applied forces. Subluxation is produced by forces greater than those causing a sprain and less than those producing posterior dislocation.

Sprain

1. During an epileptic seizure the shoulder is forcefully adducted and internally rotated.

2. The posterior capsule is stretched—some fibers are torn but its continuity is intact.

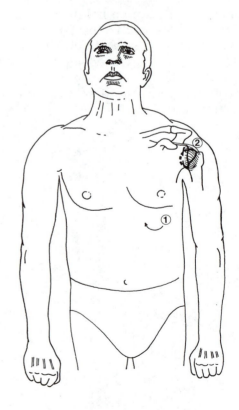

Subluxation

1. Violent internal rotation levers the head backward and outward, partially out of the glenoid fossa.

2. The posterior capsule is partially torn, thus permitting a subluxation.

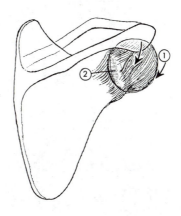

Posterior Dislocation

1. Violent internal rotation levers the humerus completely out of the glenoid fossa.

2. The posterior capsule is severely torn, thus permitting a posterior dislocation.

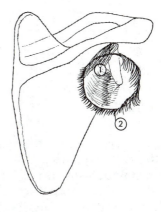

MANAGEMENT OF SPRAINS AND SUBLUXATIONS OF THE GLENOHUMERAL JOINT

Acute Anterior Sprain or Subluxation

REMARKS

The torn tissues (ligaments and capsule) must not be allowed to heal in the relaxed state.

Immobilization must be complete and continuous for at least three weeks in order to insure adequate soft tissue healing.

Inadequate healing favors repeated subluxations and eventually a neuromuscular imbalance resulting in recurrent subluxations or dislocations or in frozen shoulder. Recurrent subluxations or dislocations are most likely to develop after acute injury in patients in the second and third decades of life.

It is more likely that frozen shoulder will follow acute injury sustained in patients more than 40 years of age; consequently, immobilization should not be prolonged in the older patient after shoulder trauma.

Velpeau Immobilization

1. Place cotton pad in the axilla.
2. Encircle the arm and chest with a 15-cm cotton bandage.
3. Apply a triangular sling.

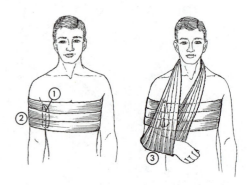

Stockinette-Velpeau Immobilization (Gilchrist)

A relatively simple and comfortable means of immobilizing the shoulder is by the use of a long stockinette.

Take a 10-cm stockinette 3 meters in length, and

1. Cut a 15-cm slot along one folded crease approximately one third from the end. Pass the patient's hand into the slot and down into the long end of the stockinette so that the slot fits in the axilla.

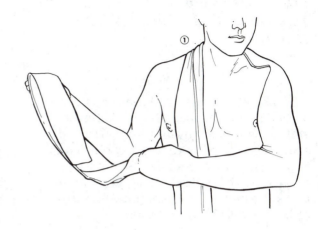

2. With the patient's arm in internal rotation and the forearm across the waist, the long end of the stockinette is passed around the opposite end of the abdomen and across the back. The short end is passed around the patient's neck, looped about the wrist, and secured with a safety pin.

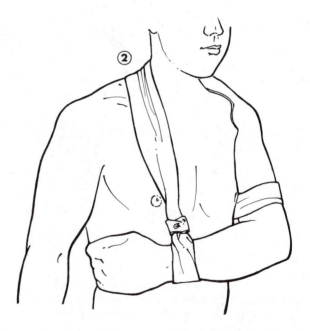

Stockinette-Velpeau Immobilization (Gilchrist) (Continued)

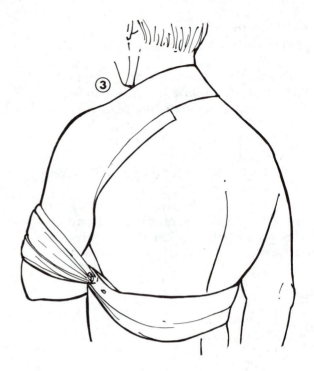

3. The stockinette end that has been passed across the back is pulled tightly and is wrapped around the affected arm and secured with a safety pin. The flap created by the axillary slot may be taped over the deltoid region to prevent the stockinette from slipping forward or backward off the shoulder.

4. A 2.5 cm transverse cut is made in the stockinette to free the patient's hand. This slot may be reinforced with a tape applied loosely around the wrist.

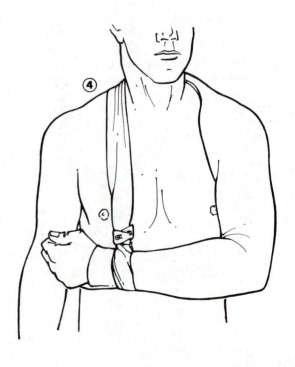

Subsequent Management

Maintain immobilization for at least three weeks.

Avoid abduction or external rotation of the shoulder but encourage active use of the hand and fingers.

After three weeks, remove the Velpeau sling and begin range-of-motion exercises.

Discourage forceful use of the arm, particularly in sports, for at least six weeks after the injury.

If the patient is more than 45 years of age, the risk of developing a frozen shoulder is higher, and the immobilization period should be long enough only to relieve pain (seven to ten days).

Note: Immobilization for recurrent injury is of little value other than to relieve pain symptoms.

Acute Inferior or Superior Subluxation

REMARKS

Inferior subluxation results when the supraspinatus muscle is weakened or torn and no longer supports the humeral head in its normal relationship with the glenoid. Most commonly this is seen in hemiplegia following a cerebrovascular accident. Sling support of the dependent paralyzed arm prevents this complication.

Prolonged immobilization of the shoulder for a fracture of the humeral neck also leads to supraspinatus atrophy and inferior subluxation of the shoulder. These fractures are best treated with early institution of range-of-motion exercises to prevent muscle atrophy and soft tissue contractures produced by immobilization.

Occasionally, the inferior subluxation has resulted from a gross disruption of the supraspinatus insertion. The usual mechanism is a fall from a height, e.g., a scaffold, in which the patient catches his body weight with one arm and avulses the rotator cuff insertion by hyperabducting the shoulder (see page 599). Gross disruption to this degree is sufficient to allow inferior shoulder subluxation and should be treated by prompt surgical repair of the rotator cuff.

Superior subluxation or displacement may also occur after a reduction of a dislocation associated with rotator cuff disruption. The superior displacement results from deltoid pull unopposed by the rotator cuff, which ordinarily would fix the humeral head in the glenoid (see page 606).

605

Types of Inferior Subluxation

SUBLUXATION FROM HEMIPLEGIA

1. Hemiplegia after a cerebrovascular accident will frequently result in inferior subluxation when the weight of the arm hangs on paralyzed rotator cuff muscles.

2. The subacromial space is widened as the result of the inability of the supraspinatus muscle to support the humeral head.

Note: This complication is best prevented by sling support and range-of-motion exercises for the paralyzed limb.

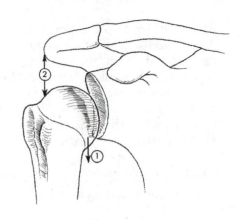

SUBLUXATION AFTER FRACTURE

1. Following a surgical neck fracture of the humerus, prolonged immobilization or

2. Hanging cast treatment will cause supraspinatus atrophy and inferior subluxation.

Note: Begin range of motion for these fractures as soon as pain subsides (seven to ten days).

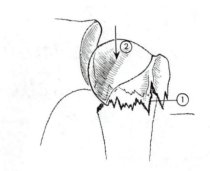

SUPERIOR AND INFERIOR SUBLUXATION FROM HYPERABDUCTION INJURY

Hyperabduction mechanism is produced by a fall when the victim catches his body weight with one shoulder. The resultant rotator cuff avulsion causes either superior or inferior subluxation and should be repaired surgically.

1. If the rotator cuff tendon is torn during dislocation, upward displacement will be evident on the postreduction x-ray as the deltoid pulls without the stabilizing effect of the supraspinatus.

2. If the x-ray is taken with the patient holding weight, the inferior displacement indicates rotator cuff support has been lost.

Note: In evaluating for inferior or superior subluxation, be sure the x-ray is centered on the shoulder, because upward or downward angulation of the beam may produce apparent "subluxation."

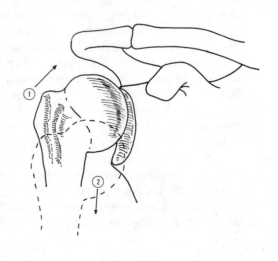

Pathologic Picture of Subluxation After Dislocation

1. The cuff is avulsed from its attachment.
2. The head rests inferiorly.

Note: This tear of the rotator cuff is confirmed by shoulder arthrogram.

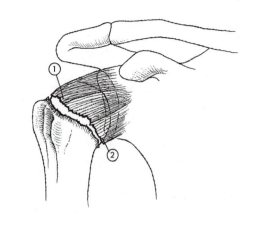

Technique of Shoulder Arthrography

1. The patient lies supine with arm by the side and internally rotated.
2. After sterile preparation, the area below and slightly lateral to the coracoid is injected with 10 ml of local anesthetic down to the neck of the scapula.
3. A 20-gauge short-beveled needle, 6 cm long, is inserted and is directed toward the glenoid.
4. The needle should enter the joint space above the axillary folds and the position should be confirmed by means of image-intensified fluoroscopy.

Note: Longitudinal traction on the arm will help open up the joint space.

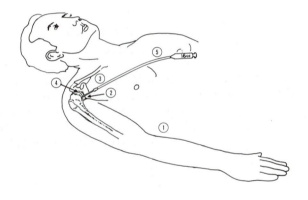

5. Use 12 ml of Reno-M-60 or a similar contrast solution mixed with 4 ml of lidocaine. Inject 2 ml first and determine by fluoroscopy that the dye is in the joint. Then inject the remaining dye.

Note: X-rays should be taken promptly after injection and should include axillary views. If the suspected tear is a chronic one, the leak may be seen only after the patient has abducted and elevated the arm.

NORMAL ARTHROGRAM

1. The glenohumeral joint does not communicate with
2. The subacromial bursa.
3. The bicipital tendon sheath is filled with dye.
4. The subscapularis bursa and
5. The axillary pouch fill with solution.

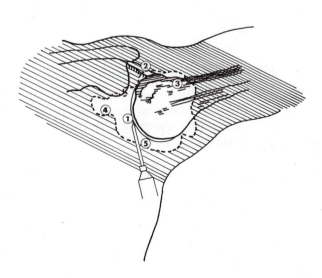

Technique of Shoulder
Arthrography (Continued)

ARTHROGRAM FOLLOWING
SUPRASPINATUS TENDON RUPTURE

1. The subacromial bursa fills with dye.

2. On 100-degree abduction the dye-filled bursa "sticks out like a sore thumb."

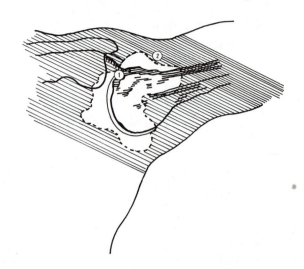

SURGICAL REPAIR OF ROTATOR CUFF (DEBEYRE, PATTE, ELMELIK)

The best approach to the torn rotator cuff is posterior using an osteotomy of the scapular spine or acromion to visualize the entire supraspinatus and rotator cuff attachment. If the tendon has retracted significantly after an old injury, the entire supraspinatus can be mobilized from its fossa and slid laterally.

Incision and Exposure

1. The patient lies on the opposite side and the skin incision runs above the scapular spine curving laterally over the acromion.

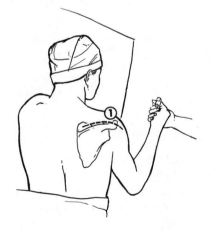

2. The trapezius is split above the spine of the scapula, and

3. The fibers of the deltoid are split downward to avoid the axillary nerve.

4. The acromion is osteotomized at its base, with care taken to avoid the suprascapular nerve and artery. The osteotomy site is opened with a self-retaining retractor to expose

5. The tear of the rotator cuff.

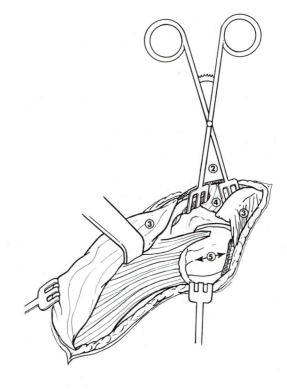

Repair

1. The torn tendon is pulled toward its normal insertion.

2. It is sutured by mattress sutures to drill holes in the bone.

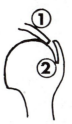

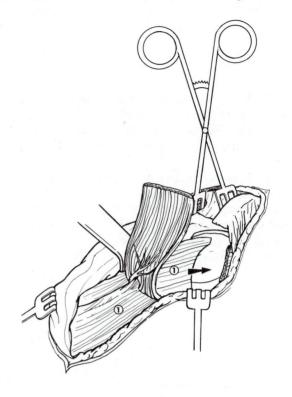

For Old Injuries with Severe Retraction

1. Elevate the supraspinatus from its fossa, making sure to preserve its nerve and blood supply.

2. Reattach the mobilized tendon to a notch created in the greater tuberosity of the humerus.

Note: After repair of the tendon the osteotomy of the acromion is fixed with a screw. The surrounding fascia and split fibers of the trapezius and deltoid are sutured.

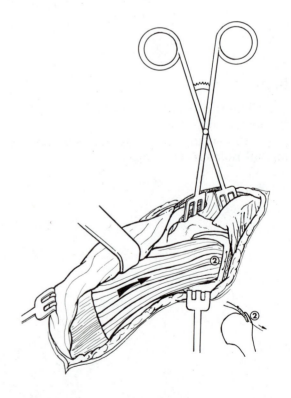

Postoperative Velpeau Immobilization

1. Place a pad of cotton in the axilla.
2. Encircle the arm and chest with 15-cm cotton bandage.
3. Support the arm in a triangular sling.

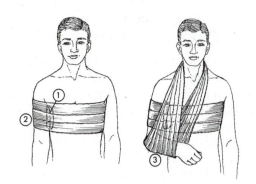

Postoperative Management

Maintain immobilization for three to four weeks.

During this period encourage motion at the elbow, wrist, and fingers.

After three to four weeks, discard all external immobilization and begin a program of range-of-motion exercises.

Start with pendulum exercises every waking hour for 5 to 10 minutes, and advance to abduction and external rotation stretching exercises (see page 139).

Allow free use of the shoulder within the tolerance of pain but do not permit strenuous sports activities for at least three months after the operative repair.

Inferior Fracture–Subluxation

Preoperative X-Ray

1. Fracture of the surgical neck.
2. Head is displaced inferiorly and rests on the glenoid rim.

OR:

1. Fracture of the surgical neck.
2. Fracture of the greater tuberosity.
3. Inferior displacement of the humeral head.

Note: The inferior displacement results commonly from (1) hemarthrosis after the fracture or (2) supraspinatus atrophy caused by prolonged immobilization or hanging cast treatment (which can be avoided by early institution of range-of-motion exercises).

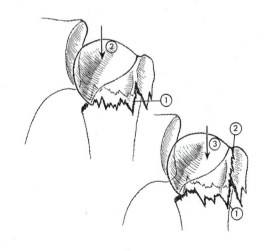

611

Stockinette-Velpeau Immobilization (Gilchrist)

A relatively simple and comfortable means of immobilizing the shoulder is by the use of a long stockinette.

Take a 10-cm stockinette 3 meters in length, and

1. Cut a 15-cm slot along one folded crease approximately one third from the end. Pass the patient's hand into the slot and down into the long end of the stockinette so that the slot fits in the axilla.

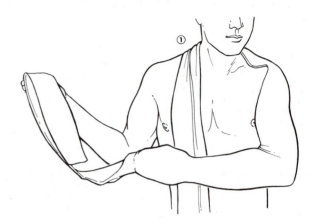

2. With the patient's arm in internal rotation and the forearm across the waist, the long end of the stockinette is passed around the opposite side of the abdomen and across the back. The short end is passed around the patient's neck, looped about the wrist, and secured with a safety pin.

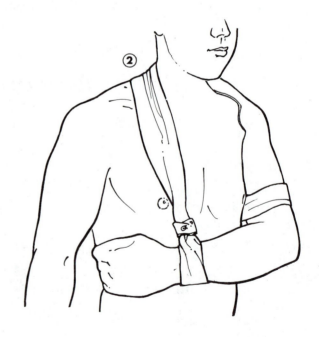

612

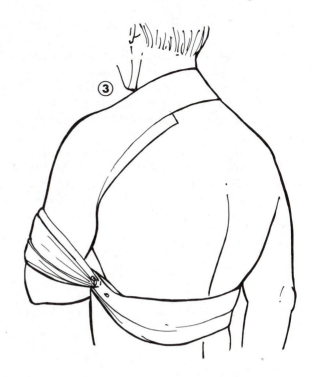

3. The stockinette end that has been passed across the back is pulled tightly and wrapped around the affected arm and secured with a safety pin. The flap created by the axillary slot may be taped over the deltoid region to prevent the stockinette from slipping forward or backward off the shoulder.

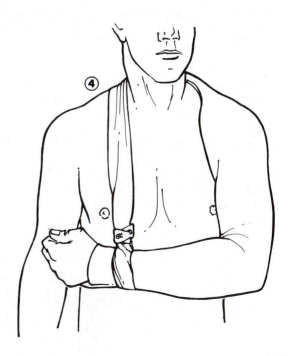

4. A 2.5-cm transverse cut is made in the stockinette to free the patient's hand. This slot may be reinforced with a tape applied loosely around the wrist.

Note: Avoid use of a hanging cast for undisplaced surgical neck fractures.

During the period of immobilization encourage motion of the elbow, wrist, and fingers.

Maintain immobilization for seven to ten days, but encourage active shoulder muscle contraction.

Satisfactory return of shoulder motion should be possible in six to eight weeks with a program of early motion exercises. Do not wait for radiographic signs of complete fracture healing to begin shoulder motion.

Institute an active exercise program beginning with pendulum exercises. Increase exercises using abduction and external rotation stretching by three weeks (see page 139).

Allow free use of the arm within tolerance of pain.

Posterior Sprain and Posterior Subluxation

REMARKS

These injuries are infrequent but they can lead to recurrent posterior dislocation (see page 600).

Treat both lesions in the same manner, by immobilization of the shoulder in extension and slight external rotation.

1. Apply a pad of cotton in the axilla.

2. Wrap a 15-cm cotton bandage around the arm and chest to maintain the shoulder in extension and neutral rotation.

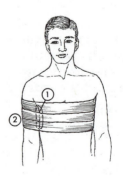
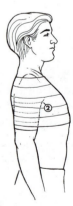

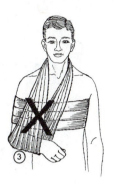

3. *Do not* use a sling, which necessitates adduction and internal rotation.

Subsequent Management

Maintain external immobilization for three weeks.

During this period encourage motion of the wrist and fingers.

Following this period institute an active program of exercises.

Begin with pendulum exercises every waking hour for five or ten minutes.

Progressively increase the exercises in range and frequency.

Allow free use of the arm within the tolerance of pain.

Strenuous activity is permissible after four to six weeks.

MANAGEMENT OF GLENOHUMERAL DISLOCATIONS

REMARKS

Although most dislocations occur after acute trauma, occasionally some individuals are able to dislocate their shoulders at will by selectively contracting muscles that cause dislocation. Management and prognosis of the voluntary shoulder dislocation differs significantly from the usual acute, involuntary dislocation.

Acute dislocations may be either anterior or posterior to the glenoid cavity. Approximately 95 per cent are anterior and 5 per cent are posterior.

Acute dislocations may occur in any age group after the first decade, but the chance of recurrence is significantly higher in patients less than 30 years of age. The recurrence rate in teenaged male athletes with dislocated shoulder often exceeds 80 per cent.

Bilateral acute dislocations may occasionally occur and are most frequently associated with epileptic seizures. They result from forceful internal rotation and adduction during the seizure causing posterior displacement.

Approximately 25 per cent of acute dislocations are associated with fractures, the most common being fractures of the greater tuberosity and the glenoid rim.

Injury to the brachial plexus and the peripheral nerves occurs quite frequently. Axillary nerve injury is a commonly associated lesion, being found in 20 to 25 per cent of cases studied by electromyography. Always check for neurologic deficit before and after reduction of the dislocation.

Posterior and medial cords of the brachial plexus are most frequently involved when the brachial plexus is injured.

Vascular injuries may also occur (1) before or during reduction, especially if reduction is carried out without adequate muscle relaxation, (2) in an elderly patient, and (3) with a chronic dislocation.

Vascular injuries may include:

1. Rupture of the axillary artery or vein, particularly near the circumflex branches.

2. Chronic arteriovenous aneurysm.

616

Always check for vascular impairment of the extremity before and after reduction.

Rotator cuff rupture is also possible in association with the dislocation and should be suspected if superior or inferior subluxation of the humeral head persists in the postreduction x-ray.

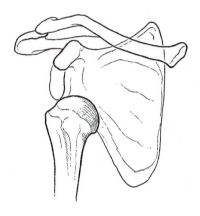

Types of Anterior Dislocations

All types of anterior dislocation should receive the same treatment.

Subglenoid dislocation (rare type).

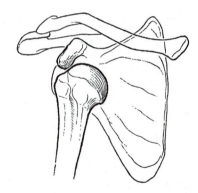

Subcoracoid dislocation (most common type).

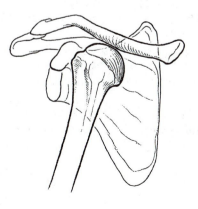

Subclavicular dislocation (rare type).

Typical Deformity of Subcoracoid Dislocation

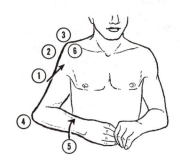

1. Arm is fixed in slight abduction and directed upward and inward.
2. Shoulder is flattened.
3. Acromion process is unduly prominent.
4. Elbow is flexed.
5. Forearm is rotated internally.
6. There is abnormal prominence in the subcoracoid region.

Reduction of Anterior Dislocations

Anesthesia is usually not necessary if the dislocation is less than two hours old. If the injury is older, however, especially in an older patient with osteoporotic bone or arteriosclerotic vessels, it is safer to perform reduction with the full muscle relaxation obtained from general anesthesia.

The common methods of reduction include the Stimson technique, the Hippocratic method, and the Kocher maneuver.

STIMSON TECHNIQUE

This should be tried first because it is the least traumatic if the patient can relax his shoulder muscles.

1. The patient is prone on the edge of the table.
2. 10-kg weights are attached to the arm, and the patient maintains this position for 10 to 15 minutes, if necessary.
3. Occasionally, gentle external and internal rotation of the shoulder aids reduction.

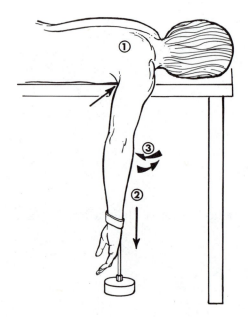

HIPPOCRATIC METHOD

1. Physician's stockinged foot is placed between the patient's chest wall and axillary folds but not in the axilla.

2. Steady traction is maintained while the patient gradually relaxes.

3. The shoulder is slowly rotated externally and adducted.

4. Gentle internal rotation reduces the humeral head.

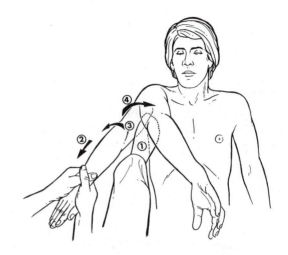

KOCHER MANEUVER

Used only if the previous methods fail. It is performed in one smooth gliding maneuver.

1. Preliminary stretching in line of bony axis of the shaft of the humerus in slight abduction. While maintaining steady traction,

2. Rotate the arm externally very gently and smoothly until 80 degrees of external rotation is achieved.

3. With the arm externally rotated, bring the elbow forward to a point near midline of trunk.

4. Rotate the arm internally and place the hand on the opposite shoulder.

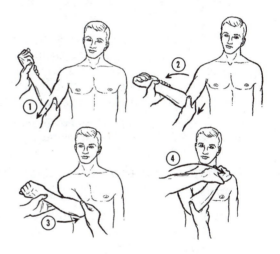

CAUTION

The Kocher method uses the arm as a lever to put the head of the humerus through a series of rotatory movements.

Great force can be expended on the soft tissue of the shoulder joint, vessels, and brachial plexus if the maneuvers are performed improperly.

Fractures of the shaft of the humerus, avulsion of the rotator cuff, and injuries to the circumflex nerve may occur.

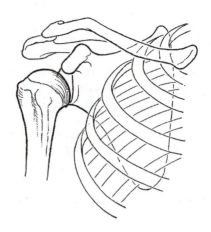

Postreduction X-Ray

The head of the humerus is in normal relation with the glenoid cavity and no fracture has occurred.

After Reduction, Check for:

1. Neurologic deficits.
2. Vascular embarrassment of the extremity.
3. Rupture of the rotator cuff.

Note: Suspect rotator cuff tear if there is superior or inferior subluxation of the reduced humeral head on x-ray.

4. Sensory loss in lesions of axillary nerve. Hypoesthesia or sensory loss in the area of distribution of the sensory branch of the axillary nerve.
5. Sensory loss in lesions of musculocutaneous nerve. Impaired sensation along the lateral border of the forearm.

Note: Paralyses of the biceps brachii, the coracobrachialis, and the brachialis muscles may be associated lesions.

Postreduction Immobilization for Young Patients

Apply a shoulder immobilizer that:
Restricts abduction.
Restricts all rotatory motions.
Restricts extension.
Allows motion at elbow, wrist, and fingers.
Permits healing of soft tissue structures and minimizes incidence of recurrence.

VELPEAU IMMOBILIZATION

1. Place cotton pad in axilla.
2. Encircle arm and chest with a 15-cm cotton bandage.
3. Apply a triangular sling.

OR

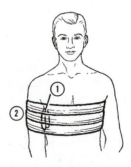
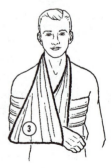

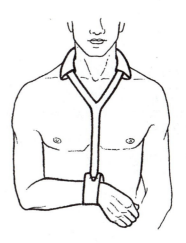

4. Use stockinette Velpeau (after Gilchrist — see page 603).

POSTREDUCTION MANAGEMENT

Encourage motion at the elbow, wrist, and fingers.

Discard apparatus after three weeks.

Institute a program of graduated motions within the limits of pain.

Begin with motions in stooped position every waking hour for five to ten minutes.

Later, add abduction and external rotation exercises (see page 139).

Allow free use of the arm within limits of pain and fatigue.

Do not permit strenuous sports activities for a minimum of three months.

Postreduction Immobilization for Middle-Aged and Elderly Patients

Apply collar and cuff that:

Allow sufficient motion to prevent a frozen shoulder.

Limit abduction and external rotation sufficiently to prevent redislocation.

Permit free active motion at elbow, wrist, and fingers.

POSTREDUCTION MANAGEMENT

Institute gravity-free exercises in stooped position immediately (five or ten minutes four times daily).

Encourage use of limb within painless arcs of motion.

For the first two weeks restrict abduction against gravity to 45 degrees.

During the third and fourth weeks permit abduction to the horizontal.

Discard apparatus at the end of the second week.

Now allow free use of the arm and step up the intensity of the exercises.

Recurrent dislocation is uncommon in persons older than 30 years, unless they are "loose-jointed."

Luxatio Erecta

REMARKS

This lesion is the result of a severe hyperabduction mechanism (see page 598).

It frequently is associated with significant injury to the rotator cuff.

If, after reduction, there is evidence on x-ray of inferior subluxation or superior displacement of the humeral head, surgical reattachment of the tendons, particularly of the supraspinatus tendon, should be considered (see page 606).

Prereduction X-Ray

1. Arm is in full abduction.
2. Humeral head lies inferior to the glenoid fossa.

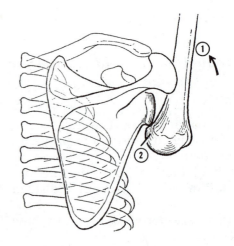

Manipulative Reduction

1. Surgeon makes steady traction upward and outward on the abducted arm.

2. Assistant makes counter traction downward.

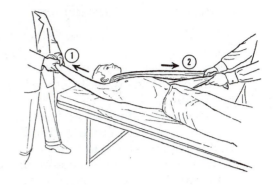

Reduction is indicated by an audible clunk.

1. Arm is then brought to the side.

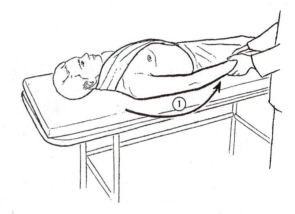

Immobilization

Apply a shoulder immobilizer (see page 603).

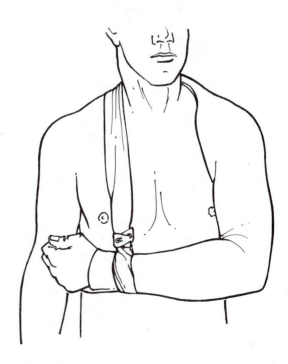

623

Postreduction Management

Encourage motion at the elbow, wrist, and fingers.

Discard apparatus after three or four weeks.

Institute a program of graduated motions within the limits of pain.

Begin with motions in stooped position every waking hour for five or ten minutes.

Later, add abduction and external rotation exercises.

Allow free use of arm within limits of pain and fatigue, but do not permit strenuous sports activities for two to three months after reduction.

Rotator cuff injury is commonly associated with this unusual dislocation and should be repaired surgically (see page 656).

Irreducible Fresh Dislocations

REMARKS

Occasionally, conservative methods fail to reduce what appears to be an uncomplicated dislocation. Do not employ forceful maneuvers in these cases, because some abnormality may be preventing reduction.

The common causes of failure are:

1. Interposition of a portion of the cuff between the humeral head and the glenoid cavity.

2. Interposition of the inferior capsule.

3. Posterior displacement of the tendon of the long head of the biceps muscle.

Surgical intervention is necessary to remove the obstructing element.

Occasionally, a chronic dislocation may be mistaken for fresh injury by an inebriated or confused patient.

Pathologic Picture

1. Reduction is not possible because the ruptured rotator cuff lies in front of the glenoid fossa like a curtain.

2. Reduction is not possible because the inferior capsule is interposed between the humeral head and the glenoid fossa.

3. Reduction is not possible because the biceps tendon is displaced posteriorly and prevents apposition of the humeral head to the glenoid fossa.

Note. A carefully obtained history should distinguish a chronic dislocation from an irreducible fresh dislocation.

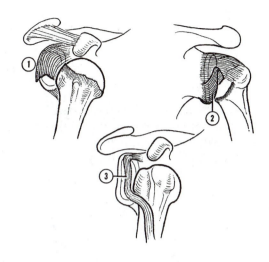

Surgical Repair

1. A 6 cm to 8 cm skin incision is made through the deltopectoral interval.

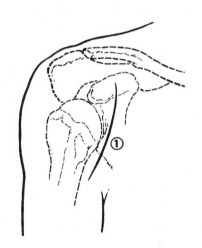

2. The deep incision is continued through the deltopectoral groove, ligating the cephalic vein if it is injured.

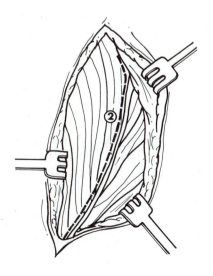

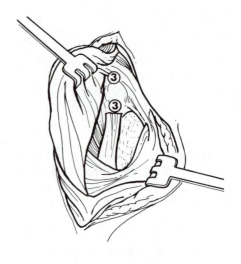

Surgical Repair *(Continued)*

3. The incision is extended laterally to detach a part of the origin of deltoid if necessary for adequate exposure. The short head of biceps may also be detached from the coracoid.

WHEN THE CUFF LIES IN FRONT OF THE HUMERAL HEAD:

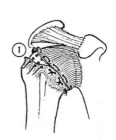

1. The cuff has been removed from in front of the glenoid fossa; dislocation has been reduced, and the cuff is reattached to the tuberosity by mattress sutures passing through drill holes in the bone.

WHEN THE BICEPS TENDON PRECLUDES REDUCTION:

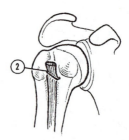

2. The biceps tendon is first replaced in its normal position, then severed at its attachment to the superior glenoid rim. Its intracapsular portion is excised, and finally it is sutured in the proximal portion of the bicipital groove.

WHEN THE CAPSULE PRECLUDES REDUCTION:

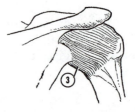

3. The inferior portion of the articular capsule is removed from in front of the glenoid cavity; next, the dislocation is reduced.

Note: A standard Putti-Platt or Magnuson repair should be performed in conjunction with any of these procedures to prevent recurrent dislocation (see page 671).

Postoperative Management

Apply a shoulder immobilizer that restricts abduction and external rotation but allows motion at the elbow, wrist, and fingers.

Discard the apparatus after three to four weeks.

Institute a program of graduated motion exercises within the limits of pain. Begin with motions in the stooped position for five to ten minutes every waking hour (see page 139).

Later, add external rotation and abduction exercises.

Allow free use of the arm within the limits of pain and fatigue.

Do not permit strenuous sports activities for a minimum of three months after surgical repair.

Old Anterior Dislocations

REMARKS

These are serious lesions and may be complicated further by treatment.

Closed reduction under general anesthesia is usually possible in dislocations less than four weeks old.

Results are better with closed than with open methods of reduction.

Open reduction is usually necessary if the dislocation is more than six weeks old or if closed methods have failed. However, old dislocations are in some instances painless and permit a fair degree of function. In elderly patients, such a lesion should be left undisturbed; if the age of the injury is uncertain or the patient's shoulder is relatively pain-free, operative treatment should be avoided.

Closed methods may be complicated by fracture of the humerus, rupture of the axillary artery, or injury to the brachial plexus. These disasters may also occur in operative reduction.

In young patients and in patients with pain or vascular embarrassment, reduction is necessary.

Regardless of the method of reduction employed, complete restoration of function is rarely achieved.

The primary obstruction to reduction is the posterior capsule, which folds over the glenoid and becomes scarred sufficiently to obstruct repositioning of the humeral head. For this reason, a posterior surgical approach to the shoulder is the most effective way of achieving reduction for chronic anterior dislocation, provided that reduction is indicated.

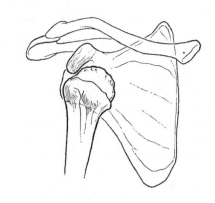

Prereduction X-Ray

Anterior dislocation less than four weeks old.

Closed Reduction

The Hippocratic method is preferred:

Employ a general anesthetic. *Complete relaxation is most essential.*

1. The physician's stockinged foot or a sling is applied between the patient's chest wall and axillary folds but not in the axilla.

2. Steady traction is maintained while the muscles are relaxed.

3. The shoulder is gently rotated externally and adducted.

4. Gentle internal rotation reduces the humeral head.

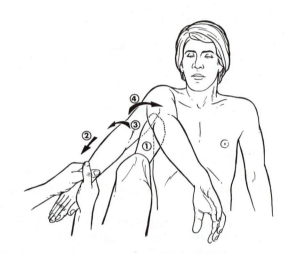

Caution: In cases of failure, try the maneuver once more. *Repeated attempts are dangerous.* Failure of closed reduction after two attempts indicates that surgical reduction will be required.

Postreduction X-Ray

The humeral head has returned to its normal anatomic position. No fracture has occurred.

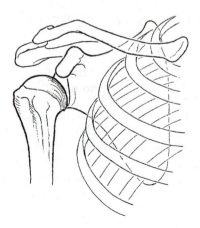

Immobilization (For Closed and Open Methods)

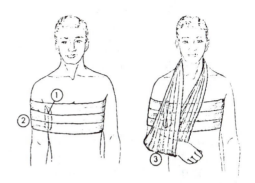

1. Place a cotton pad in the axilla.
2. Encircle the arm and chest with a 15 cm cotton bandage.
3. Apply triangular sling.

Postreduction Management (For Closed and Open Methods)

Encourage motion at the elbow, wrist, and fingers.

Discard the apparatus after three or four weeks.

Institute a program of graduated motions within the limits of pain.

Begin with motions in the stooped position every waking hour for five or ten minutes.

Later, add abduction and external rotation exercises (see page 139).

Allow free use of the arm within limits of pain and fatigue but avoid strenuous sports activities for a minimum of three months.

Obstruction to Closed Reduction

Failure to accomplish a closed reduction is due to:

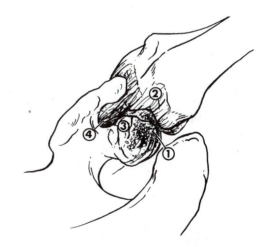

1. Bowstring of the posterior capsule forming an intra-articular scar.
2. Posterolateral fracture of humeral head is impacted against the glenoid.
3. Anterior avulsion of the glenoid labrum or fracture of the glenoid from impaction of the humeral head.
4. Stripping of the anterior capsule and subscapularis from the neck of the scapula.

Infraspinatus Repair for Chronic Anterior Dislocation via the "Back Door" Approach (Connolly Technique)

To deal with these lesions in the chronic anterior dislocation, use the "back door" approach to the shoulder.

The objectives of this posterior or "back door" approach are:

1. To remove the posterior capsule, which has become scarred down in the glenoid and prevents reduction, and
2. To avoid extensive dissection of the anterior muscles and capsule, which causes gross instability after the reduction.

629

Infraspinatus Repair for Chronic Anterior Dislocation via the "Back Door" Approach (Connolly Technique)
(Continued)

INCISION

1. With the patient on the uninvolved side, the incision runs 1 cm below the spine of the scapula out to the acromion.

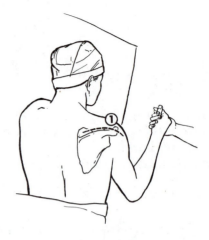

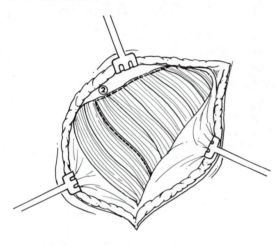

2. The deltoid is partially detached from the spine of the scapula and along its posterior margin.

REPAIR

1. The interval between the infraspinatus and the teres minor is identified, and the infraspinatus tendon and capsule are detached from the greater tuberosity.

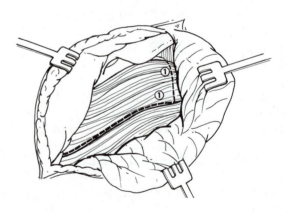

2. Scarred intra-articular capsule is excised from the glenoid cavity and freed anteriorly.

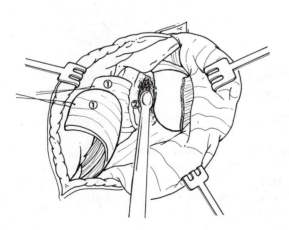

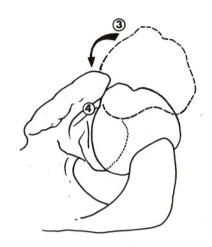

3. The humeral head is gently elevated back into the glenoid cavity while an assistant applies traction on the elbow.

4. The anterior capsule may have to be peeled off the humeral head, but the subscapularis usually can be left undisturbed.

5. Following reduction, the infraspinatus tendon is sewn into the depths of the defect that is always present with chronic dislocation.

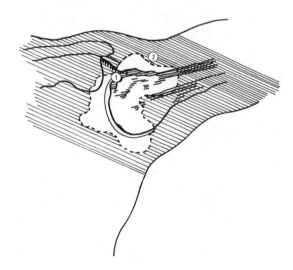

Note: Reduction is usually stable after the infraspinatus repair, and transarticular pin fixation is not necessary.

Postoperative Management

Apply a shoulder immobilizer and encourage motion at the elbow, wrist, and fingers.

Discard the apparatus after seven to ten days, depending on the stability achieved at surgery, and start circumduction exercises.

Advance to abduction and external rotation exercises.

Range of motion will be permanently limited but should be much better than it was before surgical repair.

Acute Posterior Dislocation

REMARKS

This lesion is often overlooked and occurs more frequently than generally realized. Of all acute dislocations, posterior dislocation occurs in 4 to 5 per cent.

It frequently follows epileptic seizures or occurs during electroconvulsive therapy or may result from a direct blow to the front of the shoulder during a fall.

X-rays are usually misleading because the anteroposterior view can be misinterpreted as normal. Axillary views, which are essential to make the diagnosis, may not be obtained because of the patient's pain, unless the physician personally supervises the positioning.

Clinical findings are most important in making diagnosis:

1. The limb is locked in adduction and internal rotation.

2. The coracoid process is prominent.

3. Humeral head prominence is evident under the acromion and is best noted with the arm flexed.

4. The patient cannot abduct or externally rotate the shoulder to neutral.

In fresh injuries, reduction is usually easy and prognosis is good.

Upshot X-Ray Technique for Axillary View

To make the diagnosis of a posterior dislocation, an axillary view is essential. The difficulty of obtaining this view, caused by the patient's pain, can be overcome by using the following procedure.

1. The cassette is placed above the shoulder while the x-ray beam shoots upward through the axilla.

2. Gentle abduction to 40 degrees allows visualization of the posterior dislocation.

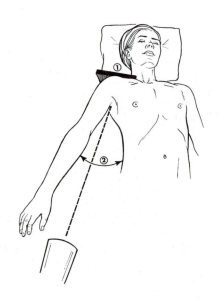

Minimal Internal Rotation of Humerus

ANTEROPOSTERIOR VIEW

1. The shaft of the humerus is rotated internally.

2. The shadow of the glenoid overlaps that of the humeral articular surface, but this may be interpreted as normal.

3. The humeral head is displaced upward in relation to the glenoid.

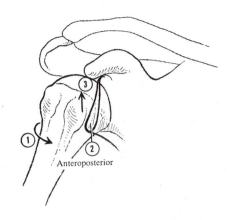

AXILLARY VIEW

This view is critical for proper diagnosis.

1. The head lies behind the glenoid.

2. The head is displaced slightly upward.

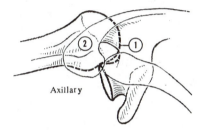

Marked Internal Rotation of Humerus

ANTEROPOSTERIOR VIEW

1. There is marked internal rotation of the shaft of the humerus.

2. The inferior portion of the glenoid fossa is exposed and is not overlapped by the spherical articular surface of the head.

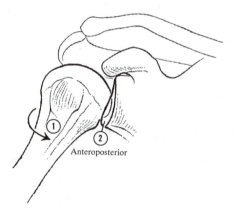

AXILLARY VIEW

This view is critical for proper diagnosis.

1. The head is behind the glenoid.

2. The head is displaced upward.

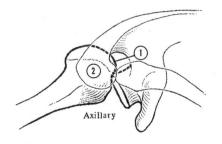

Reduction

Reduction of posterior dislocation is performed with the patient under general anesthesia.

1. Make steady traction on the arm with the elbow flexed in the long axis of the humerus.

2. An assistant mobilizes the head by pressing downward on the prominence with the thumb.

3. Adduct arm with traction maintained.

When the head reaches the glenoid brim, effect reduction with a movement that:

4. Rotates arm externally and then

5. Gently rotates arm internally.

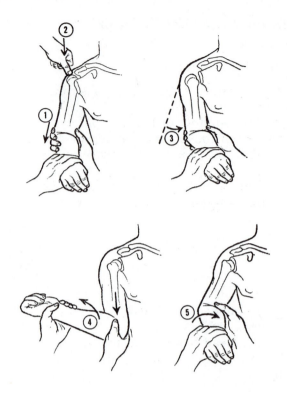

Postreduction Immobilization

1. Pad the axilla.

2. Wrap a 15 cm bias-cut bandage around the arm and forearm so that the humerus is extended and in neutral rotation.

3. Avoid the use of a sling, which adducts and internally rotates the shoulder. Use a spica cast for support.

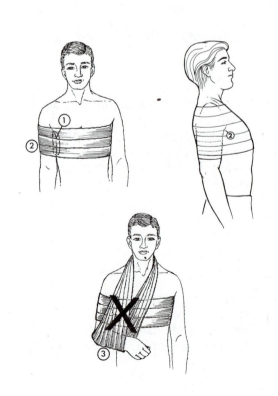

634

Spica Cast Immobilization

This method is used for very unstable reductions of posterior dislocation.

Apply plaster spica that holds arm:
Abducted 30 to 35 degrees,

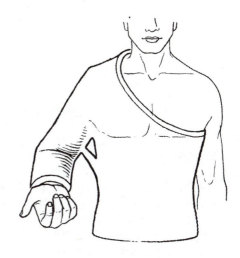

Slightly rotated externally,
Slightly behind plane of trunk.

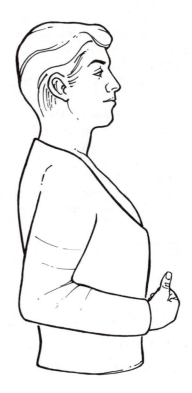

Postreduction Management

Encourage motion at wrist and fingers.
Discard apparatus after three weeks.
Institute a program of graduated motions within the limits of pain.
Begin with pendulum motions in a stooped position every waking hour for five or ten minutes.
Add abduction and external rotation exercises.
Allow free use of arm within limits of pain and fatigue.
Do not permit strenuous sports activities for a minimum of three months.

635

Old Posterior Dislocations

REMARKS

Like fresh posterior dislocation, old dislocation is difficult to recognize. Awareness of this condition is most important in establishing the diagnosis. The posterior dislocation is often erroneously diagnosed as a frozen shoulder. Occasionally it may even be bilateral.

Anteroposterior x-rays are often interpreted as normal but axillary views will consistently demonstrate the dislocation.

Old dislocations are difficult to reduce. Never attempt reduction by closed manipulative maneuvers in dislocations suspected to be more than four to six weeks old. Open reduction is the wisest choice under these conditions.

The prognosis becomes less favorable as the length of time before the diagnosis is made increases. In very old lesions there is advanced disorganization of the bone and soft tissue elements of the joints, so arthrodesis is the wisest procedure.

Basic pathology with chronic dislocations includes:

1. Bowstringing of the anterior capsule, which forms scar tissue and blocks reduction.

2. Anteromedial fracture defect in the humeral head.

3. Posterior avulsion or fracture of the labrum where the humeral head impacts.

4. Stripping of the posterior capsule and infraspinatus.

Preoperative X-Ray

ANTEROPOSTERIOR VIEW

1. The shaft of the humerus is rotated internally.

2. The shadow of the glenoid overlaps that of the humeral articular surface.

3. Slight upward displacement of the humeral head.

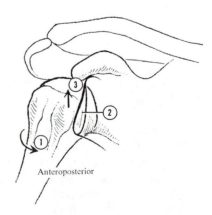

Anteroposterior

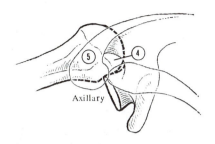

Axillary View

4. Head lies behind the glenoid.
5. Head is displaced upward.

Operative Reduction (McLaughlin Technique)

Incision

1. The vertical limb extends along the anterior border of the deltoid; it starts at the junction of the outer and middle thirds of the clavicle and terminates proximal to the deltoid tubercle.

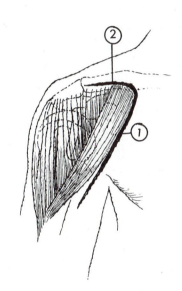

2. The horizontal limb starts at the level of the acromioclavicular joint and proceeds medially along the anterior surface of the outer third of the clavicle.

3. Deepen the vertical incision through the deltoid muscle, 1 cm from its anterior margin. If the cephalic vein is injured, it should be ligated.

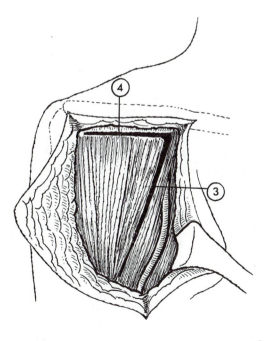

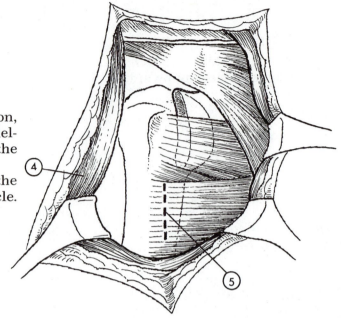

4. By sharp subperiosteal dissection, separate the clavicular head of the deltoid from the clavicle and reflect the deltoid downward and laterally.

5. Divide the proximal half of the tendon of the pectoralis major muscle.

REDUCTION

1. Divide the subscapularis tendon close to its insertion and retract the muscle medially. Protect the axillary nerve.

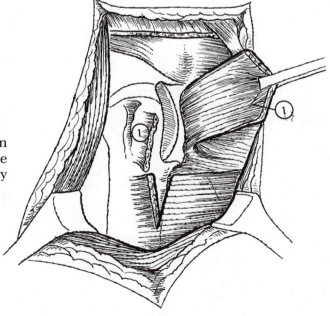

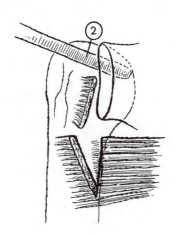

2. Place a small bone skid between the humeral head and glenoid, and disengage the posterior glenoid rim from the defect in the head.

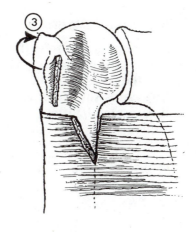

3. Externally rotate the arm to complete the reduction.

Repair

1. With a curette scarify the surfaces of the defect in the anteromedial aspect of the humeral head.

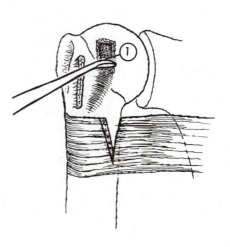

Repair (Continued)

2. Anchor the tendon of the subscapularis into the base of the defect by mattress sutures passing through drill holes in the bone.

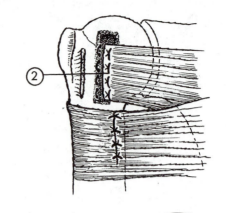

Postoperative Immobilization

1. Place a cotton pad in the axilla.
2. Encircle the arm and chest with a 15 cm cotton bandage that extends and externally rotates the shoulder.
3. Avoid sling immobilization, which internally rotates and adducts the shoulder.

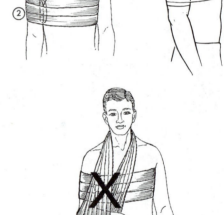

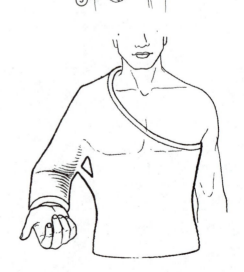

Postoperative Management

In the postoperative period, apply a plaster spica cast that holds the arm (1) abducted 30 to 35 degrees, (2) slightly rotated externally, and (3) slightly behind the plane of the trunk.

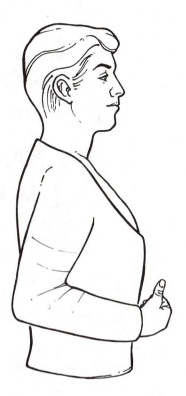

Main external immobilization for three weeks.

During this period, encourage motion of the elbow, wrist, and fingers.

After three weeks discard external immobilization.

Institute pendulum exercises on a regulated program of five to ten minutes every waking hour.

Increase gradually the range and frequency of the exercises, always within the tolerance of pain.

Add external rotation and abduction exercises.

Return to maximum level of painless function depends on the duration of the dislocation prior to reduction and upon the degree of secondary joint changes.

Note: If the joint is severely affected arthrodesis of the shoulder should be performed.

MANAGEMENT OF COMPLICATIONS OF GLENOHUMERAL DISLOCATION

REMARKS

Acute traumatic dislocation may be associated with one·or more of numerous complications.

Awareness of this possibility is most important in detecting the lesions because early detection and treatment may preclude an unfavorable result.

The most pertinent complications are:

1. Injury to the axillary artery.
2. Injury to the brachial plexus or the peripheral nerves.
3. Tear of the rotator cuff.
4. Fractures—these may involve the glenoid, humeral head, acromion, tuberosities and the neck and shaft of the humerus.
5. Recurrent dislocation.

Injury to the Axillary Artery

REMARKS

This lesion is most likely to occur in elderly patients with arteriosclerotic vessels or in patients whose shoulders are scarred by recurrent dislocation. It is not so rare that it should not be checked for and recognized promptly.

Characteristically, the shoulder swells rapidly, the patient has severe pain and paralysis of the arm, and the radial pulse is no longer palpable.

Any dislocated shoulder should be reduced by gentle manipulation, but this is especially true in elderly patients, in whom reduction is done most safely with general anesthesia.

If an old, chronically dislocated shoulder is not recognized as such and manipulation is attempted too forcefully, vascular disruption frequently occurs. Do not try to reduce a dislocation that is known or suspected to be chronic by repeated closed manipulation.

When the arterial rupture is recognized, the bleeding may be slowed by digital pressure compressing the axillary artery against the first rib. Prompt surgical exploration should then be carried out through a subclavian-axillary approach with resection of the damaged artery and vascular anastomosis or graft.

Ligation should not be done in the elderly patient, because arteriosclerotic vessels have poor collateral circulation and gangrene inevitably follows.

The types of arterial damage that may occur are:

1. Intimal damage followed by thrombosis.

2. Avulsion of a large branch from the artery; usually the subscapular or circumflex artery.

3. Rupture of the main trunk of the axillary artery.

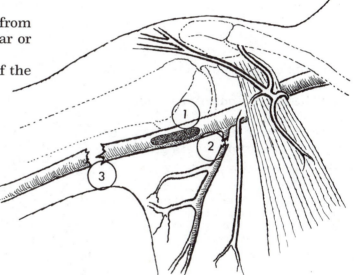

MANAGEMENT

If vascular impairment occurs, the shoulder should be reduced promptly and gently. If vascular impairment is not relieved, explore the vessels through a subclavian-axillary approach.

Prior to surgical exploration, the hemorrhage can be controlled by compressing the subclavian artery against the first rib.

The damaged vessel should be resected in its entirety; graft replacement may be necessary.

Subclavian Approach

1. With the arm abducted, incision is made from the lower border of the clavicle, down the arm and along the deltopectoral groove.

2. The pectoralis major muscle is released and is retracted inferiorly to expose the axillary vessels.

3. The pectoralis minor muscle is detached from the coracoid for greater exposure.

4. The bleeding vessel is clamped.

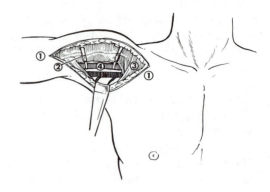

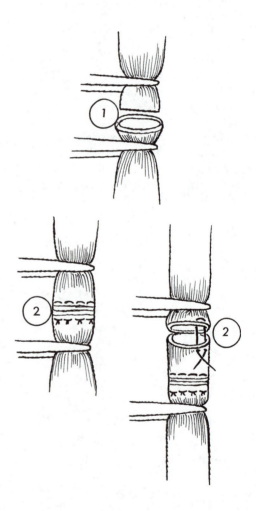

Following exposure and control of the bleeding vessel:

1. The frayed ends of the artery are resected.

2. End-to-end anastomosis is performed or a saphenous vein graft is inserted.

Note: Ligation of the vessels under these circumstances should be avoided because collateral circulation in the elderly patient is inadequate.

Injury to Nerves

REMARKS

Injury to peripheral nerves as well as to the brachial plexus may occur with acute dislocations of the shoulder.

Occurrence of nerve injury in dislocation varies in frequency from 5 per cent to 30 per cent of cases, depending on the thoroughness of the examination.

Since the axillary nerve runs along the subscapularis muscle, it is quite exposed to injury from an anterior dislocation. Electromyography will demonstrate damage to the axillary nerve in more than 30 per cent of dislocations. This is most often transitory and frequently is not associated with sensory loss.

Axillary nerve damage should be suspected in a patient who regains shoulder abduction slowly after reduction.

Occasionally the brachial plexus, particularly the medial cord, which includes the ulnar and median nerves, will be damaged. Recovery from the stretch injury to the plexus is usually spontaneous but may cause quite painful paresthesias for several months after injury.

The prognosis for recovery is good with single nerve lesions because, as a rule, the nerve deficit is temporary. The prognosis is less favorable with multiple nerve injuries, and in some cases the nerve deficit may be permanent.

The diagnosis of nerve damage may be recognized by sensory deficit, but frequently electromyography is necessary to confirm or recognize occult nerve injuries.

1. Area of hypoesthesia or sensory loss associated with injury to the axillary nerve.

2. Area of sensory loss associated with injury to musculocutaneous nerve.

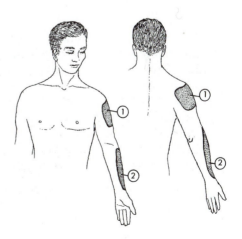

Management

For most nerve lesions, management is watchful waiting.

During this period:

1. Maintain muscle tone by active and assisted range-of-motion exercises.

2. Put shoulder, elbow, wrist, and fingers through a safe range of motion to prevent joint and muscle contraction.

3. Splint the wrist or the involved fingers to avoid passive stretching of muscles.

If return of function is progressive, continue with this treatment.

If after three months there is no clinical or electromyographic evidence of return of function, surgical exploration of the nerve should be considered.

Rupture of the Rotator Cuff

REMARKS

This complication is very rare in young adults but fairly common in older patients.

Rotator cuff disruption is very common with dislocations produced by hyperabduction or in luxatio erecta in any age group (see page 598).

Initially, rotator cuff rupture may not be recognized when the arm is immobilized after reduction.

Suspect a rotator cuff tear if there is persistent superior or inferior subluxation, especially if the patient is unable to abduct the shoulder (see page 606).

Check abduction power of the shoulder after the shoulder immobilizer is discarded; should abduction remain limited for more than two weeks, suspect a rotator cuff injury.

The principal differential diagnosis to be made for patients with these symptoms is between rotator cuff injury and axillary nerve damage. Electromyography will establish axillary nerve damage, shoulder arthrography will demonstrate the rotator cuff tear.

When the diagnosis of a cuff tear is established, surgical repair should be prompt so as to relieve the pain and decreased shoulder strength these patients usually experience.

Typical Deformity Associated with Large Tear of Cuff

1. In attempting to abduct the arm, the patient shrugs the shoulder; the deltoid contracts forcefully.

2. No abduction or weak abduction is present in the glenohumeral joint.

3. Few degrees of abduction are possible by fixing the humeral head in the glenoid cavity and rotating the scapula outward.

4. Abduction is usually weak against any resistance.

Note: In some patients the only significant manifestation of rotator cuff injury is persistent pain in the shoulder several weeks or months after reduction.

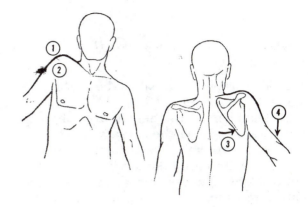

Diagnosis of Torn Rotator Cuff

Diagnosis should be confirmed by shoulder arthrogram (see page 607).

1. The subacromial bursa fills with dye or

2. On abduction, the dye-filled bursa "sticks out like a sore thumb."

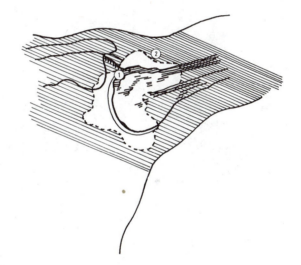

Repair of Torn Rotator Cuff

INCISION AND POSTERIOR EXPOSURE

1. The patient lies on the unaffected side, and the skin incision runs above the scapular spine, curving laterally over the acromion.

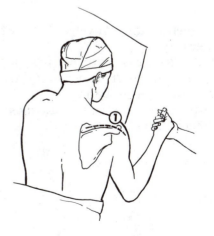

647

Repair of Torn Rotator Cuff *(Continued)*

2. The trapezius is split above the spine of the scapula and

3. The fibers of the deltoid are split downward to avoid the axillary nerve.

4. The acromion is osteotomized at its base, with care taken to avoid the suprascapular nerve and artery. The osteotomy site is opened with a self-retaining retractor to expose

5. The torn rotator cuff.

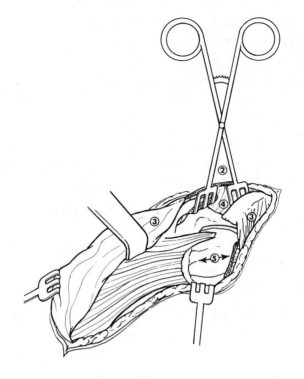

REPAIR

1. Freshen margin of retracted cuff and tuberosity.

2. With mattress sutures passing through drill holes in tuberosity, anchor detached cuff to bone.

3. With interrupted sutures, close other defects in cuff.

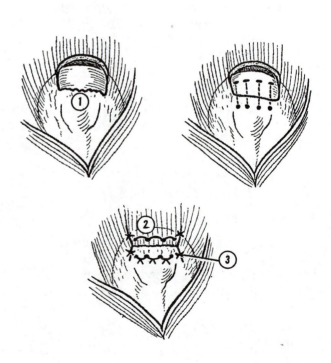

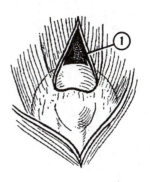

OR:

If retracted rotator cuff cannot be pulled down to the tuberosity, but some side-to-side approximation can be achieved:

1. Freshen margins of rotator cuff.

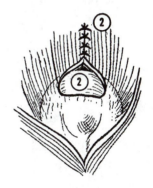

2. By interrupted sutures, approximate edges of cuff, beginning at the apex of tear and up to the point of tension. A triangular hiatus now remains in cuff.

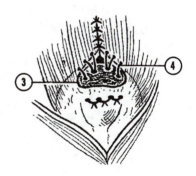

3. Remove articular cartilage from humeral head immediately below the cuff defect.

4. Reattach margins of cuff to edge of bone defect by mattress sutures passing through drill holes in the bone.

Repair with Free Biceps Graft (After Neviaser)

This method is used for massive avulsions of the rotator cuff with retraction.

1. Separate adhesions between the bursa and the rotator cuff.

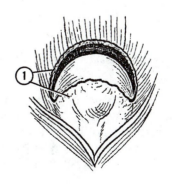

Repair with Free Biceps Graft (After Neviaser) (Continued)

2. Remove the intra-articular section of the biceps tendon and suture the distal portion of the tendon into the bicipital groove.

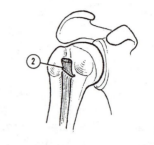

3. Section the tendon graft longitudinally and open it in book-like fashion.

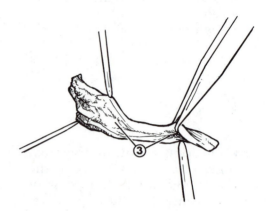

4. Suture the free graft to the cuff edges with the glistening surface of the graft facing the joint.

Note: Closure should be airtight. Test by injecting sterile saline into the joint away from suture lines.

Freeze-dried cadaver rotator cuffs have also been used to repair massive ruptures.

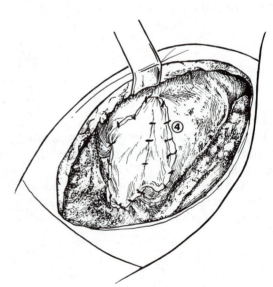

Postoperative Management

Fix the osteotomy with a screw.

Close the wound by suturing the trapezius and deltoid fasciae, which brings together the osteotomy of the acromion spine. Apply a Velpeau dressing, padding the axilla and using a sling support.

On the first postoperative day the patient should shrug and elevate the shoulder frequently during his waking hours.

After three weeks, remove the Velpeau dressing and use sling support for one week.

Start the patient on circumduction exercises, and advance to external rotation and abduction exercises.

Explain to the patient that improvement in strength will continue for many months after the repair and that pain relief should be the most significant benefit from this procedure.

Fractures Complicating Dislocations

REMARKS

Virtually all shoulder dislocations produce impaction of the humeral head and damage to the glenoid labrum. As the shoulder dislocates, the violent response of the shoulder muscles impacts the humeral head against the glenoid, producing a compression fracture of the posterolateral aspect of the head as well as a tear or fracture of the glenoid. This defect may be quite large, especially with the violent muscle contractions in seizure disorders.

In older patients, the rotator cuff contraction produces an avulsion of its insertion on the greater tuberosity of the humerus. Avulsion of the greater tuberosity fragment indicates that the force of dislocation is absorbed posteriorly rather than anteriorly. Consequently, the anterior capsule and muscle structures are relatively undamaged, and recurrence of the dislocation is infrequent.

Complete shattering of the humeral head may occur as a result of overvigorous attempts to reduce the dislocation.

HUMERAL HEAD IMPACTION FRACTURES

REMARKS

In most dislocations the violent reaction of the rotator cuff muscles impacts the humeral head against the glenoid labrum. In anterior dislocation this results in:

1. Posterolateral humeral head defect.
2. Avulsion of the anterior labrum or
3. Fracture of the glenoid.

Posterior dislocations are associated with

1. Anteromedial defect or complete fracture of the lesser tuberosity.
2. Avulsion of the posterior labrum.
3. Posterior fracture of the glenoid.

X-Ray Technique for Visualizing Posterolateral Fracture Defect

Because the anterior bone structures of the humerus obscure the posterolateral defect, the x-ray beam must be tangential to the superior surface of the head in order for the posterior defect to be visualized.

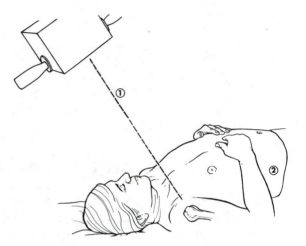

1. The tube is angled 30 degrees from the perpendicular.

2. The patient's shoulder is abducted slightly and is internally rotated so that the arm rests on the chest.

3. The posterolateral defect may vary from a subtle flattening to a deep compression fracture of the humeral head.

Note: Humeral head impaction fractures require no treatment other than that necessary for the dislocation.

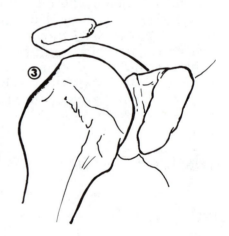

FRACTURE OF THE GREATER TUBEROSITY

REMARKS

The violence of the rotator cuff response to the dislocation may produce an avulsion fracture of the greater tuberosity rather than an impaction fracture of the head.

This is especially likely with dislocations in patients over 40 years of age and may be one of three types:

Type I: The tuberosity follows the humeral head.

Type II: The tuberosity retains its normal relation to the scapula.

Type III: The tuberosity is retracted under the acromion.

Severe damage of the rotator cuff may accompany all three of these fractures. If anatomic reduction is not achieved, surgical repair of the fracture and rotator cuff rupture should be undertaken.

TYPE I AND TYPE II FRACTURE-DISLOCATIONS

Prereduction X-Rays

TYPE I

1. The greater tuberosity has followed the humeral head.

2. The humeral head occupies a position at a distance from the glenoid fossa.

In this fracture-dislocation, the cuff is severely stretched or may be ruptured. Check for rupture.

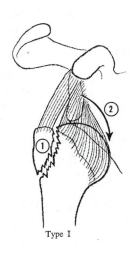

Type I

TYPE II

3. The greater tuberosity is in its normal position in relation to the glenoid fossa.

4. The humeral head is displaced from the glenoid cavity.

If reduction fails, suspect posterior displacement of the biceps tendon or interposition of the cuff and the tuberosities in front of the head. Closed reduction is usually possible, provided that the greater tuberosity has not retracted under the acromion (type III fracture).

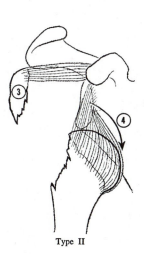

Type II

653

Manipulative Reduction

HIPPOCRATIC TECHNIQUE

1. Physician's stockinged foot is placed between the patient's chest wall and axillary folds but not in the axilla.

2. Steady traction is maintained while the patient gradually relaxes.

3. The shoulder is slowly rotated externally and adducted.

4. Gentle internal rotation reduces the humeral head.

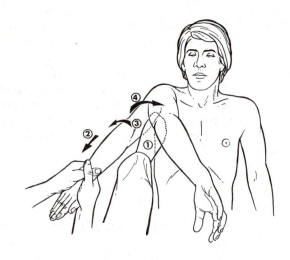

ALTERNATE METHOD

1. Use general anesthetic for muscle relaxation. Make steady traction on the arm in the plane in which it lies in relation to the trunk.

2. Then, with traction maintained, swing arm to the adducted position. This usually effects a reduction; if not,

3. Gently rotate arm externally and internally while traction is maintained.

4. After reduction, lay the arm across the chest.

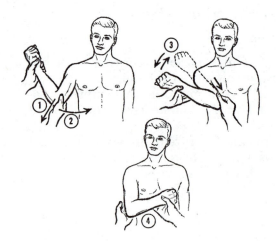

POSTREDUCTION X-RAY

1. Head is reduced.

2. Tuberosity is in its normal position.

Note: Displacement of the tuberosity more than 8 mm is likely to cause impingement against the acromion.

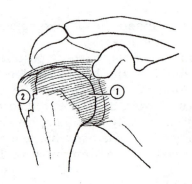

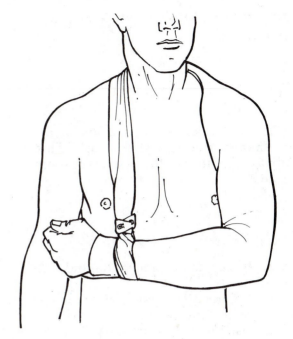

IMMOBILIZATION

Apply a shoulder immobilizer (see page 603).

POSTREDUCTION MANAGEMENT

Encourage motion at elbow, wrist, and fingers.

Discard apparatus after three or four weeks.

Institute program of graduated motions within limits of pain.

Begin with motions in stooped position every waking hour for five or ten minutes. Later, add abduction and external rotation exercises.

Allow free use of arm within limits of pain and fatigue.

Do not permit strenuous sports activities for a minimum of three months.

Indications for Operative Repair

The majority of Type I and Type II fracture-dislocations reduce and heal well by closed methods. The tuberosity fragments should be restored anatomically with no more than 8 to 10 mm of separation in order to prevent rotator cuff weakness and impingement on the undersurface of the acromion.

Any persistent weakness for six to eight weeks after reduction of the injury without evidence of axillary nerve paralysis warrants investigation with shoulder arthrogram because of the likelihood of rotator cuff disruption, which requires surgical repair.

Persistent tuberosity displacement of more than 1 cm also indicates a need for open reduction (see page 657). This displacement probably will be caused by one of several complications.

Indications for Operative Repair (Continued)

POSSIBLE COMPLICATIONS

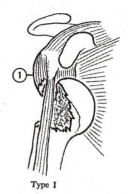

IN TYPE I

1. Dislocation with avulsion of attachment of portion of the cuff. (This always includes the supraspinatus tendon.)

Type I

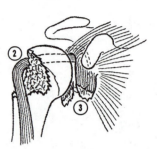

IN TYPE II

2. Biceps is displaced behind the head.
3. Tuberosities and cuff drop in front of glenoid cavity.

Reposition of head in glenoid cavity is impossible.

Type II

TYPE III FRACTURE-DISLOCATION

Prereduction X-Ray

1. Humeral head is dislocated anteriorly.
2. Greater tuberosity is retracted under the acromion process.

Note: Because of the gross disruption of the rotator cuff in this type of injury, open reduction should be the primary method of reduction.

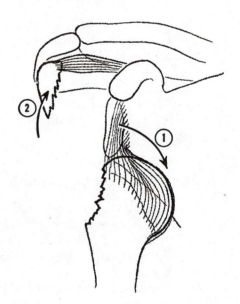

Type III

Surgical Management

Open reduction is used for Type III fracture-dislocations and also for Types I and II with persistent displacement of the tuberosity after closed reduction.

656

Surgical Management
(Continued)

Incision and posterior exposure

1. The patient lies on the unaffected side. The skin incision runs above the scapular spine, curving laterally over the acromion.

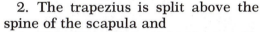

2. The trapezius is split above the spine of the scapula and

3. The fibers of the deltoid are split downward to avoid the axillary nerve.

4. The acromion is osteotomized at its base with care taken to avoid the suprascapular nerve and artery. The osteotomy site is opened with a self-retaining retractor.

5. The displaced fracture or rotator cuff is easily visualized.

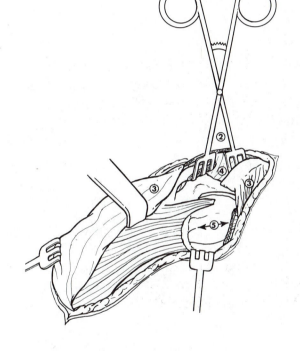

Reduction and repair

1. Disengage the biceps tendon from its posterior position and sever its proximal attachment to the glenoid rim.

2. Remove the cuff from between glenoid cavity and humeral head.

3. Reduce the dislocation.

Surgical Management
(Continued)

4. By interrupted sutures through the adjacent soft tissue, fix the tuberosities and cuff in their normal anatomic positions.

5. Cut away intracapsular portion of biceps tendon, and staple the end to the shaft of the humerus

Or

6. Fix the greater tuberosity to the shaft by a transfixion screw or heavy wire.

Then:

7. Approximate the torn edges of the cuff with interrupted sutures.

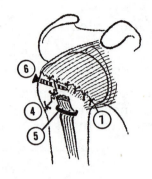

Alternative repair method

1. Grasp the retracted tuberosity and cuff with towel clip and pull it down to its normal anatomic position.

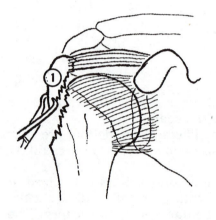

2. Anchor the tuberosity to bone and adjacent soft tissue with heavy wire sutures drilled through the bone.

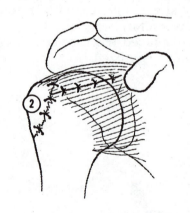

3. A Kirschner wire bow is effective for tightening the wire attachment.

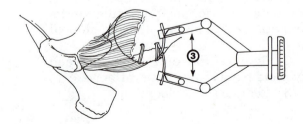

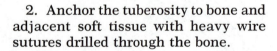

Postoperative Management

The osteotomy of the scapula is fixed with a screw and closed by repairing the trapezius and deltoid fasciae.

The shoulder is then immobilized with a Velpeau dressing.

On the first postoperative day the patient should start shrugging and elevating his shoulder every hour.

After three weeks the Velpeau is discarded and the arm is supported with a sling.

The patient starts with circumduction and pendulum exercises and advances to external rotation and abduction exercises.

The return of motion and shoulder function will take a good deal of time and effort on the part of the patient, and he should be instructed to persist in the range-of-motion exercises.

FRACTURES OF THE HEAD AND NECK OF THE HUMERUS WITH DISLOCATION

REMARKS

These are serious injuries that usually occur in middle-aged and elderly patients.

Occasionally, closed reduction of an impacted dislocation in a young patient without adequate muscle relaxation will produce a completely displaced fracture-dislocation and subsequent disruption of the circulation to the humeral head. This serious complication can be prevented by avoiding overvigorous manipulation of the shoulder dislocation.

Also, always consider that reduction may be difficult because the dislocation is chronic. Suspect chronic dislocations in alcoholics or epileptic patients.

Keep in mind that the brachial plexus and axillary vessels may be injured at the time of fracture-dislocation or may be traumatized during overvigorous closed manipulation. Operative reduction offers the safest method of handling this complex problem.

Reduction of the humeral head with repair of the tuberosity fragments is feasible only if the soft tissues remain attached for blood supply.

If the dislocated articular surface is deprived of blood supply, avascular necrosis is inevitable, and either resectional arthroplasty or prosthetic replacement should be employed.

Operative repair is especially difficult if it is delayed over two weeks, because scar formation and pericapsular bone formation as well as softening of the bone fragments will occur.

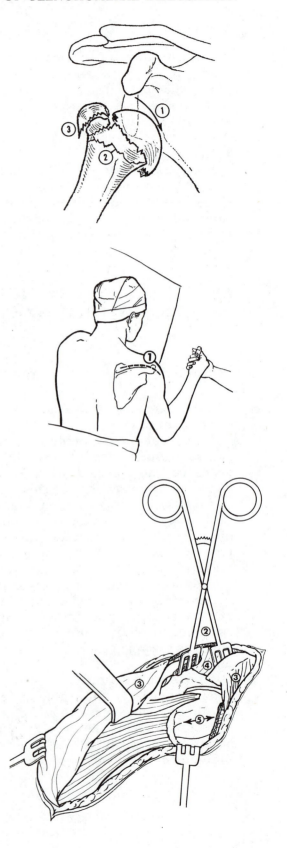

Prereduction X-Ray

1. Dislocation of head.
2. Fracture of neck.
3. Fracture of tuberosities.

Operative Repair

INCISION AND POSTERIOR EXPOSURE

1. The patient lies on the unaffected side. The skin incision runs above the scapular spine, curving laterally over the acromion.

2. The trapezius is split above the spine of the scapula and
3. The fibers of the deltoid are split downward to avoid the axillary nerve.
4. The acromion is exposed at its base with care taken to avoid the suprascapular nerve and artery. The osteotomy site is opened with a self-retaining retractor to expose the rotator cuff.
5. The displaced fragments and rotator cuff are easily visualized.

REDUCTION AND REPAIR

1. Pull distally on the arm in the axis of the body.

2. Gently lever the head into the glenoid cavity, taking care to preserve the periosteal and soft tissue attachments to the head fragments. Gentle rotation may be necessary to reduce the head fragment.

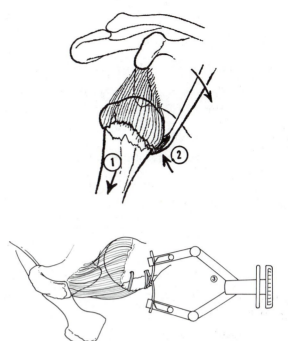

3. Secure the rotator cuff and tuberosity fragments to the shaft with several heavy wire sutures tied by a Kirschner wire tightener.

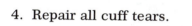

4. Repair all cuff tears.

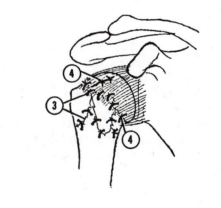

ALTERNATIVE METHOD I: RESECTIONAL ARTHROPLASTY

Employed when proximal fragment has been deprived of blood supply or cannot be reduced.

1. Excise the articular surface fragment to perform a resectional arthroplasty.

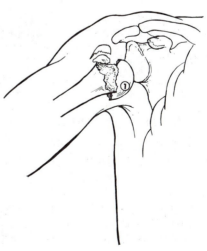

Operative Repair (Continued)

2. Reattach the rotator cuff fragments to the surgical neck by heavy wire sutures tightened with a Kirschner wire tightener.

3. Reduce the shaft and repaired rotator cuff fragments into the glenoid, and stabilize the joint by reattaching any torn capsule.

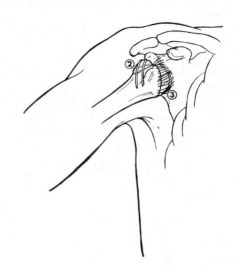

ALTERNATIVE METHOD II: PROSTHETIC ARTHROPLASTY

Employed when a prosthesis is available and the fracture has not involved a significant amount of the surgical neck.

Remove the humeral head.

4. Attach the fragments of the tuberosity to one another and to the shaft with wire sutures passed through drill holes and all fragments.

5. Insert a Neer prosthesis. The medullary canal should be drilled to accommodate a tight-fitting stem. The articular surface of the prosthesis is retrograded 30 degrees to provide stability.

Note: Active range of motion will generally be limited. Frequently the preferred method in the elderly patient is resectional arthroplasty.

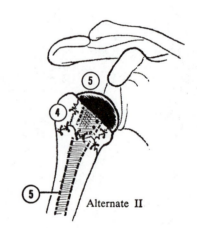

Alternate II

Postoperative Management

Fix the osteotomy of the scapular spine with a screw and close the trapezius and deltoid fasciae.

Apply a Velpeau dressing, padding the axilla and using a sling support.

On the first postoperative day the patient should shrug and elevate the shoulder frequently during waking hours.

Begin assisted external rotation exercises by the fourth day.

After three weeks, remove the Velpeau dressing and use sling support for one week.

Start with circumduction exercises, and advance to abduction exercises (see page 139).

Explain to the patient that improvement in strength will continue for many months after the repair and that pain relief should be the most significant benefit of this procedure.

OTHER FRACTURES COMPLICATING DISLOCATION

REMARKS

The lesions discussed here are rare but may be a cause of severe pain or disability after reduction.

In general, the fracture component can be disregarded and the patient can be treated in the same manner as with an uncomplicated dislocation.

Fracture of the Coracoid Process and Subcoracoid Dislocation

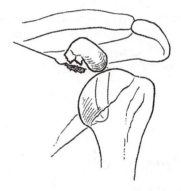

Fracture of the Acromion and Subcoracoid Dislocation

Note: This may be associated with rotator cuff disruption. Suspect tendon rupture if there is persistent weakness of abduction after recovery from the initial injury.

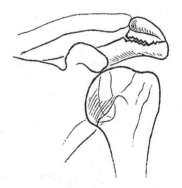

Management

Treat these injuries as uncomplicated anterior dislocations.

The fracture component may generally be disregarded provided that tendon rupture is not associated.

INTRATHORACIC DISLOCATION OF THE HUMERAL HEAD

REMARKS

This is indeed a rare lesion but it may occur.

The humerus may be driven between the ribs of the upper thoracic cage.

When the arm descends the ribs may snap off the head, leaving it in the thorax.

The entire cuff is avulsed from the humerus with or without bone fragments.

The patient may or may not show signs of respiratory difficulty.

The unusually great distance between the head and the shaft of the humerus, as seen on x-ray, may be a clue to the nature of the lesion.

Appearance on X-Ray

1. Upper end of the shaft of the humerus lying in front of the glenoid.
2. Avulsed greater tuberosity.
3. Humeral head at a great distance from the glenoid fossa.

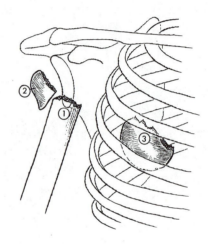

Management

REMARKS

If the diagnosis is made before operation, seek the help of a thoracic surgeon.

Use endotracheal anesthesia.

INCISION

1. Make an S-shaped incision on the anterior aspect of the shoulder beginning at the inferior margin of the acromioclavicular joint.

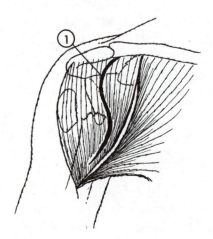

2. Develop the interval between the deltoid and the pectoralis major, and retract the cephalic vein and the pectoralis major medially; this brings into view the upper end of the shaft of the humerus.

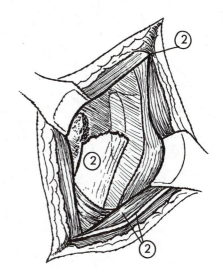

EXPOSURE AND EXTRACTION

1. Extend the skin incision along the inferior margin of the outer third of the clavicle.

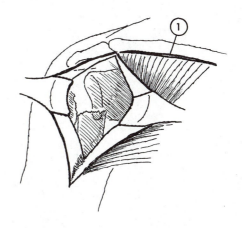

2. By subperiosteal dissection, detach the pectoralis major from the clavicle and retract it medially. This exposes the upper chest wall and the defect made by the humerus.

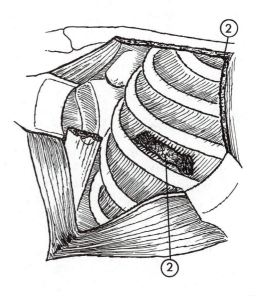

665

Management (*Continued*)

3. By digital examination in the defect locate the humeral head.

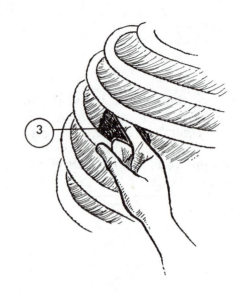

4. Extract the head from the thoracic cavity.

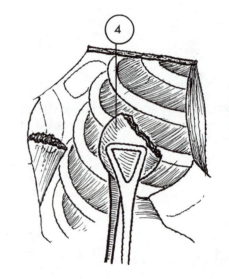

Repair

1. Place a rubber tube in the apex of the thoracic cavity and pass it out through the anterior chest wall. Place the tube in an underwater seal drainage.

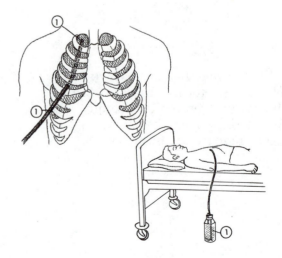

2. Remove loose fragments from the cuff.

3. Reattach the rotator cuff to the upper end of the humerus by mattress sutures passing through drill holes in the bone.

4. The biceps tendon is anchored to the upper end of the shaft of the humerus.

Note: Later prosthetic replacement may not be necessary if the patient regains a satisfactory, painless range of motion.

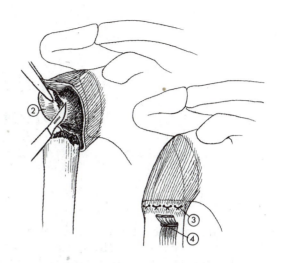

Immobilization

1. Place a cotton pad in the axilla.
2. Encircle the arm and chest with a 15-cm cotton bandage.
3. Apply a triangular sling.

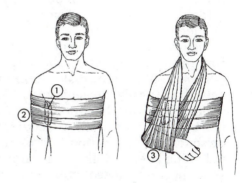

Postoperative Management

Remove the chest tube after 36 to 48 hours if the lung has expanded.

Immobilize the arm for 10 to 14 days. During this period, encourage motion at the elbow, wrist, and fingers.

Begin pendulum exercises and shoulder shrugging exercises while the arm is supported. Increase the exercises in range and frequency, and work on abduction and external exercises when the shoulder immobilizer is discarded. Advise the patient that full return of shoulder function will take many months of hard work and exercises.

Recurrent Dislocation of the Shoulder

REMARKS

The major factor determining whether a shoulder dislocation will recur is the age of the patient at the time of the initial dislocation. The degree or duration of postreduction immobilization has little bearing on recurrence rate.

The common dislocation in a teenaged male athlete has an 80 to 90 per cent probability of recurring within two years.

Dislocation with a fracture of the glenoid has an equally high chance of recurrence.

Dislocation in a 45-year-old man, which is usually associated with a fracture of the greater tuberosity, has only a 15 per cent chance of recurrence. Recurrent dislocation in older patients is quite infrequent except in naturally "loose-jointed" individuals.

Disruption of the anterior capsule and subscapularis support may not be sufficient to allow recurrent dislocation but will permit sudden episodes of subluxation and pain that significantly disable the individual. This is especially likely in a young athlete who has "wrenched" a shoulder and subsequently experiences episodes of subluxation. These transient recurrent subluxations should be recognized as real problems for the patient and should be treated appropriately.

Approximately 5 per cent of recurrent dislocations are posterior. Characteristically, the position of forward elevation and internal rotation with or without adduction, i.e., the "pushup position," results in the posterior recurrence. This relatively infrequent problem may be confused with recurrent anterior dislocation and may be treated by inappropriate surgical procedures.

An anteromedial fracture defect in the humeral head indicates that the luxation is posterior; treatment should be surgical repair of the damaged posterior glenoid capsule and infraspinatus support structures. Flattening of the anteromedial aspect of the head or fracture of the lesser tuberosity should alert the surgeon to the likelihood of a posterior dislocation.

Voluntary dislocation is a special and difficult problem demanding careful analysis. The young patient frequently acquires the ability to dislocate a lax or injured shoulder at will by stabilizing the scapula against the thorax and activating only half of the deltoid or rotator cuff force couples. The resultant overpull of part of the shoulder muscle complex may dislocate the humerus posteriorly, anteriorly, or inferiorly with respect to the glenoid.

The majority of patients with voluntary dislocations respond well to muscle strengthening exercises. If surgical treatment becomes necessary, a combination of procedures are needed, rather than one standard operation. Before recommending surgical repair of a voluntary dislocation, the physician should carefully evaluate the patient for emotional or psychiatric problems, which occur in about a third of instances and frustrate treatment of any type.

ETIOLOGY OF RECURRENT DISLOCATION

Injury from Primary Traumatic Dislocation

REMARKS

Among the lesions that are produced by initial dislocation and lead to recurrence are:
1. Detachment of portions of labrum.
2. Tearing of the capsule from the labrum and neck of the scapula.
3. Relaxation of the capsule with formation of a pouch into which the head displaces.
4. Erosion of the anterior or posterior rim of the glenoid.
5. Defects in the humeral head that engage the rim of the glenoid and lever the head out of the joint.
6. Neuromuscular imbalance, particularly involving the subscapularis in its role as prime dynamic anterior stabilizer of the shoulder.

All these lesions add to the instability of the shoulder and increase the likelihood of recurrence.

If the capsular attachment to the glenoid is torn, shoulder subluxation is likely.

Complete anterior dislocation follows stretching and loss of control of the capsule and subscapularis muscles.

Anatomic Variations in Glenohumeral Ligaments and Synovial Recesses

In addition to the trauma produced by the initial dislocation, many anatomic variations or areas of weakness in the shoulder capsule contribute to potential shoulder instability.

Sometimes, unusual arrangements of the glenohumeral ligaments and synovial recesses are the cause:

Anatomic Variations in Glenohumeral Ligaments and Synovial Recesses (Continued)

1. One synovial recess above the middle glenohumeral ligament.

2. One synovial recess below the middle glenohumeral ligament.

3. Two synovial recesses, one above and one below the middle glenohumeral ligament.

4. One large synovial recess above the inferior glenohumeral ligament; the middle ligament is absent.

5. The middle ligament comprises two small synovial folds.

6. Complete absence of synovial recesses.

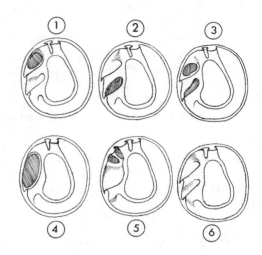

In many shoulders the synovial recess or recesses are very large and the ligaments are small or even absent so that no capsular walls exist to restrict forward displacement of the humeral head.

The anterior capsular wall is adequate.

1. Well-formed middle glenohumeral ligament.

2. Well-formed inferior glenohumeral ligament.

3. Small subscapularis recess.

4. The labrum is continuous with the capsule.

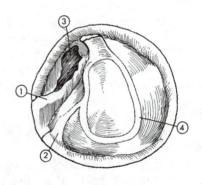

The anterior capsular wall is inadequate.

1. The middle glenohumeral ligament is poorly developed, comprising a small synovial strap.

2. The subscapularis recess is large.

3. The inferior ligament is small.

4. Only a small portion of the labrum inferiorly is continuous with the capsule.

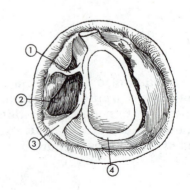

670

SURGICAL REPAIR FOR RECURRENT ANTERIOR DISLOCATION

Shoulder stability may be restored by repairing the damaged capsular and labral attachments to the glenoid (Bankart operation), by imbricating capsule and shortening the stretched out subscapularis (Putti-Platt procedure), by lateral transfer of the subscapularis (Magnuson operation), or by a number of other effective procedures.

Since most kinds of operative repair are effective in preventing recurrence in 95 to 97 per cent of cases, the surgeon should choose a method that (1) can be done expeditiously, (2) does not require screw or staple fixation likely to cause future problems for the patient, and (3) decreases external rotation and abduction range as little as possible.

In most instances, a modified Magnuson repair will meet these objectives, including the primary one of preventing recurrence.

Appearance on X-Ray

1. Large defect in upper and outer aspect of the humeral head.

When present this lesion may be difficult to demonstrate unless x-ray is taken with the arm in 50 to 80 degrees of internal rotation (see page 652).

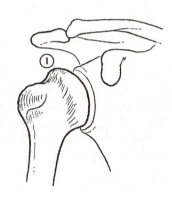

Magnuson Repair, Modified

This is the procedure of choice for most cases of recurrent dislocation.

INCISIONS

1. A 6-cm to 8-cm skin incision is made through the deltopectoral interval.

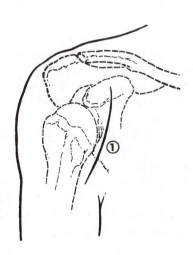

671

Magnuson Repair, Modified
(Continued)

2. The deep incision is continued through the deltopectoral groove, ligating the cephalic vein if it is injured.

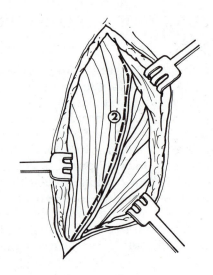

3. The incision is extended laterally to detach the origin of the deltoid if necessary for adequate exposure. The short head of the biceps may also be detached from the coracoid.

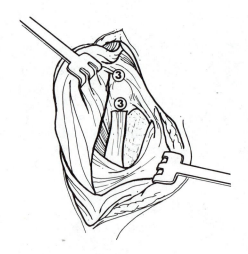

4. Identify the subscapularis muscle by externally rotating the arm, and make a 3-cm incision in the interval between the subscapularis and supraspinatus muscles.

5. A second incision of the same size is made along the lower border of the subscapularis muscle.

6. Incise the subscapularis tendon between the two incisions along the anterior lip of the bicipital groove. (Do not cut the biceps tendon.)

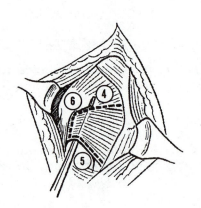

EXPOSURE

1. Separate the subscapularis tendon from the underlying capsule.

2. Dissect and free both the capsule and the subscapularis tendons at least back to the glenoid labrum, and inspect the joint for loose bodies or other defects.

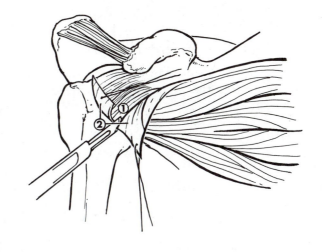

REPAIR

1. Rotate the arm internally and with a sharp osteotome remove the top layer of cortical bone lateral to the bicipital groove and inferior to the original insertion of the subscapularis muscle.

2. With the arm rotated internally, approximate the freed capsule and subscapularis tendon to the raw area, and fix these structures with sutures through drill holes in the bone.

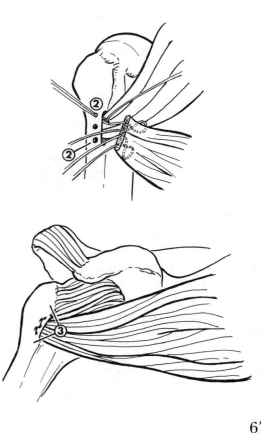

3. Approximate the capsule and the subscapularis tendons to surrounding inferior capsule and to supraspinatus tendon. Repair should accomplish a buttress by moving the subscapularis tendon and the capsule both laterally and inferiorly.

Note: Closure is routine after reattaching the biceps tendon to the coracoid process and deltoid to the clavicle.

Postoperative Immobilization

1. Place a cotton pad in the axilla.
2. Encircle the arm and trunk with a 15-cm cotton bandage.
3. Apply a triangular sling.

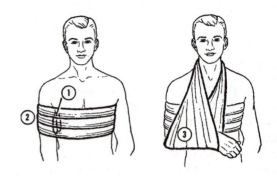

Postoperative Management

Fix the arm to the side in a position of internal rotation for four weeks.

During this period allow motion at the elbow and encourage motion at the wrist and in the fingers.

At the end of four weeks, discard the sling and bandage and begin pendulum exercises in ever-increasing arcs on a regulated regimen (five to ten minutes every waking hour).

At first, forceful external rotation of the arm is prohibited; after the fifth week active external rotation of the arm within the patient's tolerance is encouraged.

Now add abduction and external rotation exercises.

Full restoration should be achieved by the eighth week. Some permanent restriction of external rotation is always present; this does not interfere with normal function.

Alternative Incision (After Leslie and Ryan)

REMARKS

The axillary approach provides ample exposure to perform this operation and precludes cosmetically poor scars on the anterior aspect of the shoulder.

This approach is very useful in women, but exposure may be difficult in heavily muscled men.

INCISION

1. Arm is in abduction and external rotation.
2. Make an incision traversing the center of the axilla beginning at the upper border of the pectoralis major.
3. Undermine widely the skin and subcutaneous tissue all around the incision.

Note: This is a very important step in order to be able to retract the tissues sufficiently both anteriorly and superiorly.

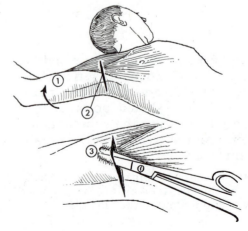

674

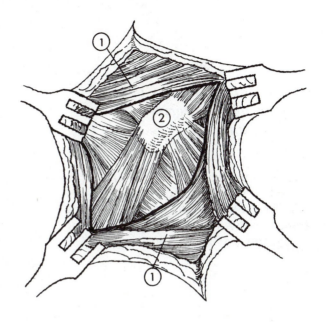

EXPOSURE

1. Develop the interval between the deltoid and the pectoralis major muscles.

2. Expose the coracoid process.

From this point on the operation is the same as that through the anterior deltopectoral approach (see page 671).

RECURRENT ANTERIOR SHOULDER SUBLUXATION

REMARKS

This most frequently occurs in a young athlete who has "wrenched" a shoulder and experiences repeated transient attacks of the shoulder "going out." Because these brief episodes are not obvious dislocations and do not require reduction, the diagnosis frequently remains in doubt and the patient continues with his disability.

A typical history of injury to the shoulder by forceful abduction and external rotation, e.g., in wrestling or football, followed by repeated painful episodes whenever the shoulder is used in certain positions should prompt the physician to suspect shoulder subluxation.

Occasionally a subluxing bicipital tendon will cause these symptoms, but the usual etiology is disruption of the capsular attachment to the anterior glenoid and labrum.

Occasionally, special x-ray views (West Point View) are helpful in detecting areas of damage to the inferior glenoid, but usually the diagnosis must be based on the history and on the pain that can be reproduced in the subluxating position.

West Point View for Glenoid Injuries with Anterior Subluxation

TECHNIQUE

1. The patient is prone with the involved shoulder raised by pads.

2. The x-ray beam is angled 25 degrees downward and 25 degrees medially, toward the axilla.

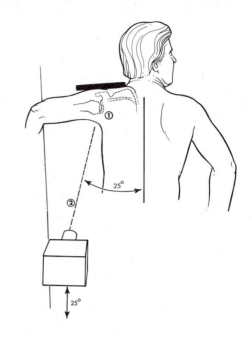

APPEARANCE ON X-RAY

1. Resultant tangential axillary view of the glenoid may show small anterior fragmentation associated with subluxation.

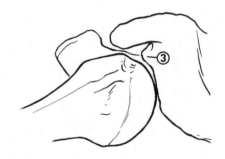

Management

Exercises to strengthen shoulder control may be helpful and should include:

1. Abduction.

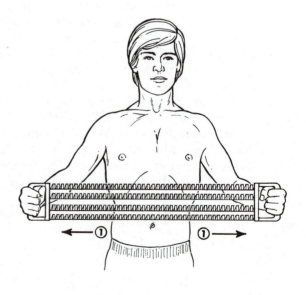

2. External rotation.

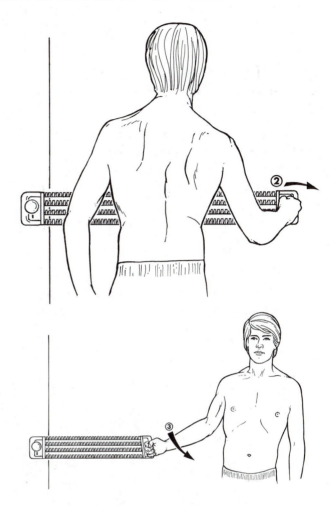

3. Internal rotation.

If symptoms of instability persist despite adequate exercise program, Magnuson repair should be performed (see page 671).

RECURRENT POSTERIOR DISLOCATION

Diagnosis

Posterior dislocation should be considered in a differential diagnosis of any patient with shoulder instability.

1. Characteristically, it occurs with forward elevation and internal rotation (pushup position).

2. Fractures of the lesser tuberosity or flattening of the anteromedial head indicate a posterior dislocation.

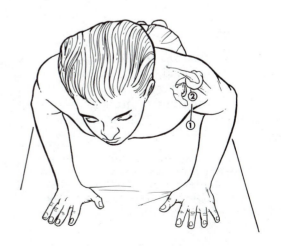

Surgical Repair by Glenoplasty and Infraspinatus Transfer (After Scott)

1. Patient lies on the unaffected side. Incision runs along the spine of the scapula and the tip of the acromion.

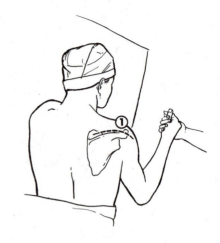

2. The deltoid muscle is detached carefully and is reflected inferiorly.

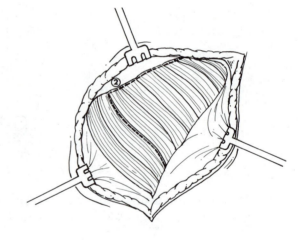

3. Overhanging 2 to 3 cm of the acromion is excised for exposure and for later use as a bone graft.

4. The infraspinatus muscle is detached from its insertion on anatomic neck and is retracted medially.

Note: The deltoid muscle should not be retracted below the teres minor so as not to damage the axillary nerve. The infraspinatus muscle should not be retracted too far medially so as to avoid injury to the suprascapular nerve.

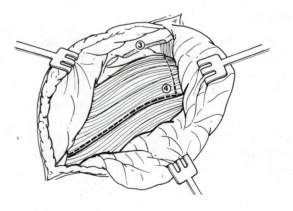

1. The capsule of the shoulder is opened in parallel with the infraspinatus muscle, and the humeral head and glenoid cavity are well visualized.

2. If the posterior labrum is detached, the capsule may be reflected medially to perform intracapsular osteotomy; otherwise a glenoid osteotomy is performed extracapsularly.

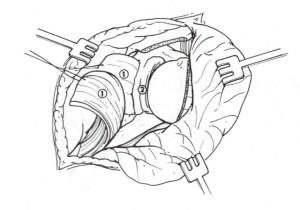

3. A broad osteotome is used to cut from the supraglenoid tubercle inferiorly to the origin of long head of triceps.

4. When it is possible to spring open the osteotomy 1 to 2 cm, the stability of the shoulder is then checked.

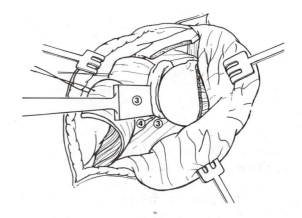

5. Graft previously obtained from the acromion is trimmed to fit and is impacted into the osteotomy site.

6. Repair of the posterior capsule and

7. Lateral transfer of the infraspinatus muscle adds to posterior stability.

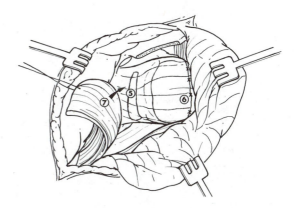

Postoperative Management

Fix the patient's arm to the side with the shoulder extended and slightly externally rotated by means of a shoulder wrap or spica cast for three weeks.

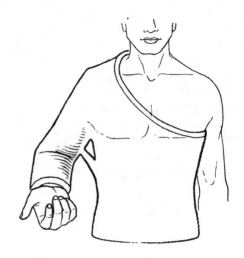

During this period allow motion at the elbow, wrist, and fingers.

At the end of three weeks discard the external support and begin a program of pendulum exercises in ever-increasing arcs every waking hour.

The patient should avoid doing pushups for three months so as to allow healing of the osteotomy.

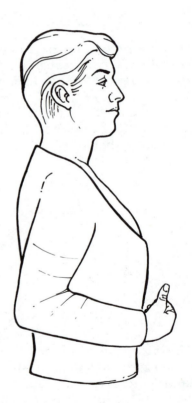

VOLUNTARY DISLOCATION

REMARKS

Voluntary dislocations are infrequent but usually occur in adolescents who may voluntarily and spontaneously dislocate their shoulders. This usually occurs after a mild injury and is characteristically painless posterior, inferior, or anterior displacement of the humeral head.

This maneuver is accomplished by voluntarily suppressing muscles necessary for stabilizing the humeral head in the glenoid, e.g., the rotator cuff muscles, while forcefully contracting muscles responsible for displacement, e.g., the anterior deltoid muscles.

Appearance on X-Ray

1. Painless posterior subluxation produced by the action of the deltoid and pectoralis major muscles.

2. Axillary view with the shoulder subluxed shows no evidence of bony damage or glenoid fracture.

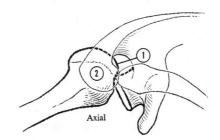

Axial

Management

A majority of these patients will respond to a program of progressive muscle-strengthening exercises (see page 676).

A careful psychiatric evaluation of these patients may also reveal that some have serious emotional and psychiatric problems underlying this self-manipulation.

A small percentage of these young patients will eventually require carefully selected combined operative repairs if the subluxations become painfully disabling.

The likelihood of recurrence after surgery is extremely high unless the individual's emotional and physical problems are carefully analyzed and managed with due caution.

SUMMARY: PITFALLS OF MANAGING SUBLUXATIONS AND DISLOCATIONS OF THE SHOULDER

The major pitfalls pertain to both the diagnosis and the treatment of this injury.

Acute anterior dislocation is obvious both clinically and radiographically.

Acute and recurrent anterior subluxations may not be obvious unless the physician considers the possibility.

Any young athlete with pain and vague symptoms of shoulder instability should be thoroughly evaluated for shoulder subluxation.

A posterior dislocation is overlooked initially in approximately half of patients owing to subtle physical and radiographic findings. Suspect a posterior shoulder dislocation in any patient with a shoulder "frozen" in internal rotation and adduction after an injury.

Injuries to the surrounding muscles and tendons are common with shoulder dislocations. Suspect a rotator cuff injury in any patient with shoulder dislocation over the age of 30. An inferior subluxation of the humeral head usually results from disuse atrophy and intra-articular hematoma rather than direct rotator cuff injury. Superior migration of the humeral head or persistently displaced fracture of the tuberosity after reduction indicates rotator cuff involvement.

If shoulder arthrography confirms the diagnosis of rotator cuff disruption, operative repair is best accomplished via a posterior approach after osteotomizing the spine of the scapula to visualize the entire supraspinatus tendon.

Reduction of a dislocated shoulder should be done with adequate muscle relaxation and with gentle, steady traction. Forceful manipulation may fracture the humeral head or rupture adjacent vascular structures, particularly in the elderly patient.

Recurrence of the shoulder dislocation is common in young athletic individuals. Prolonged shoulder immobilization after reduction does not significantly alter this susceptibility. Recurrent dislocation is infrequent in persons more than 30 years old unless they are "loose-jointed." Prolonged immobilization of more than one to two weeks should be avoided in the patient older than 30.

Most recurrent shoulder dislocations are anterior but a posterior recurrent dislocation is possible. Characteristically, the posterior dislocation is associated with the "pushup" position of internal rotation and adduction.

The direction of the recurrent dislocation or subluxation should be carefully ascertained by history and physical. Radiographic changes in the posterolateral or anteromedial head or the glenoid rim are helpful in confirming direction of the shoulder instability.

Voluntary shoulder dislocations are notoriously difficult to manage surgically. Most will respond to appropriate exercise therapy. Selective surgical procedures may occasionally be used for the young patient with symptomatic voluntary shoulder dislocation that is not responsive to a conscientious exercise program.

The shoulder is the most commonly dislocated large joint. Management of this common dislocation requires anticipation of the common pitfalls.

REFERENCES

Codman, E.: The Shoulder. Brooklyn, New York, G. Miller & Co., Medical Pub., Inc., 1934.

Connolly, J.: Humeral head defects associated with shoulder dislocations – their diagnostic and surgical significance. Instruct. Course Lec., 21:42, St. Louis, C. V. Mosby Co, 1972.

Debeyre, J., Patte, D., and Elmelik, E.: Repair of ruptures of the rotator cuff of the shoulder. J. Bone and Joint Surg., 47-B:36, 1965.

Gilchrist, D. K.: A stockinette-velpeau for immobilization of the shoulder girdle. J. Bone and Joint Surg. 49-A:750, 1967.

Inman, V. T., Saunders, J. B., and Abbott, L. C.: Observations on the function of the shoulder joint. J. Bone and Joint Surg., 26:1, 1944.

Jardon, O. M., Hood, L. T., and Lynch, R. D.: Complete avulsion of the axillary artery as a complication of shoulder dislocation. J. Bone and Joint Surg., 55-A:189, 1973.

Kraulis, J., and Hunter, G.: The results of prosthetic replacement in fracture-dislocations of the upper end of the humerus. Injury, 8:129, 1976.

Leslie, J., and Ryan, T.: The anterior axillary incision to approach the shoulder joint. J. Bone and Joint Surg., 44-A:1193, 1962.

McLaughlin, H.: Posterior dislocation of the shoulder. J. Bone and Joint Surg., 34-A:584, 1952.

Neer, C. S.: Replacement arthroplasty for glenohumeral arthritis. J. Bone and Joint Surg. 56-A:1, 1974.

Neviaser, J. S.: Arthrography of the Shoulder. The Diagnosis and Management of the Lesions Visualized. Springfield, Ill., Charles C Thomas, Pub., 1975.

Neviaser, J. S., Neviaser, R. J., and Neviaser, T. J.: The repair of chronic massive ruptures of the rotator cuff of the shoulder by use of a freeze-dried rotator cuff. J. Bone and Joint Surg., 60-A:681, 1978.

Roukous, J., Feagin, J., and Abbott, H.: Modified axillary roentgenogram. A useful adjunct in the diagnosis of recurrent instability of the shoulder. Clin. Orthop., 82:84, 1972.

Rowe, C. R., Pierce, D. S., and Clark, J. G.: Voluntary dislocation of the shoulder. J. Bone and Joint Surg., 55-A:445, 1973.

Scott, D. J.: Treatment of recurrent posterior dislocations of the shoulder by glenoplasty. J. Bone and Joint Surg., 49-A:471, 1967.

FRACTURES OF THE HUMERUS

FRACTURES OF
THE UPPER END OF THE
HUMERUS

REMARKS

For the most part, fractures of the upper end of the humerus occur from indirect mechanisms in the same age group as femoral neck fractures and Colles' fractures, i.e., the elderly. They are "fragile bone" types of fracture.

Most proximal humeral fractures (80 per cent) occur in osteoporotic patients who fall on the outstretched hand with the elbow extended. The resultant axial and torsional loading is transmitted up to the humerus and shoulder and produces characteristic fractures.

Bone is weakest in torsional strength and is most likely to fail from the indirect force of twisting. Yamada has shown in evaluating mechanics of torsional failure that the direction of the fracture line consistently is determined by the direction of the twist.

Fractures produced by external twisting of the arm run in an oblique or spiral fashion from the distal medial cortex to the superior lateral cortex.

Fractures produced by internal torsion run in a distal lateral to proximal medial direction.

The mechanisms of fracture also determine the displacement. Internal torsion characteristically causes medial displacement of the distal fragment. External torsion produces superolateral displacement of the distal fragment and sometimes anterior dislocation of the head fragment.

Fractures that are produced by direct loading tend to occur in younger, more active patients.

Direct bending can produce a typical transverse fracture of the midshaft of the humerus. This can occur from a fall directly on the abducting distal humerus that locks the proximal humerus in the glenoid. The bending moment is then applied to the midshaft and produces a characteristic transverse fracture.

Another common direct mechanism is a fall on the upper arm. A severe direct blow to the shoulder, as in a fall from a height, may cause a severe comminution or a fracture-dislocation of the proximal humerus.

The prognosis for satisfactory healing after severe direct injuries is significantly worse than after moderate indirect injuries to the humerus.

Occasionally, direct injuries to the shoulder may fracture the anatomic neck with sufficient damage to the blood supply to cause ischemic necrosis of the head. The initial x-ray may not reflect the severity of damage, and only on later x-rays will disruption of the articular surface become evident.

Understanding these implications of the injury aids in anticipating potential problems and providing appropriate treatment.

INDIRECT MECHANISMS

External Torsional Fracture

An elderly patient falls
1. On the outstretched arm with the elbow extended.
2. The direction of twist is external.

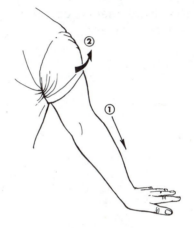

3. A typical fracture from external torsion results from failure that begins in the distal medial cortex and runs to the proximal lateral cortex.
4. The distal fragment is displaced superiorly and laterally by the force vectors.

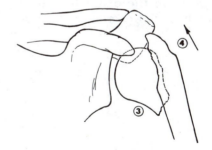

1. Extreme external torsion may produce a three-fragment or four-fragment fracture and
2. Anterior dislocation of the humeral head.

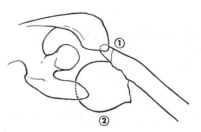

External Torsional Fracture
(Continued)

1. External torsion in the younger patient causes a fracture of the distal humerus.

2. Characteristically the failure line runs from the distal medial cortex to the proximal lateral cortex.

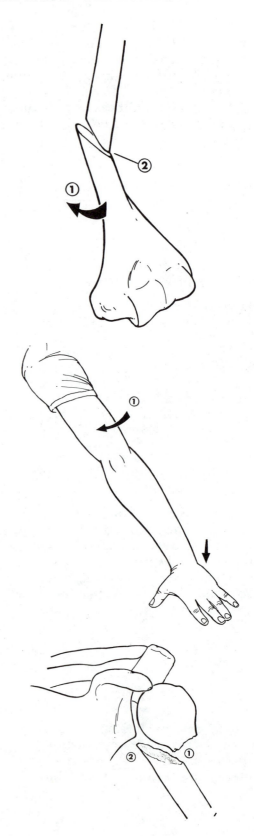

Internal Torsional Fractures

1. Failure resulting from internal torsion runs from the distal lateral to the proximal medial cortex of the humerus.

2. The force vectors displace the distal fragment medially.

1. A spiral oblique fracture of the midshaft may result from internal torsional loading.

2. The failure line begins in the distal lateral cortex and runs to the proximal medial cortex.

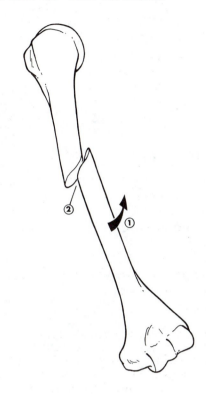

DIRECT MECHANISMS

Bending Fractures

1. The victim falls on the distal humerus and forcefully abducts the arm.

2. The proximal humerus is locked in the glenoid.

3. The bending moment produces a typical transverse fracture of the midshaft of the humerus.

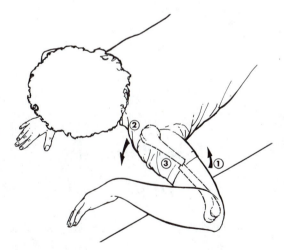

689

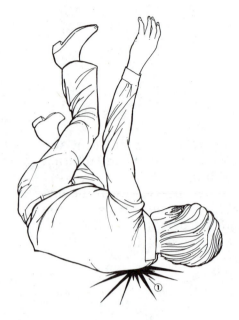

Direct Violence to the Shoulder

1. A direct blow on the shoulder, as in a fall from a horse, may violently fracture one or all of the four major anatomic structures in this region. These include

2. The anatomic neck,
3. The greater tuberosity,
4. The lesser tuberosity, and
5. The surgical neck.

Note: With fractures of the greater tuberosity from direct injury to the shoulder, always check carefully for anterior dislocation of the shoulder. When the lesser tuberosity has been fractured from a direct injury, check thoroughly for posterior shoulder dislocation.

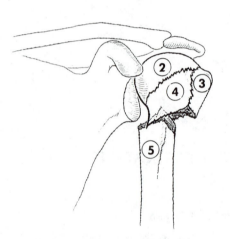

Management of Fractures of the Upper End of the Humerus

REMARKS

The objectives in treating fractures of the upper end of the humerus are to maintain shoulder function and to achieve fracture union. The latter objective is usually reached more readily than the former.

690

Fractures of the surgical neck most often should be treated as soft tissue injuries that also happen to involve bone. To avoid persistent loss of shoulder function or a frozen shoulder, treat these fractures more on the basis of clinical symptoms than of radiographic signs.

The majority of surgical neck fractures require no reduction. Rarely, the displacement and angulation will be sufficient to impair range of motion unless reduction is accomplished.

Union of fracture of the anatomic neck, for the most part, is uncomplicated. Damage to the circulation in this region may sometimes be sufficient to result in ischemic necrosis of the subchondral bone.

Fractures of the lesser tuberosity should prompt consideration and evaluation for associated posterior dislocation of the shoulder.

Fractures of the greater tuberosity demand accurate reduction and assessment of the rotator cuff function to insure restoration of painless, active abduction. Generally, displacement of more than 1 cm that persists after reduction indicates the need for open reduction with internal fixation.

Fractures or fracture-dislocations that produce displacement of two or more anatomic parts are best treated by open reduction and internal fixation to permit maximal restoration of shoulder function as well as fracture union.

Early restoration of shoulder motion is essential to restore the balance between the deltoid and rotator cuff muscles and to avoid shoulder muscle contractures. This can best be achieved in most cases by de-emphasizing the skeletal injury and giving primary treatment to the soft tissue injury.

For purposes of management, fractures of the upper end of the humerus are divided into two groups:

1. Fractures requiring no reduction.
2. Fractures requiring reduction.

FRACTURES REQUIRING NO REDUCTION

Appearance on X-Ray

Compression fracture of the greater tuberosity.

Note: Occasionally this fracture will involve the bicipital groove and produce a bicipital tendinitis (see page 703).

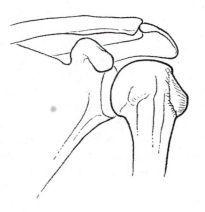

Appearance on X-Ray (Continued)

Fracture of the greater tuberosity with minimal displacement; the fragment is avulsed from the humerus. Displacement of more than 8 to 10 mm should be corrected surgically to restore normal rotator cuff function and prevent a painful arc from impingement of the displaced fracture under the acromion.

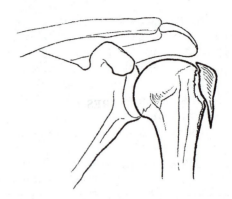

A portion of the humeral head with its articular surface is impacted into the remaining humeral head.

Note: These fractures occur during electroconvulsive therapy. Posterior dislocation should be ruled out on the basis of axillary x-rays whenever fractures occur in this area.

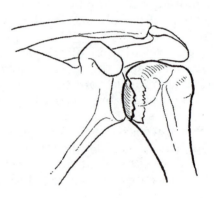

Impacted external torsional fracture of the surgical neck of the humerus in an elderly patient. The proximal fragment is in a position of slight varus or internal torsion. The normal head–neck angle is 140 degrees; a change of 25 degrees above or below this angle does not preclude good function. The angle shown here measures 120 degrees.

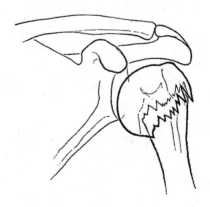

692

Impacted internal torsional fracture of the surgical neck of the humerus; the proximal fragment is in externally rotated, valgus position. The angle measures 160 degrees.

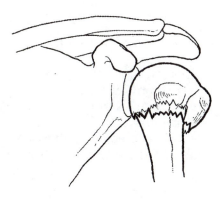

Impacted fracture of the anatomic neck of the humerus with severe comminution of the head and tuberosities. This type usually results from direct injury, and the degree of damage may not be immediately evident until complications ensue.

This fracture may result in traumatic arthritis or ischemic necrosis. Early mobilization is important to minimize painful stiffening.

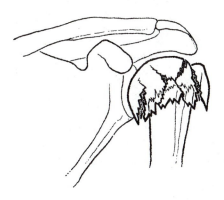

Fracture of the anatomic neck with minimal displacement.

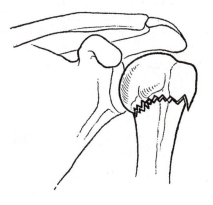

Appearance on X-Ray *(Continued)*

External torsional fracture of the surgical neck with only moderate displacement; the proximal fragment is in slight internal torsion. The head–neck angle is 155 degrees and therefore acceptable if it should heal in this position.

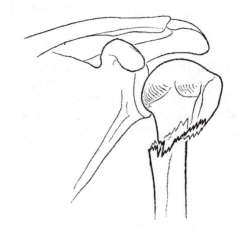

A displaced surgical neck fracture produced by internal torsion is impacted with displacement. The medial displacement of the distal fragment does not require disimpaction since shoulder function will not be impaired by healing in this position.

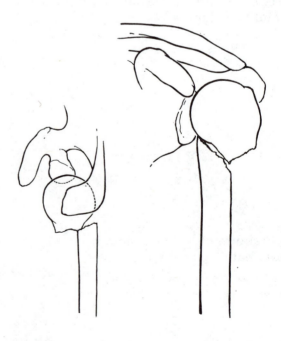

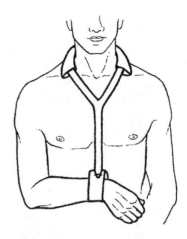

Immobilization

Collar and cuff.

Management

These fractures should not be treated by cumbersome fixation devices such as abduction splints, casts, hanging casts, or braces. Excellent results are possible if collar and cuff is employed and range-of-motion exercises are started when the acute pain subsides.

Do not wait for radiographic signs of fracture union to commence range-of-motion exercises.

Treat these injuries with emphasis on the soft tissue rather than the bony damage. Start motion when the pain of the acute injury subsides. Begin with pendulum exercises in the stooped position for three to five minutes every waking hour.

Increase range of motion and the period of exercises progressively as the pain subsides. Discard the collar and cuff after three weeks, and allow the patient to wear a sling only during sleeping hours for comfort. Progress to abduction and external rotation exercises, and concentrate on restoring full passive range of motion.

Functional range of shoulder motion should be possible within six to eight weeks after instituting exercise therapy.

Once full range of passive motion is achieved, begin resisted exercises to regain strength.

Complete recovery requires many weeks of persistent exercises to regain both motion and strength.

FRACTURES REQUIRING REDUCTION

FRACTURES OF THE GREATER TUBEROSITY

REMARKS

Retraction of the greater tuberosity under the acromion is comparable to rupture of the cuff.

For this lesion closed methods are ineffectual. Open methods give the best results.

If the greater tuberosity has been displaced downward and outward and is allowed to heal in this position, marked limitation of abduction and a painful arc will result from impingement under the acromion.

Best results are obtained when the greater tuberosity is replaced in its anatomic position by open methods.

If the tuberosity fragment is just a shell or is very small, excise it and reattach the tendon to bone.

Preoperative X-Rays

The greater tuberosity has retracted under the acromion.

The greater tuberosity is displaced outward more than 8 to 10 mm.

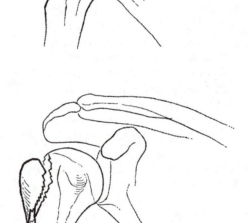

A painful arc occurs when the rotator cuff is displaced and is pinched between the acromion and humeral head on abduction.

Operative Management

INCISION AND EXPOSURE

1. With the patient on his opposite side a longitudinal incision is made above the scapular spine.

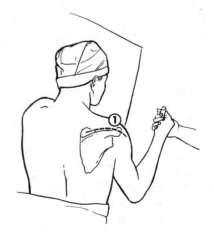

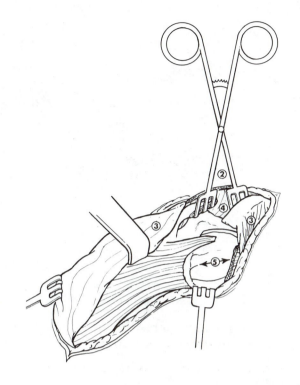

2. The trapezius and

3. The deltoid are split longitudinally.

4. The acromion is osteotomized at its base, with care taken to avoid the suprascapular nerve, to expose the

5. Displaced rotator cuff.

REDUCTION IF THE TUBEROSITY IS RETRACTED UNDER THE ACROMION

1. Grasp the retracted tuberosity and cuff with a towel clip and pull it down to its normal anatomic position.

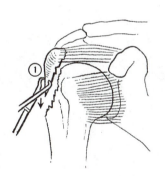

2. Fix the tuberosity to the adjacent soft tissue by interrupted wire sutures.

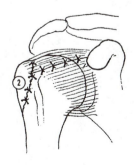

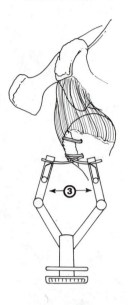

Operative Management
(Continued)

3. Use Kirschner wire tightener to fix fragments.

REDUCTION IF THE TUBEROSITY IS DISPLACED DOWNWARD AND OUTWARD

1. Replace the tuberosity to its normal position.

2. Fix the fragment with wire sutures passed through drill holes in the humeral head.

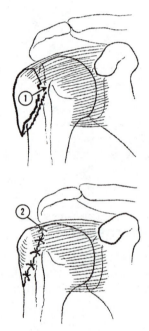

The repair should be airtight. Test for leakage by injecting sterile saline into the glenohumeral joint.

The osteotomy of the scapular spine is fixed with a screw.

The trapezius and deltoid fascia are repaired.

Postoperative Management

Immobilize the shoulder postoperatively with a Velpeau dressing or a shoulder immobilizer, but encourage the patient to begin active shoulder shrugging exercises on the first postoperative day.

Start circumduction exercises and daily motion of the elbow, wrist and fingers within the first five to seven days.

Add abduction and external rotation to regain passive range of motion.

When full range of passive motion has been achieved, add active resisted exercises to regain strength.

Full functional recovery may take four to six months, and the patient must be encouraged to persist in his muscle strengthening exercises.

FRACTURE OF THE GREATER TUBEROSITY IN WHICH THE BONE FRAGMENT IS SMALL OR JUST A SHELL

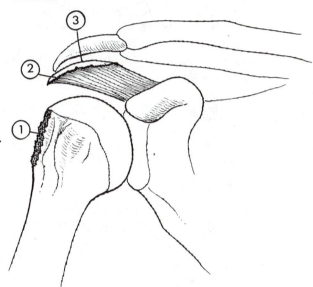

Preoperative X-Ray

1. Fracture of the greater tuberosity.

2. Fragment is just a sliver of bone.

3. Fragment lies under the acromion.

Surgical Management

1. Excise the bony fragment.

2. Reattach the tendon to the head of the humerus by interrupted sutures passing through drill holes in the bone.

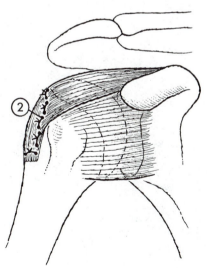

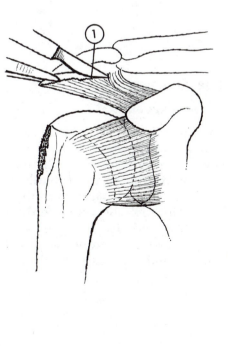

FRACTURE OF THE LESSER TUBEROSITY

REMARKS

This avulsion fracture is unusual as an isolated injury. It is most frequently encountered in comminuted fractures of the upper end of the humerus and in posterior dislocations of the humeral head.

When it occurs as an isolated fracture, the displaced fragment usually lies between the coracoid process and the head of the humerus, acting as a bony block to motions of the arm.

The fragment should be restored to its normal position by operative methods.

If the fragment is small, excise it and reattach the subscapularis tendon to the shaft of the humerus.

Preoperative X-Ray

The lesser tuberosity is avulsed and is pulled medially by the subscapularis muscle.

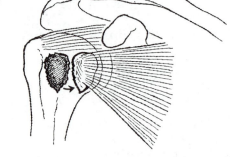

Operative Treatment

INCISION AND EXPOSURE

1. Make an S-shaped incision on the anterior aspect of the shoulder.

2. Deepen the incision through the deltoid 1 cm from its anterior border and retract the deltoid mass laterally.

3. Retract the cephalic vein and the remaining strip medially.

4. Identify the fragment of the lesser tuberosity and the subscapularis muscle.

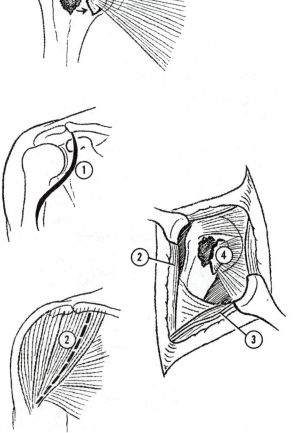

REDUCTION

1. Grasp the lesser tuberosity and the attached tendon with a towel clip.

2. With the arm in a position of internal rotation, pull the fragment into its normal position.

3. Anchor the fragment in place by interrupted sutures passing through drill holes made in the detached fragment and in the edges of the defect in the humerus.

Note: If the bicipital tendon is involved in the fracture fragment, fix it in its groove (see page 704).

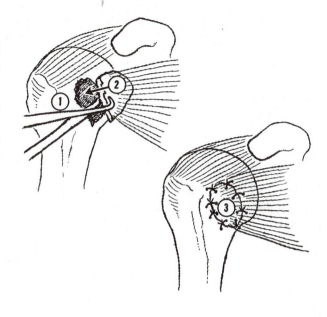

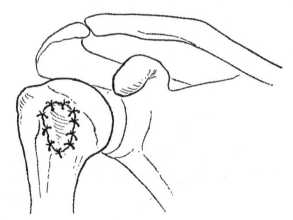

Postoperative X-Ray

The lesser tuberosity now occupies its normal anatomic position.

Postoperative Management

Apply a Velpeau or a shoulder immobilizer.

By the end of the third week, begin pendulum exercises in the stooped position for three to five minutes every waking hour.

Refrain from forceful external rotation exercises.

Increase the range of motion and the period of exercises progressively as the pain subsides.

Discard the shoulder immobilizer after three weeks and permit wearing of a triangular sling at night.

Begin abduction and external rotation exercises until full range of passive motion is achieved.

Encourage free use of the arm within the limits of pain.

After passive range of motion has been restored, work on active muscle strengthening.

Full restoration of function should be achieved in ten to twelve weeks.

FRACTURE OF THE LESSER TUBEROSITY IN WHICH THE BONE FRAGMENT IS SMALL

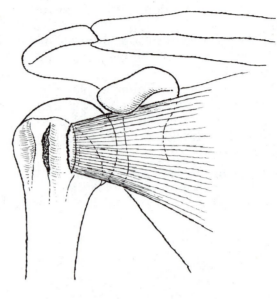

Preoperative X-Ray

The subscapularis has avulsed a small sliver of bone and pulled it medially.

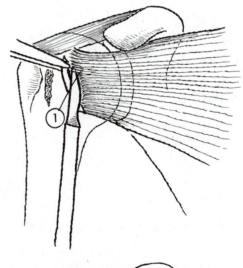

Operative Treatment

1. Excise the bony fragment.

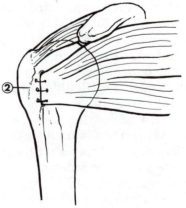

2. Reattach the subscapularis tendon to the shaft of the humerus with sutures to holes drilled in the defect.

Complications of Undisplaced Fractures (Initially Requiring No Reduction)

REMARKS

Compression fractures of the greater tuberosity may disrupt the bicipital groove sufficiently to cause bicipital tendinitis and pain after fracture healing. This can be alleviated by excising the intracapsular portion of the tendon and closing any defect in the rotator cuff.

Occasionally, undisplaced fractures of the humeral head or anatomic neck, sustained usually from a direct blow to the shoulder, will produce ischemic necrosis of the subchondral bone and traumatic arthritis. Pain after this injury may be sufficient to require prosthetic arthroplasty.

BICIPITAL TENDON INJURY

Appearance on X-Ray

Healed compression fracture of the greater tuberosity with disruption of the bicipital groove.

Note: In this particular case there was severe pain and limitation of motion caused by an associated bicipital tenosynovitis.

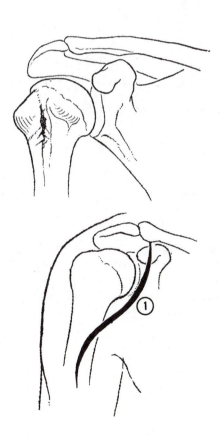

Operative Management

INCISION AND EXPOSURE

1. Make an S-shaped incision on the anterior aspect of the shoulder.

Operative Management
(Continued)

2. One cm from the anterior border of the deltoid, deepen the incision through the deltoid and retract the deltoid mass laterally.

3. Retract the cephalic vein with the remaining strip of muscle medially.

4. Identify the biceps tendon.

5. Divide the transverse ligament.

6. Open the cuff along the coraco-humeral ligament, and sever the biceps tendon at its insertion into the glenoid rim.

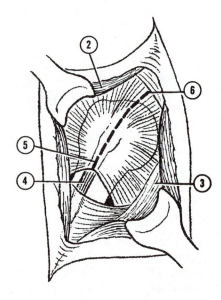

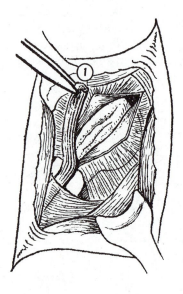

REPAIR

1. Excise the intracapsular portion of the tendon.

2. Suture the proximal end of the remaining tendon into drill holes in the shaft immediately below the tuberosities and in the bicipital groove.

3. Close the defect in the rotator cuff.

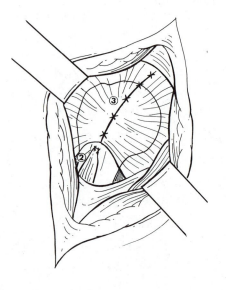

Postoperative Management

Apply a triangular sling.

Start pendulum exercises (three to five minutes every waking hour) on the second day.

As pain subsides, increase the intensity of the exercises.

Add abduction and external rotation exercises.

Encourage immediate free use of the arm and discard the sling after the first week.

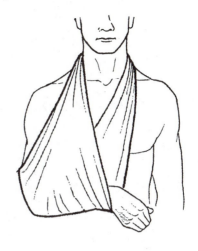

AVASCULAR NECROSIS

Appearance on X-Ray

A healed compression fracture of the head of the humerus has resulted in collapse of the subchondral bone and avascular necrosis.

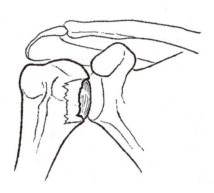

Management

1. If pain is severe, the humeral head is replaced with a Neer prosthesis.

2. The stem of the prosthesis fits snugly in the shaft.

3. The head is slightly retroverted and the rotator cuff is reattached to its normal insertion.

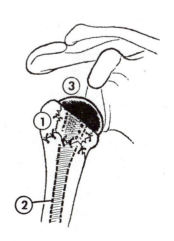

Anatomic and Surgical Neck
Fractures with Marked Displacement

REMARKS

These lesions are more common in adults than in children.

Reduction is required only in unimpacted fractures with marked separation of fragments and in fractures with severe angular deformity.

Prereduction X-Rays

DISPLACED FRACTURE OF THE ANATOMIC NECK

1. Fracture of the anatomic neck of the humerus.

2. Displacement has resulted in a varus angulation.

3. Acceptance of this deformity will significantly impair shoulder abduction.

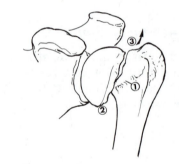

COMMINUTED FRACTURE OF THE SURGICAL NECK

1. Comminuted internal torsional fracture of the surgical neck of the humerus.

2. The head is completely separated from the shaft, and the distal fragment is displaced medially.

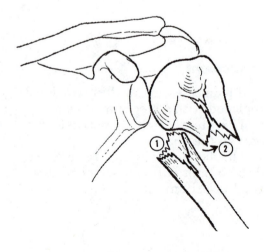

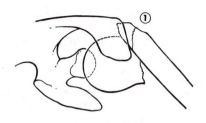

1. A comminuted external torsional fracture. The distal fragment displaces superiorly and laterally.

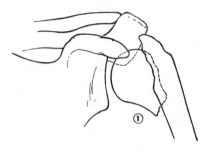

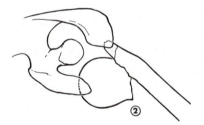

2. These external torsional fractures should be evaluated carefully with axillary views to determine whether the head fragment has dislocated anteriorly.

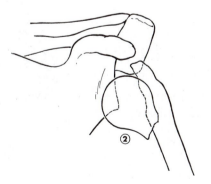

MANIPULATIVE REDUCTION

Complete muscle relaxation is essential. This is best attained by general anesthesia.

1. With the patient in a recumbent position, the operator makes steady traction on the arm in line with the long axis of the body.

2. While traction is maintained, the arm is adducted across the anterior surface of the thorax and is flexed in relation to the frontal plane of the body. This restores the length of the humerus.

3. Operator then places the other hand in the axilla, and while firm pressure is made on the head fragment with the thumb, the shaft fragment is pushed outward.

4. After the fragments are aligned, traction is released, gradually engaging the fragments.

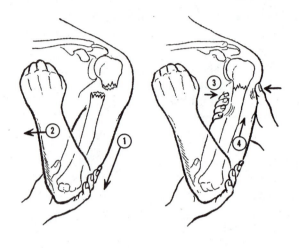

Postreduction Immobilization

Apply collar and cuff.

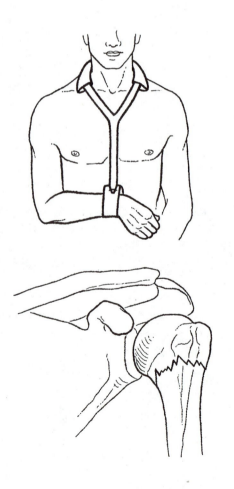

Postreduction X-Rays

ANATOMIC NECK FRACTURE

The fragments are engaged and in near normal alignment.

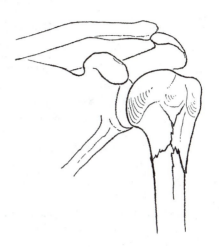

SURGICAL NECK FRACTURE

The fragments are engaged and in near anatomic alignment.

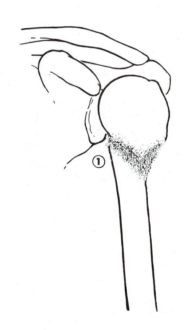

1. Perfect anatomic reduction is not essential for fractures of the surgical or anatomic neck, provided that the rotator cuff function is not impaired. Bayonet apposition may be quite satisfactory.

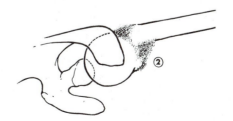

2. Axillary view of a surgical neck fracture healed in bayonet apposition demonstrates excellent functional range of motion without impingement on the acromion.

Postreduction Management

The arm is kept at the side for seven to ten days to permit the pain to subside before motion of the glenohumeral joint is instituted.

Begin pendulum exercises in the stooped position for three to five minutes every waking hour.

Increase the range of motion and the period of exercises progressively as the pain diminishes.

The collar and cuff may be discarded after three weeks and a triangular sling may be worn only during sleeping hours. Begin abduction and external rotation exercises by the end of the third week and concentrate on restoring passive range of motion.

When full range of passive motion is achieved, add active exercises to regain strength.

Restoration of most function should be achieved by twelve weeks, but the patient must persist in active exercises to regain full strength.

Failure to start early active motion exercises after this type of injury leads to long-standing pain and disability from shoulder stiffness.

ALTERNATE METHOD: HANGING CAST TREATMENT

The vast majority of proximal humeral fractures do not require hanging cast immobilization because this may readily distract the fracture.

The hanging cast may occasionally be useful for fractures produced by external rotation mechanism with superior and lateral displacement of the distal fragment.

Avoid prolonged use of a hanging cast, for more than one to two weeks, because it tends to distract this type of fracture.

1. An external torsional type of fracture has occurred with superior and lateral displacement of the distal fragment.

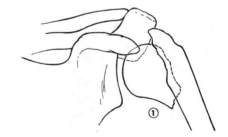

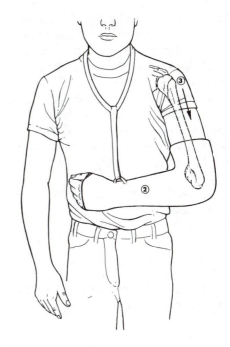

2. Hanging cast treatment is used for two weeks to pull lightly on the upward displacement.

3. The traction aligns the surgical neck fracture in near anatomic position.

Subsequent Management

The cast should be removed within the first two weeks to avoid distracting the fracture. A hand sling would then be sufficient immobilization once the fracture reposition has been achieved.

Encourage the patient to begin early circumduction exercises while in the hanging cast as well as while in the hand sling.

ALTERNATE METHOD: SKELETAL TRACTION

Gentle manipulation and gravity traction from the arm weight are sufficient to reduce and hold most humeral fractures.

Occasionally, if the patient must be kept in bed for reasons other than the fracture, traction may be employed, but as a general rule skeletal traction should be avoided.

1. Traction is made by use of a threaded pin or wire through the base of the olecranon. Drill from the ulnar aspect to the radial side to avoid impaling the ulnar nerve.

2. Begin traction with the arm in a flexed, adducted position to disimpact the fracture, and gradually abduct to no more than 60 degrees so as to align the distal fragments with the proximal fragments.

3. Apply sufficient traction to maintain alignment.

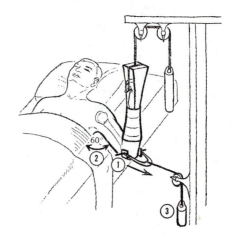

CAUTION

Avoid too much traction. Fracture must not be distracted.

Postreduction Management

After two to three weeks sufficient healing occurs to assure maintenance of reduction without traction.

The fragments now move in unison on internal and external rotation of the arm.

Now take off all apparatus and permit the patient to wear a collar and cuff.

Start motion immediately with pendulum exercises in the stooped position three to five minutes every waking hour.

Increase the range of motion and the period of exercises progressively as the pain decreases.

Discard the collar and cuff after three weeks, and permit wearing of a triangular sling only during sleeping hours.

Add abduction and external rotation exercises, and concentrate on restoring a full passive range of motion.

Encourage free use of the arm at all times within the limits of pain. Restoration of most function should be achieved by ten to twelve weeks, but the patient must persist in active exercises for many months to regain full strength.

ALTERNATE METHOD: OPEN REDUCTION

Operative treatment is indicated principally when the proximal humeral fragment has been fractured into two or more pieces and the rotator cuff attachment has been disrupted (see page 696).

Operative fixation is also necessary for nonunions, which, ironically, are most often produced by previously inadequate internal fixation. Internal fixation should not be used merely because closed reduction of the surgical neck fracture is not anatomic. Fixation in this area is difficult, and the results from operative treatment are usually less satisfactory than with closed methods emphasizing early functional exercise.

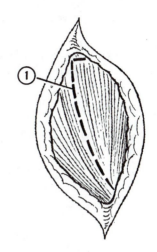

Operative Procedure

1. The fracture is exposed through the anterior deltoid splitting incision.

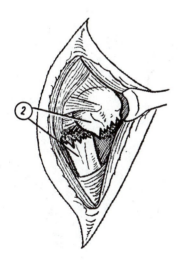

2. The fragments are levered into place and

3. Fixed with an Arbeitsgemeinschaft für Osteosynthesefragen T-shaped plate.* One screw is drilled into each tuberosity.

Note: If open reduction is for nonunion, supplement fixation with autogenous bone graft from the iliac crest.

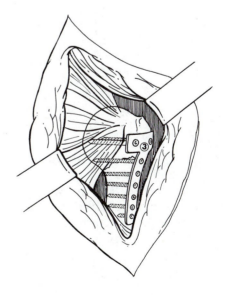

*Available from Synthes Ltd., P. O. Box 529, Wayne, PA 19087.

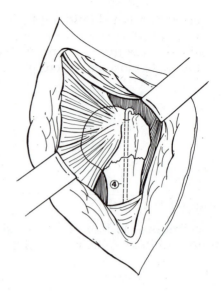

Operative Procedure (Continued)

4. If the humeral head will not hold screws, use an intramedullary Rush pin.

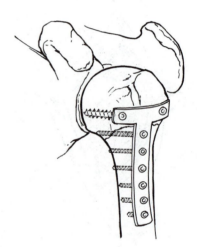

Postreduction X-Rays

The fragments are held by the T-shaped plate fixing the head to the shaft.

The plate need not be removed unless it produces symptoms from impingement.

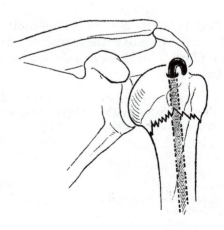

AFTER RUSH PIN FIXATION

Alignment is maintained by Rush intramedullary nail.

The Rush pin usually has to be removed at three to four months because of impingement under the acromion.

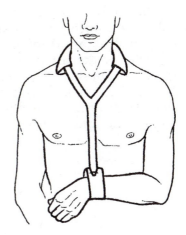

Postoperative Immobilization

Apply a collar and cuff or Velpeau immobilizer.

Postoperative Management

Start motion immediately, at first with pendulum exercises in the stooped position for three to five minutes every waking hour.

Increase the range of motion and the period of exercises progressively as the pain diminishes.

Discard the collar and cuff after three weeks and permit the use of a triangular sling during sleeping hours.

Encourage the free use of the arm at all times within limits of pain.

Add abduction and external rotation exercises by the third week to regain passive range of motion.

When full range of passive motion has been achieved, add active exercises to regain strength.

The Rush pin usually must be removed by the fourth month because of impingement; for this reason the T-shaped plate is preferable.

Fractures of the Anatomic Neck of the Humerus

REMARKS

These fractures are rare injuries in adults and occur because of failure through the old epiphyseal line or the anatomic neck.

They frequently heal in a malunited position and can cause impingement on the undersurface of the acromion during abduction.

The injury is more common in children and is discussed in Chapter 2 (epiphyseal injuries, page 158).

An adult fracture through the anatomic neck is very likely to disrupt blood flow to the articular segment and avascular necrosis follows a large number of these injuries.

Surgical intervention is likely to add to the vascular injury and can be avoided by brief use of the hanging cast to pull the displaced distal fragment into alignment with the head fragment.

Appearance on X-Ray

ANATOMIC NECK FRACTURE IN AN ADULT

1. The fracture line runs through the old epiphyseal line, which is also the point of vascular entry into the humeral head. The distal fragment displaces superiorly and laterally and will impinge on the acromion during shoulder abduction.

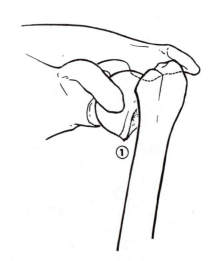

EPIPHYSEAL FRACTURE IN THE CHILD

1. Type II epiphyseal fracture has occurred.

2. There is a triangular fracture of the metaphysis.

3. The shaft fragment of the humerus is displaced upward in relation to the head fragment.

Note: These fractures are reduced by the manipulative techniques described in Chapter 2 (see page 159).

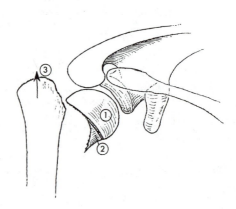

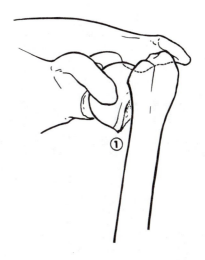

Management of Adult Anatomic Neck Fractures

1. The objective of treatment is to reduce the superior displacement of the distal fragment without further impairing blood supply to the head fragment.

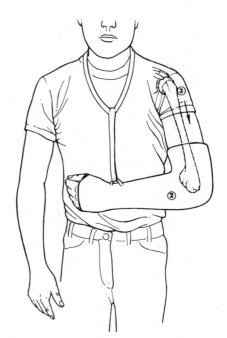

2. A lightweight hanging cast is used to pull the distal fragment inferiorly.

3. Some medial displacement of the distal fragment is acceptable, as it will not impinge on the acromion during shoulder motion.

SUBSEQUENT MANAGEMENT

Remove the hanging cast after seven to ten days to avoid fracture distraction.

Then support the fractured shoulder in a collar and cuff or a hand sling.

Start active shoulder circumduction exercises within the first week and advance to abduction-external rotation exercises by four to six weeks.

Advise the patient that segmental collapse of the humeral head from vascular damage is quite possible. If symptoms become sufficiently painful, prosthetic replacement may be necessary.

FRACTURES OF THE
SHAFT OF THE HUMERUS

REMARKS

Most fractures of the humeral shaft result from direct violence in vehicular accidents, falls, or gunshot wounds. Occasionally, indirect twisting injuries from throwing a ball or arm wrestling will produce the fracture.

Most commonly, this injury affects active adults rather than elderly patients, and typically the injury produces transverse fractures in the midshaft of the humerus.

These fractures typically are caused by bending mechanisms applied to the distal end of the humeral shaft while the proximal end is locked in the glenoid (see page 689).

At one time fractures of the humeral shaft were prime candidates for nonunion, particularly when excessive external immobilization with spica casts or "airplane splints" was used or inadequate internal fixation added to the fracture disease. Elaborate attempts at fracture reduction and external immobilization are unnecessary and sometimes detrimental to healing. The concept of functional muscle control of the fracture, using devices that permit fracture alignment without inhibiting functional muscle activity, has diminished the frequency of nonunion significantly.

Humeral shaft fractures, like femoral shaft fractures, remain surrounded by a richly vascularized envelope of muscle, so fracture reduction is accomplished simply with the aid of gravity and muscle balance. Early muscle function achieved through active muscle contraction and control maximizes the evanescent burst of primary external callus that restores structural strength to the humeral fracture.

Because of the effectiveness of closed treatment, operative intervention is unwarranted, except in the patient with multiple fractures, for the occasional fracture with radial nerve injury, and for the fracture that is clinically nonunited for longer than ten to twelve weeks.

If operative treatment is necessary, fixation must be secure. Compression plate methods offer the best security, particularly for the usual transverse fracture in the midhumerus.

For fractures in the flared distal third of the humerus, crossed intramedullary Rush pins provide good fixation.

The most common complication is radial nerve injury, which occurs in 15 to 20 per cent of humeral fractures. This is most often a benign neurapraxia that recovers spontaneously. Approximately one in five cases does not recover, however.

Permanent nerve damage is most likely to result from open fractures or penetrating injuries. The occasional fracture at the junction of the mid third and distal third of the humerus with varus angulation frequently may entrap the radial nerve and may cause permanent damage if the nerve is not released. A nerve injury under these circumstances or without electromyographic evidence of return by eight to twelve weeks warrants surgical exploration.

Union of the humeral shaft fracture should be clinically evident by ten weeks. If fracture motion is still demonstrable by the end of ten weeks, open reduction and plate fixation should be done promptly. Delaying internal fixation necessitated by nonunion only increases the disuse atrophy of bone and muscle, causing internal fixation to be more difficult and the ultimate functional rehabilitation of the patient to be much less successful.

Open reduction and plate fixation are frequently indicated for the victim of polytrauma. The patient with a forearm or lower limb fracture will recover more readily and completely if the humeral shaft fracture can be stabilized internally.

For the vast majority of humeral shaft fractures, simple closed reduction methods are most appropriate and most likely to succeed. Shortening and angulation of most humeral shaft fractures cause minimal functional or cosmetic problems and are not generally indications for operative intervention.

Fractures with Minimal or No Displacement or Angulation

Appearance on X-Ray

1. Transverse fracture of the shaft with minimal displacement.
2. Slight oblique fracture of the shaft with good contact of bone fragments and minimal angulation.
3. Comminution of the shaft with good alignment and minimal separation of fragments.

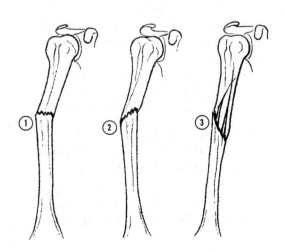

Initial Immobilization

1. Pad axilla.
2. Wrap arm against chest in position that maintains reduction.
3. Support arm with a sling for angulated fractures and encourage active elbow muscle contraction.

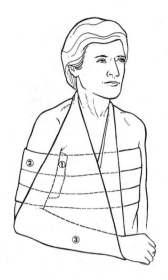

Initial Immobilization for Angulation

1. The assistant makes mild steady downward traction.
2. Apply directly to the skin a long slab of plaster (10 cm wide). The slab extends from the level of the acromion down the lateral aspect of the arm, around the elbow, and up the medial aspect of the arm to the axilla.
3. The slab is maintained in position by a cotton elastic bandage.
4. Place a pad of cotton in the axilla.
5. Place the arm in a triangular sling.

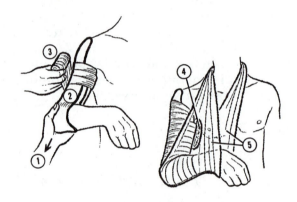

Subsequent Immobilization: Simple Hand Sling (Spak Method)

To maximize the primary healing response after the initial immobilization (three to five days), use a collar and hand sling giving no support to the elbow or forearm on the fracture side.

1. With the elbow flexed at right angles, the patient grips the lower end of the sling.
2. If the patient cannot maintain grip, fix sling to hand with adhesive tape but do not wind sling around hand.
3. Instruct the patient in circumduction shoulder exercises and allow progression to shoulder elevation.

Note: Until strength returns, a temporary support for the limb may be necessary at night using either a pillow or splint.

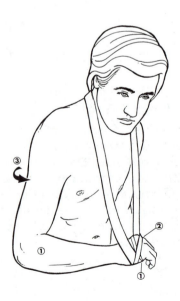

Alternate Method of Immobilization: Functional Cast Sleeve (After Sarmiento)

This may be used as a supplement to the Spak sling method.

1. Plaster cast or prefabricated polypropylene brace extends medially from 2.5 cm below the axilla to about 1 cm above the medial epicondyle, and

2. Extends laterally from below the acromion to just above the lateral epicondyle.

3. Sleeve allows complete range of elbow and shoulder motion.

4. Velcro straps on brace permit removal for cleaning and adjustment as edema subsides.

Note: Sling support is used until patient regains active elbow muscle control.

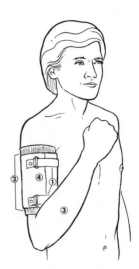

SUBSEQUENT MANAGEMENT

A shoulder harness may be attached to the proximal portion of the cast sleeve and may be looped around the neck to prevent slippage.

Encourage the patient to exercise all joints of the fractured limb actively and passively.

Within the first week after application of the sleeve or hand sling, begin pendulum exercises with the elbow extended. This will frequently correct any residual angulation.

By six to eight weeks the sleeve or sling may be discarded, when there is clinical and radiographic evidence of union.

Fractures with Marked Displacement or Angulation

Appearance on X-Ray

1. Transverse fracture with complete displacement and overriding of fragments.

2. Oblique fracture with serration of bone ends.

3. Comminuted fracture with marked angulation.

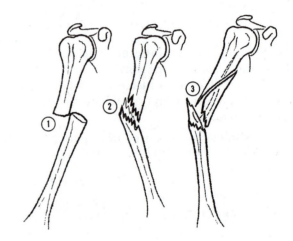

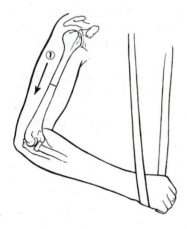

Management

Manipulative reduction is unnecessary if:

1. The weight of the arm and

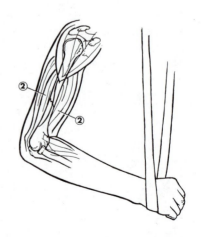

2. The surrounding muscular envelope are permitted to work for instead of against reduction.

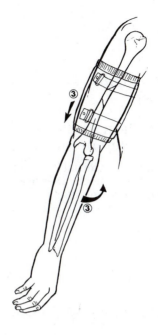

3. Pendulum exercises with elbow in extension will correct any residual deformity.

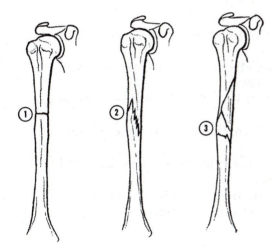

X-Rays One Week After Beginning Active Elbow Extension

1. The fragments are engaged and in acceptable alignment.
2. The serrated ends of the fragments are engaged. Contact is good. Alignment is excellent.
3. Angulation has been corrected. Contact of the fragments is adequate.

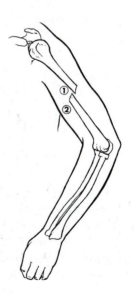

Acceptable Reduction

1. 1 to 2 cm of shortening or
2. Angulation of 5 to 10 degrees will

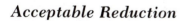

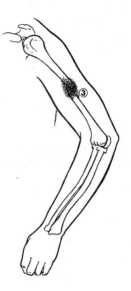

Acceptable Reduction
(Continued)

3. Heal without significant cosmetic or functional impairment.

Note: Healing by external callus is prompt when functional muscle exercises are incorporated into treatment.

Subsequent Management

Encourage the patient to exercise all the joints of the fractured limb actively and passively.

If the patient regains muscle control and elbow extension, the fracture deformity and angulation will frequently correct.

The humeral sleeve or cast may need to be changed or adjusted as swelling subsides.

External support may be discarded when the fracture is clinically united, usually by six to eight weeks.

Have the patient continue to work at achieving full passive range of motion and resisted active exercises.

Recovery of full shoulder and elbow function may take three to five months. Encourage the patient to persist with the exercises.

Torsional-Varus Deformity of Distal Humeral Fractures

Fractures of the distal humerus may be forced into an internal torsional-varus deformity. This results from treatment with methods such as the hanging arm cast which maintains the forearm against the patient's trunk thereby internally rotating the distal fragment.

Techniques which support the limb but encourage elbow motion alleviate the tendency of the distal fragment to rotate internally.

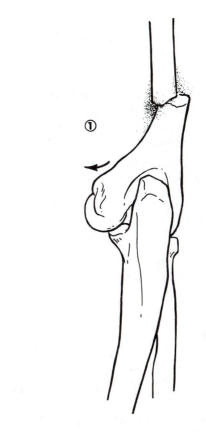

1. Internal torsion results from positioning the forearm continuously against the chest. Tilting of the internally rotated distal fragment produces a varus angulation.

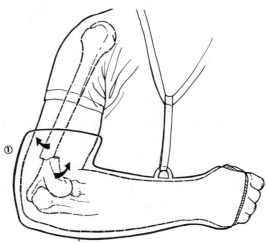

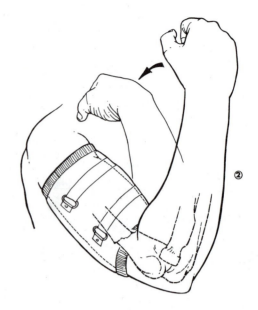

2. If the fracture is treated by allowing active elbow motion, the distal fragment becomes aligned in the axis of elbow joint motion.

Note: Torsional deformities of the distal humerus are not as functionally significant as are torsional deformities of the distal femur. Corrective osteotomy is usually not necessary.

Radial Nerve Involvement in Fractures of the Shaft of the Humerus

REMARKS

Radial nerve injuries occur most frequently in association with mid-shaft fractures. The nerve lesion usually is a benign neurapraxia that recovers spontaneously.

Radial nerve injury associated with a gunshot wound or an open fracture of any kind is least likely to recover spontaneously. Operative exploration of the open fracture and the nerve is warranted.

Occasionally, the radial nerve will be injured by a spiral fracture in the distal third of the humerus with a characteristic radial angulation and overriding of the distal fragment. At this level the nerve penetrates the intermuscular septum and consequently has little mobility. Closed reduction of this type of fracture with nerve involvement may worsen the nerve injury. Open fracture reduction with neurolysis is the safest method of managing combined injuries at this level.

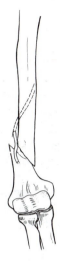

Since 15% to 20% of humeral shaft fractures will involve the radial nerve, always check for nerve injury before and after treatment, and record the findings.

The clinical features of radial palsy are:
1. Wrist drop.
2. Loss of supination of forearm,
3. Loss of extension of the fingers and thumb, and
4. Sensory deficits on dorsum of forearm, hand, and thumb.

The majority of radial nerve injuries from humeral fractures recover spontaneously, but approximately one in five does not recover.

In most instances the period of observation for spontaneous recovery should be at least 12 weeks, which allows time for fracture consolidation. If there is no clinical or electromyographic indication of nerve regeneration by that time, neurolysis is indicated.

Fractures of the Shaft of the Humerus in Polytrauma

REMARKS

Displaced humeral shaft fractures frequently occur in victims of polytrauma, including cerebral concussion, hemothorax, abdominal injuries, or multiple fractures, which prevent mobilization of the victim.

Temporary skeletal traction may be necessary to align the fracture while the patient is in bed, but fracture distraction must be avoided. Traction should be discontinued as soon as the patient can be mobilized. Humeral fractures associated with arterial injuries may also be safely immobilized after arterial repair by means of light skeletal traction.

A simple hand sling support or a humeral cuff may then be employed until the fracture heals.

Humeral shaft fractures, when combined with major fractures in other long bones such as the forearm, femur, or tibia, frequently require plate fixation to permit prompt patient mobilization and rehabilitation.

Humeral fractures in severely confused, agitated or psychotic patients may require early internal fixation to prevent inadvertent penetration of the fracture ends through the skin.

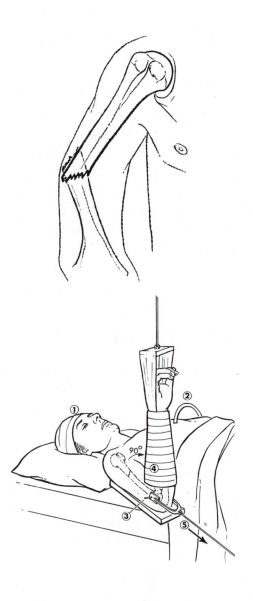

Prereduction X-Ray

Oblique fracture of the humerus with angulation and overriding in a patient who suffered a hemothorax and cerebral concussion.

Temporary Immobilization in Skeletal Traction

1. While the patient recovers from his head injury,

2. And as long as the chest tubes are in place, preventing immobilization of the arm against the chest,

3. A threaded Kirschner wire is used for traction and is inserted through the upper end of the ulna.

4. The forearm is suspended with the elbow flexed 90 degrees.

5. Traction is made in line with the humerus and with the arm in slight abduction.

CAUTION

Start with 5 lb (2.3 kg) of weight and take a check x-ray within 24 hours. Adjust the amount of weight so that the alignment is maintained but the fragments are not distracted.

Secondary Immobilization

As soon as the head and chest injuries allow the patient to be mobilized, remove all the traction apparatus and apply a humeral sleeve cast or brace.

1. Plaster cast or prefabricated polypropylene brace extends medially from 2.5 cm below the axilla to slightly above the medial epicondyle, and

2. Extends laterally from below the acromion to just above the lateral epicondyle.

3. Sleeve allows complete range of elbow and shoulder motion.

4. Velcro straps on brace permit removal for cleaning and adjustment as the edema subsides.

Note: A sling support is used until the patient regains active elbow muscle control.

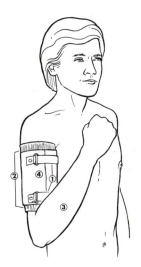

Subsequent Management

Encourage the patient to exercise all joints of the fractured limb actively and passively.

Within the first week after application of the sleeve, begin pendulum exercises with the elbow in extension. This will frequently correct any residual angulation.

By six to eight weeks, the external support may be discarded, when there is clinical and radiographic evidence of union.

Postreduction X-Ray

1. The fragments are satisfactorily reduced and have not been distracted.

2. Union has occurred by primary external callus evident at six weeks.

Note: Healing by external callus occurs promptly when functional muscle exercises are incorporated into treatment.

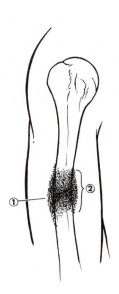

FRACTURES OF THE SHAFT OF THE HUMERUS ASSOCIATED WITH MULTIPLE LONG BONE FRACTURES

REMARKS

This is one of the few exceptions to the generally effective rule regarding closed treatment for most humeral shaft fractures. Internal fixation of the humeral shaft fracture in a patient with multiple long bone fractures permits prompt mobilization and functional restoration.

Open reduction and internal fixation of upper limb fractures may be combined with closed or open treatment of long bone fractures in the lower limb.

Preoperative X-Rays

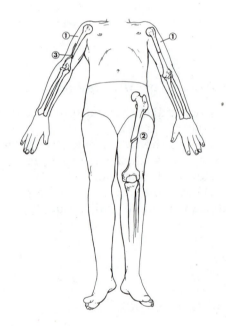

1. Bilateral humeral shaft fractures combined with

2. Fracture of the left femoral shaft.

3. The angulated fracture of the distal third of the humerus caused radial nerve paralysis.

Note: Open reduction and internal fixation of both humeral fractures permit mobilization of the patient in a cast brace for femoral fracture within four weeks after injury.

The fracture of the midshaft of the humerus is treated by plate fixation. The angulated distal third fracture is immobilized with intramedullary Rush pin and cerclage wiring after decompression of the radial nerve.

730

OPERATIVE FIXATION

Fracture of the Middle Third of Humerus

INCISION AND EXPOSURE

1. Use an anterolateral incision (after Henry), running lateral to the biceps and cephalic vein.

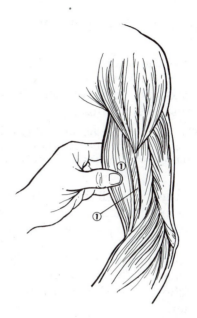

2. The brachialis is split, and wide exposure is possible with the elbow flexed.

3. The fracture is exposed with minimal periosteal stripping.

4. Radial nerve is one fingerbreadth below the deltoid eminence.

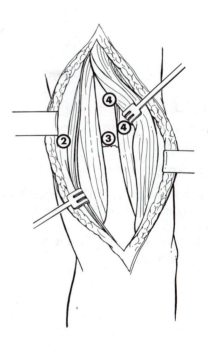

Fracture of the Middle Third of Humerus (Continued)

FIXATION OF TRANSVERSE MIDSHAFT FRACTURE

1. Identify the fracture and after removing any interposed soft tissue apply a six-hole compression plate. Avoid periosteal stripping.

Note: The plate should be applied to the lateral or posterior surface depending on which is the convex surface of the fracture.

2. Bend the plate slightly if necessary before application to prevent any malalignment once compression is applied.

3. Arbeitsgemenschaft für Osteosynthesefragen compression technique is followed precisely to achieve rigid fixation.*

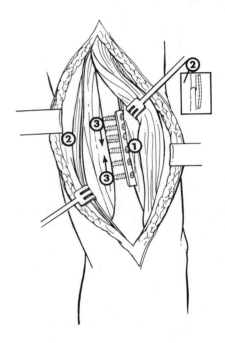

Fracture of Distal Third of Humerus with Radial Nerve Involvement

INCISION AND EXPOSURE

1. Henry's anterolateral approach is used to expose the radial nerve proximal and

2. To follow it to the fracture site, where it is entrapped.

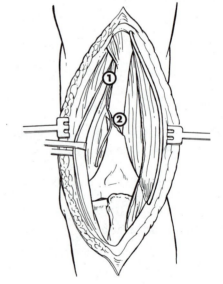

---

*Equipment available from Synthes Ltd., P.O. 529, Wayne, PA 19087.

REDUCTION

1. Angulated fracture is reduced while the nerve is protected.

2. Two Rush pins are passed simultaneously through both condyles and across the fracture site, with the sled runner striking the opposite cortex.

3. Bending the pins slightly helps them conform to the contour of the lower humerus.

4. Cerclage wires may be added for additional support. Radial nerve is completely free of fracture.

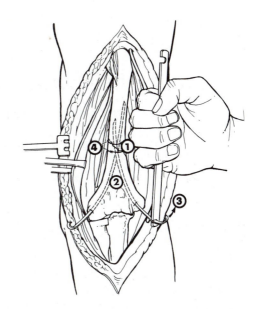

POSTOPERATIVE IMMOBILIZATION

Use arm immobilizer for three to five days after operation, until swelling subsides.

Encourage active range of motion to the shoulder, elbow, and hand within the first postoperative day.

When the patient has active control of elbow motion, encourage full extension.

When triceps strength has returned, crutch walking may be started to aid in the management of the fractured femur.

The fractured femur is treated in this patient by closed reduction and cast-brace application.

Fixation of the humeral fracture allows the patient to become ambulatory within the first month after injury.

Delayed Union or Nonunion of Fractures of the Shaft of the Humerus

REMARKS

Humeral fracture union should be evident after eight to ten weeks of closed treatment, provided that the patient has carried out the functional exercises as described.

If for some reason the patient has been inhibited from using the arm and fracture motion is still evident ten weeks after injury, internal fixation should be employed.

To delay for five to six months in deciding about inevitable operative treatment only increases the difficulty of fixation and diminishes the amount of function returned.

A compression plate or neutralization plate with screws is the most effective method of fixing the humeral fracture for nonunion.

Nonunions with bone defects should also be treated by cancellous grafting.

The plate is applied to the convex side of the angulated nonunion. Frequently, this requires placement on the posterior cortex.

1. Nonunion of a transverse mid-shaft fracture at four months.

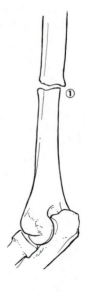

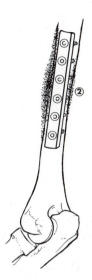

2. Union after compression plating and cancellous graft.

1. Nonunion of a spiral oblique fracture at four months.

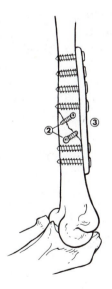

2. Union after lag screws and
3. Neutralization plate applied posteriorly on convex surface.

Fracture of the Supracondyloid Process

REMARKS

This is a rare lesion, but because of the proximity of the median nerve, symptoms of median nerve neuritis may obscure the lesion.

The supracondyloid process is a bony prominence of varying size situated on the anteromedial aspect of the humerus 5 to 7 cm above the medial epicondyle. Between this process and the medial epicondyle stretches a fibrous band from which a portion of the pronator teres muscle arises.

Through the interval between the humerus and the fibrous band pass the brachial artery and the median nerve.

Fracture of the supracondyloid process causes locking and pain and may cause irritation of the median nerve. Fracture is usually the result of direct trauma.

Treatment of fracture is by excision of the fragment.

1. Supracondyloid process.
2. Fibrous band.
3. Brachial artery and median nerve.

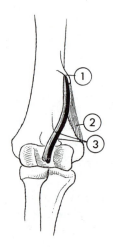

SUMMARY: COMPLICATIONS AND PITFALLS OF FRACTURES OF THE HUMERUS

The major complications from proximal humeral fractures are due to their effects on surrounding soft tissue.

The common fractures of the surgical neck that are produced by indirect torsional mechanisms usually heal promptly. It is the disrupted rotator cuff or the stiffened shoulder capsule that frequently requires a prolonged time for recovery.

The first pitfall to avoid in managing these injuries is that of incomplete assessment. Always consider the likelihood of rotator cuff disruption or, occasionally, a complete humeral head dislocation in association with a proximal humeral fracture.

The vast majority of surgical neck fractures are not associated with significant complications and can be treated with a program emphasizing functional exercise and deemphasizing radiographic appearance. Avoid the pitfall of treating on the basis of radiographic evidence and immobilizing the shoulder unnecessarily, which superimposes capsular contracture and shoulder stiffness on the healing process.

The tendency to treat fractures of the humeral shaft by attempted rigid external immobilization has been a major pitfall in the past. Devices such as airplane splints, which immobilize muscles more than fracture fragments, have contributed significantly to a high nonunion rate. Recognition that these fractures will heal despite less than rigid fixation has been of fundamental importance in diminishing the occurrence of nonunion significantly.

Devices such as simple hand slings or arm splints encourage functional use of muscles surrounding the fracture. This muscle function promotes fracture alignment and prompt healing by the process of external callus formation.

If one uses closed methods and functional treatment, operative intervention is rarely needed for humeral shaft fractures. When internal fixation is chosen, it should be for specific objectives and functional purposes rather than for subjective or esthetic interpretation of radiographic appearances. Internal fixation of a humeral fracture should be done only when the surgeon can achieve the goal of rigid fracture immobilization without risking the pitfall of infected nonunion.

REFERENCES

Henry, A. K.: Extensile Exposure. 2nd edition. Baltimore, Williams & Wilkins, 1962, pp. 15–38.

Holstein, A., and Lewis, G. B.: Fractures of the humerus with radial-nerve paralysis. J. Bone and Joint Surg. 45–A:1382, 1963.

Horak, J., and Nilsson, B. E.: Epidemiology of fracture of the upper end of the humerus. Clin. Orthop. 112:250, 1975.

Loomer, R., and Kokan, P.: Non-union in fractures of the humeral shaft. Injury, 7:274, 1976.

Mast, J. W., Spiegel, P. G., Harvey, J. P., et al.: Fractures of the humeral shaft. Clin. Orthop. 112:254, 1975.

McKibbon, B.: The biology of fracture healing in long bones. J. Bone and Joint Surg. 60–B:150, 1978.

Muller, M. E., Allgower, M., and Willenegger, H.: Manual of Internal Fixation. Heidelberg, Springer-Verlag, 1970.

Neer, C. S.; Displaced proximal humeral fractures. J. Bone and Joint Surg. 52–A:250, 1975.

Rush, L. V.: Atlas of Rush Pin Technics. Meridan, Miss., The Berivon Company, 1955, pp. 178–193.

Sever, J. W.: Nonunion in fracture of the shaft of the humerus. J.A.M.A. Vol. 104, no. 5, 382, 1935.

Sarmiento, A., Kinman, P. B., Galvin, E. G., et al.: Functional bracing of fractures of the shaft of the humerus. J. Bone and Joint Surg. 59–A:596, 1977.

Spak, I.: Humeral shaft fractures. Acta Orthop Scand. 49:234, 1978.

Weber, B. G., and Cech, O., eds.: Pseudoarthrosis: Pathophysiology, Biomechanics, Therapy, and Results. New York, Grune & Stratton, 1976, pp. 108–119.

Yamada, H.: Strength of Biological Materials, edited by F. G. Evans. Huntington, N.Y. Robert E. Krieger Publishing Co., 1973, pp. 1–73.

FRACTURES AND DISLOCATIONS IN THE REGION OF THE ELBOW

FRACTURES OF THE LOWER END OF THE HUMERUS

REMARKS

Fractures in this region are caused most often by an indirect injury to the elbow resulting from a fall on the outstretched, extended arm.

In Children. The vast majority of distal humeral fractures occur in children and are classified as supracondylar fractures.

Ninety-five per cent of these fractures are displaced posteriorly, but occasionally a flexion moment will displace the distal fragment and elbow anteriorly.

In addition to anterior or posterior displacement, the distal fragment may be tilted medially (varus) or laterally (valgus). Analysis of the initial displacement helps to determine the position needed for immobilization after reduction.

The most deceptive fracture and the second in frequency is a lateral condylar fracture in a child (see page 771). Because of the pull of attached muscles, even slight displacement is likely to result in non-union and growth deformity of the elbow. Open reduction and internal fixation are indicated more often and with greater validity for this fracture than for any other fracture in children.

Occasionally, injuries to a child's distal humerus will produce a type I or type II epiphyseal separation (see page 150). This rare injury, which can be treated readily by closed methods, must be distinguished from the lateral condylar fracture, which is a type IV epiphyseal fracture and usually requires internal fixation to insure proper healing.

A major cause of confusion about humeral fractures in children is the irregular development of ossification centers about the elbow.

In case of doubt in the differential diagnosis of a fracture line vs. an epiphyseal line on a radiograph, compare with a radiograph of the other elbow.

Frequently, the only initial radiographic evidence of a fracture is the "fat pad sign," the radiolucent line produced when fracture hematoma elevates the fat pad in the olecranon fossa.

Even without definite radiographic signs, if a young patient has pain localized to the elbow after injury, the limb should be protected with a splint until subsequent x-rays confirm or rule out the possibility of fracture.

The third most common distal humeral injury in children results from an abduction force on the elbow that produces tension on the flexor group of muscles and avulses the medial epicondyle. This injury is often associated with a dislocation of the elbow, which may cause the epicondylar fragment to be trapped within the joint. Most of these fractures are relatively undisplaced. Wide displacement to the level of the joint should prompt suspicion of either entrapment in the joint or complete fracture of the unossified medial condyle, either of which would require open reduction.

Oblique fractures of the medial condyle are the least common elbow fracture in children, but occasionally they may result from avulsion pull of the flexor origin when a valgus strain is applied to the elbow. These avulsion injuries are frequently unstable and carry a definite risk of nonunion unless stabilized with internal fixation.

A recently recognized, but frequently perplexing fracture of the lower end of the humerus is the "little leaguer's elbow." This is most commonly seen in the adolescent baseball pitcher who traumatizes the immature epiphyses by repetitive throwing and avulses the medial epicondyle or compresses and fractures the subchondral bone of the lateral condyle or radial head.

In Adults. Distal humeral fractures in adults are produced most frequently by direct violence, e.g., sideswipe injury to the elbow resting on a car window. The result is an intercondylar T-shaped fracture, in which the articular surface may be extremely comminuted. The prognosis for this type of fracture in adults is poorer than in children, at least in terms of restoration of function.

Reduction in traction and early range-of-motion exercises are the most effective treatment techniques for intercondylar T fractures in the adult.

Fractures of the capitellum usually occur in adults when the radial head is thrust upward against the condyle, shearing off its articular surface. Operative excision of the loose fragments is the treatment of choice for these injuries.

APPEARANCE OF INDIVIDUAL OSSIFICATION CENTERS ABOUT THE ELBOW

1. The secondary ossification center for the capitellum appears earliest and should be ossified by two years.

2. The radial ossification center is evident by six years.

3. The internal or medial epicondyle is evident by seven years.

4. The trochlea ossification center appears at ten years.

5. The lateral or external epicondyle is seen at eleven years.

Note: When in doubt about the difference between normal epiphyseal line and a fracture line, compare with an x-ray of the opposite, uninjured elbow, and look for elevation of fat pads indicating fracture hemorrhage.

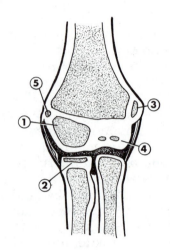

TYPES OF FRACTURES OF THE LOWER END OF THE HUMERUS

Undisplaced Fracture

Undisplaced fractures may frequently be manifested only by a fat pad sign caused by posterior hemorrhage.

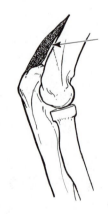

742

Extension Type of Fracture

The distal fragment is displaced upward and backward in 95 per cent of supracondylar fractures.

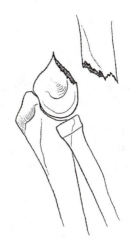

Flexion Type of Fracture

The distal fragment is displaced forward in about 5 per cent of supracondylar fractures as the result of a flexor moment about the elbow.

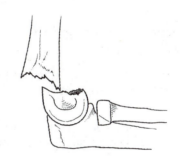

Supracondylar Fractures with Displacement

Supracondylar fracture with posterior and medial displacement causing varus tilt and cubitus varus deformity. This is the commonest type of fracture deformity.

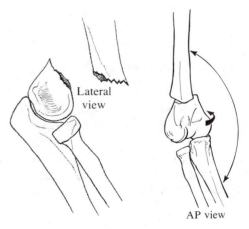

Lateral view

AP view

743

Supracondylar Fractures with Displacement (Continued)

Supracondylar fracture with posterior and lateral displacement causing valgus tilt and cubitus valgus deformity.

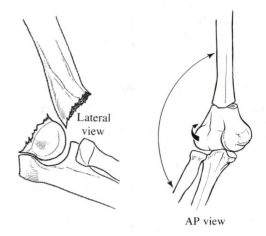

Lateral view

AP view

Lateral Condylar and Distal Epiphyseal Fractures

Lateral condylar fracture with capitellum avulsed by pull of extensor muscles.

Note: Radial head no longer articulates with capitellum. This is a type IV epiphyseal fracture.

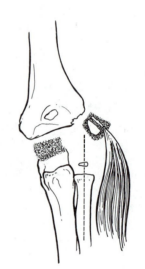

Epiphyseal Fracture of the Lower Humerus

Unlike avulsion of the capitellum in lateral condylar fracture, the articulation of the capitellum with the radius is retained. This is a type I epiphyseal fracture, and treatment is the same as for supracondylar fracture.

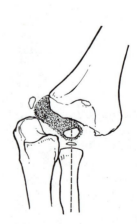

744

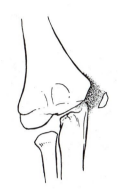

Medial Epicondylar and Condylar Fractures

Medial epicondylar fracture may rarely include the trochlea or medial condyle.

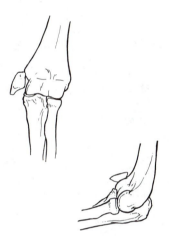

Fracture of the medial condyle with displacement and anteromedial rotation.

OTHER FRACTURES OF THE DISTAL HUMERUS IN ADOLESCENTS AND ADULTS

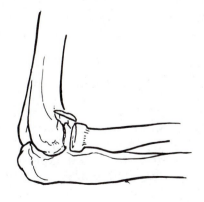

Shear Fracture of Capitellum in Adult

745

Intercondylar Fractures in Adults

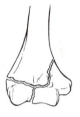
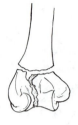
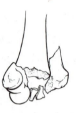

Little Leaguer's Elbow

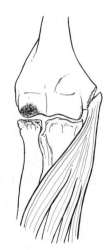

Complications of Fractures of the Lower End of the Humerus

Fractures about the elbow carry more than their share of complications, both early and late.

Treat these injuries with due caution.

Early Complications

Nerve injuries. Elbow fractures may produce neurapraxia of the median, ulnar, or radial nerves, most of which are temporary.

Vascular injuries. Extensive antecubital swelling may eventually produce ischemic contracture of the forearm muscles and ischemic neuropathy. This can be a permanent and severe complication.

Late Complications

Nonunion. This is especially likely with lateral or medial condylar fractures with any displacement.

Malunion or changes in the carrying angle are most commonly associated with supracondylar fractures.

Loss of elbow motion. Loss of flexion is more serious and disabling than loss of extension.

Myositis ossificans. Soft tissue calcification may follow overvigorous passive stretching to regain motion after injury.

Progressive ulnar nerve palsy. This results from a cubitus valgus deformity after a lateral condylar fracture.

Instability of the elbow. This may occur with overvigorous surgical treatment or with nonunion of condylar fractures.

Supracondylar Fractures

REMARKS

This fracture is most common in children less than eleven years of age and affects boys three times more often than girls.

Posterior displacement (extension type) occurs in 95 per cent of injuries and anterior displacement (flexion type) occurs in 5 per cent.

About one third of supracondylar fractures have little or no displacement and offer no difficulty in reduction and treatment. The rest are associated with varying degrees of displacement and require considerable thought and effort to treat adequately.

A few undisplaced supracondylar fractures may have no definitive radiographic signs of injury other than an elevated posterior fat pad from fracture hematoma. These fractures are treated symptomatically with splint support.

Achievement of fracture union is no problem in supracondylar fractures. The major objective in treating these injuries is to prevent complications, particularly from vascular injury or loss of carrying angle.

The most serious complication is Volkmann's ischemic contracture.

Ten per cent of children lose the distal radial pulse temporarily after supracondylar fractures because of extensive antecubital swelling. This circulatory impairment is rarely due to direct injury to the brachial artery. Reducing the fracture, avoiding elbow flexion greater than a right angle, and elevating the swollen limb in traction will eliminate obstruction to venous return and will prevent secondary obstruction of arterial inflow.

747

Rarely, if fracture reduction worsens the vascular impairment, the brachial artery may actually be entrapped by the fracture fragments, requiring open reduction.

Although temporary loss of a radial pulse is common, failure to correct impending Volkmann's ischemia will have dire consequences (see page 826). Refusal to actively extend the fingers and a complaint of forearm pain with passive extension of the fingers are the most reliable signs of impending Volkmann's ischemia.

The most common complication (occurring in up to 60 per cent of cases) of supracondylar fracture is loss of carrying angle, cubitus varus (or gunstock) deformity. The opposite complication of increased carrying angle, or cubitus valgus, may also occur but is much less of a cosmetic deformity.

Treatment of supracondylar fractures is made difficult by overdependence on radiographic interpretation of the reduction. Postreduction x-rays of a flexed elbow are useless in determining the carrying angle. Analysis of the mechanics of initial fracture displacement and attention to the details of forearm positioning after reduction are essential to correct cubitus varus or cubitus valgus deformity.

Medially displaced supracondylar fractures are most prone to tilt into cubitus varus and should be immobilized with the forearm pronated to tighten the brachioradialis and common extensor muscles and to close the fracture laterally. The less common laterally displaced fracture should be immobilized with the forearm supinated to close the fracture medially and to prevent increased cubitus valgus.

Persistent posterior displacement after reduction will be remodeled by normal flexion-extension motion of the elbow, but persistent tilt causing cubitus varus deformity may require corrective osteotomy.

NORMAL CARRYING ANGLE

Clinical Appearance

The angle is readily discerned when:

1. The shoulder is rotated externally,

2. The elbow is extended, and

3. The forearm is supinated.

4. Line is from center of humeral head to center of elbow joint to center of wrist.

Note: Flexion of the elbow prevents adequate measurement of this angle.

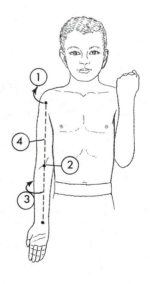

Appearance on X-ray

1. Line parallels the long axis of the humerus.

2. Line parallels long axis of the ulna.

3. Angle formed is the "carrying" or cubitus angle.

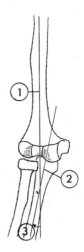

Variations of Normal Carrying Angle (Smith)

Girls: Range 0 to 12 degrees (average 6.1 degrees).

Boys: Range 0 to 11 degrees (average 5.4 degrees).

Nine per cent of normal children have no carrying angle (cubitus rectus).

Forty-eight per cent of normal children have a carrying angle of 5 degrees or less.

Typical Varus Deformity

1. Clinical appearance.

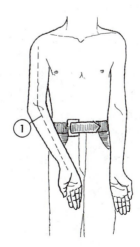

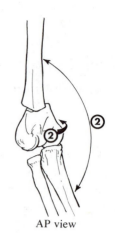

Typical Varus Deformity (Continued)

2. Radiographic appearance of varus deformity with a medially displaced fracture and tilt of the distal fragment.

AP view

TYPES OF SUPRACONDYLAR FRACTURES

TYPICAL DEFORMITY OF SUPRACONDYLAR FRACTURE

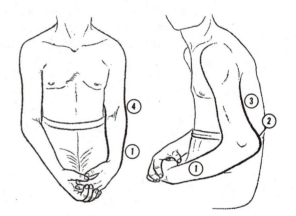

Without Lateral Displacement or Angulation

1. The forearm appears shortened.
2. The end of the elbow is unduly prominent.
3. A concavity is formed in the region of the triceps tendon.
4. In the front view no medial or lateral displacement exists.

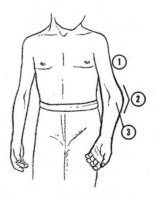

With Medial Displacement of the Distal Fragment – Leading to Varus Deformity

1. The arm appears shortened.
2. The normal carrying angle of the elbow is reversed (cubitus varus).
3. The end of the elbow is unduly prominent.

MECHANISM OF FRACTURE WITH POSTERIOR DISPLACEMENT

Typically the mechanism is a fall on the outstretched hand with

1. The elbow hyperextended and the forearm supinating or

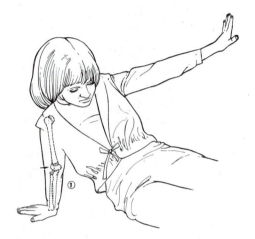

2. The elbow hyperextended and the forearm pronating.

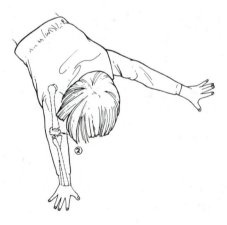

1. Hyperextension of the elbow results in posterior displacement of the distal supracondylar fracture fragment.

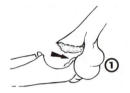

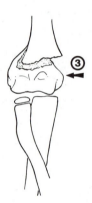

2. Forced supination causes medial displacement of the distal fragment.

3. Forced pronation results in lateral displacement of the distal fragment.

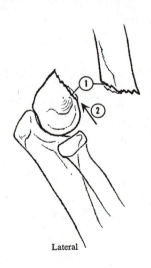

PREREDUCTION X-RAYS OF SUPRACONDYLAR FRACTURE

With Medial Tilt Leading to Cubitus Varus Deformity

LATERAL VIEW

1. The distal fragment is widely separated from the shaft of the humerus.

2. The distal fragment is displaced upward and backward.

Lateral

ANTEROPOSTERIOR VIEW

3. The distal fragment is displaced medially and

4. The distal fragment is tilted inward (cubitus varus).

Note: This is the most common deformity and should be immobilized with the forearm pronated.

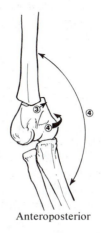

Anteroposterior

With Lateral Tilt — Leading to Cubitus Valgus Deformity

ANTEROPOSTERIOR VIEW

1. The fracture line is transverse and the distal fragment is displaced laterally.

2. The lateral displacement causes valgus tilt.

3. The result is an increased carrying angle.

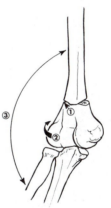

AP view

LATERAL VIEW

4. The distal fragment is displaced up and back.

Note: The key factor in reduction is to correct the medial or lateral tilt so as to prevent alteration of the carrying angle. Some residual anterior or posterior displacement may be accepted, because elbow motion will remodel displacement in this plane.

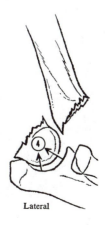

Lateral

753

EPIPHYSEAL SEPARATION OF THE LOWER END OF THE HUMERUS

REMARKS

The peak incidence for this injury occurs in the age group of newborn to 2.5 years.

The diagnosis may be difficult when it occurs in infants and young children with no or small ossification centers.

Child abuse (someone twisting the child's arm) may be the etiology in about one-third of cases.

Another mechanism is a fall from a height onto an outstretched and supinated arm causing posterior and medial displacement of the epiphysis.

Three groups of injuries have been identified by DeLee and coworkers, all of which are either Type I or Type II epiphyseal injuries.

Group A (Newborn to Nine Months Old)

1. The elbow is displaced postero-medially.

2. There is no ossification center in the capitellum or no Thurston-Holland fracture fragment from the metaphysis.

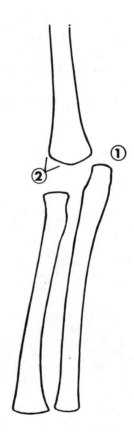

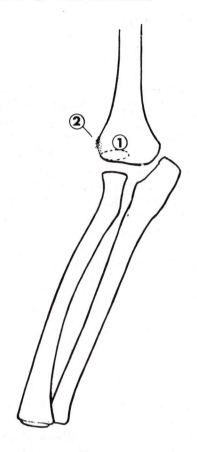

Group B (Seven Months to Three Years Old)

1. The ossification center has developed in the capitellum and is displaced with the radius and ulna.

2. There may or may not be a small metaphyseal fragment.

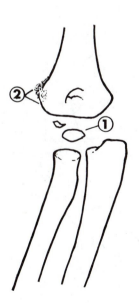

Group C (Three to Seven Years Old)

1. The ossification center is well developed in the capitellum and displaced with the radius.

2 There is a large Thurston-Holland fragment fractured off the metaphysis.

DIAGNOSIS

Clinically the elbow is swollen markedly and appears dislocated. The major problem in the diagnosis of this injury is due to the fact that the cartilaginous ossification centers may not be present. A knowledge of when ossification centers develop is essential (see page 742).

Comparative x-rays should be taken of both elbows, but in the very young infant the diagnosis may be based entirely on clinical examination.

The key to interpretation of the injury is disruption of the normal relationship between the proximal radius and the capitellum. If a line drawn through the proximal radius passes through the capitellum, the elbow may be normal or there may have been either a supracondylar fracture or an epiphyseal separation.

If the line drawn through the radius on x-ray does not pass through the capitellum, then either the elbow is dislocated or a fracture of the lateral condyle has occurred.

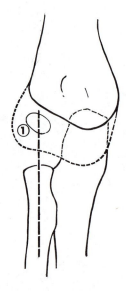

Normal Elbow

1. In a normal infant's elbow the line through the long axis of the radius must pass through the capitellum regardless of the position of the elbow.

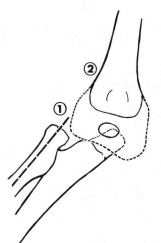

Elbow Dislocation

1. With the elbow dislocated, the axis of the proximal radius passes laterally or rarely medially to the capitellum.

2. There is no Thurston-Holland sign or metaphyseal fracture fragment evident.

Lateral Condylar Fracture

1. The capitellar fragment is fractured and is displaced laterally to the axis of the radius.

Note: Epiphyseal separations are most commonly mistaken for this injury and frequently undergo unnecessary operative intervention unless the difference between the Type I or II epiphyseal injury and this Type IV epiphyseal injury is kept in mind.

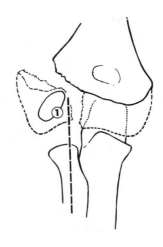

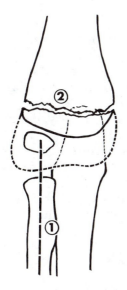

Supracondylar Fractures

1. The radiocapitellar line is maintained.
2. The fracture line is usually evident above the physis.

Epiphyseal Separation

1. There is maintenance of the normal radiocapitellar alignment on both the anteroposterior and lateral x-rays.

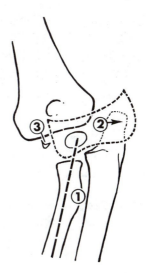

757

Epiphyseal Separation
(Continued)

2. Consistently, the epiphysis and capitellum are displaced medially and posteriorly.

3. There is usually a fracture fragment from the metaphysis, i.e., the Thurston-Holland sign.

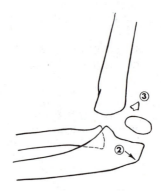

MANAGEMENT

Closed reduction is the treatment of choice for these epiphyseal Type I and II injuries. Open reduction is not indicated.

If the elbow is markedly swollen, it is best elevated and managed in Dunlap's traction (see page 767).

For fresh fractures, gentle reduction and correction of the immediate displacement are all that is necessary. The fracture then is reduced and managed essentially the same as supracondylar fractures. The child should be hospitalized for at least one to two days to monitor circulation closely.

If the child is not seen until two to three weeks after injury, callus is present and no attempts should be made at correction.

Cubitus varus deformity may occur but it is less common after these injuries than after a supracondylar fracture, particularly if the injury is immobilized in pronation.

Immobilization should be no longer than three weeks, since some measurable loss of motion is found with prolonged immobilization.

MANAGEMENT OF EXTENSION FRACTURES — SUPRACONDYLAR AND TRANSCONDYLAR FRACTURES — AND OF EPIPHYSEAL SEPARATIONS OF THE LOWER END OF THE HUMERUS

REMARKS

Before reduction is attempted, always check for:

1. Radial pulse — if absent, determine if circulation to hand is adequate.

2. Status of soft tissues of elbow, forearm, and hand.

3. Motor and sensory deficits of the radial, median, and ulnar nerves.

4. Signs of forearm muscle ischemia, such as pain on passive finger extension.

Fractures with little or no displacement are readily treated by the method of manipulative reduction discussed in this section.

Fractures with wide displacement should be subjected to one attempt at manipulative reduction. If it fails, use an alternate method such as lateral traction or overhead traction, also discussed in this section.

MANIPULATIVE REDUCTION

Although minimally displaced fractures may be reduced without using an anesthetic, general anesthesia is preferable for most fractures with displacement.

1. The assistant fixes the arm of the patient.

2. With one hand, grasp the patient's wrist and make steady firm traction in the line of the long axis of the limb with the forearm in the neutral position.

3. While traction is maintained, correct any lateral displacement with the other hand. If the distal fragment is displaced laterally it is pushed inward; if it is displaced medially it is pushed outward.

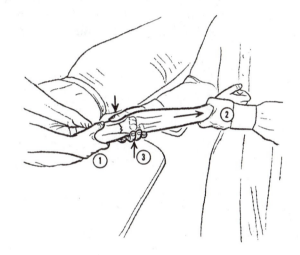

1. After the length is restored and the angular deformity is corrected, maintain traction with one hand.

2. Place the thumb of the other hand over the anterior surface of the end of the proximal fragment and the fingers behind the distal fragment.

3. While traction is maintained,

4. The elbow is flexed beyond a right angle.

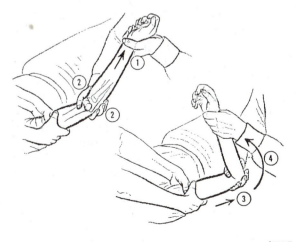

Postreduction Checks

The optimum position of flexion is 10 degrees beyond a right angle.

If this position obliterates the pulse, decrease the flexion until a full bounding pulse returns.

Check the position of the fragments by x-ray; this may or may not give any reliable information.

Check for medial angulation of the distal fragment.

Outline the bony prominences, medial epicondyle, the olecranon and the lateral epicondyle, on the normal side with the elbow flexed the same amount as on the affected side. They form an almost symmetrical equilateral triangle and are aligned with the long axis of the humerus.

Outline the bony prominences on the affected side, compare the two sides, and determine if there is any medial angulation or tilt of the distal fragment from the long axis of the humerus. Typically, the olecranon moves medially with cubitus varus.

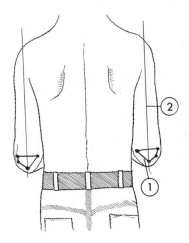

The angular deformity is corrected if:

1. The ends of the elbows are symmetrical and

2. The bony prominences are normally aligned with the long axis of the humerus.

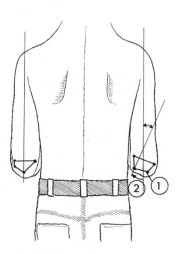

Now proceed with immobilization of the fracture.

An angular deformity still exists if:

1. The ends of the elbows are asymmetrical and

2. The distal fragment (the bony prominences) tilts medially from the long axis of the humerus. The olecranon has moved medially, indicating cubitus varus deformity.

Postreduction X-Ray

1. The normal relation of the distal fragment to the shaft of the humerus is restored. (The normal angle is 45 degrees.)

2. The medial displacement of the distal fragment has been corrected.

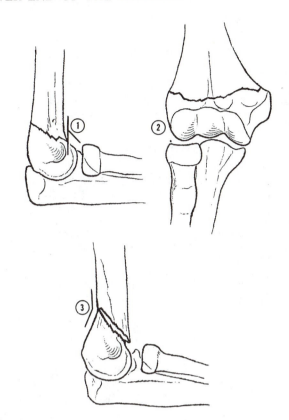

3. Some persistent posterior displacement of the distal fragment may be accepted provided that the varus tilt is corrected.

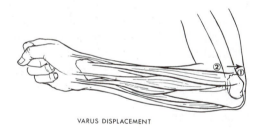

Postreduction Forearm Position

X-rays will not adequately indicate the degree of tilt. The only way to insure against cubitus varus or cubitus valgus deformity is by using the position of the forearm to close the fracture gap.

1. Medial (varus) displacement of the distal fragment produces cubitus varus deformity.

2. Immobilization with forearm pronation tightens the extensor origin and closes the lateral fracture gap, preventing cubitus varus deformity.

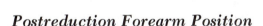

VARUS DISPLACEMENT

1. Lateral (valgus) displacement of the distal fragment produces cubitus valgus deformity.

2. Immobilization with the forearm supinated tightens the flexor-pronator group and closes the fracture gap medially, preventing cubitus valgus deformity.

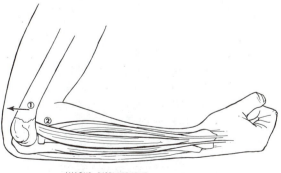

VALGUS DISPLACEMENT

761

Immobilization

1. Flex the elbow to 90 to 100 degrees.

2. Check radial pulse to insure that the flexion does not obliterate circulation.

3. Immobilize laterally displaced fractures in supination to prevent cubitus valgus.

4. Immobilize medially displaced fractures in pronation to prevent cubitus varus.

Note: Do not apply a circular cast immediately because of the risk of antecubital swelling after reduction.

5. Elevate the limb with a triangular sling.

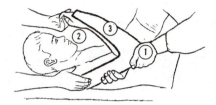

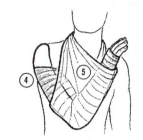

Postreduction Management

The patient should be hospitalized for at least 48 hours.

The radial pulse should be checked at regular intervals by the physician and nursing personnel.

Although the radial pulse may be lost in 10 to 15 per cent of cases, active and passive finger motion without pain indicates that ischemic muscle injury is unlikely.

Pain on passive extension of the fingers indicates the need for prompt treatment of impending ischemia (see page 161).

In the absence of radial pulse Doppler flowmeter or photoplethysmography can be used to monitor distal flow.

Immediately after reduction, elevate the arm on pillows and apply cold (ice bags).

With diminution of swelling (after five to seven days) flexion may be increased and another plaster slab applied.

Repeat x-rays at time of splint change. Some redisplacement of the distal fragment posteriorly may occur without necessitating remanipulation.

Subsequent Management

The plaster slab immobilization is continued for four to five weeks. By the end of five weeks the limb can be supported in a sling and the patient begins active range-of-motion exercises.

Do not employ physical therapy or other modalities to stretch the elbow passively, because passive stretching only impedes recovery and leads to myositis ossificans.

By six weeks the patient is allowed free use of the arm.

Maximum restoration of function is achieved only after several months.

ALTERNATE METHOD: OVERHEAD TRACTION

REMARKS

Indications:

Failure to obtain reduction by manipulative maneuvers.

Failure to retain the normal position of the fragments without the use of traction.

Swelling so great that the necessary flexion of the elbow required to maintain reduction of fragments impairs circulation of the arm and hand. (The radial pulse becomes faint or is obliterated.)

Note: These indications apply to all fractures of the lower end of the humerus (supracondylar, transcondylar, epiphyseal separations and comminuted fractures).

Overhead traction is advantageous in that it treats the swelling of the arm by elevation and allows reduction by direct visualization of the bony landmarks and their alignment.

Remember that reduction is determined primarily by visual rather than radiographic evaluation.

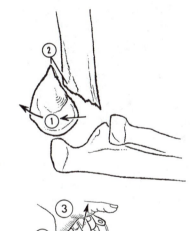

Prereduction X-Ray

1. The distal fragment is displaced outward and backward.

2. Marked obliquity of the line of fracture prevents engagement of the fragments by manipulative maneuvers.

Reduction by Overhead Traction

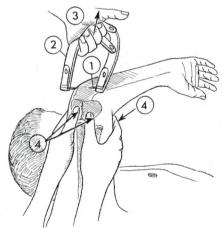

1. Pass a 2-mm to 3-mm threaded Kirschner wire through the upper end of the ulna, 2 cm from the tip of the olecranon. Insert from the ulnar side to avoid impaling the nerve.

2. Attach to the wire a traction bow.

3. While steady traction is made on the bow in the long axis of the humerus by an assistant,

4. Push the distal fragment forward with both thumbs while the fingers make counter pressure on the proximal fragment.

Reduction by Overhead Traction (Continued)

ALTERNATE METHOD

1. A useful technique that avoids the risk of ulnar nerve damage is to insert a winged traction screw.*

2. Holes in the wing permit application of traction so as to correct either varus or valgus deformity.

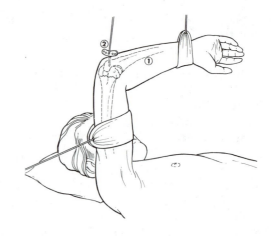

Position of Patient in Bed

1. Patient is in the supine position and weights are applied to make overhead traction.

2. Apply enough weight to suspend the arm. The shoulder girdle should be under tension but should not be lifted off the level surface of the mattress.

Note: Too much weight may cause distraction of the fragments; also, neurovascular complications may be precipitated by excessive traction.

3. Place the forearm in a balanced suspension apparatus using a sling; the forearm is midway between pronation and supination.

4. The elbow is flexed 90 degrees.

5. The hand overhangs the opposite shoulder.

6. Make counter traction on the proximal fragment with a sling around the lower part of the arm; 1 to 2 lb (.45 to .90 kg) of weight pulling backward usually is sufficient.

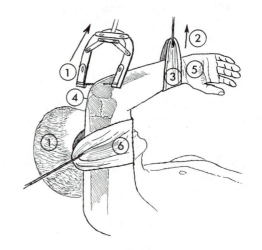

---

*Available from Zimmer-U.S.A., Warsaw, Indiana, 46580.

Correction of Medial (or Lateral) Angulation of Distal Fragments

1. Palpate the bony prominences on the back of the elbow and mark their center points with ink (olecranon, medial and lateral epicondyles).

2. Align the prominences with the long axis of the humerus so that they conform to the apearance of the prominences on the normal side. This corrects any medial or lateral tilt.

3. To maintain the corrected alignment it may be necessary to attach the rope to the handle of the traction bow in an eccentric position.

Note: This visual alignment method is more accurate than radiographic determination of reduction with the elbow flexed.

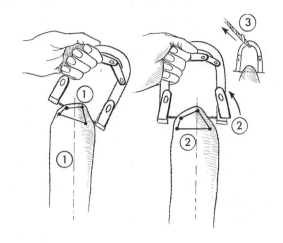

Care During Traction Period

Check the traction apparatus constantly and make the necessary adjustments.

Do not apply too much weight.

In the case of preexisting circulatory embarrassment check the radial pulse or use flowmeter measurement at frequent designated intervals for the first 24 hours and record observations.

Maintain traction for five to seven days, until pain and swelling at the fracture site have subsided.

Postreduction X-Ray

1. The lateral displacement and angulatory deformity have been corrected.

2. The distal fragment still exhibits slight backward projection. (This amount of displacement is compatible with normal function.)

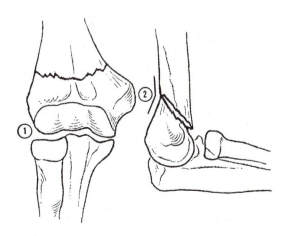

765

Postreduction Management

After five to seven days, under general anesthesia, the traction apparatus may be removed and fracture reduction evaluated visually and radiographically.

Apply a longarm plaster cast over the arm in slight flexion above a right angle.

The forearm is pronated to correct any medial (varus) displacement.

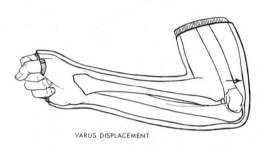

VARUS DISPLACEMENT

For lateral (valgus) displacement the forearm is supinated.

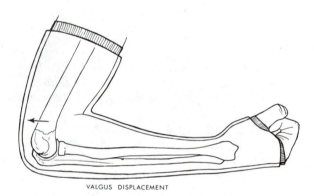

VALGUS DISPLACEMENT

Remove the cast by four to five weeks after injury and place the arm in a triangular sling while the patient regains active elbow motion.

Encourage graded active exercises of the elbow within the tolerance of pain. *Do not* permit forceful passive stretching of the elbow.

After five or six weeks from the time of reduction, allow free use of the arm.

In children, maximum restoration of function is achieved in three to five months. In adults, this period is longer by several months.

ALTERNATE METHOD: LATERAL (DUNLOP) TRACTION

REMARKS

This method may be used instead of overhead skeletal traction. It has certain advantages:

1. It allows adequate venous drainage of the limb without the necessity of inserting a traction pin.

2. It may be used as a temporary immobilizing method to permit swelling to subside prior to reduction.

Its disadvantages are:

1. It usually does not permit fracture reduction by positioning.

2. The alignment of the elbow bony landmarks may not be visualized.

Dunlop Traction

1. The arm is suspended laterally.

2. Skin traction is made on the forearm. (Use foam rubber strips secured by a cotton elastic bandage.)

3. Counter traction is applied by a sling over the front of the arm attached to 1 or 2 lb (.45 to .90 kg) of weight.

Note: This counter traction is never applied if there is clinical evidence of circulatory embarrassment or marked swelling.

4. The side of the mattress is elevated.

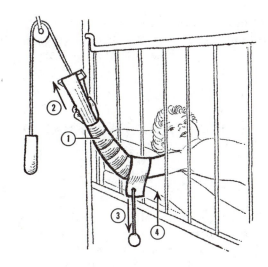

Care During Traction Period

Check the traction constantly and evaluate the distal circulation for any signs of impending ischemia.

X-rays may be taken after 24 to 48 hours, but do not rely on traction alone to reduce the fracture.

By three to four days, after swelling has subsided, fracture may be manipulated as previously described (see page 759).

Do not wait more than five days to do this, since healing may advance rapidly and an unacceptable position may be unalterable if manipulative reduction is delayed.

Postreduction Management

Apply a long arm cast with the elbow flexed 10 to 20 degrees. The forearm is pronated to correct varus displacement or supinated to correct valgus deformity.

Remove the cast after four to five weeks.

Place the arm in a triangular sling.

Encourage graduated active exercises of the elbow within the tolerance of pain.

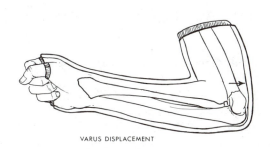

VARUS DISPLACEMENT

Postreduction Management
(Continued)

Do not permit forceful passive stretching of the elbow.

After five or six weeks from the time of reduction, allow free use of the arm.

In children maximum restoration of function is achieved in three to five months. In adults this period is longer by several months.

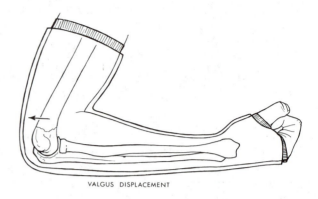

VALGUS DISPLACEMENT

SUPRACONDYLAR FRACTURE WITH FORWARD DISPLACEMENT

REMARKS

In general, soft tissue damage is less extensive than in the extension type of fracture.

Reduction is achieved by traction in extension and lateral pressure on the displaced distal fragment.

Prereduction X-Ray

1. The distal fragment is displaced forward.

2. The distal fragment is displaced outward.

3. The distal fragment with the bones of the forearm is tilted so that the carrying angle of the elbow is increased.

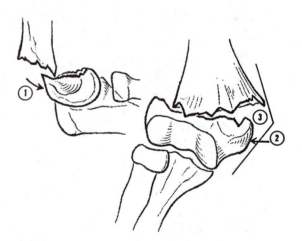

MANIPULATIVE REDUCTION

The patient is under general anesthesia.

1. Steady traction is made in the line of the limb by an assistant.

2. The arm is fully extended.

3. The forearm is in supination.

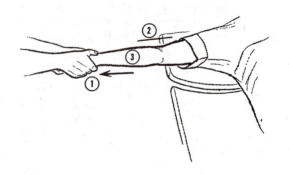

768

While traction is maintained, correct the lateral displacement by

1. Making firm inward pressure on the displaced distal fragment with one hand while

2. Steadying the lower end of the proximal fragment with the other hand.

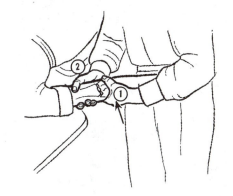

Immobilization

1. Apply a long plaster slab 10 cm wide along the posterior aspect of the arm and forearm.

2. The elbow is extended fully.

3. The forearm is in full supination.

4. Fix the plaster slab with a 7.5-cm cotton elastic bandage.

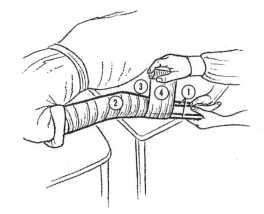

Postreduction X-Ray

1. The distal fragment is restored to its normal anatomic position.

2. The lateral displacement and angulatory deformity are corrected.

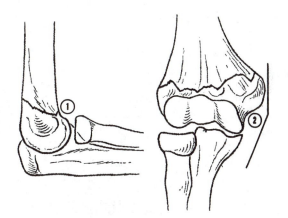

Postreduction Management

Remove the plaster after three weeks in children, after four weeks in adults.

Place the arm in a triangular sling.

Begin a program of graduated active exercises.

Never employ passive stretching of the elbow joint.

Allow free use of the arm after four or five weeks.

ALTERNATE METHOD: FOR ADULTS AND THE AGED (AFTER SOLTANPUR)

REMARKS

Immobilization of the older patient's elbow in extension for the period necessary to heal this fracture may result in permanent limitation of motion.

For the older patient, apply a cast in two stages, thereby allowing fracture reduction and immobilization in flexion. This method takes advantage of the fact that the displaced fracture fragment behaves as part of the forearm.

Technique of Reduction

STAGE I

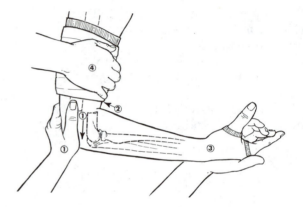

1. The surgeon grasps the condyles and pulls distally to disengage the fracture fragments.
2. The elbow is flexed to slightly less than 90 degrees.
3. The limb is wrapped in cast padding by an assistant.
4. A circular cast is applied around the upper arm only.

STAGE II

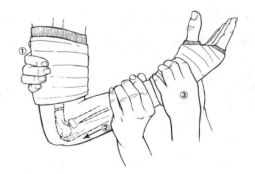

When the upper arm cast has set.
1. The surgeon supports the upper arm and
2. Pushes the patient's hand, forearm, and condylar mass downward to reduce the fracture with the aid of the forearm.
3. Assistant completes the long arm plaster cast.

Postreduction Management

Confirm the position by x-ray and recheck within a week.

The plaster cast may be discarded by six weeks and the arm may be placed in a sling.

Begin a program of active exercises.

Do not permit passive stretching of the elbow joint.

Lateral Condylar Fractures
(After Flynn and coworkers)

REMARKS (See also page 163)

Lateral condylar fractures are type IV epiphyseal fractures and tend to be displaced by the pull of the forearm extensor muscles.

Fractures with less than 2 mm of displacement usually heal within six weeks. If a fracture line is still evident after six weeks, immobilization must be continued for as long as twelve weeks.

Displacement of more than 3 mm may occur even during cast immobilization and should be treated with internal fixation.

Established nonunions in good position that are symptomatic while the elbow is still immature may be salvaged by internal fixation that spares the physis of the condylar fragment.

Operative correction of malunited fractures, however, is not indicated in the growing elbow.

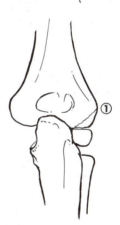

Lateral Condylar Fracture
Displaced Less than 2 mm

1. Fracture line was still evident after six weeks of immobilization.

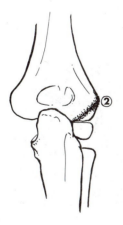

2. Immobilization was necessary for twelve weeks until union was complete.

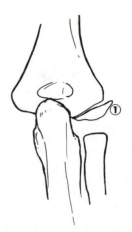

Lateral Condylar Fracture
Displaced More than 3 mm

1. Closed reduction was attempted.

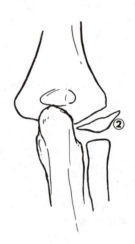

2. Displacement worsened in cast owing to pull of the extensor muscles.

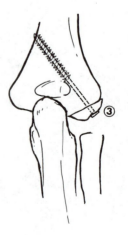

3. Internal fixation with screw was performed for this nonunion in good position.

4. An old malunited condylar fracture in poor position should be left alone until growth is completed. Surgical attempts to replace it will traumatize the physis and cause further damage.

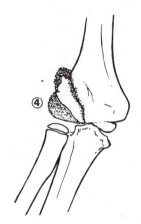

Postreduction Management

After closed or open reduction, immobilize the fracture in a long arm cast with the wrist extended and the forearm supinated to close the fracture gap and diminish the pull of the attached muscles. Take x-rays two or three times during the first two weeks to insure that displacement has not recurred.

Maintain the immobilization for six weeks; then remove the cast and evaluate the healing response carefully by x-ray.

If complete healing of the fracture gap is not evident at six weeks, immobilize in a cast for six weeks longer.

Do not rely on lack of pain symptoms or lack of fracture mobility to indicate healing. There must be complete closure of the fracture gap on x-ray before the fracture can be considered healed.

Only when the x-ray shows solid union, which may take ten to twelve weeks, should active elbow motion be allowed.

If internal fixation with a pin or screw has been employed, remove the fixation and begin active motion.

Fractures of the Medial Condyle and Medial Epicondyle

REMARKS

Fractures of the medial epicondyle are discussed along with apophyseal and epiphyseal fractures (see page 169).

Fracture of the medial condyle is a rare injury that has a definite risk of nonunion. It is caused by a fall on the outstretched hand producing a valgus stress on the elbow.

If the avulsed fragment is only slightly displaced and is not rotated, closed treatment is possible.

If the avulsed fragment is displaced and rotated, open reduction and internal fixation are necessary.

In a widely displaced fracture of the medial epicondyle in a child younger than 8 years in whom the ossification center of the trochlea has not yet appeared, suspect that a large portion of the cartilaginous trochlea is included with the medial epicondyle.

Satisfactory anatomic restoration is possible only with open reduction of these displaced injuries.

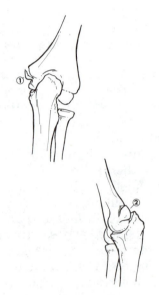

Slightly Displaced Fracture

1. Fracture line is oblique from capitulotrochlear groove to the medial supracondylar ridge above the epicondyle.

2. The medial condyle is avulsed but is not rotated or tilted anteriorly.

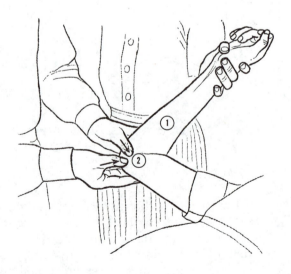

Closed Reduction

1. Flex the elbow 90 degrees and pronate the forearm and flex the wrist to relax the common flexor muscles.

2. Press directly over both condyles to compress them.

3. Apply a long arm cast with the elbow at 90 degrees, the forearm in full pronation, and the wrist in 30 degrees of flexion.

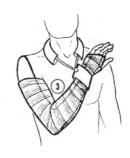

Displaced Fracture

1. Fracture line is rotated medially.
2. Fragment has tilted anteriorly.

For technique of open reduction and internal fixation, see page 173.

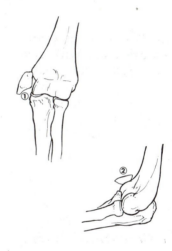

Displaced Medial Condylar Fracture in a Child That Was Misdiagnosed as Medial Epicondyle Fracture

1. Anteroposterior x-ray in an 8-year-old child demonstrates what appears to be a widely displaced separation of the medial epicondyle that could be treated by closed methods.
2. Injury actually included a large portion of the unossified trochlea and required open reduction.

Note: Since the trochlear ossification center appears on x-ray only after the age of 10–12 years, suspect that a widely displaced medial epicondyle fracture may significantly involve the trochlea.

For technique of open reduction and internal fixation, see page 173.

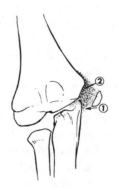

Postreduction X-Rays

1. Displaced, rotated condylar fracture is reduced and is fixed with a threaded screw through bony portion.

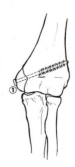

2. Displaced medial epicondyle and trochlea fractures are fixed with two smooth Kirschner wires buried under the skin.

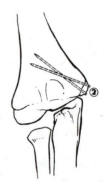

Postreduction Management After Closed or Open Treatment

Immobilize the fracture in a long arm cast with the elbow flexed 90 degrees, the forearm pronated, and the wrist flexed 30 degrees to diminish muscle pull.

Take x-rays weekly for several weeks to insure that displacement has not occurred.

Remove the cast at six weeks and evaluate healing response carefully on radiographs.

If complete healing of the fracture gap is not evident at six weeks, immobilize the elbow in a cast for four to six weeks longer.

Do not rely on the patient's lack of pain symptoms as indication of healing. There must be closure of the fracture gap on x-ray before the fracture can be considered healed.

When x-ray shows solid union, which may take ten to twelve weeks with closed treatment, begin active elbow motion.

Little Leaguer's Elbow

REMARKS

These avulsion or fatigue-compression fractures of the adolescent athlete's elbow have been growing in frequency with the increasing emphasis on competitive organized sports programs.

Acceleration of the baseball pitcher's forearm causes a valgus strain on the elbow, which, if repeated often enough, may avulse the medial epicondyle or fatigue fracture the subchondral bone of the capitellum or the radial head.

The little leaguer's bone structure cannot withstand the extreme loading produced by repetitive hard throwing.

Similar fatigue problems may also occur in the shoulder.

Loose bodies produced by these injuries rarely require operative excision. The most effective treatment is preventive. Adolescent athletes should avoid overuse of the throwing elbow and should be warned to rest the elbow if throwing causes pain.

Persistent elbow pain in the adolescent throwing athlete should not be attributed to soft tissue strain, because there is frequently significant underlying bony damage.

1. Extreme valgus strain is applied to the elbow during forearm acceleration and rotation while throwing.

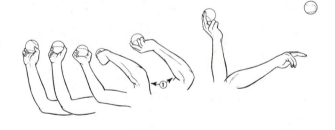

2. Avulsion of the medial ligament or compression of the radiohumeral joint results from overly repetitive throwing in this manner.

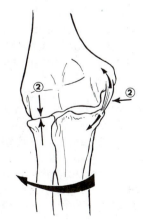

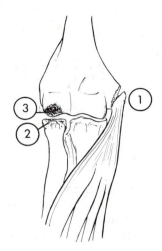

1. Avulsion fracture of the medial epicondyle in an adolescent pitcher is the most common injury and may be mistaken for elbow strain.

2. A fatigue fracture of the radial head or

3. Osteochondritis dissecans may result from radiohumeral compression.

Fracture of the Capitellum in the Adult

REMARKS

Injuries to the capitellum occur commonly from a fall on the outstretched arm.

This injury usually fractures the radial head but may damage the capitellum by direct transmission of the force through the radial head, which acts like a piston and shears off the capitellum into the radial fossa.

Injuries of this type are deceiving because they may appear minor but can cause significant limitation of elbow motion. A true lateral x-ray will demonstrate the free osteochondral fragment displaced anterosuperiorly into the radial fossa.

There are two types of injuries to the capitellum, (1) a complete anterior displacement of the capitellar fragment and (2) a partial decortication or bruising that may be associated with a radial head fracture.

Operative treatment with excision of the fragment is more effective than attempted anatomic reduction.

The trochlear-ulnar articulation allows excision of the entire capitellum and radial head as well, if necessary for comminuted fractures, without causing valgus instability of the elbow.

Even a portion of the anterior trochlear surface may be excised with the capitellar fragment without compromising elbow stability, provided that the posterior trochlear surface is intact.

The fracture line may rarely involve the posterior trochlea as well as the capitellum; in essence it is then a transcondylar fracture.

Excision of fracture fragments should be avoided in a child, because it inevitably results in angulatory growth deformities.

Types of Fractures of the Capitellum

1. Impact of the radial head drives the capitellar fragment anteriorly into the radial fossa. This is the most frequent type of injury and blocks flexion.

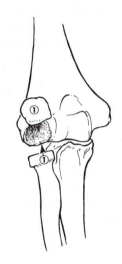

2. Impact of the radial head "bruises" the articular cartilage of the capitellum and may form a type of osteochondritis dissecans. This may not displace and may be manifested only by a persistent block of elbow extension or symptoms of a loose body. It may also only be seen during arthrotomy for removal of the fractured radial head.

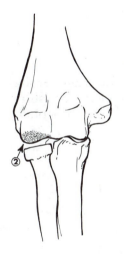

Preoperative X-ray – Shear Fracture of the Capitellum

1. Fracture is not evident on the anteroposterior x-ray but the lateral x-ray, showing capitellar fragment displaced into the radial fossa, is diagnostic.

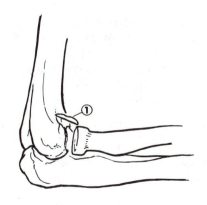

779

Operative Management

INCISION AND EXPOSURE

1. The Kocher lateral J approach is used with an incision from the supracondylar ridge to 5 mm distal to the radial head.

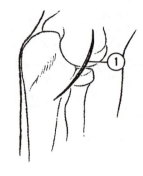

2. Develop the interval between the anconeus muscle and the extensor carpi ulnaris muscle.

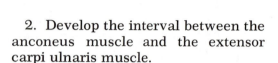

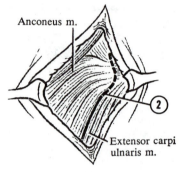

Anconeus m.

Extensor carpi ulnaris m.

3. Deepen the incision through the capsule and extend the capsular incision proximally along the epicondylar ridge.

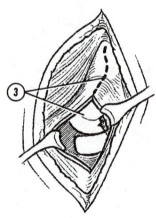

EXCISION

1. Clean all debris from the inside of the joint and from the lower surface of the capitellum.

2. Remove the capitellar fragment.

3. If the radial head is fractured, it may also be removed.

Note: Obtain an intraoperative x-ray to insure that all fragments have been excised. Also check the stability of the elbow joint in extension.

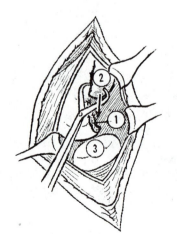

Postoperative X-Ray

A sizable capitellum fragment may be removed without impairing the stability of the elbow. Excision is usually preferable to internal fixation in comminuted fractures.

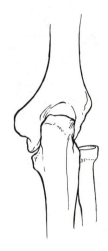

Postoperative Management

The arm is immobilized in a posterior splint with the elbow flexed 90 degrees.

Active range of motion is begun at five to seven days, when the wound edema and pain have subsided.

Avoid passive stretching exercises and intensive physical therapy.

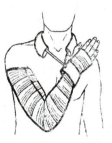

Intercondylar T Fracture of the Humerus in the Adult

REMARKS

The lesions are infrequent in comparison with supracondylar fractures in children.

They occur most often in adults more than 40 years of age.

The mechanism of injury is direct trauma to the elbow that drives the olecranon against the humeral articular surface and splits the distal end.

The fracture may be one of three general types depending on the degree of condylar displacement.

Minimally displaced fractures without rotational deformity can be treated by closed reduction and cast immobilization.

Fractures with rotational deformity or severe comminution are best treated by skeletal traction.

The best results are obtained if the fracture fragments are reasonably aligned and there is minimal soft tissue damage.

Since open reduction and internal fixation entail wide exposure and further trauma to soft tissues, they are rarely indicated and should be reserved for fractures that cannot be reduced by traction.

Before internal fixation is begun, there should be reasonable expectation that the fixation achieved will produce sufficient stability for active range of motion.

TYPES OF INTERCONDYLAR T FRACTURES (RISEBOROUGH AND RADIN)

Type I

T-shaped intercondylar fracture with trochlear and capitellar fragments separated but not appreciably rotated in the frontal plane.

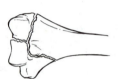

Type II

Separation and significant rotational displacement; this is the most common type.

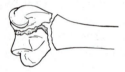

Type III

T-shaped intercondylar type fracture with severe comminution of articular surfaces and wide separation of condyles.

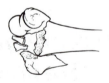

MANAGEMENT OF INTERCONDYLAR T FRACTURE IN THE ADULT

Type I

PREREDUCTION X-RAY

Fracture with minimal rotational deformity.

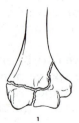

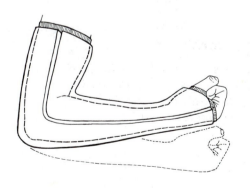

REDUCTION

1. If elbow is swollen, elevate the limb for two or three days to eliminate edema.

After the period of elevation:

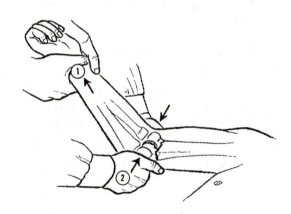

1. An assistant makes steady traction with the elbow extended 135 degrees, and

2. The surgeon makes firm lateral pressure on the condyles.

POSTREDUCTION MANAGEMENT

Immobilize the fracture in a bivalved cast for three to four weeks. (Immobilization for a longer time promotes permanent stiffness.)

Begin gentle active range-of-motion exercises, but protect the limb in the bivalved cast when the patient is not actively exercising the elbow.

Clinical and radiographic evidence of fracture union is usually sufficient that the plaster may be discarded by the end of the seventh or eighth week.

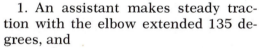

783

Type II

PREREDUCTION X-RAY

1. Fragments are separated and there is significant rotational displacement and deformity.

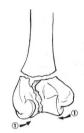

MANAGEMENT BY SKELETAL TRACTION

1. The patient is on a firm bed fitted with a lateral traction apparatus.

2. Elevate the side of the bed slightly for counter traction.

3. Pass a 3-mm Kirschner wire through the olecranon from medial to lateral sides, taking care to avoid the ulnar nerve, and apply 5 to 8 lb (3 to 4 kg) of traction.

4. Rotational deformity of the condyles can be corrected by rotation of the forearm.

5. Abduct the shoulder approximately 70 degrees.

Note: Check reduction by x-ray. If alignment is not satisfactory after two to three days, manipulate the fracture under general anesthetic as described for type I. Keep the arm in traction after manipulation.

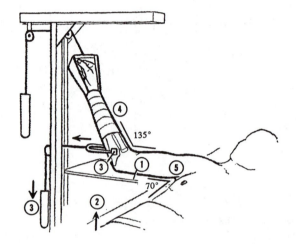

POSTREDUCTION X-RAY

The Kirschner wire through olecranon corrects the rotational displacement, although the fracture is incompletely reduced.

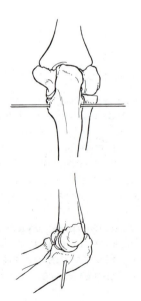

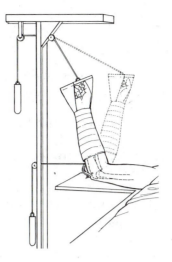

POSTREDUCTION MANAGEMENT

Continue traction for three weeks. Use of a Salvatori traction bow* allows elbow motion while in traction.

After three weeks of traction, protect the joint with a bivalved cast for three weeks while the patient continues actively exercising every hour.

Satisfactory functional restoration is likely with a guarded exercise program despite the failure to restore the joint to anatomic normal.

Type III

PREREDUCTION X-RAY

Severe comminution of articular surface with rotational displacement of the condyles.

Note: These fractures may be open injuries, which should be treated with immediate debridement followed by a Kirschner wire traction technique.

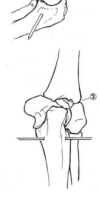

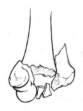

X-RAYS DURING TRACTION

1. Condyles have been approximated and rotational malalignment has been corrected by rotation of the forearm.
2. Distraction of the fracture fragment should be avoided.

*Available from Wright Corporation, Memphis, Tennessee.

Type III *(Continued)*

POSTREDUCTION MANAGEMENT

Continue traction for three weeks. Use of Salvatori traction bow* allows elbow motion while in traction.

After three weeks of traction, protect the joint with a bivalved cast for three weeks while the patient continues actively exercising every hour.

Satisfactory restoration is likely with a guarded exercise program despite failure to restore the joint to anatomic normal.

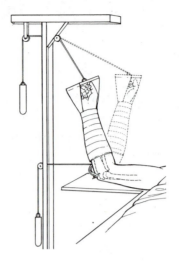

OPERATIVE TREATMENT

REMARKS

Operative treatment gives poorer results for these fractures than does skeletal traction and early range-of-motion exercises.

When traction or closed manipulation completely fails to reduce the fracture, operative fixation is also likely to fail, and the patient will have an even worse functional disability.

Rarely, if rotation of the condyles cannot be corrected by forearm rotation or other closed methods, open reduction and internal fixation may be useful. Adequate fixation of the condylar fragments must be achieved to permit active range of elbow motion soon after operation.

Surgical Procedure

POSITION OF PATIENT

1. Patient is in the prone position.
2. The forearm hangs over the end of an arm board.

The arm is draped separately.

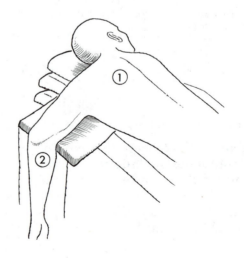

---

*Available from Wright Corporation, Memphis, Tennessee.

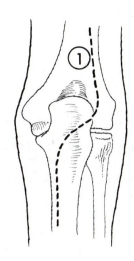

INCISION AND EXPOSURE

1. Begin the incision on the postero-lateral aspect of the arm 8 to 10 cm proximal to the tip of the olecranon. Continue the incision distally to the level of the elbow joint, then gently curve it obliquely downward across the base of the olecranon, and continue it directly downward along the crest of the ulna for 8 cm.

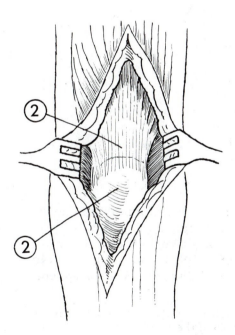

2. Expose the aponeurosis of the triceps as far distally as its insertion on the olecranon, and expose the olecranon as far distally as its base.

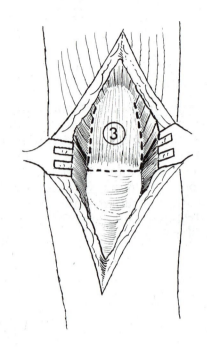

Surgical Procedure (Continued)

3. Outline the tongue-shaped aponeurosis of the triceps and by sharp dissection detach it from its insertion on the olecranon.

4. Reflect the triangular aponeurotic flap proximally.

5. With a sharp fine osteotome divide transversely the olecranon 0.5 cm from its tip; discard the excised portion.

Note: Subsequently in the operation the aponeurosis of the triceps will be attached to the remaining portion of the olecranon. This tendon-to-bone suture allows earlier and safer mobilization of the elbow than bone-to-bone approximation held with a screw. Removal of the olecranon fragment may also allow more complete elbow extension when fracture heals.

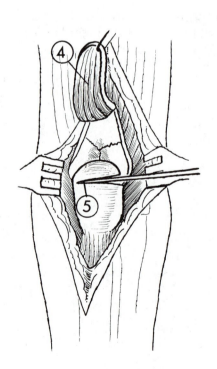

TECHNIQUE OF FIXATION

1. First achieve provisional transcondylar Kirschner wire fixation of the intra-articular fragments.

2. Next, use a lag screw introduced parallel to the axis of the elbow joint from the capitellum into the trochlea.

3. Once the condyles have been fixed, use two crossed lag screws that grip the opposite far cortex.

4. Alternatively, two small semitubular plates can be used to give more rigid fixation and to allow earlier postoperative range of motion.

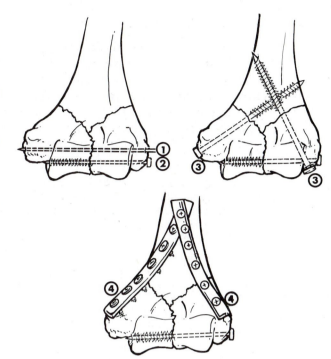

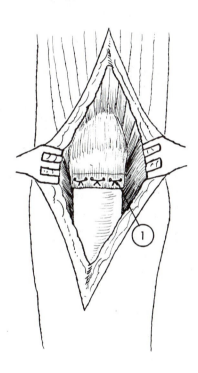

1. Following radiography to determine adequacy of reduction, reattach the aponeurosis of the triceps to the base of the olecranon by mattress sutures passing through drill holes in the bone.

Note: Before reattaching the triceps, flush out the joint with saline to remove all debris.

Postoperative Immobilization

1. Apply a posterior plaster slab from axilla to the metacarpophalangeal joint.

2. Fix the plaster slab with 10-cm cotton bandage.

3. The elbow is flexed 90 degrees.

4. The forearm is turned in neutral position and the arm is supported in a triangular sling.

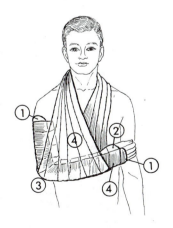

Postoperative Management

After five to seven days, remove the plaster splint and begin active range-of-motion exercise to the elbow within the limits of the sling.

After two to three weeks, the elbow may be exercised actively out of the sling to increase the range and frequency of exercise according to the tolerance of the patient. After the fifth or sixth week discard the sling.

Maximum restoration of motion will be slow in coming.

Never apply passive stretching to the elbow to improve the range of motion.

Note: If internal fixation is inadequate or insecure, but reduction has been accomplished, postoperative resumption of olecranon traction and an exercise program will sometimes be useful adjuncts to operative treatment.

DISLOCATIONS OF THE ELBOW JOINT

Posterior Dislocations of the Elbow Joint

REMARKS

Except for the shoulder, the elbow is the joint most frequently dislocated, and in children less than 10 years of age, elbow dislocation occurs more often than any other luxation.

Generally the radius and the ulna, which are firmly bound together by the annular ligament and interosseous membrane, displace posteriorly as a unit.

Occasionally displacement occurs laterally, medially, or anteriorly, but the vast majority of dislocations are posterior.

Considerable violence is absorbed by the elbow during dislocation, and 30 to 40 per cent of dislocations are associated with fractures of adjacent structures.

The most common associated fracture in children (less than 14 years of age) is avulsion of the medial epicondyle. In adults associated fracture may involve the coronoid process or the radial head, the capitellum, or the olecranon.

Because elbow dislocations traumatize the anterior brachial muscle, myositis ossificans may complicate the injury, particularly if passive exercise is inflicted on the patient.

Emphasis on active rather than passive range-of-motion exercises to regain elbow motion has diminished the occurrence of this complication significantly.

Dislocated elbows are always at risk of vascular injury. The frequency of vascular impairment (one to three per cent) after dislocation is not as high as with supracondylar fractures, but the results may be equally catastrophic.

Because of the extent of trauma from elbow dislocation, simple posterior plaster slabs are preferable to circular casts for temporary immobilization after reduction. Close follow-up is essential after reduction, with the patient either remaining in the hospital or returning to the surgeon's office within 24 hours of cast application.

Nerve injury, most often a temporary neurapraxia, may also complicate management. The ulnar and median nerves are damaged usually by the same injury that disrupts the brachial artery.

Reduction of the elbow dislocation is usually quite simple. It is the management of the common complications, particularly of associated fractures and vascular and nerve injuries, that makes the difference between good and mediocre care.

As with any dislocation or subluxation, elbow dislocation may be subject to recurrence if bony, ligamentous, and muscular support structures are disrupted sufficiently. Most elbows are quite stable after reduction, but the degree of instability can only be evaluated by testing the range of joint motion subsequent to reduction.

Rarely, a patient will be seen with a chronically dislocated elbow that can be reduced by traction and closed technique if it is less than four weeks old. Dislocations older than four weeks require extensive open procedures, which are indicated primarily for persistent and severe pain.

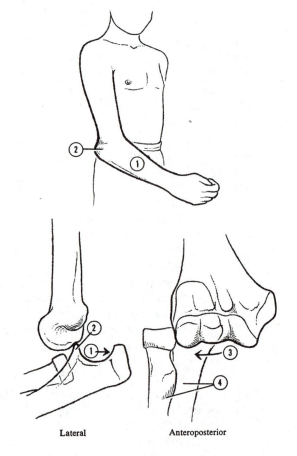

Lateral   Anteroposterior

Typical Deformity (Uncomplicated Posterior Dislocation)

1. The forearm appears to be shortened.
2. The olecranon is very prominent.

Prereduction X-Ray

LATERAL VIEW

1. Both bones of the forearm are displaced backward and are behind the humerus.
2. The coronoid process of the ulna impinges on the posterior aspect of the humerus in the olecranon fossa.

ANTEROPOSTERIOR VIEW

3. In this instance both bones are displaced radially.
4. The radius and ulna maintain their normal anatomic position in relation to each other.

Note: Always check carefully prior to reduction for alteration in distal CMS (circulation, motor, sensory) function.

Anesthesia for Reduction

Local anesthesia may be quite effective for the usual patient with elbow dislocation. For the extremely anxious patient, use general anesthesia.

1. Insert 20-gauge needle into the joint proximal to the dislocated radial head.

2. Aspirate hemarthrosis.

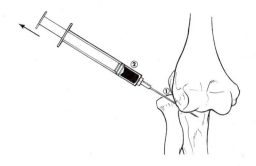

3. Inject 10 cc of 0.5% bupivacaine (Marcaine). Wait 10 minutes for anesthesia and then carry out reduction.

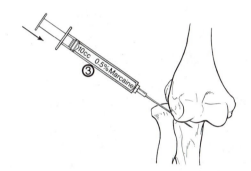

Manipulative Reduction

1. While an assistant holds the arm and makes steady counter traction,

2. Grasp the wrist with one hand and make steady traction on the forearm in the position in which it lies.

3. While traction is maintained, correct any lateral displacement with the other hand.

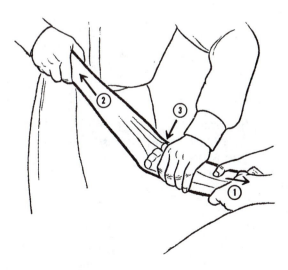

Manipulative Reduction (*Continued*)

THEN:

1. While traction is maintained,
2. Gently flex the forearm.

Note: With reduction a click is usually felt and heard as the olecranon engages the articular surface of the humerus.

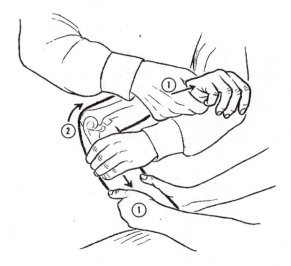

Evaluation of Stability

Following reduction,

1. Gently move the elbow through its normal range to check stability in extension.
2. If the elbow is unstable in extension, several diagnoses are possible: (a) in a child, entrapment of the medial epicondyle, (b) in an adult, unstable fracture of the radial head or the olecranon, or (c) posterolateral disruption of the capsule.

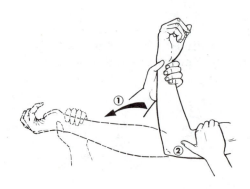

Postreduction X-Ray

1. The articular surface of the humerus is in its normal position in relation to the ulna.
2. Both bones have been restored from a lateral position to their normal positions in relation to the humerus.

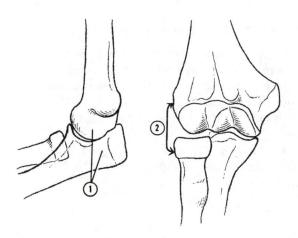

Immobilization

1. Apply a posterior plaster slab from the upper arm to the base of the fingers.

2. Flex the elbow as much as the swelling will permit without embarrassing the circulation of the arm.

3. Fix the plaster slab with a cotton elastic bandage.

4. Suspend the arm with a collar and cuff.

Note: Avoid the use of a circular cast, which would add considerably to the risk of ischemic muscle injury. Always check carefully after reduction for alteration in distal CMS (circulation, motor, sensory) function.

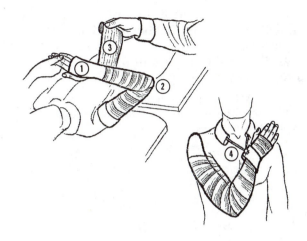

Postreduction Management

Observe the patient carefully for the first 24 to 36 hours for signs of circulatory impairment.

If the elbow was stable immediately after reduction, allow gentle active exercises as soon as swelling subsides, usually by three to five days.

If the elbow was unstable after reduction and no fracture was evident, treat for soft tissue disruption by immobilization for three to four weeks. If instability is due to fracture, open reduction may be necessary to permit range-of-motion exercises.

Emphasize the patient's need for active exercise after immobilization is discarded.

Never permit passive stretching of the elbow, which has been implicated as a cause of myositis ossificans in the brachialis muscle.

Anterior Dislocation of the Elbow Joint

REMARKS

This lesion is very rare.

It is usually associated with a fracture of the olecranon.

There is severe soft tissue trauma.

795

Prereduction X-Ray

1. The olecranon is in front of the anterior surface of the lower end of the humerus.

2. The radial head is in front of and proximal to the external condyle.

Note: Always check carefully prior to reduction for alteration in distal CMS (circulation, motor, sensory) function.

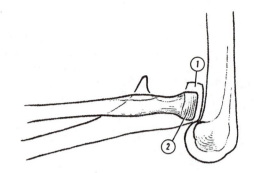

Manipulative Reduction

Reduction is performed with the patient under local or general anesthesia (see page 793).

1. An assistant grasps the arm and makes counter traction.

2. The operator grasps the wrist with one hand and makes traction in the line of the arm, and

3. With the other hand makes firm steady pressure downward and backward on the upper end of the forearm. A click usually indicates that reduction is achieved.

4. The arm is flexed to 45 degrees beyond a right angle.

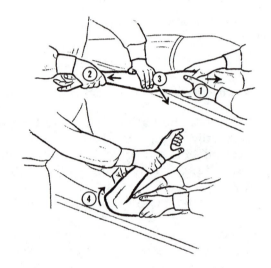

Evaluation of Stability

Following reduction,

1. Gently move the elbow through its normal range to check stability in extension.

2. If the elbow is unstable in extension, several diagnoses are possible: (a) in a child, entrapment of the medial epicondyle, (b) in an adult, unstable fracture of the radial head or the olecranon, or (c) posterolateral disruption of the capsule.

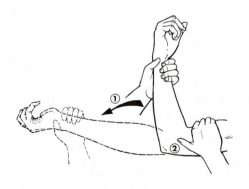

Immobilization

1. Apply a posterior plaster slab from the upper arm to the base of the fingers.

2. Hold the arm at an angle of 135 degrees.

3. Encircle the arm and slab with a cotton elastic bandage.

4. Support the arm in a triangular sling.

Note: Avoid the use of a circular cast, which would add considerably to the risk of ischemic injury. Always check carefully after reduction for alteration in distal CMS (circulation, motor, sensory) function.

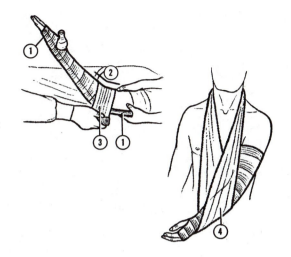

Postreduction Management

Observe the patient carefully for the first 24 to 36 hours for signs of circulatory impairment.

If the elbow was stable immediately after reduction, allow gentle active exercises as soon as swelling subsides, usually by three to five days.

If the elbow was unstable after reduction and no fracture was evident, treat for soft tissue disruption by immobilization for three to four weeks.

If instability is due to fracture, open reduction may be necessary to permit early range-of-motion exercise.

Emphasize the patient's need for active exercise after immobilization is discarded.

Never permit passive stretching of the elbow, which has been implicated as a cause of myositis ossificans in the brachialis muscle.

Lateral Dislocation of the Elbow Joint

REMARKS

This lesion is rare and is usually associated with extensive soft tissue trauma.

The medial ligaments are disrupted.

797

Typical Deformity

1. The elbow is broadened.
2. The axis of the forearm is displaced laterally in relation to the humerus.
3. The forearm is pronated.
4. The internal condyle is unduly prominent.
5. The olecranon is lateral to the external condyle.
6. The head of the radius may be prominent and readily palpable.

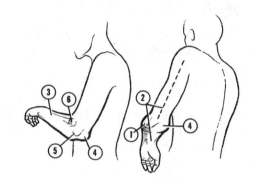

Prereduction X-Ray

1. The olecranon fossa is displaced lateral to the external condyle.
2. The forearm is pronated.
3. The radial head lies above the level of the olecranon.

Note: Always check carefully prior to reduction for alteration in distal CMS (circulation, motor, sensory) function.

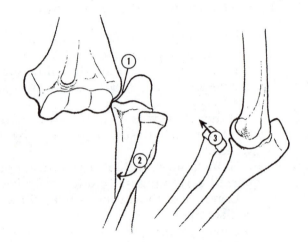

Manipulative Reduction

Reduction is performed with the patient under local or general anesthesia (see page 793).

1. An assistant steadies the arm.
2. The operator with one hand makes moderate traction at the wrist with the elbow short of complete extension.
3. The other hand first forces the upper end of the ulna (A) downward, (B) outward, and (C) backward.

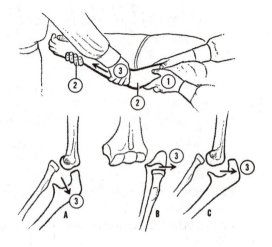

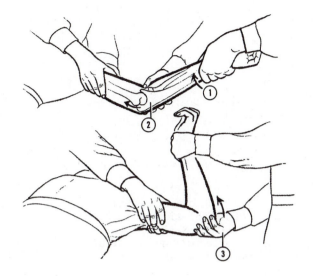

THEN:

1. The operator supinates the forearm and

2. Pushes the ulna around the end of the humerus and

3. Flexes the elbow to a point permitted by soft tissue swelling.

Evaluation of Stability

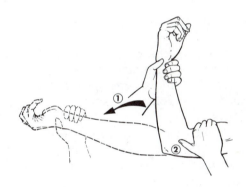

Following reduction,

1. Gently move the elbow through its normal range to check stability in extension.

2. If the elbow is unstable in extension, several diagnoses are possible: (a) in a child, entrapment of the medial epicondyle, (b) in an adult, unstable fracture of the radial head or the olecranon, or (c) medial and lateral disruption of the capsule.

Postreduction X-Ray

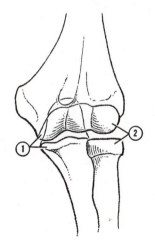

1. The olecranon fossa articulates with the trochlea.

2. The radial head articulates with the capitellum.

Immobilization

1. Apply a posterior plaster slab from the upper arm to the base of the fingers.

2. Flex the elbow as much as the swelling will permit without embarrassing the circulation of the arm.

3. Fix the plaster slab with a cotton elastic bandage.

4. Suspend the arm with a collar and cuff.

Note: Avoid the use of a circular cast, which would add considerably to the risk of ischemic muscle injury. Always check carefully after reduction for alteration in distal CMS (circulation, motor, sensory) function.

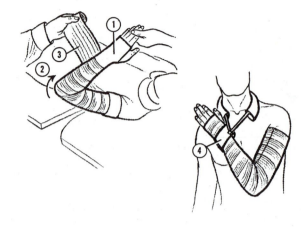

Postreduction Management

Observe the patient carefully for the first 24 to 36 hours for signs of circulatory impairment.

If the elbow was stable immediately after reduction, allow gentle active exercises as soon as swelling subsides, usually by three to five days.

If the elbow was unstable after reduction and no fracture was evident, treat for soft tissue disruption by immobilization for three to four weeks. If instability is due to fracture, open reduction may be necessary to permit early range-of-motion exercise.

Emphasize the patient's need for active exercise after immobilization is discarded.

Never permit passive stretching of the elbow, which has been implicated as a cause of myositis ossificans in the brachialis muscle.

Medial Dislocation of the Elbow Joint

REMARKS

This is a rare lesion and the amount of medial displacement of the forearm bones varies.

Generally, the radial head follows the ulna; occasionally, it may maintain its normal position in relation to the capitellum.

Soft tissue damage is usually severe, including rupture and tearing of the lateral ligaments.

Typical Deformity

1. The elbow is broadened.
2. The long axis of the forearm is displaced inward.
3. The external condyle is unduly prominent.

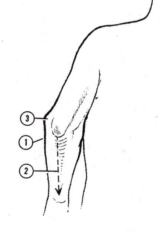

Prereduction X-Ray

1. Both bones of the forearm have shifted medially.
2. The head of the radius rests on the trochlea.
3. The olecranon fossa is medial to the internal condyle.

Note: Always check carefully prior to reduction for alterations in distal CMS (circulation, motor, sensory) function.

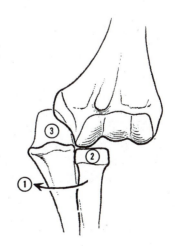

Manipulative Reduction

Reduction is performed with the patient under local or general anesthesia (see page 793).

1. While an assistant holds the arm steady,

2. Grasp the wrist with one hand and make moderate traction in the line of the forearm with the elbow just short of complete extension.

3. While traction is maintained, with the other hand force the upper end of the ulna downward and outward; a click usually indicates complete reduction.

4. Release traction on the forearm and bring the forearm into as much flexion as soft tissue swelling will permit without embarrassing the circulation of the forearm and hand.

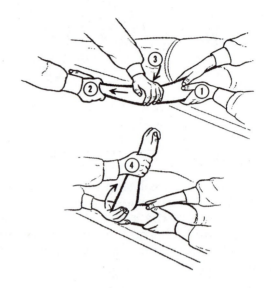

Evaluation of Stability

Following reduction,

1. Gently move the elbow through its normal range to check stability in extension.

2. If elbow is unstable in extension, several diagnoses are possible: (a) in a child, entrapment of the medial epicondyle, (b) in an adult, unstable fracture of the radial head or the olecranon, or (c) medial and lateral disruption of the capsule.

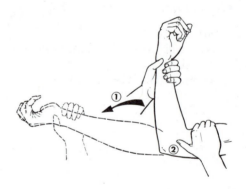

Postreduction X-Ray

1. The olecranon fossa of the ulna is in normal relation to the trochlea.

2. The radial head articulates with the capitellum.

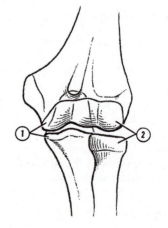

Immobilization

1. Apply a posterior plaster slab from the upper arm to the base of the fingers.

2. Flex the elbow as much as the swelling will permit without embarrassing the circulation of the arm.

3. Fix the plaster slab with cotton elastic bandage.

4. Suspend the arm with a collar and cuff.

Note: Avoid the use of a circular cast, which would add considerably to the risk of ischemic muscle injury. Always check carefully after reduction for alteration in distal CMS (circulation, motor, sensory) function.

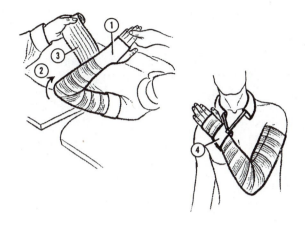

Postreduction Management

Observe the patient carefully for the first 24 to 36 hours for signs of circulatory impairment.

If the elbow was stable immediately after reduction, then allow gentle active exercises as soon as swelling subsides, usually by three to five days.

If the elbow was unstable after reduction and no fracture was evident, treat for soft tissue disruption by immobilizing three to four weeks.

If instability is due to fracture, open reduction may be necessary to permit early range-of-motion exercise.

Emphasize the patient's need for active exercise after immobilization is discarded.

Never permit passive stretching of the elbow, which has been implicated as a cause of myositis ossificans in the brachialis muscle.

Divergent Dislocation of the Elbow Joint

REMARKS

This lesion is extremely rare and occurs only if the annular and interosseous ligaments, which bind the radius and ulna, are completely disrupted. The two bones may then be displaced in an anteroposterior or a medial-lateral direction.

803

Anteroposterior Type

1. The distal end of the humerus lies between the two forearm bones.
2. The ulna is behind the humerus.
3. The radius is in front of the humerus.

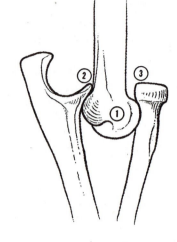

Medial-Lateral Type

1. The distal end of the humerus lies between the forearm bones.
2. The ulna is displaced medially.
3. The radius is displaced laterally.

Note: Always check carefully prior to reduction for alteration in distal CMS (circulation, motor, sensory) function.

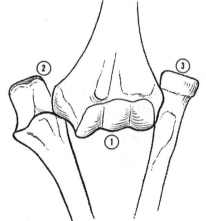

Manipulative Reduction

ANTEROPOSTERIOR TYPE

1. While an assistant steadies the arm,
2. Make steady traction on the extended forearm with one hand and
3. Backward pressure on the ulna with the other hand. When the sigmoid engages the trochlea,
4. Make firm downward pressure on the radial head and
5. Flex the arm to the limit permitted by the soft tissue swelling and the supinated forearm.

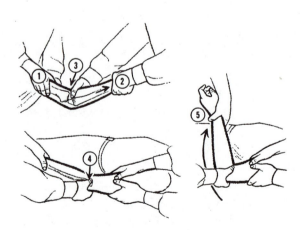

LATERAL TYPE

1. While an assistant steadies the arm,

2. Make steady traction on the extended forearm with one hand and

3. Downward pressure on the upper end of the forearm with the other hand; then,

4. Squeeze together the radius and the ulna and

5. Flex the forearm to a point permitted by the soft tissue swelling.

6. Supinate the forearm.

Note: Evaluate stability by passive flexion and extension of the elbow. Disruption of the soft tissues to the degree sufficient to produce this dislocation usually necessitates performing reconstructive procedures after the swelling of the acute injury has subsided. Always check carefully after reduction for alteration in distal CMS (circulation, motor, sensory) function.

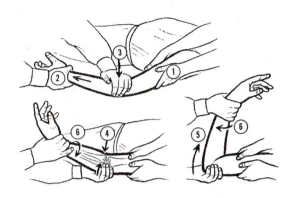

Immobilization

1. Apply a posterior plaster slab from the upper arm to the base of the fingers.

2. Flex the elbow as much as swelling will permit without embarrassing the circulation of the arm.

3. Fix the plaster slab with a cotton elastic bandage.

4. Suspend the arm with a collar and cuff.

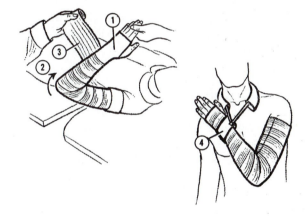

Postreduction Management

The injury that has caused gross instability of the radius and ulna usually requires secondary reconstruction of the annular ligament when the swelling subsides.

If the elbow proves stable after reduction, continue immobilization for four to five weeks.

Institute exercises for the shoulders and fingers immediately.

Remove the plaster slab at five weeks and allow only active elbow exercise.

Use the sling for temporary support but discard this by seven to ten days and allow free use of the arm.

Never permit passive stretching, which promotes development of myositis ossificans.

FRACTURES ASSOCIATED WITH DISLOCATIONS OF THE ELBOW JOINT

REMARKS

Approximately 30 per cent of elbow dislocations will have associated fractures, most commonly avulsion fractures of the medial epicondyle in the child or of the coronoid process in the adult. In general, these fractures should be ignored and the patient should be treated for the primary problem of dislocation.

Immobilization for more than five to seven days is unnecessary; in fact, prolonged immobilization (four to six weeks) to achieve x-ray union of minor avulsion fractures associated with dislocations may cause significant and prolonged elbow stiffness, even in young children.

Results of elbow dislocation associated with fracture tend to be worse in both children and adults than are results of dislocation alone. One reason is the severity of the initial injury. Another major factor is overtreatment of the fracture by either operative intervention or prolonged external immobilization.

The major consideration in a child with an avulsion fracture of the medial epicondyle is whether the fragment has displaced into the joint or whether it includes a portion of the unossified trochlea. Gross displacement of an epicondylar fragment to the level of the elbow joint raises these possibilities as well as the need for operative repair. Minimally displaced epicondylar fractures should be treated symptomatically and should not necessitate prolonging immobilization for more than one to two weeks.

The combination of an elbow fracture and dislocation becomes especially complex in an adult. Overvigorous surgical treatment, such as excision of a fractured radial head, may add to the elbow's instability. Radial head fractures associated with dislocations may be ignored temporarily while the patient is allowed to test elbow stability for a few weeks after injury with active exercise. If such a "trial by motion" demonstrates that the radial head fracture causes significant symptoms of limitation of motion, it can be excised four to six weeks after injury.

Fractures of the coronoid process associated with dislocation should never be excised, because excision inevitably causes recurrence of the dislocation. A "trial by motion" is also useful for coronoid fractures to assess elbow instability before embarking on any surgical interventions.

Treat fractures associated with elbow dislocation cautiously. Nothing is gained by early excision of fracture fragments and much (elbow stability) may be lost.

A fracture of the olecranon, which by its nature causes the elbow to be unstable, is the major indication for early operative intervention. For this fracture-dislocation, fixation of the ulna is necessary to reduce the dislocation.

Posterior Dislocation of the Elbow and Fracture of the Coronoid Process

REMARKS

Fracture of the coronoid frequently complicates posterior dislocation of the elbow.

The fracture should be ignored.

Reduction of the dislocation and immobilization in acute flexion usually result in healing of the fracture with no dysfunction.

Prereduction X-Ray

1. Posterior dislocation of the ulna and radius.

2. Fracture of the coronoid process with moderate displacement due to pull of the brachialis muscle.

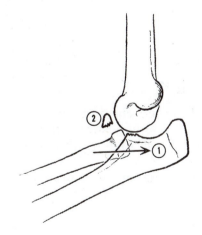

Manipulative Reduction

Note: Before reduction, aspiration of the elbow will relieve pain from hemarthrosis, and a local anesthetic may also be instilled (see page 793).

1. An assistant steadies the arm.
2. The operator makes steady traction in the line of the elbow.
3. While pressure is made over the anterior aspect of the lower arm,
4. The forearm is flexed acutely.

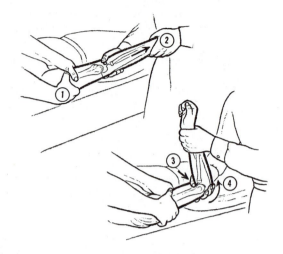

Evaluation of Stability

Following reduction,

1. Gently move the elbow through its normal range to check stability in extension.
2. If elbow is unstable in extension, it must be immobilized for three to four weeks to allow for healing of the anterior disruption. Ordinarily, the fracture of the coronoid process does not affect postreduction stability or require prolonged immobilization.

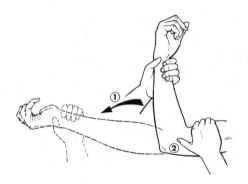

Postreduction X-Ray

1. The radius and the ulna are in their normal anatomic positions in relation to the distal end of the humerus.
2. The fragments of the coronoid are in apposition.

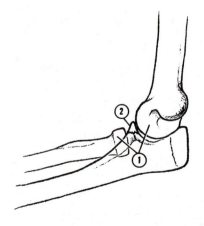

Immobilization

1. Apply a posterior plaster slab from the axilla to the base of the fingers.

2. The forearm is in acute flexion.

3. The forearm is fully supinated.

4. Suspend the arm with a collar and cuff sling.

Note: Avoid the use of a circular cast, which would add considerably to the risk of ischemic muscle injury. Always check carefully before and after reduction for alteration in distal CMS (circulation, motor, sensory) function.

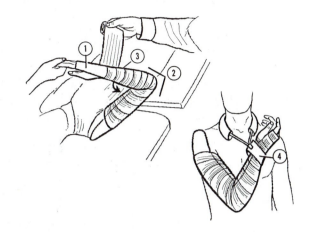

Postreduction Management

Observe the patient carefully for the first 24 to 36 hours for signs of circulatory impairment.

If the elbow was stable immediately after reduction, allow gentle active exercises as soon as swelling subsides, usually in three to five days.

If the elbow was unstable after reduction, treat for soft tissue disruption and immobilize the elbow in flexion for three to four weeks.

Emphasize the patient's need for active exercises after immobilization is discarded.

Never permit passive stretching of the elbow, which has been implicated as a cause of myositis ossificans in the brachialis muscle.

Dislocation of the Elbow with Fracture of the Radial Head

REMARKS

Associated fracture of the radial head is relatively common in elbow dislocations in the adult. In contrast to a capitellar fracture, which displaces superiorly into the radial fossa, radial head fracture displaces distally when associated with an elbow dislocation (see also page 778).

The dislocation should be reduced promptly, whereas the radial head fracture should, in general, be ignored.

Aspirate the elbow at the time local anesthetic is instilled, and evaluate the ranges of elbow motion and forearm rotation after reduction.

Usually the elbow is quite stable and motion is not affected by the radial head fracture. If this is the case, immobilize the elbow for three to five days with a sling and allow the patient to test the elbow with a trial by motion.

If the radial head fragment proves to be blocking motion it may be excised electively, but if the elbow is unstable removal of the fragment too early will increase the elbow's instability. This is especially likely if there is also a fracture of the coronoid process.

The additional trauma inflicted on the elbow during excision of the radial head also tends to add to the likelihood of myositis ossificans.

Little can be gained and much can be lost by early aggressive surgical excision of a radial head fracture associated with elbow dislocation.

Prereduction X-Ray

1. Posterior dislocation of the elbow.
2. Fracture of the radial head with displacement of the fragments.

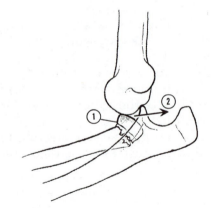

Manipulative Reduction

Note: Aspiration of the elbow will relieve pain from hemarthrosis and allow instillation of local anesthetic (see page 793).

1. While an assistant holds the arm and makes steady countertraction,
2. Grasp the wrist with one hand and make steady traction on the forearm in the position in which it lies.
3. While traction is maintained, apply direct pressure to the radial head fracture.

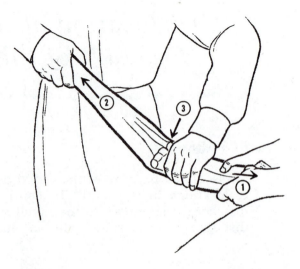

810

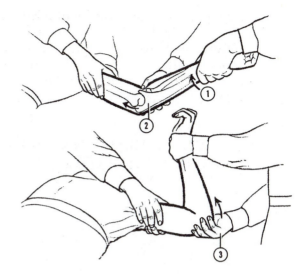

1. Supinate the forearm with direct pressure over the radial head.

2. Push the ulna upward around the end of the humerus.

3. Flex the elbow after reduction of the dislocation to point permitted by soft tissue swelling.

Evaluation of Stability

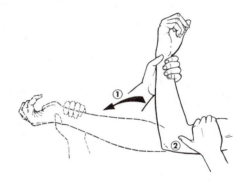

1. Test the stability of the elbow reduction and radial head fracture by gentle flexion and extension after reduction.

2. If elbow is unstable, suspect associated fracture of the coronoid process.

Postreduction X-Ray

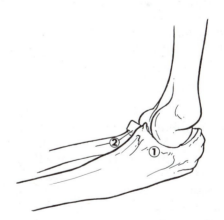

1. Elbow dislocation is reduced.

2. The radial fracture remains angulated at 30 degrees.

Note: Always check carefully before and after reduction for alteration in distal CMS (circulation, motor, sensory) function.

Postreduction Management

If the elbow reduction was stable on testing, immobilize the elbow in a sling for three to five days until swelling subsides. Following this allow the patient to begin active exercises.

Avoid immediate excision of a radial head fracture, especially if there is injury to the brachialis insertion to the coronoid process.

Rarely, a displaced radial head fragment may produce persistent symptoms after trial by motion. It may then be excised electively after disruption from the acute injury subsides, usually after five to seven weeks.

OPERATIVE EXCISION OF DISPLACED, SYMPTOMATIC RADIAL HEAD FRACTURE

Preoperative X-Ray

1. Radial head fragment has displaced sufficiently to block elbow flexion. This is rare.

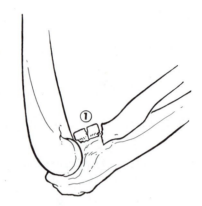

Operative Excision

The operation is done with the patient's arm resting on his chest and the elbow flexed.

INCISION AND EXPOSURE

1. Make an oblique incision extending downward from the lateral epicondyle to the ulna in the interval between the extensor carpi ulnaris and the anconeus muscles.

2. Deepen the incision through the fascia and between the anconeus and extensor carpi ulnaris. This exposes the capsule.

3. Make a longitudinal incision in the capsule to expose the radial head and capitellum.

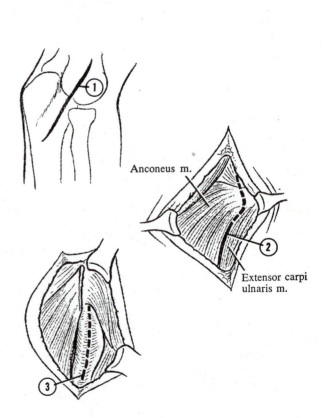

Anconeus m.

Extensor carpi ulnaris m.

EXCISION

1. Identify the orbicular ligament and divide the periosteum immediately above it. Don't strip any of the periosteum from the bone.

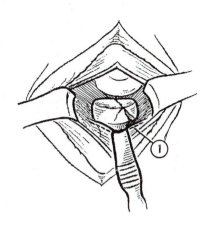

2. Cut the bone with a thin sharp osteotome immediately above the orbicular ligament.

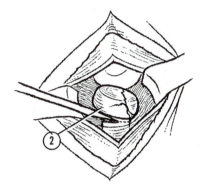

REPAIR

1. Remove any loose pieces of bone and trim away any tags of periosteum attached to the end of the neck.

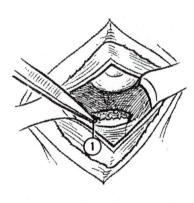

2. Cover the raw stumps of the neck with a purse-string suture passed in the surrounding soft tissue.

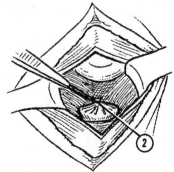

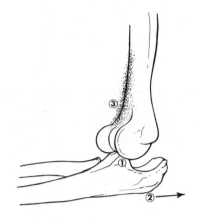

CAUTION

1. Avoid excising any loose fragments from the coronoid process along with a radial head fracture, because this may lead to:
2. Posterior subluxation or
3. Myositis ossificans.

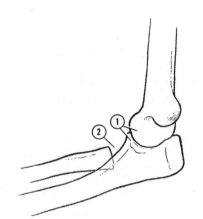

Postreduction X-Ray

1. The articular surfaces of the distal end of the humerus and the ulna are in normal anatomic position.
2. The radial head has been resected.

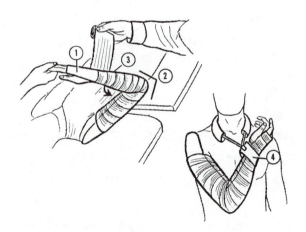

Immobilization

1. Apply a posterior plaster slab from the axilla to the base of the fingers.
2. Flex the forearm as much as is permitted by soft tissue swelling without embarrassing the circulation.
3. Supinate the forearm fully.
4. Suspend the arm with a collar and cuff sling.

Postreduction Management

Maintain plaster immobilization for five to seven days, until postoperative swelling subsides.

Now place the arm in a triangular sling and allow the patient to begin active range of motion.

Discard the sling after seven to ten days.

Avoid passive stretching of the elbow, which has been implicated as a cause of myositis ossificans in the brachialis muscle.

Forward Dislocation of the Elbow with Fracture of the Olecranon

REMARKS

Generally there is anterior subluxation or dislocation of both bones of the forearm. Usually, the radius retains its relationship with the ulna because of the orbicular ligament attachment and moves forward with the ulna.

Occasionally the ligamentous support will be completely disrupted and the radius will dislocate separately from the ulna.

The radial nerve as well as the ulnar nerve may be injured. Always check for nerve as well as circulatory deficit. The injury is reduced readily by applying traction to the extended forearm. Maintenance of reduction requires internal fixation of the fracture in adults.

In children, closed treatment usually permits stable reduction. (See also discussion of Monteggia's fracture, page 959.)

Prereduction X-Ray

1. Comminuted fracture of the olecranon.

2. The radius and ulna have moved together to an anterior position.

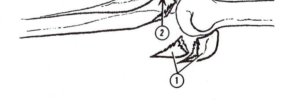

Operative Reduction

EXPOSURE

1. Make a posterolateral incision 7 to 8 cm long beginning 2.5 cm above the olecranon and extending downward along the outer border of the ulna.

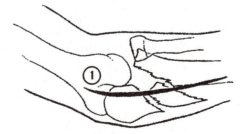

815

Operative Reduction
(Continued)

2. The fracture site is exposed by sharp dissection; loose fragments of bone and blood clots are removed from between the fragments.

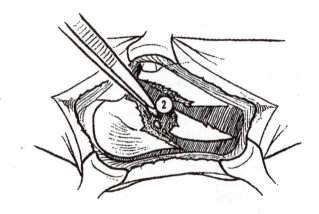

REDUCTION

1. The fracture and dislocation are reduced by traction on the extended forearm.

2. The fragments are held in apposition by towel clips.

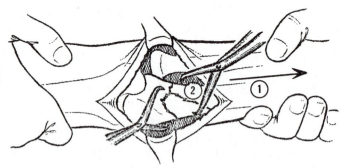

3. The arm is laid across the patient's chest, flexed at 90 degrees.

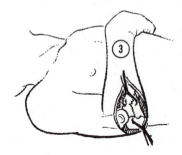

4. Two smooth Steinmann pins are passed through the olecranon fracture and are bent proximally.

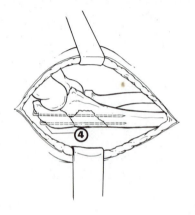

FIXATION

1. Drill a 2-mm to 3-mm hole in the shaft distal to the fracture.

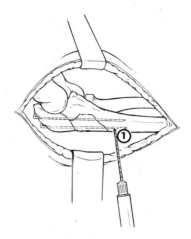

2. Pass a 20-gauge wire through the holes in a figure of eight. This is a tension wire to neutralize the pull of the triceps and to close the fracture through the articular surface.

3. Tighten the wire over the Steinmann pins with a wire tightener.

Note: Test the stability of fixation by flexing and extending the elbow. Obtain an intraoperative x-ray to determine the completeness of reduction.

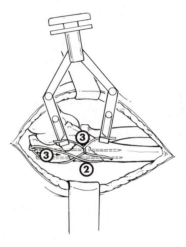

Intraoperative X-Ray

1. The fragments of the olecranon are in normal anatomic alignment.

2. The ulna and radius are in normal positions in relation to the articular surface of the humerus.

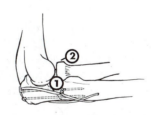

Postoperative Immobilization

1. Apply a bivalved cast or splint.

2. Begin active range of elbow motion when the swelling subsides.

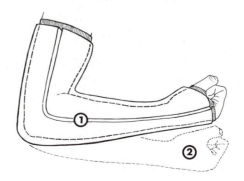

Postreduction Management

The fixation should be sufficiently rigid to permit active range of motion in the elbow within one to two weeks.

Use the protection of the bivalved cast or splint when the patient is not exercising.

Have the patient work especially to regain full extension.

The splint may be changed to a position with the elbow extended at three weeks.

Discard the protective splint by five to six weeks if the fracture position is stable.

Avoid passive stretching of the elbow.

Note: Recovery is slow and the patient must persist in the exercises. The internal fixation need not be removed unless it causes irritation of overlying soft tissues.

Anterior Displacement of the Radius and Ulna (Sideswipe Fracture) with Multiple Fractures

REMARKS

Generally the lesion comprises:
1. Fracture of the shaft of the humerus.
2. Fracture of the olecranon.
3. Fracture of the shaft of the ulna.
4. Anterior displacement of the radius and ulna.

Note: Occasionally the shaft of the radius is fractured or the radial head may be fractured or dislocated

The prime concern is reduction of the dislocation and maintenance of the position.

Lag screw fixation of the olecranon and tension band plating of the ulna shaft fracture generally give effective stability.

Closed treatment is usually possible for the humeral fracture, provided that elbow motion is allowed.

Prereduction X-Ray

1. Fracture of the olecranon.
2. Fracture of the shaft of the ulna.
3. Fracture of the shaft of the humerus.
4. Forward displacement of the radius and ulna.

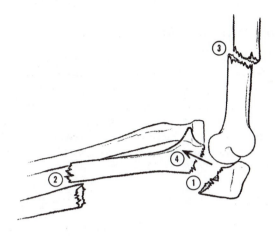

Operative Reduction

1. Make an 8-cm incision directly over the fracture site of the shaft of the ulna.

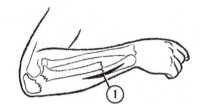

2. Expose the fragments.

3. Make a second posterolateral incision beginning immediately over the tip of the olecranon and extending downward along the outer margin of the ulna.

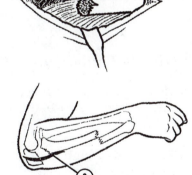

4. Expose the olecranon fracture.

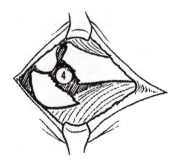

Operative Reduction

1. Reduce the olecranon fracture and radial head dislocation and keep the fracture reduced by holding it with a tenaculum or towel clip.

2. Insert one or preferably two lag screws across the olecranon fracture to stabilize the proximal injury.

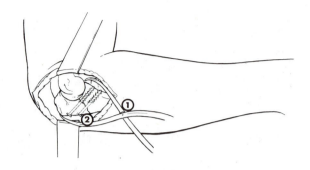

3. Apply a semitubular plate with at least three screws on each side of the fractured shaft to stabilize the distal fracture.

Note: When there is much comminution a primary cancellous bone graft may also be utilized.

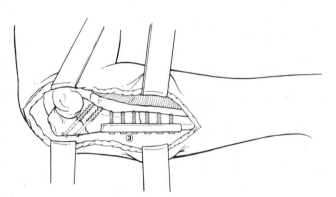

Treat the fracture of the humerus as a separate injury by applying a humeral cast that permits elbow motion within the first seven to ten days.

Immediately Postoperative Immobilization

This is a temporary immobilization for the arm and the forearm to be used until active exercises may be instituted.

1. Apply a long plaster slab extending from the axilla along the posterior aspect of the arm, around the elbow (flexed 90 degrees) and up on the anterior aspect of the arm.

2. Apply a second plaster slab to the forearm in the form of a sugar tong extending around the elbow to the base of the fingers. Fix the slabs with cotton elastic bandages.

3. Support the arm in a triangular sling.

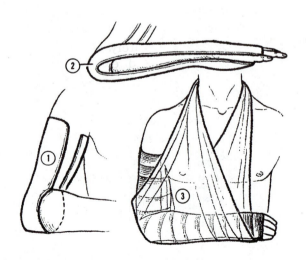

Postimmobilization Management

Maintain the plaster support for three to five days until the postoperative swelling subsides.

Next, place the arm in a humeral cast and the forearm in a sling and allow active range of motion exercises.

Discard the sling by four to six weeks if reduction remains stable. Avoid passive stretching of the elbow.

The humeral cast may be discarded generally by eight to ten weeks when the humeral fracture has consolidated.

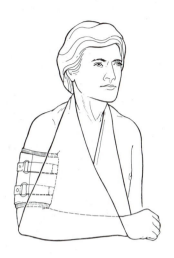

Fracture-Dislocation with Forward Displacement of the Forearm Bones and Rupture of the Orbicular Ligament of the Radius

REMARKS

This lesion is best managed by:

1. Immediate reduction of the forward dislocation of the forearm bones.

2. Reduction and stabilization of the olecranon fracture by tension band wiring.

3. Primary repair of the orbicular ligament; if this is not possible, the ligament should be reconstructed.

Note: This injury is frequently associated with motor paralysis of the radial nerve. Evaluate the motor nerve function carefully, particularly wrist and finger extension, before operation. This injury is usually a neurapraxia and can be corrected by prompt reduction of the fracture-dislocation.

Prereduction X-Ray

1. Fracture of the olecranon.
2. Forward displacement of the ulna and radius.
3. Displacement of the radius from the ulna indicative of a torn orbicular ligament.

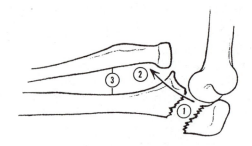

Operative Reduction
(Speed and Boyd)

1. Make a 12-cm incision on the posterolateral aspect of the elbow beginning 2.5 cm above the tip of the olecranon on the lateral margin of the triceps tendon.
2. Extend the incision distally along the dorsal margin of the shaft of the ulna.

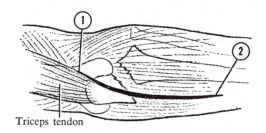

Triceps tendon

3. By subperiosteal dissection, elevate the anconeus and supinator muscles and displace them laterally.

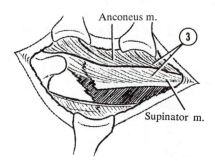

Anconeus m.

Supinator m.

4. Reflect the supinator from the upper fourth of the radius; this exposes the lateral surface of the ulna and the upper fourth of the radius.
5. By sharp dissection inward the entire olecranon can be exposed.
6. Dissect from the forearm a strip of deep fascia 1 cm wide and 10 cm long. The proximal end is left attached to the ulna.

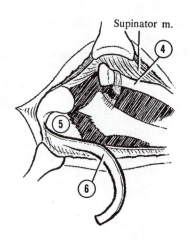

Supinator m.

1. Pass the strip of fascia around the neck of the radius from below.

2. Reduce the fracture of the olecranon and stabilize the fragments with two Steinmann pins and tension band wiring (see page 816).

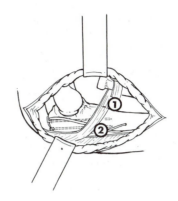

3. Reduce the dislocation of the radial head and pull the orbicular ligament tight and suture it tightly to itself around the neck of the radius.

Note: If the radial head is fractured, it may be removed through this incision and the orbicular ligament may be repaired, if necessary, to stabilize the radial shaft.

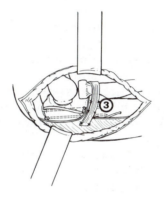

Postreduction X-Ray

1. The fragments of the olecranon are accurately aligned by the Steinmann pins and tension band wiring.

2. The radial head is accurately opposed to the capitellum and to the ulna.

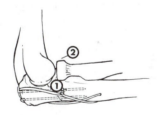

Immobilization

1. Apply a bivalved long arm cast and maintain immobilization for four weeks.

2. After four weeks begin active gentle exercises on an hourly basis. Between exercises protect the limb in a posterior splint.

Note: Return of elbow function comes slowly after this serious injury. Internal fixation need not be removed unless it causes irritation of overlying soft tissues.

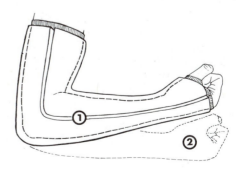

Transcondylar Fracture-Dislocation of the Elbow

REMARKS

This serious injury results from a flexion type mechanism or a direct posterior blow to the flexed elbow causing an intracapsular, transcondylar fracture.

Both distal humeral condyles are displaced as a single unit.

The radius and ulna are dislocated from the fractured condyles.

This frequently is an open injury and commonly causes significant vascular and nerve impingement. Temporary longitudinal traction on the forearm with the elbow in extension will usually restore the radial pulse.

Open reduction and internal fixation should be done promptly to reduce this unstable fracture dislocation and restore satisfactory function to the elbow.

This injury should be distinguished from supracondylar fractures in children and condylar fractures in adults without dislocation which ordinarily do not require operative fixation.

Preoperative X-Ray

1. Intracapsular, transverse fracture above the capitellum and trochlea with anteromedial rotation.

2. The radius and ulna dislocate medially in relation to the condylar fractures.

Note: Severe displacement compromises the brachial artery. The elbow should be temporarily extended to relieve any circulatory embarrassment.

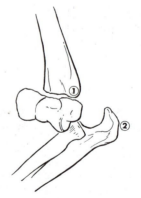

Postreduction X-Ray
(After Grantham and Tietjen)

1. The transcondylar fracture is reduced and is fixed with Steinmann pins introduced from both the medial and lateral condyles and reaching to the opposite cortex. (Lag screws may also be used.)

2. When the condyles are stabilized, the dislocation of the radius and ulna is reduced.

Note: Care should be taken to identify and free the brachial artery and any nerves involved by the fracture at the time of reduction.

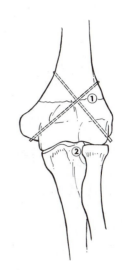

Postoperative Immobilization

The elbow is immobilized at 45 degrees of flexion by means of a posterior splint.

Radial pulse and circulation are monitored closely for the first two days after injury.

Remove the sutures and posterior splint when swelling has subsided, usually by ten days.

If the elbow fracture-dislocation was stable, the patient may begin active exercises by ten days.

If the reduction was unstable, immobilization must be continued for six to eight weeks, but a stiff elbow is likely to result.

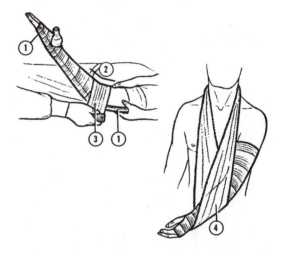

VASCULAR AND NEURAL COMPLICATIONS ASSOCIATED WITH FRACTURES AND DISLOCATIONS OF THE ELBOW JOINT

Vascular Complications

MECHANISM OF INJURY

REMARKS

Vascular complications occur so commonly with direct and indirect injury to the elbow that the circulation should be assumed to be impaired until proven otherwise.

Vascular damage is frequently associated with open fractures and dislocations, which are usually produced by direct blunt trauma, e.g., gunshot wounds, or by penetrating injuries, e.g., glass lacerations of the antecubital region.

The most specific signs of direct arterial injury are pulsatile bleeding from the wound or rapid swelling after injury. Direct violence to the elbow producing these signs warrants close examination for evidence of distal circulatory impairment and prompt exploration of the vessels if evidence is found.

Supracondylar fracture, produced by an indirect mechanism from a fall on the outstretched hand, most often causes circulatory impairment secondary to antecubital swelling rather than to direct arterial insult. Prompt elevation of the limb in traction after a supracondylar fracture will permit venous drainage through the antecubital region and will prevent strangulation of neurovascular structures.

Rarely, reduction of the supracondylar fracture will cause arterial insufficiency and loss of radial pulse owing to impalement of the brachial artery. Be alert to this possibility after reduction, because it indicates the need to decrease elbow flexion and possibly to explore the artery.

Elbow dislocation, particularly open dislocation, is more likely than supracondylar fracture to lacerate the brachial artery directly. Loss of radial pulse with signs of impending ischemia that persist after reduction of the elbow dislocation indicates the need for surgical exploration of the artery without delay.

Direct Injuries

These cause direct arterial damage:

1. Glass laceration is the most common cause of arterial injury in this area, with or without fracture.

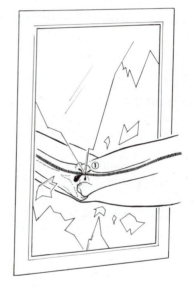

1. Direct blunt trauma to the elbow causing
2. Open fracture or dislocation commonly damages brachial artery.

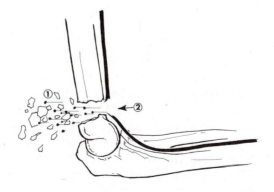

Supracondylar Fracture

This damages the circulation indirectly, through swelling.

1. Artery is usually intact.

2. Soft tissue swelling from the fracture occludes the venous return from the forearm. When venous pressure within the forearm compartment approaches the diastolic pressure,

3. Arterial flow is occluded and neuromuscular ischemia ensues.

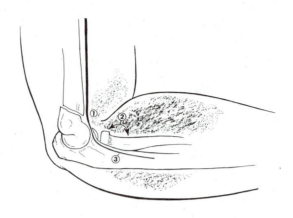

4. Rarely, neurovascular structures are actually entrapped by the fracture and circulation is worsened by reduction.

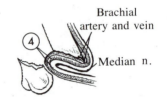

Brachial artery and vein

Median n.

Elbow Dislocation

The brachial artery is most likely to be damaged with open dislocation.

1. Wide displacement of ulna from humerus.

2. This is usually associated with an open wound and direct injury to the antecubital region.

3. The lacertus fibrosis is torn.

4. The common flexor muscles are avulsed.

5. The extreme force of dislocation tears the artery.

6. The median nerve may also be injured or entrapped.

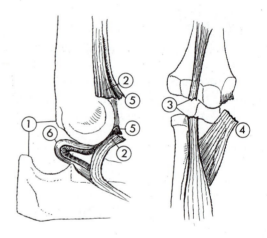

DIAGNOSIS OF ARTERIAL INJURIES IN THE UPPER LIMB: THE "P" SIGNS

REMARKS

The most specific sign of arterial injury is pulsatile bleeding or rapid swelling. Even a history of pulsatile bleeding associated with an open or penetrating wound to the elbow should indicate the diagnosis.

The earliest sign of impending, progressive ischemia of the forearm muscle is pain on passive extension of the patient's fingers. Ischemic muscle causes pain, whether in the heart or in the forearm, by the accumulation of cellular breakdown products, particularly potassium, which provoke pain impulses and further muscle contraction. Passive stretching of the fingers brings the irritated, ischemic state of the muscle to clinical attention.

The absence of a radial pulse may or may not be significant, particularly after indirect injury, e.g., supracondylar fracture. Noninvasive methods of measuring blood flow such as the Doppler flowmeter technique, give the most reliable, objective information and should be readily available to evaluate all questionable cases.

Invasive arteriography may occasionally be helpful in evaluating elbow injuries in the adult, but after supracondylar fracture in a child, this arterial study itself may produce sufficient vasospasm to impair peripheral circulation.

The other "P" signs of arterial injury besides pulsatile bleeding, pain, and pulselessness are paresthesias and paralysis indicative of peripheral nerve ischemia. Partial ischemia causes the nerve to be hyperirritable and produces painful paresthesias. Total ischemia causes nerve conduction to cease promptly. The diagnosis of arterial injury should be made long before these clinical signs develop.

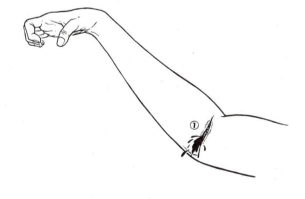

"P" Signs of Arterial Injury

1. Pulsatile bleeding or rapid swelling about the elbow is most specific.

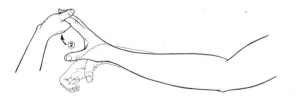

2. Pain on passive extension indicates impending forearm muscle ischemia.

"P" Signs of Arterial Injury (*Continued*)

3. Pulselessness should be evaluated by Doppler flowmeter.

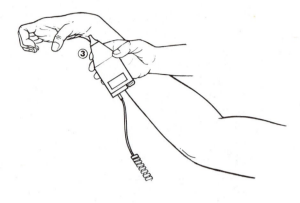

4. Paresthesia and paralysis due to nerve ischemia are early signs only with a sudden major arterial interruption such as axillary artery thrombosis.

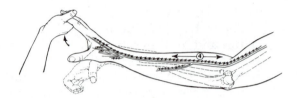

Note: In crush injuries to the arm, distal radial flow may be normal despite progressive development of forearm compartment syndrome. If the forearm is tense and swollen and the patient has pain with passive finger extension, measure intracompartmental pressure in both volar and dorsal compartments with a needle manometer to evaluate the need for fasciotomy (see page 64).

MANAGEMENT

REMARKS

If flowmeter measurements indicate significant impairment of circulation, the next step depends on the nature of the injury to the vessels.

In direct injuries, lacerations, open dislocations, or penetrating wounds to the elbow, the likelihood of significant arterial injury is so high that surgical exploration should not be delayed.

Arteriorrhaphy or vein grafting is usually necessary with direct injury to the vessel, depending on the extent and nature of the damage. Ligation of the brachial artery, which has sometimes been recommended, carries a 25 per cent risk of producing peripheral gangrene, especially in the adult.

In an indirect injury, most typically a supracondylar fracture in a child, with less than six hours of ischemia, a period of elevation and traction for one to two hours will usually diminish swelling sufficiently to permit adequate distal flow.

Forearm fasciotomy is indicated when circulation does not return after elevation or if signs of impending ischemia are present for six hours or more after supracondylar fracture.

The fasciotomy must completely decompress the ischemic muscles and nerves to prevent residual contracture.

Direct measurement of intracompartmental pressures in both the volar and dorsal compartments of the forearm with needle manometer is valuable to determine the effectiveness of fasciotomy (see page 64).

In approximately half the cases, a dorsal fasciotomy should be performed in addition to the volar fasciotomy.

Arterial repair is usually unnecessary after indirect injury, except for the rare situation of impalement of the artery by the fractured bone.

MANAGEMENT OF CIRCULATORY IMPAIRMENT WITHIN SIX HOURS OF SUPRACONDYLAR FRACTURE

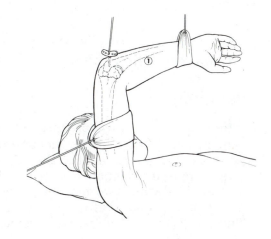

Ten to fifteen per cent of supracondylar fractures will cause loss or diminution of radial pulse and swelling of the forearm.

Most cases respond to elevation and traction.

1. Use skeletal traction or

2. Side arm traction.

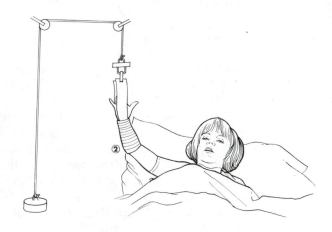

Subsequent Management

Circulatory impairment should be relieved in one to two hours. Monitor the radial pulse closely by Doppler flowmeter, and continue traction until swelling subsides (three to five days).

When the swelling has diminished, the fracture may be reduced under light anesthesia and the skeletal pin may be removed (see page 759).

1. Apply a posterior slab with
2. The elbow flexed 90 degrees.
3. The forearm is pronated or supinated, depending on the initial (varus or valgus) displacement of the fracture.
4. A collar-and-cuff sling supports the arm.

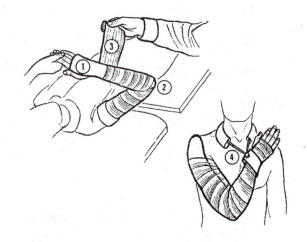

MANAGEMENT OF ISCHEMIA SIX HOURS OR MORE AFTER SUPRACONDYLAR FRACTURE: OPERATIVE MANAGEMENT

REMARKS

Indications for prompt surgical intervention are loss of pulse, as demonstrated by flowmeter measurement, after direct injury, laceration, open fracture, or gunshot to the elbow.

Indirect injuries, such as supracondylar fracture in which distal flow is not regained after two hours of elevation or in which ischemia is still manifest six hours after injury should be surgically explored. The objective is to decompress the forearm by fasciotomy while exploring the brachial artery.

Permanent neuromuscular damage will ensue if the limb is completely ischemic for more than six hours.

Preoperative Care

Avoid direct application of ice to the ischemic forearm, because temperatures below 65° F (18.1° C) may inflict cold injury on top of the ischemic injury.

Use intravenous broad-spectrum antibiotics preoperatively and postoperatively for a total of 36 hours or longer if indicated by the degree of wound contamination and muscle injury.

Life-threatening cardiorespiratory and central nervous system injuries must be cared for and shock must be treated prior to embarking on the peripheral artery exploration.

Avoid systemic heparinization. Local injection of heparin (10,000 units in 100 cc saline) into the divided or traumatized artery at the time of exploration gives adequate anticoagulation.

Techniques of Fasciotomy for Indirect Injuries

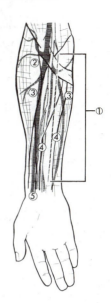

1. Incision should extend from elbow to wrist. Avoid placing incision directly over distal tendons and nerves.

2. Incise deep fascia as far distally as necessary to evacuate hematoma and decompress the forearm muscles.

3. Open epimysium if the muscles are still tight.

4. Decompress the deep muscle compartments and nerves.

5. Monitor the distal radial artery flow by palpation or flowmeter, and explore the brachial artery if the distal flow is still inadequate.

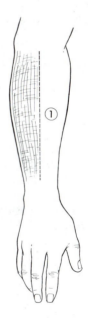

1. Dorsal fasciotomy should also be done if the volar decompression does not produce sufficient lowering of dorsal compartment pressure.

What to Do with the Brachial Artery

Surgery of the arterial lesion should be carried out by a vascular consultant if at all possible.

The findings to be expected include segmental or diffuse arteriospasm, severe contusion with thrombosis, and complete laceration of the vessel.

Local arteriospasm may respond to topical 2.5 to 5 per cent Papavarine.

Most often the vessel should be opened by a small arteriotomy and a Fogarty catheter should be used to dilate the area of spasm and to remove the thrombosed intima.

Resection with end-to-end anastomosis may be effective for laceration or contusion of the vessel, but be certain that all the damaged area is resected prior to repair, because the extent of vascular damage may be greater than is initially apparent. Use a reversed saphenous vein graft if there is any tension on the anastomosis.

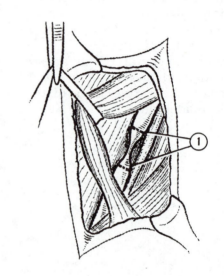

ARTERIOSPASM

1. The segment of brachial artery shows marked arteriospasm.

2. A Fogarty catheter is passed across the site of spasm to dilate the vessel and
3. To remove the thrombus causing the vasoconstriction.

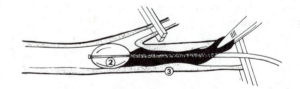

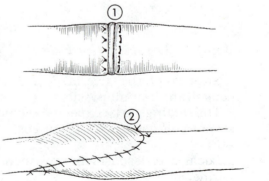

RECONSTITUTION OF THE ARTERY BY ANASTOMOSIS

1. End-to-end anastomosis.
2. Another type of anastomosis suitable for small arteries.

Management of the Fracture

Supracondylar fracture associated with ischemic injury may be immobilized by percutaneous Kirschner wires.

1. The Kirschner wires are introduced through the lateral epicondyle.

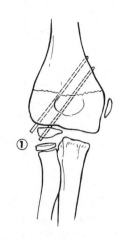

2. The limb is supported in a posterior splint with slight elbow flexion.

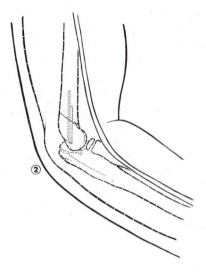

Postoperative Management

If the circulation has been restored by fasciotomy, elevation of the limb will help venous return.

Continue to monitor distal flow with hourly flowmeter measurements for the first 24 to 36 hours.

Fasciotomy incision may be closed by seven days, as soon as the swelling subsides. A secondary closure is preferable to skin grafting in the forearm.

The patient may begin gentle active range-of-motion exercises after three weeks, protecting the limb in a sling when not exercising.

The fixation wires may be removed at six to eight weeks after fracture.

Neural Complications

Neural injuries are more common complications of elbow fractures and dislocations (10 to 20 per cent of cases) but cause less permanent impairment than vascular disruptions. Neural injuries are often concomitant with vascular injuries.

The radial and median nerves are most frequently involved.

Two or all three nerves may be implicated.

Partial lesions are by far more common than complete lesions.

The median nerve may be displaced posteriorly in posterior dislocations and in supracondylar fractures with wide separation of the fragments. In this position it may prevent reduction.

The median nerve is known for its ability to escape injury in supracondylar fractures, even with marked displacement of the fragments.

As a rule, spontaneous recovery occurs in partial lesions.

Neurologic deficit without vascular embarrassment is not an indication for operation.

Exploration of the nerve or nerves may rarely be indicated, if there is no clinical or electromyographic evidence of recovery within six to eight weeks after fracture.

RECURRENT DISLOCATION OF THE ELBOW JOINT

REMARKS

Recurrent dislocation is a surprisingly infrequent sequela (1 to 2 per cent of injuries) from elbow luxation. It should be distinguished from chronic and congenital dislocation.

Recurrent dislocation is most likely to follow injury to the child's lax elbow and may be associated with displaced fragments after medial epicondylar or other fractures.

The second most common cause of instability is laxity of the postero-lateral capsule. This capsule with its ligament structure ordinarily stabilizes the elbow in full extension but is susceptible to avulsion from its superior attachment at the time of dislocation.

Careful testing of stability after initial reduction of the elbow and radiographic assessment of fracture fragments, especially in a child's medial epicondylar fracture, will demonstrate the occasional dislocation likely to recur.

Not all elbow instability requires surgical treatment.

Subluxation of the radial head may be easily reduced by the patient and may cause only occasional problems of "locking" which should not be mistaken for osteochondritis dissecans.

In the typical case of recurrent dislocation in a child or adolescent, recurrence is infrequent and may cease as normal growth tightens the capsule and ligament structure.

Surgical repair is indicated for dislocations recurring frequently with trivial injury in the older adolescent and adult.

The simplest, most direct way of improving stability is by repairing the lateral ligamentous and capsular laxity (Osborne and Cotterill).

Surgical Repair (after Osborne and Cotterill)

INCISION AND EXPOSURE

1. An incision is made on the lateral side of the elbow from the lateral epicondyle distal to the annular ligament.

2. The elbow is opened behind the lateral ligament, and any fragments of bone are removed.

3. The bone of the lateral condyle is cleared of soft tissue and is scarified.

4. Two transverse drill holes are made in the lateral condyle and heavy nylon sutures are passed through these holes.

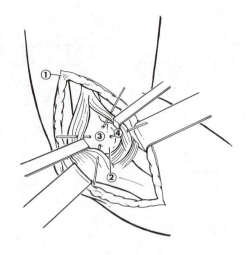

REPAIR

1. The posterolateral capsule is tied down tightly into the scarified site by the suture.

Note: A similar repair may occasionally be necessary for an unstable medial ligament.

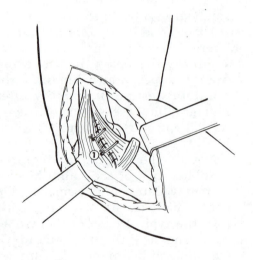

Postoperative Management

Apply a plaster splint with the elbow flexed 40 degrees.

The splint is removed at four weeks and the patient is allowed to begin active range-of-motion exercises.

Avoid any passive stretching exercises.

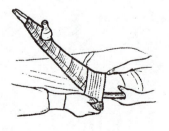

OLD UNREDUCED DISLOCATIONS OF THE ELBOW JOINT

REMARKS

This is a serious and difficult lesion to manage. It usually occurs in individuals who have neglected to obtain medical care because of alcoholism, psychosis, or geographic distance.

Chronic traumatic dislocation may rarely be seen in children, but congenital dislocation is more common and is usually bilateral.

If it can be reliably determined that the dislocation is less than four weeks old, closed reduction using skeletal traction should be attempted.

If the injury is more than four weeks old, open reduction is necessary, and the result is likely to be a permanently stiff elbow.

Open reduction should be reserved for children and adults with significant preoperative pain who are likely to benefit from the extensive operation to achieve reduction.

Elbow arthroplasty, either resectional or replacement, should be considered as an alternative to open reduction in the older adult with chronic symptomatic dislocation.

Total elbow arthroplasty must be reserved for the patient likely to cooperate with long-term postoperative care, which frequently rules out a number of patients presenting with chronic dislocation.

The management of this problem requires astute judgment of the patient's needs as well as careful operative technique.

CLOSED REDUCTION OF UNREDUCED DISLOCATION

This method can be used for dislocations less than four weeks old.

Reduction in Traction

1. Olecranon pin is inserted, and
2. Traction is begun with elbow in extension.

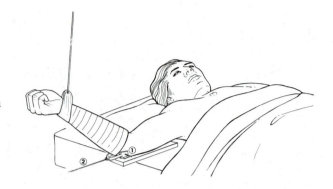

3. When radius and ulna have been pulled to the level of the humerus, the position in traction is slowly changed and elbow flexion is accomplished.

Note: General anesthesia is necessary to achieve the flexion-reduction. If reduction in traction fails, open reduction may be carried out.

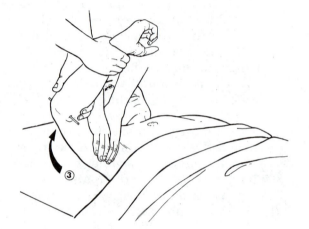

Immobilization after Reduction in Traction

Remove the traction pin and
1. Apply a posterior plaster slab from the axilla to the base of the fingers.
2. The forearm is in acute flexion.
3. The forearm is supinated.
4. Suspend the arm with a collar-and-cuff sling.

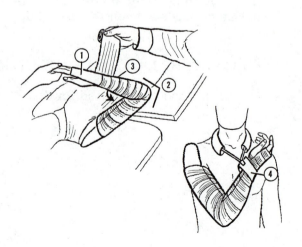

Postreduction Management

Maintain fixation by plaster for three weeks.

Now place the arm in a triangular sling holding arm at 90 degrees flexion.

Discard the sling after seven to ten days.

Institute active exercises for the elbow.

Avoid passive stretching of the elbow.

OPEN REDUCTION OF UNREDUCED DISLOCATION

REMARKS

This method may occasionally be useful in cases in which reduction by traction has failed.

It is especially applicable to children with old, symptomatic, unreduced dislocations.

In general, the results are not as good in adults as they are in children.

The procedure should not be carried out when there is evidence of myositis ossificans. In this instance, the patient should be allowed to regain whatever motion he can with active exercises for several months. If the result is still unsatisfactory because of pain and severe limitation of motion, an arthroplasty may be considered (see page 845).

Surgical Procedure (Technique of Speed)

Note: This technique employs a V–Y lengthening of the triceps to achieve reduction. Temporary transarticular pin fixation is also used.

INCISION AND EXPOSURE

1. Make an incision over the posterolateral aspect of the arm beginning 10 cm above the olecranon in the midline; extend the incision to the tip of the olecranon. Then continue outward over the external condyle of the humerus and the head of the radius, and for 5 cm on the forearm.

2. By sharp dissection, elevate the edges of the incision, exposing the insertion of the triceps muscle and the posterior aspect of the elbow.

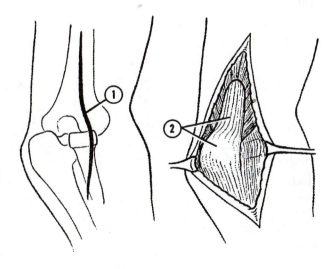

Surgical Procedure (Technique of Speed) (Continued)

1. Dissect out the proximal end of the tendinous aponeurosis of the triceps muscle and reflect it downward.

2. Make an incision in the midline of the triceps muscle down to the humerus, extending from 8 cm up the shaft to the reflection of the capsule around the articular surface.

3. Strip free by subperiosteal dissection the distal end of the humerus, anteriorly and posteriorly, from all muscular attachments.

4. Separate, close to the bone, the attachments of the joint capsule around the humeral condyles.

Note: On the ulnar side, identify the ulnar nerve and retract it out of its groove.

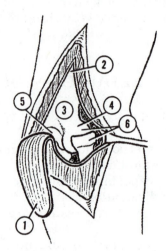

5. Remove all excess callus and fibrous tissue from the olecranon fossa and posterior aspect of the humerus.

6. Carry out the dissection laterally far enough to expose the complete capitellum and the head of the radius.

7. Lateral view used to exhibit the extent of the dissection that is occasionally necessary in order to effect a reduction.

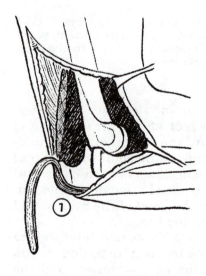

REDUCTION

Reduction is achieved by:

1. Rotating the forearm while

2. Downward and backward pressure is made over the capitellum to engage the radial head on the capitellum.

3. The coronoid process is then slipped forward over the trochlea to complete the reduction.

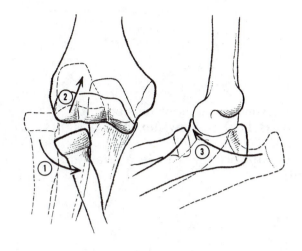

FIXATION

1. Transfix the olecranon to the humerus with a heavy, smooth Steinmann pin.

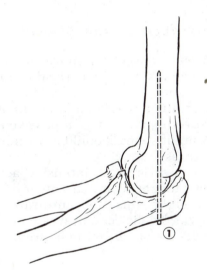

2. Approximate the muscles and periosteum on the posterior aspect of the humerus.

3. Suture the fascia over the head of the radius.

4. Suture the aponeurosis of the triceps with a V–Y lengthening to overcome the shortening produced by the chronic dislocation.

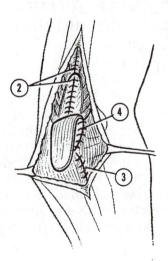

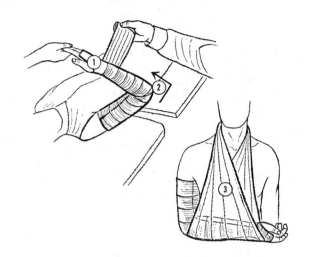

Immobilization

1. Apply a posterior plaster slab.
2. Hold the elbow flexed at a right angle.
3. Support the arm in a triangular sling.

Postreduction Management

After two weeks, remove the transfixion wire and place the arm in a triangular sling during the day and in the posterior plaster splint during the night.

Institute a regulated program of active exercises.

Never employ forceful passive maneuvers to increase motion.

A night splint should be worn for two or three months to prevent contractures.

Progress is slow; intensive active exercises, always within the patient's tolerance of pain, must be continued for months.

In adults, this procedure rarely produces a satisfactory result, especially if the dislocation was more than six weeks old. In general, better results are obtained in children.

ALTERNATE METHOD: RESECTIONAL ELBOW ARTHROPLASTY

REMARKS

Resectional arthroplasty often produces better results for old unreduced dislocations in adults than open reduction.

Elbow resectional arthroplasty at present is preferable to artificial joint replacements for symptomatic problems of chronic dislocations. The operation usually affords good relief of pain and a useful increase in both hinge motion and forearm rotation of the elbow.

The major complication of resectional arthroplasty is elbow instability, which can be diminished by a period of transarticular pin fixation and cast immobilization following the operative procedure.

Because of this tendency to instability, arthroplasty should be avoided in persons who do heavy labor or who are crutch dependent (i.e., rheumatoid arthritis patients).

Do not perform this operation in the presence of traumatic myositis ossificans; wait until the process has subsided completely.

Resectional Arthroplasty of the Elbow Joint

INCISION AND EXPOSURE

1. Make a posterolateral incision beginning 10 cm above the olecranon in the midline; it continues to the tip of the olecranon and then continues laterally over the external condyle of the humerus and the radial head onto the forearm for 5 cm.

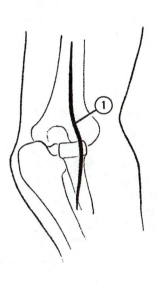

2. Elevate by sharp dissection the edges of the incision sufficiently to expose the insertion of the triceps, the posterior aspect of the elbow, and the posterior aspect of the upper end of the ulna.

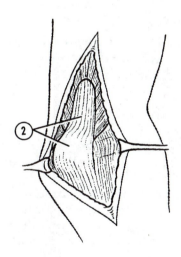

Resectional Arthroplasty of the Elbow Joint (Continued)

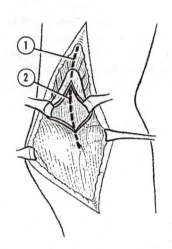

1. Divide longitudinally in the midline the triceps muscle and its aponeurosis.

2. Deepen the incision through the periosteum of the humerus and the posterior capsule and then along the lateral border of the olecranon process.

3. Strip by subperiosteal dissection the triceps muscle from the lower end of the humerus for 5 cm.

4. Subperiosteal dissection is continued on each side, dividing all muscular and capsular attachments to the humeral condyles and exposing the humeral condyles and the radial head.

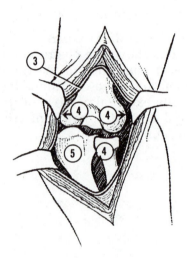

Note: During dissection on the inner side of the joint, the ulnar nerve should be identified, removed from its bed, and retracted to a safe position.

5. By subperiosteal dissection, expose the olecranon and the upper end of the shaft of the ulna.

With a sharp osteotome and power drilling:

1. Remove bone from the lower end of the humerus at the level of the epicondyle.

2. Excise a sufficient amount of bone from the olecranon, coronoid process, and radial head to permit reduction but still allow an articulation.

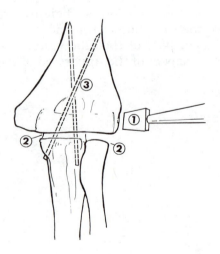

3. Maintain reduction by smooth Steinmann pins that cross from the olecranon into the humerus.

After thoroughly irrigating the wound with antibiotic solution, close the ligamentous and capsular layers snugly.

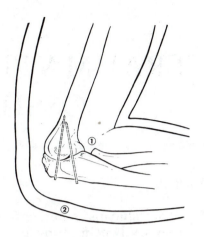

Immobilization

1. Maintain the elbow in 90 degrees of flexion and in neutral rotation by means of the two Steinmann pins.

2. Use a posterior plaster-of-Paris splint for additional immobilization.

Postoperative Management

Remove the cast and Kirschner wire fixation at four weeks and apply a triangular sling.

The patient continues in a sling for an additional two months while gradually exercising the elbow.

Institute an intensive program of active exercises.

Range of motion will slowly improve for many months after the operation.

TRAUMATIC MYOSITIS OSSIFICANS

Myositis ossificans is poorly named, because it is neither a myositis nor a primary bone-forming process. Rather, this lesion is characterized by a fibrous, osseous, and cartilaginous metaplasia in soft tissue that may or may not involve bone and periosteum.

This reactive lesion is apt to follow trauma to the anterior aspect of the elbow, as a result of extensive initial injury, overly aggressive surgical intervention, or passive stretching "therapeutic" exercises.

Radiographic evidence of this process is evident usually by three to four weeks after the injury but may take four to six months to completely mature.

Myositis ossificans has become less common after elbow fractures and dislocations than in the past, as the hazards of overvigorous passive stretching have become known.

The relationship of the brachialis muscle substance to the anterior capsule makes the muscle area a prime location for reactive calcification. Any insult to this area during the recovery phase is likely to exacerbate the calcification response to trauma.

In elbow dislocation, surgical excision of fragments performed immediately after injury often may provoke myositis ossificans.

Passive stretching exercises also incite calcification and subsequent blockage of elbow motion. Early (within three to five days) active motion within the patient's tolerance is a more physiological method of regaining elbow function and less likely to promote reactive calcification.

Myositis ossificans should not be confused with calcification in the medial or lateral capsule, which is seen frequently on x-ray after recovery from elbow dislocation but does not usually affect motion (see also page 89).

Appearance on X-Ray

1. Massive calcification in the region of brachialis muscle following dislocation.

2. This calcification is not sharply demarcated and exhibits no lamellae of ossified bone.

Note: This is usually seen within three to four weeks after the injury but takes up to four to six months to completely mature.

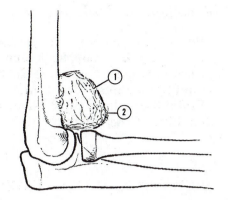

MANAGEMENT

Early reduction of the dislocation and fracture minimizes formation of reactive myositis ossificans.

Avoid all passive stretching of the elbow.

Allow the patient to use the arm freely and actively but always within the limits of painless motion.

Prohibit any form of vigorous physical therapy, especially massage and manipulation or weight lifting to stretch the elbow.

With this program the area of hematoma in the brachialis muscle will gradually resorb and the bony mass will generally shrink in size.

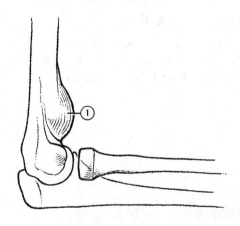

X-Ray After Active Exercise

1. After active exercise the bony mass is reduced considerably in size.

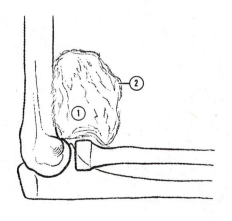

X-Ray After Passive Stretching

1. The ossification has enlarged in the brachialis anticus region.

2. The mass has become poorly demarcated and irregular in shape.

Management While the Process Is Still Active

Put the arm at complete rest for seven to ten days in a posterior plaster slab holding the elbow at 90 degrees of flexion.

After this period, remove all fixation and allow free use of the arm within the painless arcs of motion.

Prohibit any form of physical therapy, especially massage or passive stretching of the elbow.

OPERATIVE MANAGEMENT

Indications

Operative intervention is justified only after the bone is mature and only if the lesion acts as a mechanical block to normal function of the elbow.

Wait at least six months before advising operative excision.

Preoperative X-Ray

1. The bone on the anterior aspect of the elbow is smooth and regular, and it exhibits mature bony lamellae.

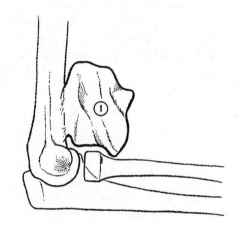

Postoperative X-Ray

1. The bony mass has been completely removed. Mechanical blocking of the joint has been eliminated.

Note: Recurrences of bone formation are not likely to occur if the operation is delayed until the new bone has become mature; on the other hand, violent reformation of new bone may take place if surgical interference occurs during the immature phase of the myositis ossificans process.

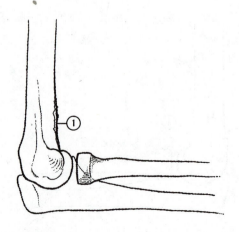

OTHER FRACTURES, DISLOCATIONS, AND INJURIES ABOUT THE ELBOW

Fractures of the Olecranon and Separation of the Olecranon Epiphysis

REMARKS

Anatomic reduction of fractures of the olecranon is essential for good function and triceps strength. In this respect a fractured olecranon affects elbow function much like a fractured patella affects knee function.

Operative reduction is indicated in any fracture in which the fragments separate when the forearm is brought to 90 degrees of flexion. This applies even if the fragments are in apposition when the arm is extended.

Operative excision is feasible for comminuted fractures, but most can be reduced and held with internal fixation.

Separation of the olecranon epiphysis encountered in a patient between the ages of 10 and 16 years is comparable to fracture of the olecranon and is treated in a like manner.

FRACTURES OF THE OLECRANON WITHOUT DISPLACEMENT

Appearance on X-Ray

1. Complete oblique fracture of the olecranon with no displacement of the fragments.

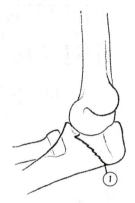

2. Comminuted fracture of the olecranon with no displacement of the fragments.

Note: X-ray taken with elbow flexed 90 degrees shows no displacement and indicates that triceps aponeurosis is intact and prolonged immobilization is unnecessary.

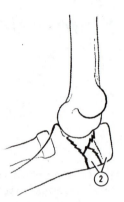

Immobilization

Apply a posterior splint with the elbow in slight (30 degrees) flexion to relax the triceps.

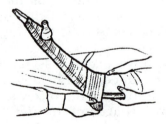

Postimmobilization Management

Treat this undisplaced fracture symptomatically.

When the swelling and the initial pain of the injury subside, usually by five to seven days, begin guarded exercises through range of elbow motion.

Splint may be discarded after three weeks, but the patient should avoid heavy lifting or pushing with the arm for three months.

FRACTURES OF THE OLECRANON WITH DISPLACEMENT

Appearance on X-Ray

1. Complete oblique fractures with separation of the fragments.

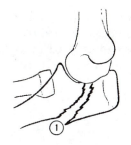

2. Comminuted fracture with separation of fragments. As much as 60 per cent of the comminuted olecranon may be excised without disturbing stability, but internal fixation is usually preferable to operative excision.

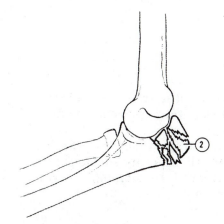

3. Separation of the olecranon epiphysis.

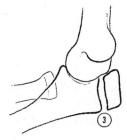

Operative Reduction

1. Make a posterolateral incision 8 cm long, beginning 2.5 cm above the olecranon and extending downward along the outer border of the ulna.

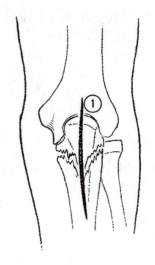

2. Remove loose fragments of bone and blood clots from between the main fragments.

3. Make a transverse drill channel just distal to the fracture surface of the distal fragment if tension-band wiring is planned.

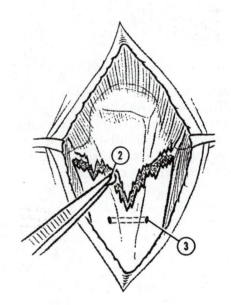

Fixation

1. The fragments are held in apposition by a tenaculum.

2. The fracture is fixed with two lag screws or

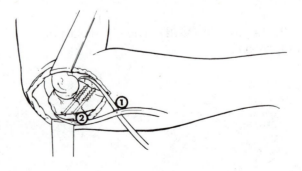

854

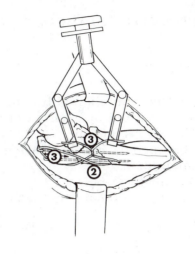

2. Two Steinmann pins and

3. A tension-band wire fixation to neutralize the pull of the triceps.

Note: Test stability of fixation by flexing and extending the elbow. Obtain intra-operative x-ray to determine completeness of reduction.

Intraoperative X-Ray

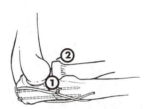

1. The fragments of the olecranon are in normal anatomic alignment.

2. The ulna and the radius are in normal position in relationship to the articular surface of the humerus.

Immobilization

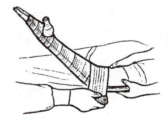

Apply a posterior plaster splint.

Immobilize the elbow in slight (30 degrees) flexion.

Note: Elevate the limb for three days postoperatively, until swelling subsides.

Postreduction Management

Begin guarded active exercises when swelling has subsided and incision has healed (five to seven days).

Continue with wearing of the protective splint for three weeks whenever the patient is not exercising the elbow.

Splint may be discarded after three to four weeks, depending on stability of fixation.

The patient should avoid heavy lifting or pushing with the arm for at least three months.

ALTERNATE METHOD: EXCISION OF THE OLECRANON

REMARKS

Isolated comminuted fractures without injury to ulnar or radial head may be treated by excision of the olecranon and secure reattachment of the triceps tendon.

This method is useful when internal fixation has failed because of comminution.

As much as 60 to 70 per cent of the olecranon may be excised, provided that the remaining portion of the articulation is undamaged.

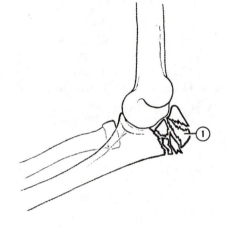

Appearance on X-Ray

1. Severe comminution of the proximal half of the olecranon.

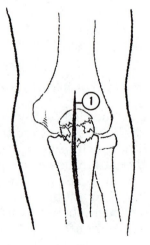

Excision of the Olecranon

1. Expose the fracture site through an 8-cm posterolateral incision.

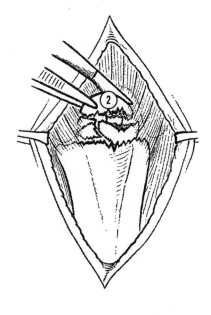

2. By sharp dissection remove the fragments of bone.

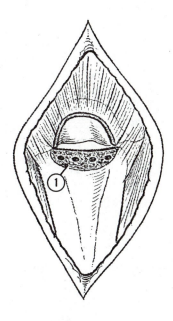

1. Trim the remaining proximal surface of the ulna and make several drill holes in the ulna.

2. Approximate the triceps tendon to the raw surface of the ulna with nonresorbable mattress sutures passed through the drill holes.

3. Anchor the edges of the triceps tendon to the adjacent soft tissues on each side of the ulna.

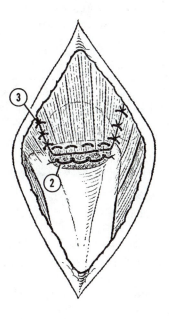

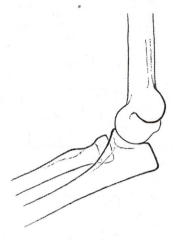

Postexcision X-Ray

All bony fragments have been removed; the end of the ulna is smooth.

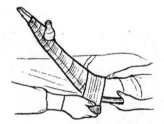

Immobilization

1. Apply a posterior splint with
2. The elbow in slight (30 degrees) flexion to relax the triceps.

Postoperative Management

Remove the cast at the end of three weeks.
Apply a triangular sling for seven to ten more days.
Institute a program of active exercises for the elbow, and do not permit passive forceful movements.

Fractures of the Head and Neck of the Radius (in Adults)

REMARKS

These fractures are most often produced by an indirect mechanism, usually a fall on the outstretched hand with the elbow extended and the forearm supinated. Alternately, a direct blow to the lateral aspect of the elbow may fracture the exposed radial head.

The force transmitted along the radius impacts the radial head against the capitellum with the result that the weaker radial head or radial neck fractures.

Most often the fracture remains undisplaced or displaces distally. If fracture fragments displace into the radial fracture, the capitellum has usually been fractured rather than the radial head.

In adults the radial articular surface is frequently involved, while in children the weaker radial physis or plate fails without involving the articular surface.

The most common fracture, the undisplaced type, is best treated symptomatically by aspiration of the hemarthrosis, temporary sling support, and prompt resumption of active exercise to regain elbow motion.

Although closed reduction of the displaced fracture in an adult is useless, it is the treatment of choice for the angulated fracture of the radial neck in a child.

The adult's displaced fracture may be treated by an early trial of motion, followed by operative excision for the occasional fracture in which loose fragments impede motion.

Operative excision of bone fragments should be avoided in a child's immature elbow because growth arrest and deformity as well as limitation of elbow motion inevitably follow bone excision.

Occasionally the distal radioulnar joint is disrupted at the time of or subsequent to the proximal radial fracture. Silastic replacement of the proximal radius is useful to stabilize the injured proximal and distal joints under these circumstances.

X-Ray Diagnosis of Radial Head Fractures

These are common fractures and frequently are not recognized on cursory x-ray examination.

Any adult who falls and complains of pain in the elbow should be considered to have a radial head fracture until proved otherwise.

1. Most often these are linear cracks which may be seen only with an oblique view of the proximal radial head.

Note: Fragments that displace superiorly are produced by fractures of the capitellum and not from radial head fractures (see page 778).

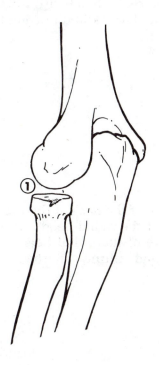

TYPES OF FRACTURES TREATED BY A TRIAL OF MOTION (AFTER ADLER AND SHAFTAN)

1. Fissure fracture of the head of the radius and fracture of the neck without displacement of fragments.

2. Fracture of the neck of the radius without displacement of the radial head.

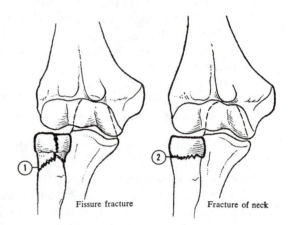

Fissure fracture   Fracture of neck

1. Marginal fracture of the lateral portion of the radial head with some outward displacement of the fragment.

2. Marginal fracture of the medial portion of the radial head with inward displacement. The radio-ulnar joint is involved.

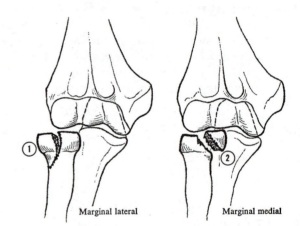

Marginal lateral   Marginal medial

1. Fracture of the neck of the radius with tilting of the radial head.

2. Fracture of the radial head with impaction and tilting of the fragment.

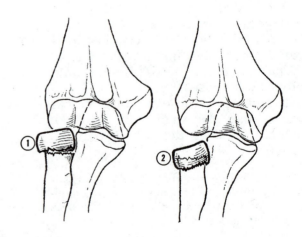

1. Severe comminution of the radial head with displacement of the fragments.

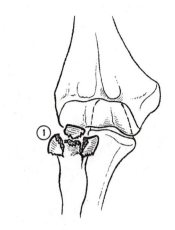

Immediate Management

Aspirate the elbow to relieve pain from hemarthrosis as well as to evaluate motion.

1. An 18-gauge needle is introduced superior to the radial head.
2. Blood is withdrawn.

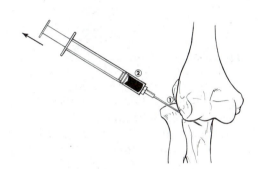

3. 0.5% Marcaine is injected.

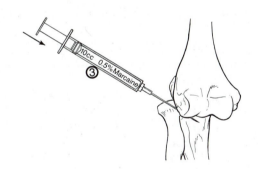

1. Test motion by flexion-extension and rotation of the elbow.
2. If fragments block motion in full flexion, they should be excised, but usually elbow motion is good.

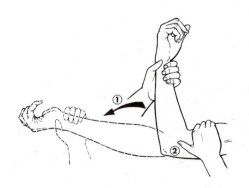

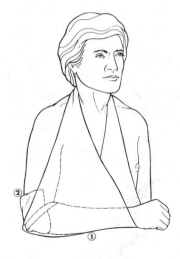

Immediate Immobilization

1. Support the elbow in a sling.
2. For the first 48 hours, apply ice to the radial region to relieve pain.

Trial by Motion

When the pain subsides, the patient may begin forearm rotation exercises with the arm in a sling.

By five to seven days, the pain will have subsided sufficiently to allow active flexion and extension exercises.

If extension is slow to return, the patient should use a night splint with the elbow in maximum extension.

SURGICAL EXCISION OF THE RADIAL HEAD

Indications

Objective clinical evidence of limitation of flexion from fracture fragments during the acute assessment under local anesthetic or after eight weeks of trial by motion is the major indication for excision of the radial head.

Rarely, the patient will desire excision of radial head fragments because of elbow crepitance, which is usually painless.

Surgical Procedure

1. Make an oblique incision extending downward from the lateral epicondyle to the ulna in the interval between the extensor carpi ulnaris and the anconeus muscles.

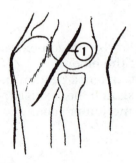

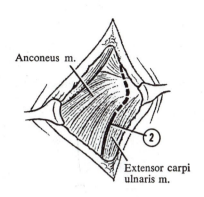

2. Deepen the incision through the fascia and between the anconeus and the extensor carpi ulnaris. This exposes the capsule.

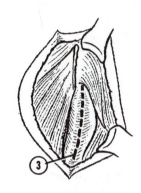

3. Make a longitudinal incision in the capsule to expose the radial head and the capitellum.

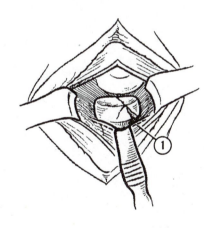

1. Identify the orbicular ligament and divide the periosteum immediately above it. Do not strip any of the periosteum from the bone.

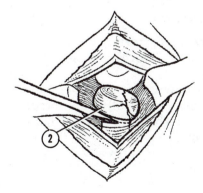

2. Cut the bone with a thin sharp osteotome immediately above the orbicular ligament.

Surgical Procedure (Continued)

1. Remove any loose pieces of bone and trim away any tags of periosteum attached to the end of the neck.

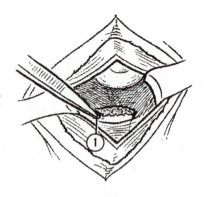

2. Close the capsule and ligamentous tissues over the resected end of the radius.

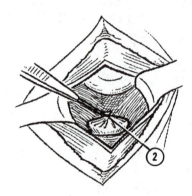

Immobilization

1. Apply a posterior plaster slab from the axilla to the base of the fingers.
2. The elbow is flexed 90 degrees.
3. The forearm is fully supinated.
4. Suspend the arm with a collar-and-cuff sling.

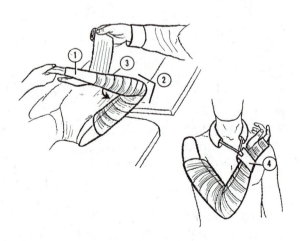

864

Postoperative Management

Discard the plaster splint after three to five days, when swelling has subsided.

Institute active progressive motion within the patient's tolerance of pain to restore flexion-extension, pronation, and supination. Support the limb with a triangular sling when the patient is not exercising.

Avoid forceful stretching of the joints.

COMMINUTED FRACTURE OF THE RADIAL HEAD WITH DISLOCATION OF THE DISTAL RADIOULNAR JOINT

REMARKS

This is a rare acute lesion. The dislocation at the distal radioulnar joint may be overlooked.

It is produced by a severe longitudinal compression force that drives the radius upward.

Disruption of the distal joint permits the shaft of the radius to be displaced further upward than normal with fracture.

Similarly, symptomatic instability of the distal radial joint may frequently follow excision of the proximal radius.

Always suspect this combination when a patient with a fracture of the radial head complains of pain in the wrist.

In these patients excision of the radial head will increase the proximal shift of the radius and aggravate the deformity at the wrist. This can be especially disabling in the laborer.

To stabilize both the proximal and distal ends of the radius, replace the radial head with a silastic prosthesis.

The distal radioulnar joint should be reduced and fixed before the radial head is replaced.

Appearance on X-Ray

1. There is severe comminution and mushrooming of the radial head.
2. The radial shaft is displaced upward against the capitellum.

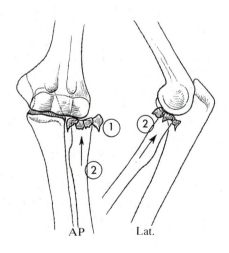

AP   Lat.

865

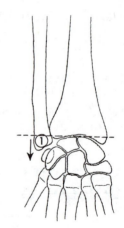

Appearance on X-Ray (*Continued*)

1. The styloid process is at a lower than normal position in relation to the ulna.

Note: Normally the styloid process of the radius extends 1 cm beyond that of the ulna.

MANAGEMENT

Reduction and Fixation of the Distal Radioulnar Joint

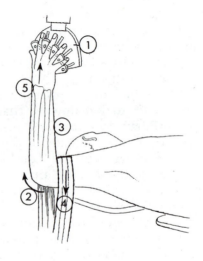

The patient assumes the supine position on a fracture table.

1. Apply finger traction apparatus.
2. The elbow is flexed 90 degrees.
3. The arm is fully supinated.
4. Make counter traction with a muslin bandage secured to the bottom of the table.
5. Now apply finger traction until the radial styloid is distal to the ulnar styloid.

1. While traction is continued and an assistant holds the wrist in ulnar deviation,

2. Pass a threaded wire 2 mm through the ulna into the radial styloid. The wire enters 4 to 5 cm proximal to the tip of the ulnar styloid and is directed slightly forward toward the radial styloid, making an angle with the ulna of about 45 degrees.

3. Cut the wire below the level of the skin.

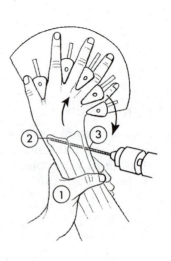

Note: Before cutting the wire take x-rays to determine the exact position of the wire. If it is not correctly placed withdraw it and reinsert it.

Postreduction X-Ray

1. Radial length is restored. The radial styloid is distal to the ulnar styloid.

2. The transfixion wire maintains the normal position of the radius and prevents any proximal migration.

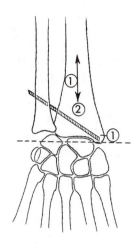

Swanson Silastic Replacement of the Radial Head

1. Make an oblique incision extending downward from the lateral epicondyle to the ulna in the interval between the extensor carpi ulnaris and the anconeus muscles.

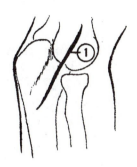

2. Deepen the incision through the fascia and between the anconeus and the extensor carpi ulnaris. This exposes the capsule.

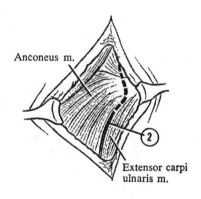

Anconeus m.

Extensor carpi ulnaris m.

3. Make a longitudinal incision in the capsule to expose the radial head and the capitellum.

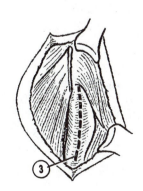

Swanson Silastic Replacement of the Radial Head (Continued)

1. Identify the orbicular ligament and divide the periosteum immediately above it. Do not strip any of the periosteum from the bone.

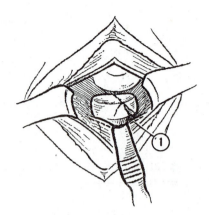

2. Cut the bone with a thin sharp osteotome immediately above the orbicular ligament.

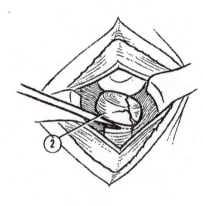

1. Remove any loose pieces of bone. Trim away any tags of periosteum attached to the end of the neck.

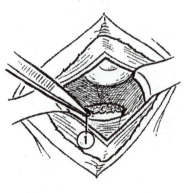

2. Insert a silastic prosthesis into the intramedullary canal of the proximal radial shaft.

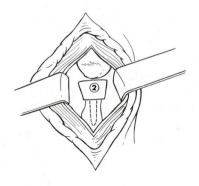

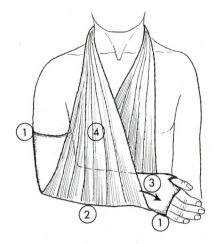

Postoperative Management

1. A cast is applied from the middle of the arm to the metacarpal head.
2. The forearm is in midposition.
3. The wrist is in a neutral position and is deviated toward the ulna.
4. The arm is supported in a triangular sling.

Encourage the patient to exercise shoulder, elbow, and fingers immediately.

At the end of two weeks remove the cast and the wire. (The wire can be removed under local anesthesia.)

Institute a regulated program of exercises to restore flexion, extension, pronation, and supination at the elbow and full motion in the wrist and fingers.

Avoid any forceful stretchings of the elbow joint.

Maximum restoration of function is attained only after many months. Progress is usually very slow.

Fractures of the Head and Neck of the Radius in Children

REMARKS

The mechanism of this injury is essentially the same as that in the adult; however, the nature of the bony damage is different in children, in that the articular surface of the radial head is rarely involved. The fracture is usually through the epiphyseal physis or distal to it in the neck.

An indirect mechanism produces the lesions. The child falls on the outstretched hand with the elbow extended and the forearm supinated. Upon striking the ground two forces act: one travels up the radius driving the radial head against the capitellum; the other is a valgus strain at the elbow forcing the capitellum to tilt the radial head downward and outward.

The direction of the tilting of the radial head depends upon the rotational position of the radius at the moment the hand makes contact with the ground. Also, the momentum of the body plays a role in the degree of displacement of the radial head.

The concomitant valgus strain may result in avulsion of the medial epicondyle or strain or rupture of the medial ligament or fracture of the upper third of the ulna.

Various degrees of tilting of the radial epiphysis from the horizontal are encountered. These are classified as follows:

0 to 30 degrees — minimal displacement.

30 to 60 degrees — moderate displacement.

More than 60 degrees — complete displacement. (The epiphysis is off the shaft and lies parallel to it.)

Another, more unusual mechanism of injury to the radial epiphysis is the result of a temporary dislocation of the joint which reduces spontaneously. In the process the capitellum shears off the radial epiphysis and causes the epiphysis to rotate posteriorly 90 degrees.

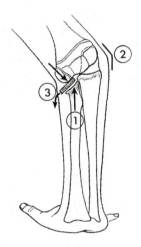

Mechanism of Injury

1. The force travels up the radius, driving the head against the capitellum as the hand strikes the ground.

2. The normal valgus angle of the elbow plus the momentum of the body and the direction of the arm create a valgus strain at the elbow.

3. The capitellum tilts the radial head downward and outward.

Concomitant Lesions on the Medial Side of the Elbow

Avulsion of the medial epicondyle.
Strain or rupture of the collateral ligament.
Fracture of the olecranon.

Unusual Type of Backward Rotation of the Radial Epiphysis

1. The radial epiphysis is rotated 90 degrees backward, as seen on the lateral and anteroposterior views.

Note: This lesion is reduced by open operation.

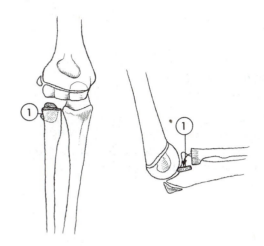

MANAGEMENT

REMARKS

The type of treatment employed is governed by the degree of displacement.

In general, tilts up to 20 degrees are accepted. These require nothing more than a sling for 10 to 14 days followed by free use of the arm. With growth, realignment of the epiphysis with the shaft takes place. In fact, in very young children almost normal realignment may occur even with severe displacements.

All displacements over 20 degrees should be subjected to manipulative reduction — even those with complete displacement, because occasionally reduction is achieved.

Even after an initially successful manipulative reduction, the position may be lost and open reduction may become necessary.

Failure to reduce the angulation to less than 20 degrees warrants open reduction with internal fixation.

Among complications that should be anticipated are premature fusion of the upper radial epiphysis with secondary cubitus valgus, avascular necrosis of the radial head, ectopic bone formation, and residual loss of rotation as the result of proximal radioulnar scarring.

The major factor in the result appears to be the age at which the injury is sustained and the completeness of reduction. Fractures in younger children that are adequately reduced, either by closed or open technique, heal with the best results.

Prereduction X-Ray of a Displaced Upper Radial Epiphysis

1. In the lateral view, the radial head is tilted forward.
2. In the anteroposterior view, the radial head is tilted outward.

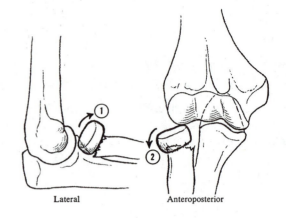

Lateral   Anteroposterior

Manipulative Reduction

1. An assistant steadies the arm.
2. The operator grasps the wrist of the extended forearm with one hand and the elbow with the other; the forearm is adducted.
3. The thumb is placed over the displaced radial epiphysis.

Note: Rotate the forearm so that the most prominent portion of the displaced head is in a lateral position and is superficial (between the extensor muscles and the anconeus).

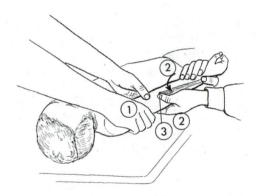

1. While the forearm is adducted,
2. The thumb makes firm pressure upward and inward on the radial epiphysis.
3. Next the forearm is supinated and
4. Flexed acutely.

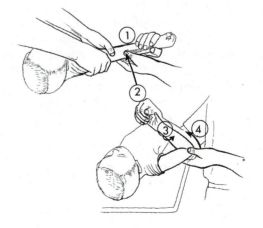

872

Postreduction X-Ray

1. In the lateral view, the forward tilt of the epiphysis is corrected.

2. In the anteroposterior view, the outward tilt of the epiphysis is corrected.

3. In both views, the articular surface of the epiphysis is parallel to that of the capitellum.

Note: If the reduction is not anatomic but the tilt of the fragment has been decreased to less than 20 degrees, it may be accepted.

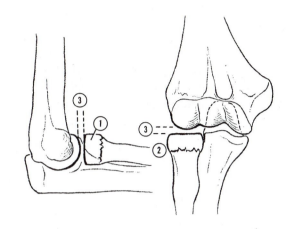

Immobilization

1. Apply a posterior plaster slab from the axilla to the base of the fingers.

2. The forearm is at right angles in midposition.

3. Suspend the arm with a collar-and-cuff sling.

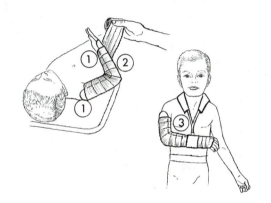

Postreduction Management

Discard the posterior plaster slab after two weeks.

Apply a triangular sling for one week.

After removal of the plaster, institute active progressive motion within the patient's tolerance of pain to restore flexion, extension, pronation, and supination.

Avoid forceful stretching of the joint.

Note: Maximum restoration of function is attained only after many months. Progress is usually very slow.

OPERATIVE REDUCTION

Indication

Operative reduction is necessary in all instances in which manipulative reduction fails to restore an acceptable alignment of the displaced fragments. The angulation of the epiphysis should not exceed 20 degrees.

Surgical Procedure

INCISION

1. Make an oblique incision extending downward from the lateral epicondyle to the ulna in the interval between the anconeus and the extensor carpi ulnaris.

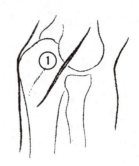

2. Deepen the incision through the fascia and between the anconeus and the extensor carpi ulnaris. This exposes the capsule.

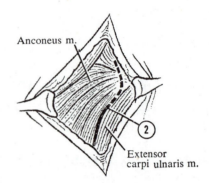

3. Make a longitudinal incision in the capsule to expose the radial epiphysis and the capitellum.

Note: The posterior intraosseous nerve, which runs through the supinator muscle but a fingerbreadth from the radial head in children, must be carefully protected during this exposure.

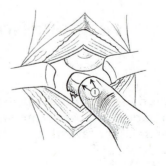

REDUCTION

1. The surgeon places his thumb over the displaced radial epiphysis and pushes upward and backward until the articular surface of the epiphysis is parallel to that of the capitellum.

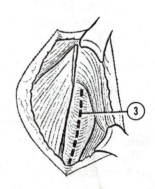

FIXATION

1. If the radial head fragment is completely detached and unstable after reduction, fix it in position with two Kirschner wires introduced posteriorly and lateral to the lateral condylar of the humerus.

2. The ends of the wires are bent and are buried subcutaneously for later removal.

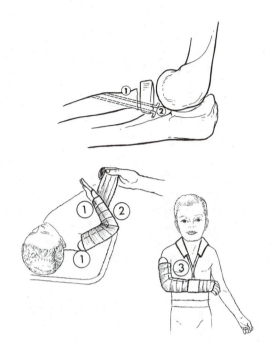

Immobilization

1. Apply a posterior plaster slab from the axilla to the base of the fingers.

2. The forearm is at right angles and in midposition.

3. Suspend the arm with a collar-and-cuff sling.

Postreduction Management

Discard the posterior plaster slab after three weeks.

Apply a triangular sling for one to two weeks.

After removal of the plaster, institute progressive motion within the patient's tolerance to restore flexion-extension, pronation, and supination.

If Kirschner wire fixation was used, the wire(s) may be removed at three weeks for the epiphyseal fracture but will need to stay in longer for radial neck fracture.

Avoid forceful stretching of the joint.

Note: Maximum restoration of the function is obtained only after many months. Progress is frequently very slow.

PROGNOSIS FOLLOWING FRACTURES OF THE RADIAL EPIPHYSIS

The major factors that influence prognosis are the adequacy of reduction and the age of the patient at the time of injury.

Although premature fusion of the upper radial epiphysis occurs fairly often, significant shortening or angulation is rare and is never severe enough to require osteotomy.

Avoid excising the radial head for any of the complications resulting from proximal radial epiphyseal fractures, because impairments (in function and growth) are magnified by bone loss in the immature elbow.

Fractures of the Coronoid Process

REMARKS

Isolated fracture of the coronoid process may occur, although the injury is usually associated with a posterior dislocation of the elbow.

The fragments vary in size from small chips to large segments of the coronoid process; the former lesions are of little significance.

Occasionally fragments are displaced into the joint cavity causing blocking of the joint. These require excision from the joint cavity.

CHIP FRACTURE AND FRACTURE WITH MINIMAL DISPLACEMENT

Appearance on X-Ray

CHIP FRACTURE

1. Small chip of the coronoid process is avulsed and displaced slightly anteriorly.

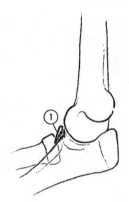

LARGER FRAGMENT

2. Triangular fragment of bone is detached from the coronoid process; the displacement is minimal.

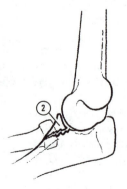

Immobilization

No reduction is necessary.

1. Apply a posterior plaster slab from the axilla to the base of the fingers.

2. The forearm is in acute flexion.

3. The forearm is in full supination.

4. Suspend the arm with a collar-and-cuff sling.

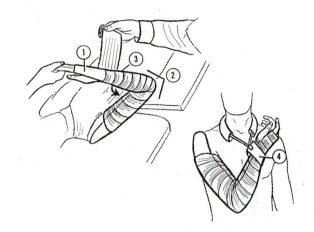

Postimmobilization Management

Maintain the plaster fixation seven to ten days.

Now place the arm in a triangular sling holding the arm at 90 degrees flexion.

Discard the sling after seven to ten days.

Institute active exercises for the elbow.

Avoid passive stretching of the elbow.

FRACTURES OF THE CORONOID WITH DISPLACEMENT OF FRAGMENTS

Prereduction X-Ray

1. Large triangular fragment is displaced anteriorly.

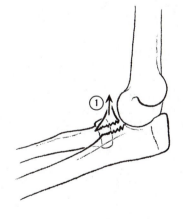

Manipulative Reduction (Under Local or General Anesthesia)

1. The physician makes firm pressure directly over the coronoid with the thumb of one hand while
2. With the other hand he forces the forearm into acute flexion.

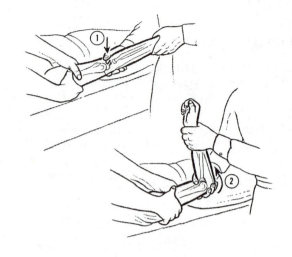

Postreduction X-Ray

1. Fragment is restored to its normal anatomic position.

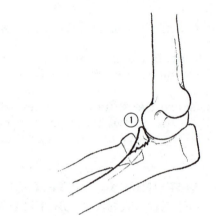

Immobilization

1. Apply a posterior plaster slab from the axilla to the base of the fingers.
2. The forearm is in acute flexion.
3. The forearm is fully supinated.
4. Suspend the arm with a collar-and-cuff sling.

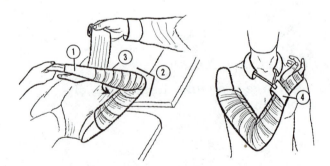

Postreduction Management

Maintain plaster fixation for three to four weeks.

Now place the arm in a triangular sling holding the arm in 90 degrees flexion.

Discard the sling after seven to ten days.
Institute active exercises for the elbow.
Avoid passive stretching of the elbow.

Note: Occasionally fragments of bone will be displaced into the joint cavity, causing blocking of the joint. These fragments must be removed. Caution—Do not remove coronoid fracture fragments associated with an elbow dislocation, or the elbow will redislocate.

Subluxation of the Radial Head in Children (Nursemaid's Elbow)

REMARKS

This is a relatively common disorder in children between the ages of one and four years; frequently it is at first not recognized.

Sudden traction on the extended forearm is the usual mechanism producing the lesion (nursemaid's elbow).

X-ray examination fails to depict the lesion.

The diagnosis is made from the history and the clinical manifestations. These are:

Sudden traction on the extended forearm.
Sudden onset of pain.
The arm dangles at the side and is held in pronation.
The child resists any movements of the elbow, although flexion and extension are free.
Supination is limited and painful.
Neurologic examination is negative.

The disorder is undoubtedly the result of stretching of the orbicular ligament that allows some fibers to slip between the capitellum and the head of the radius.

Up to the age of five the circumference of the cartilaginous radial head is the same as that of the neck so that when the arm is forcefully hyperextended or suddenly pulled, the radial head slips below the upper orifice of the annular ligament.

By eight years of age the radial head is larger than the neck, and subluxation does not occur.

Because of the strength of the annular ligament, isolated dislocation of the radial head does not occur in the adult without fracture of the ulna.

Manipulative Reduction

Generally no anesthesia is required.

1. Grasp the wrist with one hand with the forearm extended and

2. With the other grasp the elbow with the thumb resting over the radial head.

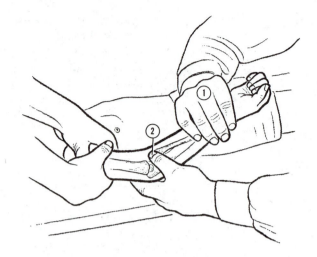

1. As the forearm is fully supinated,

2. Firm pressure is made on the radial head and

3. The forearm is pushed directly upward.

Note: Free, painless supination of the forearm is indicative of a successful reduction.

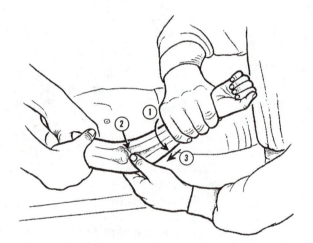

Immobilization

1. Apply a collar and cuff.

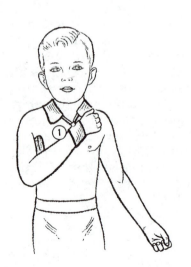

880

Postreduction Management

Discard the collar and cuff at the end of one week.
Allow free use of the arm.
Avoid traction or hyperextension movements at the elbow.

Posterior Dislocation of the Radial Head in the Newborn Infant

REMARKS

This rare lesion is secondary to a difficult delivery, usually breech presentation. Most often the distal humeral epiphysis is damaged by this mechanism of injury.

A clue to the diagnosis is the attitude of the arm.

The child holds the arm adducted and internally rotated and the forearm pronated.

Careful palpation of the radial head indicates its posterior and lateral position.

X-ray evaluation is difficult owing to the lack of ossification centers, but the pronated position and the displacement of the radial long axis relative to the capitellum should lead one to suspect posterior dislocation.

Prereduction X-Ray

1. Ulna is in normal relation with the humerus.
2. Radius is pronated.
3. Radial head is dislocated, although this ossification center is not present at birth and the dislocation can be diagnosed only on the basis of the displaced long axis of the radius relative to the capitellum.

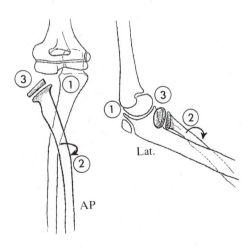

881

Reduction

1. Grasp the wrist with one hand with the forearm extended and
2. With the other grasp the elbow with the thumb resting on the radial head.

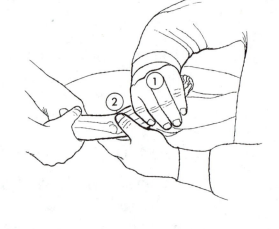

1. As the forearm is fully supinated,
2. Make firm pressure on the radial head.

Note: Maintain the forearm extended; flexion will reproduce the posterior dislocation.

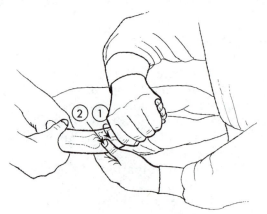

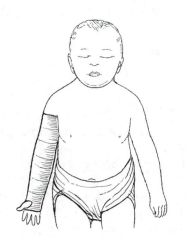

Immobilization

Apply a light long arm cast.
The forearm is extended and supinated.

Postreduction Management

Remove the cast after three weeks.
Allow free use of the arm.
No other treatment is required.

SUMMARY: COMPLICATIONS AND PITFALLS OF FRACTURES AND DISLOCATIONS OF THE ELBOW

The pitfalls and complications of these injuries about the elbow are many and should be anticipated.

The most serious complication is the vascular conpromise due most often to swelling in the antecubital region, which obstructs venous return. Because of the serious but preventable consequences of this complication, all fractures and dislocations about the elbow should be carefully assessed before reduction and observed after reduction for the P-signs of impending ischemia. Measurement with ultrasonic flowmeter and intracompartmental pressure recordings add valuable objective guides to the clinical assessment of distal perfusion and should be used routinely.

Reduction of the common supracondylar fracture is relatively simple. Prevention of cubitus varus deformity depends on the physician's understanding of the three dimensions of fracture displacement. Radiography is notoriously unreliable in assessing torsional deformities from supracondylar fractures. The physician's visual assessment of the bony landmarks about the fracture during traction and the use of forearm rotation to correct varus or valgus moments should serve as the main defenses against altered elbow carrying angle.

Elbow dislocation is a common injury that must be assessed carefully for potential forearm ischemic injury before and after treatment. Circular casts should be avoided, as should prolonged immobilization after reduction. Dislocated elbows with or without associated fractures are usually stable. If the elbow proves stable on testing after reduction, immobilization should not be prolonged longer than three to five days. Fractures of the coronoid process, the radial head, or the medial epicondyle associated with elbow dislocation should not prolong the period of immobilization after reduction. Elbow dislocations requiring surgical treatment have poor long-term results. Early operative intervention should be reserved for those few conditions, such as olecranon fractures, that cause demonstrable instability with flexion, extension, or varus-valgus testing of the elbow after reduction.

Humeral condylar fractures in children, because of their tendency to rotate during cast immobilization, most often require open reduction and internal fixation. These represent a consistent exception to the rule that children's fractures are best treated by closed methods.

Most adult condylar fractures can best be managed by closed reduction and traction techniques emphasizing early functional exercises. Internal fixation of the comminuted adult's fracture in this area is technically difficult and usually unsatisfactory. The exceptions to this are the capitellum fracture, which can be treated by excision, or the transcondylar fracture associated with the dislocation of the elbow.

Fractures of the proximal ulna should be carefully assessed for their effect on elbow stability and on triceps function. In most instances internal fixation using tension-band wiring provides excellent fixation and permits early functional elbow exercise.

Fractures of the radial head are common in adults, whereas fractures of the radial neck represent the more common injury in children. Most are relatively undisplaced and can be treated symptomatically with minimal immobilization. A period of three to five weeks should be offered the adult patient with this injury to evaluate its significance on elbow function using a "trial of motion." If the radial head fragment displaces significantly or blocks elbow motion, it may be excised. When in doubt about the necessity to excise the radial head after fracture or fracture-dislocation, the rule should be, "Wait and see."

REFERENCES

Adler, J. B., and Shaftan, G. W.: Radial head fractures, is excision necessary? J. Trauma, 4:115, 1964.

Alvarez, E., Patel, M. R., Nimberg, G., et al.: Fractures of the capitulum humeri. J. Bone and Joint Surg., 57-A:1093, 1975.

Anderson, L. D.: Speed and Boyd procedure for Monteggia fractures. In Campbell's Operative Orthopaedics, edited by A. H. Crenshaw, St. Louis, The C. V. Mosby Company, 1971, p. 666.

Arnold, J. A., Nasca, R. J., and Nelson, C. L.: Supracondylar fractures of the humerus. J. Bone and Joint Surg., 59-A:589, 1977.

Ashbell, T. S., Kleinert, H. E., and Kutz, J. E.: Vascular injuries about the elbow. Clin Orthop., 50:107, 1967.

Billet, D. M.: Unreduced posterior dislocation of the elbow. J. Trauma, 19:186, 1979.

DeLee, J. C., Wilkins, K. E., Rogers, L. F., et al.: Fracture-separation of the distal humeral epiphysis. J. Bone and Joint Surg. 62–A:46, 1980.

Dickson, R. A., Stein, H., and Bentley, G.: Excision arthroplasty of the elbow in rheumatoid disease. J. Bone and Joint Surg., 58-B:227, 1976.

El Ghawabi, M. H.: Fracture of the medial condyle of the humerus. J. Bone and Joint Surg., 57-A:677, 1975.

Elstrom, J. A., Pankovich, A. M., and Kassab, M. T.: Irreducible supracondylar fracture of the humerus in children. J. Bone and Joint Surg., 57-A:680, 1975.

Fahey, J. J., and O'Brien, E. T.: Fracture-separation of the medial humeral condyle in a child confused with fracture of the medial epicondyle. J. Bone and Joint Surg., 53-A:1102, 1971.

Flynn, J. C., Richards, J. F., and Saltzman, R. I.: Prevention and treatment of non-union of slightly displaced fractures of the lateral humeral condyle in children. J. Bone and Joint Surg., 57-A:1087, 1975.

Gelberman, R. H., Zakalib, G. S., Mubarak, S. J., et al.: Decompression of forearm compartment syndromes. Clin. Orthop. 134:225, 1978.

REFERENCES

Grantham, S. A., and Tietjen, R.: Transcondylar fracture-dislocation of the elbow. J. Bone and Joint Surg., 58-A:1030, 1976.

Holda, M. E., Manoli, A., and Lamont, R. L.: Epiphyseal separation of the distal end of the humerus with medial displacement. J. Bone and Joint Surg. 62-A:52, 1980.

Jones, E. R. L., and Esah, M.: Displaced fractures of the neck of the radius in children. J. Bone and Joint Surg., 53B:429, 1971.

Kaplan, S. R., and Reckling, F. W.: Fracture separation of the lower humeral epiphysis with medial displacement. J. Bone and Joint Surg., 53-A: 1105, 1971.

Linscheid, R. L., and Wheeler, D. K.: Elbow dislocations. J.A.M.A., 194:1171, 1965.

Lipscomb, P. R., and Burleson, R. J.: Vascular and neural complications in supracondylar fractures of the humerus in children. J. Bone and Joint Surg., 37-A:487, 1955.

Mizuno, K., Hirohata, K., and Kashiwagi, D.: Fracture-separation of the distal humeral epiphysis in young children. J. Bone and Joint Surg. 61-A:570, 1979.

Osborne, G., and Cotterill, P.: Recurrent dislocations of the elbow. J. Bone and Joint Surg., 48-B:340, 1966.

Palmer, E. E., Niemann, K. M., Vesely, D., et al.: Supracondylar fracture of the humerus in children. J. Bone and Joint Surg., 60-A:653, 1978.

Protzman, R. R.: Dislocation of the elbow joint. J. Bone and Joint Surg., 60-A:539, 1978.

Riseborough, E. J., and Radin, E. L.: Intercondylar T fractures of the humerus in the adult. J. Bone and Joint Surg., 51-A:130, 1969.

Smith, L.: Deformity following supracondylar fractures of the humerus. J. Bone and Joint Surg., 42-A:235, 1960.

Soltanpur, A.: Anterior supracondylar fracture of the humerus (flexion type). J. Bone and Joint Surg., 60-B:383, 1978.

Speed, J. S.: An operation for unreduced posterior dislocation of the elbow. South. Med. J., 18:193, 1925.

Swanson, A. B.: Flexible Implant Resection Arthroplasty of the Hand and Extremities. St. Louis, the C. V. Mosby Company, 1973.

Tullos, J. S., and King, J. W.: Lesions of the pitching arm in adolescents. J.A.M.A., 220:264, 1972.

Whitesides, T. E., Jr., Haney, T. C., Morimoto, K., and Harada, H.: Tissue pressure measurements as a determinant for the need of fasciotomy. Clin. Orthop., 113:43, 1975.

FRACTURES OF THE SHAFTS OF THE BONES OF THE FOREARM

ANATOMIC CONSIDERATIONS

Biomechanics of Forearm Rotation and of Fracture Reduction

REMARKS

The anatomic disruption produced by the injury to the forearm's two-bone-and-four-joint system must always be kept in mind in selecting treatment.

The function most often significantly impaired by forearm fracture is the unique rotatory motion necessary for positioning of the hand.

Rotation of 120 to 140 degrees is ordinarily possible in the forearm. It is limited primarily by the passive resistance of stretched muscle antagonists, by the radius impinging on muscles in the interosseous space, and by ligamentous contracture.

Ordinarily the normal lateral curve of the radius permits it to clear soft tissues during forearm rotation. If a fracture decreases the radial curve, impingement on the muscles, particularly the flexor pollicis longus and the deep finger flexors, will limit rotation.

The interosseous space is widest in neutral rotation and narrowest in full pronation and supination. Maintenance of extreme pronation or supination for long periods during fracture treatment will cause permanent contracture of muscles and ligaments between the two bones.

The interosseous membrane acts as a hinge for radioulnar rotation. Its fibers, which run from the ulna in a proximal direction to the radius, prevent the radius from being pushed upward. Superior and inferior oblique cords in the membrane run in the opposite direction so as to resist downward pull on the radius.

According to Steindler, the interosseous membrane and ligaments are less significant checks to forearm rotation than is muscle contracture. Rotation iş most likely to be maintained if permanent muscle contracture is prevented by functional exercise.

When the forearm is free, the radius rotates around the ulna. Should the radius become fixed, as in a fall on the outstretched hand, the ulna pivots around the radius. If the elbow is locked in extension, then the entire extremity rotates around the radius, exerting extreme leverage on the radioulnar joints.

The major anatomic consideration in reducing forearm fractures is to achieve proper rotational reduction. Bayonet apposition of the fracture causes less loss of rotation than does incomplete rotational realignment. The basic technique of rotational reduction is to align the mobile distal radial fragment with the fixed proximal one.

The best way to determine the rotational position of the proximal radial fragment is to compare the shape of the bicipital tuberosity with the opposite uninjured radius. In full supination, the bicipital tuberosity points toward the ulna. As the rotation of the radius changes, so does the relationship of the tuberosity to the ulna.

The upper fragment of a radial fracture does not pronate past neutral and consequently most forearm fractures should not be immobilized in a pronated position. Besides overrotating the distal fragment, forearm pronation leads to a volar displacement of the distal fragment caused by the weight of the hand as well as by the cast.

Once the distal fragment is rotated in proper relationship to the proximal one, it is frequently possible to achieve end-to-end apposition of both bones. End-to-end reduction of the ulna with corner-to-corner reduction of the radius may also be accepted if the normal radial curve is maintained. Angulation of the radius of more than 10 degrees in either a volar or an ulnar direction is likely to restrict rotation because of soft tissue impingement.

Once reduction is achieved and the initial fracture swelling subsides, rigid immobilization of the wrist and elbow is unnecessary. Purposeful, controlled, functional muscle and joint motion benefits fracture healing by contributing to the revascularization process. Functional result is also improved by minimizing scarring and contracture of the forearm muscle.

Biomechanics of Normal Forearm Rotation

1. The normal 9-degree outward curve of the radius permits rotation without soft tissue impingement.

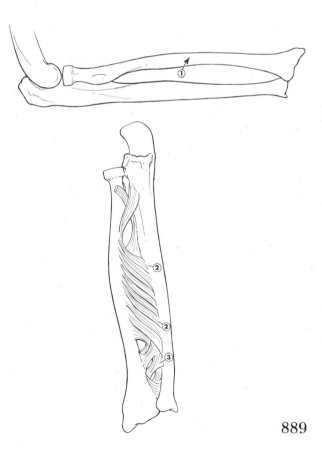

2. The interosseous membrane, which extends from the distal ulna to the proximal radius, prevents upward displacement of the radius and acts as the radioulnar hinge.

3. Superior and inferior oblique cords of the interosseous membrane resist downward pull on the radius.

Note: The major limitation of forearm rotation is due to muscle impingement rather than to the interosseous membrane.

Biomechanics of Normal Forearm Rotation (Continued)

PRONATION AND SUPINATION

1. Pronation and supination range is 120 to 140 degrees.

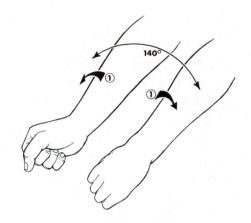

2. The principal checks to forearm rotation are tight muscles and impingement, particularly of the flexor pollicis longus on the flexor digitorum profundus.

INTEROSSEOUS SPACE

1. The interosseous space is widest in neutral rotation.

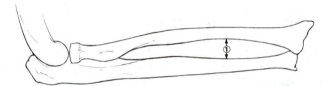

2. It is narrowest in full pronation as well as

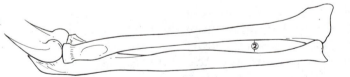

3. In full supination.

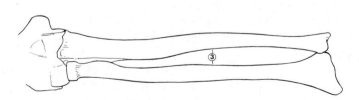

Effect of Fractures on Interosseous Space

1. Fracture of both bones of the forearm.

2. The radial arch is lost.

3. The ulnar fragments are displaced.

4. Muscles and other soft tissues between the bones would limit rotation if the fracture healed in this position.

Note: The loss of pronation is more readily accommodated by shoulder motion than is loss of supination. Many patients are not functionally impaired or do not notice loss of 40 to 50 degrees of forearm rotation, particularly of pronation.

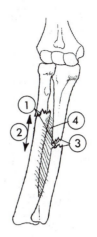

LOSS OF FOREARM PRONATION

1. With the elbow extended the axis of rotation passes through the shoulder.

2. Loss of forearm pronation is accommodated by

3. Shoulder abduction and

4. Shoulder internal rotation.

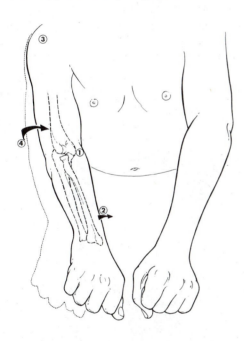

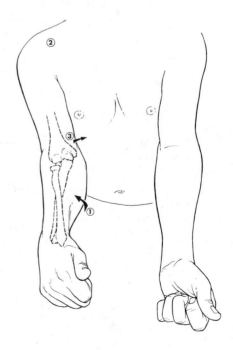

LOSS OF FOREARM SUPINATION

1. Accommodation for loss of forearm supination requires

2. Shoulder external rotation

3. With the arm adducted; adduction is limited by the trunk.

EVALUATION OF ROTATIONAL ALIGNMENT BY POSITION OF THE BICIPITAL TUBEROSITY (EVANS' TECHNIQUE)

Compare the bicipital tuberosity on the fractured side with the tuberosity on the unfractured side to determine the amount of supination necessary for alignment of the distal and proximal fragments.

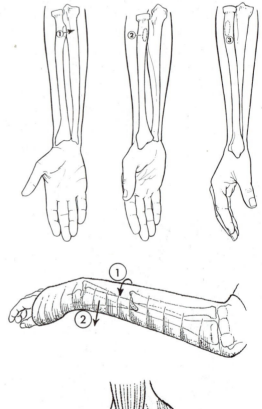

1. In full supination, the bicipital tuberosity is directed toward the ulna.

2. In 40-degree supination, the tuberosity moves posteriorly.

3. In neutral, tuberosity is almost directly posterior.

Other Factors Affecting Alignment

WEIGHT OF HAND

Immobilization of forearm fractures in full pronation should be avoided even for fractures in the distal third.

1. Full pronation.

2. Weight of the hand displaces distal fragment downward.

MUSCLE INSERTIONS

1. The strong supinators, the biceps and the supinator brevis, insert into the proximal third of the radius.

2. The pronator teres inserts into the middle third of the radius.

3. The pronator quadratus inserts into the distal third of the radius.

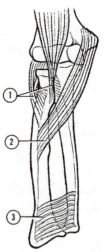

Note: The muscle contribution to rotational fracture deformity is unpredictable. Evans' rotational alignment method eliminates the need for guesswork.

ROTATORY REALIGNMENT OF FRACTURES OF THE UPPER RADIUS (EVANS' TECHNIQUE)

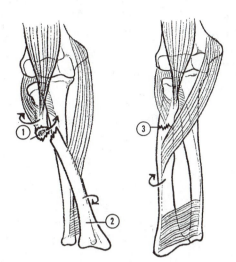

1. The proximal fragment is supinated and flexed.

2. The distal fragment is pronated and drawn inward toward the ulna.

3. Since the position of the bicipital tuberosity indicates that the proximal fragment is supinated, the fracture is reduced by supinating the distal fragment.

Note: Avoid immobilization in extreme supination, because this narrows the interosseous space. Once fracture ends are reduced or hooked together, the forearm may be rotated toward neutral position to widen the interosseous space.

ROTATORY REALIGNMENT OF MID-THIRD RADIAL FRACTURE

The amount of rotation that has occurred as a result of the fracture can be determined only by studying the position of the bicipital tuberosity (see page 892).

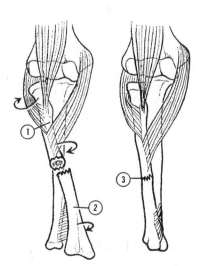

1. The proximal fragment is flexed and is supinated approximately 45 degrees as determined by the position of the bicipital tuberosity.

2. The distal fragment is pronated in relation to the proximal fragment.

3. The fracture is reduced by supinating the distal fragment approximately 45 degrees.

Note: Once the fracture ends are reduced or hooked together, the forearm may be rotated toward neutral position to widen the interosseous space.

FRACTURE DEFORMITIES

Narrowing of the Interosseous Space due to Angulation

1. Fracture of both bones.
2. Severe rotational and angular deformity.
3. The interosseous space is narrowed owing to the fracture angulation.

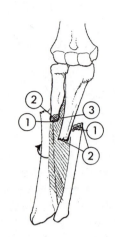

Effect of Fracture Reduction on Forearm Rotation

1. End-to-end reduction of the ulna.
2. Corner-to-corner reduction of the radius will not impair rotation as compared with rotation of the opposite forearm.

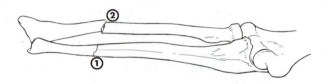

1. Fracture angulation of more than 10 degrees

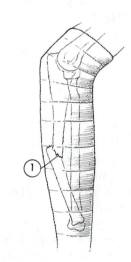

or

2. Rotational malalignment will impair forearm rotation.

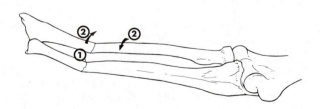

894

RADIOULNAR DISRUPTION IN ASSOCIATION WITH SINGLE-BONE FRACTURES

Most single-bone fractures of the forearm are undisplaced.

If displacement occurs, dislocation of either the proximal or distal radioulnar joint is highly likely.

1. Fracture of the ulna with anterior angulation.

2. Dislocation of the radial head.

Note: Suspect anterior dislocation of the radial head with any anterior angulation of the proximal ulna. It may not be recognized on the initial x-ray, or it may occur after the cast is applied.

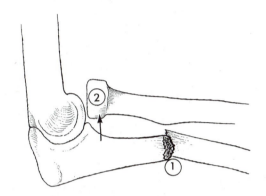

1. Fracture of the middle third of the ulna.

2. Posterior angulation.

3. Analyze x-ray carefully for posterior dislocation of radial head in association with displaced ulna fracture.

Note: This radioulnar instability should be recognized before the cast is applied.

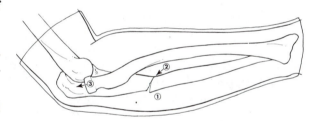

1. Fracture of the radius with angulation (anterior angulation).

2. Dislocation of the distal radioulnar joint.

Note: Failure to recognize the subluxation or dislocation of the radioulnar joint may result in pain and impairment of function that require surgical intervention.

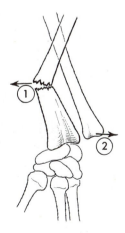

EPIDEMIOLOGY OF FRACTURES OF THE FOREARM IN ADULTS (PATIENTS OVER 17 YEARS OF AGE)

Although statistics vary from series to series, the following list represents the usual distribution of forearm fractures in adults.

Most of the fractures are produced by direct trauma.

15 per cent are open fractures.

85 per cent occur in men.

50 per cent occur under the age of 40.

85 per cent occur under the age of 60.

40 per cent of all forearm fractures are fractures of both bones.

50 per cent show some comminution.

60 per cent involve the middle third of the bones.

Mechanism of Fracture

DIRECT INJURY

The most common mechanism of injury to the forearm is the direct blow, which most frequently causes an isolated fracture of the ulna (nightstick fracture).

Greater direct violence may be sustained from motor vehicle accidents, falls, or gunshot wounds, which produce two-bone fracture or, least frequently, solitary fracture of the radius.

Direct injury may be sufficient to produce an open fracture, but the majority of forearm fractures do not communicate with the external environment.

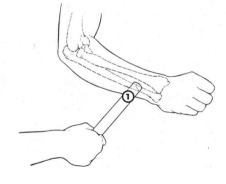

1. Solitary fracture of the ulna from a direct blow (nightstick fracture).

2. Solitary fracture of the distal radius. The distal radioulnar joint is undisturbed, provided that the radius does not shorten.

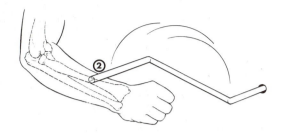

3. Gunshot fracture, both bones.

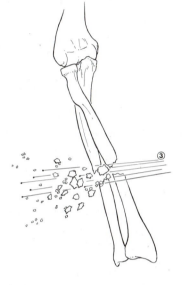

INDIRECT INJURY

The most common indirect mechanism of forearm fracture is a fall on the outstretched hand.

The vertical loading is associated with a rotatory force when the body's weight twists about the axis of the fixed radius, causing either hyperpronation or hypersupination of the forearm. Hyperpronation tends to angulate the fracture dorsally, whereas hypersupination causes the fracture to angulate in a volar direction.

Usually the radius angulates more than the ulna. The most common fracture sustained through indirect mechanism is the incomplete or greenstick fracture in a child. This quite frequently can be reduced by reversing the rotational force that produced it.

When the adult falls on the outstretched arm with the radius locked and the elbow in extension, the ulna and humerus rotate around the distal radioulnar joint. The extreme torque of this injury disrupts the distal radioulnar joint and fractures the distal radius (Galeazzi's fracture).

With the elbow slightly flexed during the fall on the outstretched hand, the torque tends to be absorbed more proximally about the elbow, producing a fracture of the ulna with dislocation of the radial head (Monteggia's fracture-dislocation).

Greenstick Fracture (in a Child) from Forceful Pronation

1. Forceful pronation causes
2. The radius to angulate dorsally as it rotates over the ulna.

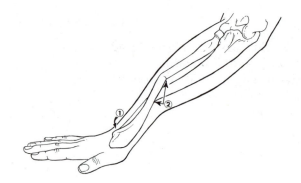

Greenstick Fracture (in a Child) from Forceful Supination

1. Force vectors from supination injury produce
2. Volar angulation of the radius to a greater degree than
3. Angulation of the ulna.

Note: This is the most common type of greenstick deformity. The greater angulation of the radius indicates that the injury occurred while the radius was rotating around the ulna.

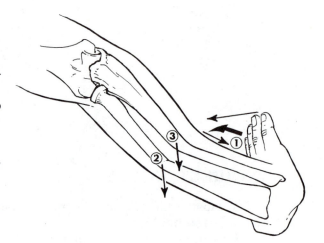

Rotational Injury Producing Galeazzi's Fracture

1. With the elbow extended and the wrist hyperextended,
2. The entire length of the humerus and ulna rotates around the fixed distal radius.
3. The distal radioulnar joint fails.
4. The radius fractures from bending or torque loading.

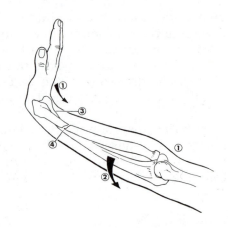

898

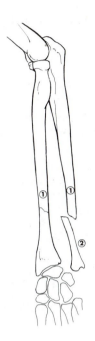

Occasionally,

1. The radius and ulna both fail.
2. The distal radioulnar joint also dislocates.

Anterior Monteggia Lesion from Elbow Hyperextension

1. A fall backward forces the forearm into supination.
2. The elbow is hyperextended.
3. Reflex contraction of the elbow flexors dislocates the radial head anteriorly.
4. The force of the injury displaces the ulna through the flexor carpi ulnaris and may displace it through the skin.

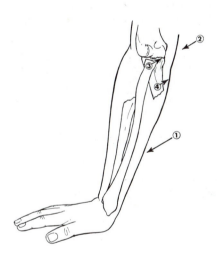

Torsional Injury Producing Anterior Monteggia Fracture-Dislocation

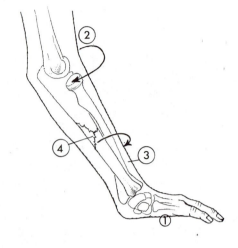

1. With the hand fixed to the ground,

2. The momentum of the fall causes the trunk and arm to rotate externally while

3. The ulna rotates internally around the fixed radius.

4. Fracture of the ulna results.

As the force continues,

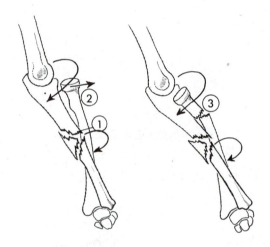

1. The radius and the proximal fragment of ulna come into contact.

2. The radial head is levered anteriorly out of the proximal radioulnar joint.

or

3. A fracture of the radius occurs in the proximal third of its shaft.

GENERAL
CONSIDERATIONS
IN TREATMENT

REMARKS

Fractures of the forearm have been common afflictions of mankind throughout all history. Judged by skeletal remains in Egyptian and New World burial grounds, forearm fractures have always been far more common than fractures of the leg, at least until our present, mechanized civilization.

The ability of early man to heal his fractures was remarkable; rate of nonunion rarely exceeded 5 per cent and was most common in the ulna according to Stewart.

Selection of treatment must be based on a proper appreciation of the fracture's biological capacity for healing.

Only recently has the technique of forearm fracture fixation been refined to the point where nonunion for surgical treatment is below the level that might have been expected had the fracture been left to heal without professional help.

Bagby, the originator of our current technique of dynamic compression plating, has pointed out that until the frequency and severity of complications inherent with any open reduction can be reduced to the level associated with closed methods, compression plating should be reserved for those situations in which its long-term results are convincingly superior.

The major advantage of internal fixation over closed treatment of forearm fractures is considered to be earlier and better functional restoration rather than a substantially higher rate of union. On the average, healing time after good operative fixation is about half that required with good closed treatment.

Methods of closed treatment, however, have also improved, particularly with the work of Sarmiento, who emphasizes functional bracing during treatment. Joint motion and muscle function permitted by this method maximize the healing response and minimize functional disability when healing is completed.

Muscle and soft tissue scarring, the inherent result of forearm fractures likely to restrict forearm function, should be minimized by functional exercise during recovery from either closed or open reduction.

Both closed and open treatment of forearm fractures require skill, patience, and a critical appreciation of the indications and limitations of both the technique and the surgeon.

Single-bone fractures without associated proximal or distal radioulnar dislocation and two-bone fractures without comminution do well with closed methods.

In the adult, fracture of the radius or ulna associated with dislocation of the adjacent proximal or distal radioulnar joint requires internal fracture fixation to permit reduction of the dislocation.

Comminuted fractures with bone loss requiring bone grafting should also be treated by internal fixation.

Except for these categories of fractures in adults, an attempt at closed reduction and functional cast or cast-brace treatment is indicated for most forearm fractures.

Forearm fractures in children have considerably different physiologic implications and must be considered separately (see page 979).

CLOSED REDUCTION AND FUNCTIONAL TREATMENT OF FOREARM FRACTURES (SARMIENTO)

REMARKS

Early functional use of muscles and joints in association with closed or open treatment will lessen the muscular scarring that inevitably follows forearm fractures and restricts motion.

Inability to achieve or maintain fracture reduction by closed methods does not preclude surgical treatment. A delay of seven to ten days to evaluate the feasibility of closed treatment makes no difference in the ultimate result if open treatment proves necessary.

The technique of reduction depends on proper rotational realignment of the distal fragment with the proximal one.

The major factor limiting forearm rotation is soft tissue impingement, brought about particularly by narrowing of the interosseous space. This space is widest in neutral rotation, which is the ideal position for immobilization of most fractures.

Avoid extremes of pronation or supination in reducing fractures, particularly pronation, which causes volar displacement of the distal fracture fragment (see page 892).

Aim for anatomic restoration of length and radial curvature. End-to-end reduction of the ulna with corner-to-corner reduction of the radius is acceptable, provided that the interosseous space has not been narrowed by angulation.

Protect and maintain the interosseous space by molding firmly between the reduced radius and ulna while the plaster sets and by avoiding extremes of pronation or supination.

Once the initial swelling of injury has subsided, a secondary or functional cast-brace may be applied to permit wrist and elbow flexion and extension.

Functional muscle and joint motion during the early stages of healing aids the healing response and minimizes residual functional disability from muscle scarring after the fracture has healed.

Functional closed treatment of forearm fractures depends on a comprehension of the anatomy of the forearm in order to judge the adequacy of reduction. The method also depends on the surgeon's appreciation of the biology of healing as well as the mechanics of fracture fixation.

Closed functional treatment requires as much skill and judgment as does operative technique. It offers the additional advantage of minimizing major complications that still can occur from any operative invasion of the fracture site.

One should not be so determined to achieve closed reduction that anatomic impairment results. Angulation of more than 10 degrees, shortening, and malrotation should not be accepted.

Initially, the fracture is treated by closed reduction under general or regional anesthesia and a standard long arm cast until swelling subsides.

By seven to fourteen days, depending on the degree of fracture swelling and instability, a functional cast-brace is applied, which permits flexion and extension of the elbow and wrist but limits rotation of the forearm.

Results obtained are in many ways superior to those from successful open reduction and internal fixation, although exact anatomic reduction is seldom obtained by the closed method.

ISOLATED FRACTURE OF THE RADIUS WITHOUT DISLOCATION OF THE RADIOULNAR JOINT

Appearance on X-Ray

1. Undisplaced fracture of the proximal half of the radius.

2. The interosseous space is preserved.

Note: The largest number of these fractures are relatively undisplaced and require no reduction. Always include the proximal and distal joints on x-ray and check carefully for dislocation.

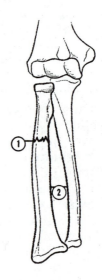

Initial Immobilization

1. Apply a circular cast from the axilla to the base of the fingers.
2. The elbow is flexed 90 degrees.
3. The forearm is supinated to align the distal fragment with the proximal fragment as determined by analysis of the bicipital tuberosity (see page 892).

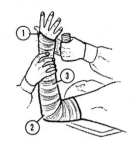

4. Avoid extreme supination, which narrows the interosseous space.
5. The cast should allow free motion of the shoulder and fingers.

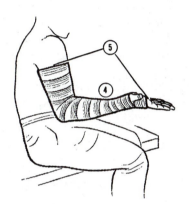

Functional Cast-Brace Treatment

When swelling and initial pain subside (usually by five to seven days), apply a functional brace.

1. Forearm is suspended in a finger-trap.
2. Plaster or orthoplast material is firmly molded to compress tissues of the interosseous space and to maintain the radial curvature.
3. Supracondylar elbow extension permits flexion and extension but limits pronation and supination.
4. Wrist hinge and hand component permit palmar flexion and dorsiflexion of the wrist.*

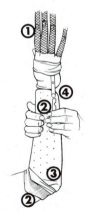

---

*Available from Zinco Industries, Inc., 3724 Park Place, P.O. Box 567, Montrose, California, 91020.

Postreduction Management

Encourage functional exercises of elbow, wrist, shoulder, and forearm muscles during the period of immobilization.

As pain subsides and confidence returns, the patient will use the fractured limb with greater vigor.

Evaluate the fracture position periodically by x-ray during the first two to three weeks after functional cast-bracing.

Most functional braces will last for the period of time required for fracture union and will not require replacement.

The average time for healing of the isolated radial fracture is approximately eleven weeks.

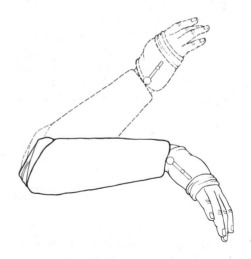

ISOLATED FRACTURE OF THE ULNA

REMARKS

This most common of forearm fractures is usually isolated and remains undisplaced. If angulation or displacement is evident, carefully evaluate the proximal and distal radioulnar joints for dislocation.

In contrast to fractures of the radius, ulnar fractures may be treated with a circumferential sleeve that is less limiting than the functional cast-brace used when the radius is fractured.

The isolated ulnar fracture, in the past, has been the forearm fracture most likely to develop nonunion when treated by conventional open or closed technique. Functional bracing of this benign-appearing but difficult fracture frequently offers a better chance for healing than even the best operative technique.

The reason for better results with closed functional treatment of ulnar fracture is uncertain, except for the improved blood supply to external callus that results from maintenance of muscle function.

Avoid overemphasizing radiographic signs of union. Dutoit and Gräbe have shown that clinical union (freedom from pain and no motion at the fracture site) consistently precedes radiologic union.

All fractures that reach clinical union will eventually unite radiographically. Prolonging immobilization until there is radiographic evidence of union is unnecessary in most reliable patients.

DuToit and Gräbe have also shown that ulna fracture angulation of 10 to 20 degrees does not affect clinical result. Fractures in the distal ulna and oblique fractures with displacement are most prone to angulation.

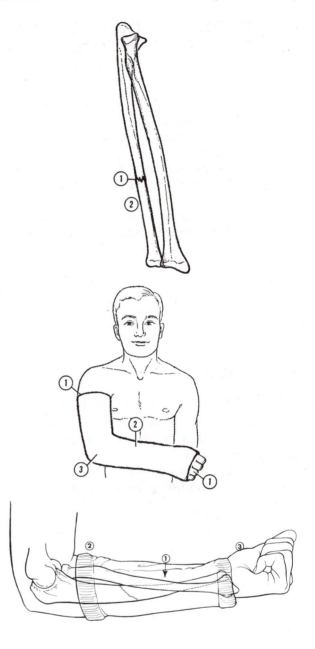

Appearance on X-Ray

1. Transverse fracture at the junction of the lower and middle thirds.

2. No angulation is evident. If angulation occurs, check carefully for dislocation of the distal or proximal radioulnar joint.

Note: Most isolated ulnar fractures are relatively undisplaced.

Initial Immobilization

Obviously this fracture needs no reduction.

1. Apply a circular cast from the axilla to the base of the fingers.

2. The forearm is in midposition.

3. The elbow is flexed at a right angle.

Functional Sleeve Application

This is applied when the swelling and pain subside (seven to ten days).

1. A plaster sleeve is molded firmly into the interosseous space.

2. The elbow and

3. The wrist are free.

Note: Alternately, an orthoplast sleeve, with Velcro straps that permit tightening of the sleeve and allow its removal for personal hygiene, may be used.

Subsequent Management

The patient is usually capable of using the arm with minimal discomfort in a few days.

The sleeve usually holds up for the entire treatment.

The time for the average ulnar fracture to heal and the sleeve to be discarded is approximately ten weeks.

Emphasize clinical rather than radiographic evidence of union. When the fracture is clinically healed, immobilization may be discontinued.

DISPLACED OR UNDISPLACED TWO-BONE FRACTURES IN THE UPPER HALF OF THE FOREARM (IN ADULTS)

REMARKS

Reduction of these fractures should be carried out with attention to rotational alignment so as to avoid fracture displacement during treatment.

Varying degrees of supination are necessary to align the distal fragment with the proximal one. However, avoid extreme supination, which closes the interosseous space.

The amount of fracture rotation is determined by radiographic study of the bicipital tuberosity compared with the opposite, intact radius (see page 892).

Prereduction X-Ray

MINIMALLY DISPLACED FRACTURE

1. Fragments of both bones are slightly angulated but firmly engaged and not displaced.

2. The interosseous space at the level of the fractures is reduced in width.

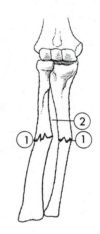

1. A tuberosity view compared with one of the opposite unfractured forearm shows that the proximal fragment is in 30 degrees of supination, which is the position for reduction of the distal fragment.

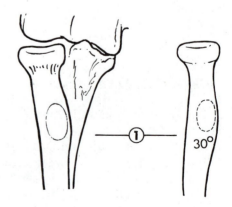

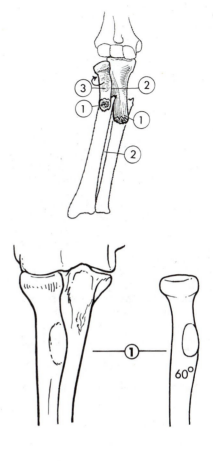

DISPLACED FRACTURE

1. Shortening has occurred.
2. The interosseous space is narrowed.
3. The proximal radial fragment is supinated.

1. A tuberosity view shows the proximal fragment is in 60 degrees of supination when compared with the opposite side, which is the position for reduction of the distal fragment.

Manipulative Reduction

Reduction is performed under general or regional intravenous anesthesia.

PREFERRED METHOD OF ACHIEVING ANESTHESIA. INTRAVENOUS REGIONAL ANESTHETIC

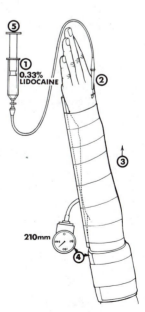

1. Mix 15 cc of 1% lidocaine and 30 cc. of normal saline to make a 0.33% solution. The dose should be 0.5 cc. of this solution per kg of body weight.
2. Insert a small butterfly needle into the hand on the fractured side, which is immobilized in a splint.
3. Elevate the limb at least 3 minutes to diminish edema.
4. Using a pretested and securely taped blood pressure cuff, stop circulation by rapid inflation to at least 210 mm.

Note: Specially designed double tourniquets may also be used.

5. Lower the arm and inject an appropriate dose of the lidocaine solution.

Manipulative Reduction
(Continued)

1. The needle is removed and after a 10-minute interval the fracture is reduced. Always keep the cuff inflated for at least 15 minutes.

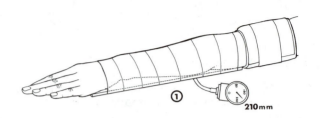

Note: When reduction is satisfactory, deflate the tourniquet for intravenous anesthetic to 80 mm Hg and after ten seconds reinflate it to 210 mm Hg. Monitor vital signs and mental status; if these are unchanged, remove the tourniquet completely. Continuing monitoring the patient's vital signs and mental status for 10 minutes following release of the tourniquet. The entire procedure requires two assistants, one to monitor the pressure of the cuff during the block and the other to assist in reduction. Minimum tourniquet time should always be in excess of 15 minutes. Resuscitation equipment should be immediately available when administering anesthetic of any type.

1. The patient assumes the supine position on the fracture table.

2. The fingers are engaged by finger traction apparatus.

3. Counter traction is made on the arm in a plane parallel to the forearm by a sling of muslin bandage anchored to a crossbar at the bottom of the table.

4. The elbow is flexed 90 degrees.

5. The forearm is supinated to the degree determined by comparison of the tuberosity views.

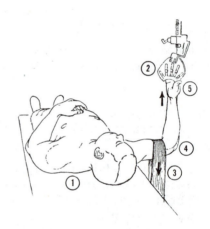

1. Strong traction is applied to the forearm through the finger traction apparatus until length is restored and angular deformity is corrected. This requires at least 10 minutes of traction.

2. After length is restored, the surgeon squeezes the volar muscle mass between the radius and the ulna, forcing the two bones apart.

Note: If, on palpation, the radius remains overlapped, it can be corrected by angulating the forearm while maintaining traction.

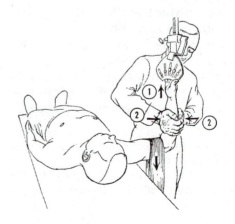

910

Postreduction X-Rays

MINIMALLY DISPLACED FRACTURE

Note: Ideally, reduction is evaluated by image-intensified fluoroscopy.

1. The angular deformities of both bones are corrected. The radial curve is normal.
2. The interosseous space is restored to normal width.

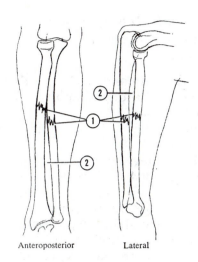

Anteroposterior   Lateral

DISPLACED FRACTURE

1. Angulatory deformity has been decreased to less than 10 degrees, although reduction is not anatomic.
2. The interosseous space is restored to normal width.

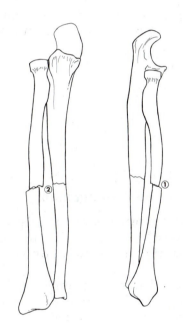

Initial Immobilization

1. While traction is maintained, apply a circular plaster cast from the axilla to the base of the fingers.
2. The forearm is supinated to the degree determined by the tuberosity views. Avoid extreme supination, which narrows the interosseous space.
3. The elbow is flexed 90 degrees.
4. Mold the cast along the volar surface of the radius.

Note: After the cast hardens, the traction is released and the muslin bandage is pulled out of the cast. If intravenous anesthesia has been used, the tourniquet can be released and the patient is monitored as described under "Preferred Method of Anesthesia."

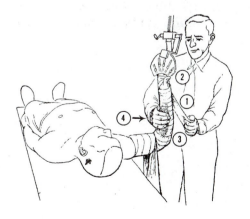

Subsequent Management: Functional Cast-Brace Treatment

When the pain and swelling subside (at seven to ten days), apply a functional cast-brace.

1. The forearm is suspended in finger-traps.

2. The plaster or orthoplast material is firmly molded to compress the tissues in the interosseous space and to maintain normal radial curvature.

3. A supracondylar elbow extension permits flexion and extension but limits forearm pronation and supination.

4. A wrist hinge and hand component permits palmar flexion and dorsiflexion.

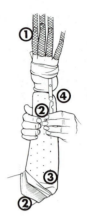

Postreduction Management

Encourage functional exercises of elbow, wrist, shoulder, and forearm muscles during the period of immobilization.

As pain subsides and confidence returns, the patient will use the fractured limb with greater vigor.

Evaluate fracture position periodically by x-rays during first 2 to 3 weeks after cast-brace application.

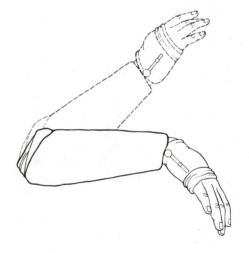

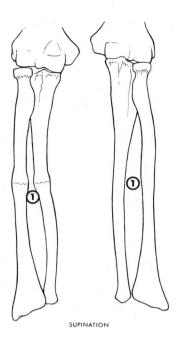

SUPINATION

Reduction is inadequate if the interosseous space becomes narrowed significantly or angulation exceeds 10 degrees. Complete overriding of the fragments is also unacceptable, although end-to-side apposition may be accepted. If the reduction is lost, remanipulate the fracture or perform open reduction and internal fixation.

Follow-up X-ray After Cast-Brace Removal

Slight bayonet or end-to-side apposition permits healing with satisfactory function that is not limited in
1. Supination or

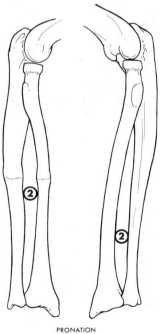

2. Pronation when compared with the opposite intact forearm.

PRONATION

Subsequent Management

Experience with the functional cast-bracing method demonstrates that immobilization of the wrist and elbow is not indispensable for healing of forearm fractures.

Allowing the patient to use the injured limb actively while still supporting the fracture with a snug brace appears to maximize the healing response.

If adequate reduction cannot be maintained during the early stages of treatment, prompt surgical intervention can be employed and the limb may then be protected postoperatively with the functional cast-brace technique.

The average time for healing of displaced two-bone fractures is 15 weeks. Clinical union, with freedom from pain and absence of motion at the fracture site, always occurs before radiographic healing, but protective splints should be continued until the fracture has consolidated on x-ray.

Functional activity during the healing minimizes soft tissue interosseous scarring and muscle contraction and resultant disability when the immobilization is discontinued.

DISPLACED OR UNDISPLACED TWO-BONE FRACTURES IN THE LOWER HALF OF THE FOREARM (IN ADULTS)

REMARKS

These fractures are managed in the same manner as fractures in the upper half of the forearm, except that the rotation should be closer to a neutral position than to supination.

Following initial reduction, a long arm cast is applied until pain and swelling subside (seven to ten days).

Subsequently, a functional cast or cast-brace is applied, and elbow and wrist motion are encouraged.

Prereduction X-Ray

UNDISPLACED FRACTURE

1. Fragments of both bones are angulated but not displaced.
2. The interosseous space between the proximal fragments is decreased in width.

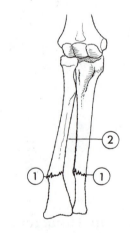

DISPLACED FRACTURE

1. Both the radius and the ulna have shortened and angulated.
2. The interosseous space is extremely narrowed.

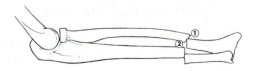

914

Manipulative Reduction

Reduction is performed under general or regional intravenous anesthesia (see page 909).

1. The patient assumes the supine position on the fracture table.

2. The fingers are engaged by the finger traction apparatus.

3. Counter traction is made on the arm in a plane parallel to the forearm by a sling of muslin bandage anchored to the crossbar at the bottom of the table.

4. The elbow is flexed 90 degrees.

5. The forearm is in neutral rotation.

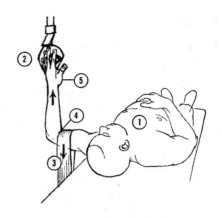

1. Apply strong traction through the finger traction apparatus until length is restored and angulation is corrected. This requires at least 10 minute of traction.

2. After length is restored, squeeze the volar muscle mass between the radius and the ulna, forcing the two bones apart.

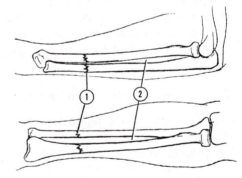

Postreduction X-Ray

UNDISPLACED FRACTURE

1. Angular deformity of both bones is corrected.

2. The interosseous space is restored to its normal width.

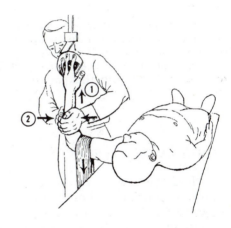

DISPLACED FRACTURE

1. The fractures are aligned but

2. Angulation should not be accepted.

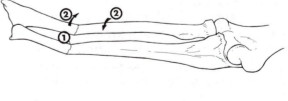

3. This is corrected by remanipulation and immobilization in neutral rotation.

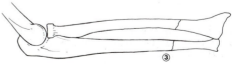

Immobilization

While traction is maintained, apply a circular cast from the axilla to the proximal palmar crease.

1. The elbow is flexed 90 degrees.
2. The forearm is in neutral position.
3. Mold the plaster along the surface of the radius.

Note: Fractures in the distal forearm require less rotation for immobilization. Especially avoid pronation, which tends to cause volar displacement of the distal fragment (see page 892).

Note: After the cast hardens, release the traction apparatus, cut the muslin sling, and pull it out of the cast. If intravenous anesthetic has been used the tourniquet can now be released, and the patient is monitored closely (see page 909).

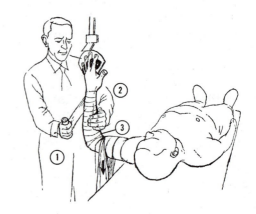

Initial Cast Treatment

Mold the cast well along the volar surface of the radius, restoring its normal concavity. This tends to force the muscles between the bones and preserves the width of the interosseous space.

Check the arm constantly for evidence of circulatory embarrassment; if any signs are noted, bivalve the cast immediately.

The cast should allow free motion at the shoulder and at the fingers.

When pain and swelling subside, apply a functional cast-brace.

Functional Cast-Brace Treatment

1. The forearm is suspended in finger-traps.
2. The plaster or orthoplast material is firmly molded to compress the tissue in the interosseous space and to maintain radial curve.
3. A supracondylar elbow extensor permits flexion and extension but limits pronation and supination.
4. Wrist hinge and hand component permit palmar flexion and dorsiflexion.*

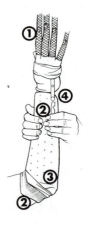

---

*Available from the Zinco Industries, Inc., 3724 Park Place, P. O. Box 567, Montrose, California, 91020.

Subsequent Management

Encourage functional exercises of elbow, wrist, shoulder, and forearm muscles during the period of immobilization.

As pain subsides and confidence returns, the patient will use the fractured limb with greater vigor.

Evaluate fracture position periodically by x-ray during the first 2 to 3 weeks after cast-brace application.

Most functional cast-braces will last for the period of time required for union and will not require replacement.

The average healing time for two-bone fractures is 15 weeks, but occasionally the process may take as long as 6 months. Functional activity allowed during this slower healing minimizes scarring and muscle contracture present when the plaster is discarded.

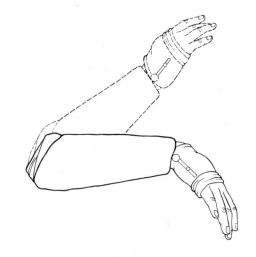

X-Ray of Two-Bone Distal Fracture after Functional Treatment

Excellent union is evident at 15 weeks, on the average, despite lack of immobilization of the wrist and elbow. Compression of the soft tissues and interosseous membrane by this snug cast or brace technique maintains fracture stability during the healing.

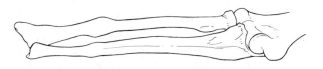

917

OPERATIVE
MANAGEMENT OF
FOREARM FRACTURES

REMARKS

A dynamic compression plate (DCP), as first described by Bagby and refined by the Swiss A.S.I.F. group, is ideal for internal fixation of forearm fractures requiring operative treatment.

Henry's anterior approach and placement of the plate on the flat volar surface are most effective for the majority of radial fractures in the distal half of the forearm.

For fractures of the proximal half of the radius, Thompson's posterior approach and dorsal application of the plate are least likely to injure the radial nerve or to block pronation of the radius.

The plate is applied after elevating the periosteum, and the fracture is reduced by fitting any loose bone fragments directly under the plate.

Use a plate sufficiently long (usually a 5-hole or 6-hole plate) to engage at least five cortices of each of the fragments. Avoid inserting screws closer than 1.0 cm from the fracture so as not to comminute the fracture.

For segmental fractures, apply two separate plates, each holding one fracture as an independent entity.

If there is dislocation of the proximal or distal radioulnar joint, stabilization of the fractured forearm bone usually also stabilizes the dislocation.

Rarely, the annular ligament of the proximal radioulnar joint will be disrupted and will require reconstruction. Also, if the distal radioulnar joint remains unstable in spite of the fracture fixation, it may be reduced and fixed by crossed Kirschner wires.

In fixation of a two-bone fracture of the forearm, both fractures should be exposed and reduced temporarily. The fracture that is less comminuted and is more likely to be securely stabilized by the plate should be fixed first.

Supplemental bone graft is usually unnecessary if loose cortical fragments are reinserted beneath the plate. For extensively comminuted fractures, e.g., gunshot fractures, bone grafting should be done at the time of plating.

Open fractures that require plate fixation because of comminution should be treated initially by thorough wound debridement and should be plated later, when there is no evidence of an infection, usually at one to three weeks.

Other than infection, the most common cause of failure of the plating technique is inadequate fracture fixation. The plate must be of adequate length to permit screw fixation of at least five cortices proximal and five cortices distal to the fracture.

The plate must be centered over the fracture to permit symmetrical compression of the fragment and to avoid angulation.

No screw should be inserted closer than 1 cm from the fracture to avoid fracture comminution and loss of fixation.

The plates need not be removed routinely except in athletes planning to return to contact sports or in patients in whom the subcutaneous presence of the plate irritates overlying soft tissues.

INDICATIONS FOR OPERATIVE MANAGEMENT

With skillful management and knowledge of rotational reduction, the majority of forearm fractures can be treated by closed methods and functional cast-bracing.

Open reduction and internal fixation should be done for fractures in which angulation cannot be reduced by closed means to less than 10 degrees and for fractures in which the interosseous space remains significantly reduced so that obstruction to radial rotation about the ulna is likely to occur.

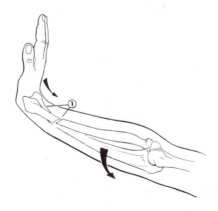

Other candidates for early internal fixation are:

1. Fracture of the radius with ulnar dislocation (Galeazzi's fracture).

2. Two-bone fracture with ulnar dislocation.

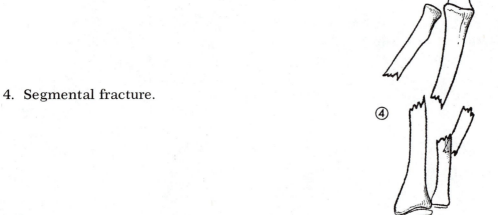

3. Fracture of the ulna with radial head dislocation (Monteggia's fracture).

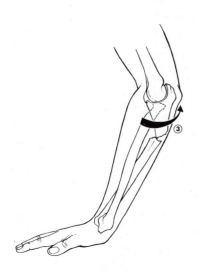

4. Segmental fracture.

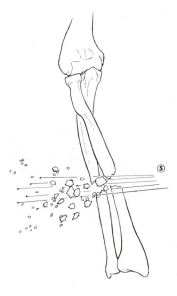

5. Comminuted or gunshot fracture with bone loss requiring bone grafting.

Fractures of the Proximal Half of the Radius

REMARKS

These may not be isolated injuries. Always check the distal radioulnar joint, because dislocation is quite possible.

Closed reduction should be attempted, but angulation of more than 10 degrees toward the ulna is unacceptable, since this is particularly likely to limit the rotation of the radius about the ulna.

The surgical approach to this region should be posterior so as to protect the radial nerve and to allow dorsal application of the plate, which is less likely to block rotation.

The dorsal interosseous nerve runs directly on the dorsal radius opposite the bicipital tuberosity. When placing a plate on the dorsal surface at this level, be sure to protect the posterior interosseous nerve and make certain that there is no soft tissue under the uppermost portion of the plate likely to include the nerve.

Preoperative X-Ray

Fracture of the proximal third of the radius.

1. The proximal fragment is supinated and displaced forward.

2. The distal fragment is pronated and drawn toward the ulna.

Note: If angulation cannot be improved by closed reduction, it should not be accepted because it would seriously limit forearm rotation. Dislocation of the distal radioulnar joint should be suspected with radial instability of this severity.

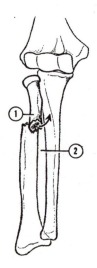

Operative Technique (Thompson Approach)

INCISION AND EXPOSURE

1. The incision runs posterior from the lateral epicondyle to the mid-forearm between the extensor digitorum communis and the extensor carpi radialis brevis, with the forearm pronated.

2. The fascia is opened and dissection is continued carefully between the extensor digitorum communis and the extensor carpi radialis brevis.

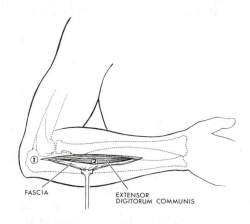

3. To protect the dorsal interosseous (radial) nerve exiting from the inferior margin of the supinator, the forearm is supinated and the supinator muscle is detached from its radial insertion.

4. Additional exposure is obtained by reflecting the abductor pollicis longus while protecting the radial nerve.

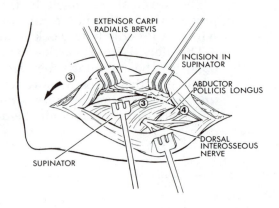

922

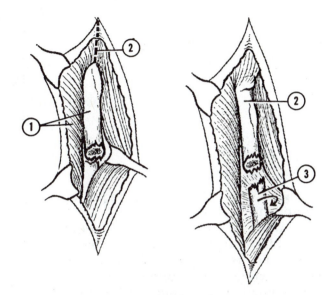

1. Expose the radius by subperiosteal dissection, retracting the supinator laterally.

2. Proximal exposure is possible up to the neck of the radius.

3. The distal fragment is exposed, and reduction is achieved by rotational positioning.

REDUCTION

1. Lever the fragments into normal anatomic alignment correcting rotation.

2. Apply a five-hole or six-hole dynamic compression plate to the dorsal surface.

3. A three-pronged Lowman clamp retains the plate in correct position, centered over the fracture.

4. Any bone fragments must be inserted under the plate, which is carefully aligned in the long axis of the bone to compress the fracture without angulation.

Note: Be careful to avoid entrapping the posterior interosseous nerve under the proximal end of the plate.

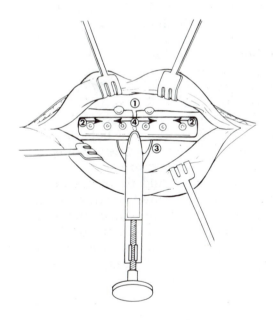

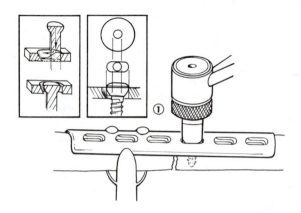

PLATE FIXATION

The A.O. or A.S.I.F. technique of fixation is followed closely.

1. A neutral drill guide is used for the initial fixation of the plate to the bone. This guide is not marked by an arrow and it centers the chamfered screw at the bottom of the obliquely inclined screw hole. A 3.2-mm hole is drilled and tapped, the first screw is inserted at least 1 cm from the fracture.

2. With the fracture anatomically reduced, the plate is pulled toward the upper fragment and a second hole is drilled with the load drill guide. This guide locates the hole 1.0 mm eccentrically from the geometric center of the hole. *The arrow of this eccentrically designed load drill guide must always point toward the fracture.*

3. As the screw is inserted eccentrically, it glides along the obliquely inclined edge of the screw hole toward the center, at the same time pushing or compressing the fracture.

4. The plate should be of adequate length to permit screw fixation of at least five cortices proximal and five cortices distal to the fracture. These remaining screw holes are drilled using the neutral drill guide.

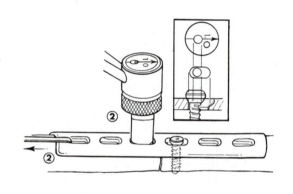

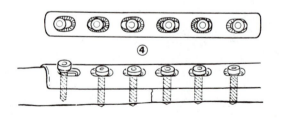

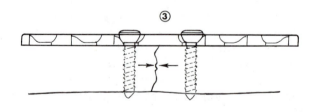

Postoperative Management

Avoid closing the fascia; tight closure over the plates can produce compartmental syndrome and ischemic necrosis.

Immobilization should be individualized according to the type of fracture, the adequacy of the fixation, and the cooperation of the patient.

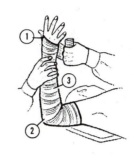

IMMEDIATE MANAGEMENT

1. Apply a compression dressing for three to five days.
2. Allow prompt commencement of exercises of the elbow and hand by removing the postoperative splint when swelling subsides.
3. Maintain rotational alignment by forearm positioning, but avoid extreme supination.

If the fracture was comminuted or if the patient is unlikely to cooperate:

Apply a functional cast-brace after the initial swelling subsides and maintain for six weeks.

Allow the patient to actively exercise shoulder, elbow, wrist, and hand. The cast-brace may usually be discarded by six to eight weeks if fracture union is evident on x-ray.

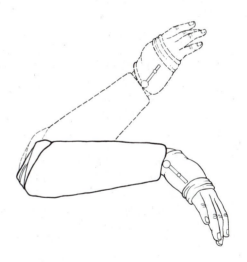

Follow-up Management

On the average the fracture line will fill in by eight weeks and all external support can be discarded.

The patient should be cautioned to avoid heavy lifting or reinjury of the forearm as it regains strength. In active individuals, a protective brace is useful during the third and fourth postoperative months.

Routine removal of the plates is not necessary except in athletic individuals who participate in contact sports or in patients in whom the subcutaneous presence of the plate(s) irritates overlying soft tissues.

Fractures of the Distal Half of the Radius With or Without Dislocation of the Distal Radioulnar Joint

REMARKS

In the early part of this century, the eponym for solitary fracture of the distal radius was the "chauffeur's fracture," because the most common mechanism was a violent, direct blow to the radius incurred while turning the crank on a motor car. Isolated, undisplaced fractures may still occur from direct blows.

Another mechanism of injury is a forceful rotation, either in a pronation or supination direction, that disrupts the distal radioulnar joint and also fractures the radius. Forceful pronation causes dorsal angulation, whereas supination causes volar angulation (see page 898).

Single-bone fracture of the distal radius or displaced radial fracture at any level should be carefully evaluated for associated dislocation of the distal radioulnar joint. Dislocation may not be evident on the initial x-ray and may show up only on subsequent studies or even after cast application (Galeazzi's fracture).

Undisplaced distal radial fractures can be treated by closed methods, avoiding pronation, which tends to cause volar displacement of the distal fragment (see page 892).

For fractures with disruption of the radioulnar joint, internal fixation is critical to permit realignment of the distal joint. The anterior approach by Henry's exposure should be used, because the plate can be applied to the flat anterior surface of the radius.

Preoperative X-Ray

SUPINATION INJURY

1. Fracture of the shaft of the radius proximal to (8 cm from) the radiocarpal joint.

2. The fragments angulate toward the ulna and

3. In a volar direction, indicating that the mechanism was a supination injury.

4. The head of the ulna is dislocated (Galeazzi's fracture).

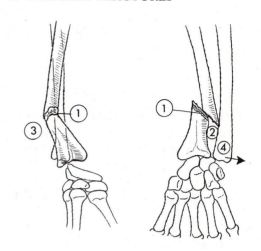

PRONATION INJURY

1. The distal fragment is pronated and displaced toward the ulna, volarly and proximally.

2. The interosseous space is markedly reduced.

3. The fracture is oblique and angulates dorsally, indicating a pronation mechanism.

Note: Fractures with this much displacement and angulation are always associated with disruption of the distal radioulnar joint.

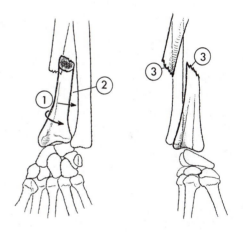

927

Operative Reduction: Dynamic Compression Plating (Exposure of Henry)

INCISION AND EXPOSURE

1. Make an incision along the anterior margin of the brachioradialis, beginning at the radial styloid process and extending proximally for the required distance.

2. Divide the deep fascia along a line slightly medial to the margin of the brachioradialis.

3. Identify the radial artery and vein between the brachioradialis (laterally) and the flexor carpi radialis (medially).

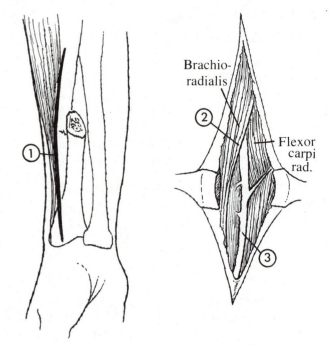

4. Identify and protect the sensory branch of the radial nerve. It lies beneath the brachioradialis.

5. Develop the interval between the brachioradialis and the extensor carpi radialis longus laterally and the flexor carpi radialis medially.

6. Now the floor of the wound is composed of the pronator quadratus, the flexor pollicis longus, and the flexor digitorum sublimis.

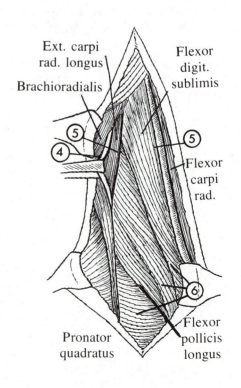

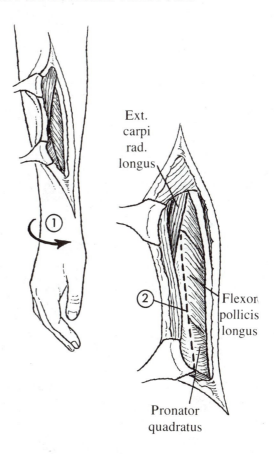

1. Pronate the forearm.

2. Incise the tissue longitudinally on a line between the origin of the pronator quadratus and the flexor pollicis longus (medially) and the tendon of the extensor carpi radialis longus (laterally).

3. Expose the shaft of both fragments by subperiosteal dissection.

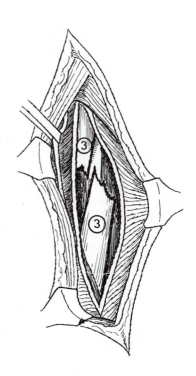

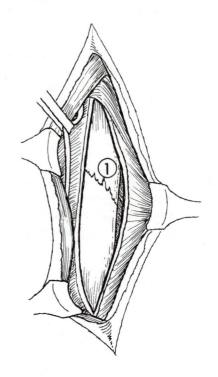

Operative Reduction: Dynamic Compression Plating (Exposure of Henry) (Continued)

REDUCTION

1. Lever the fragments into normal anatomic position.

2. Fix the fragments with a five-hole or six-hole dynamic compression plate on the volar side of the radius, maintaining reduction with a three-prong Lowman clamp.

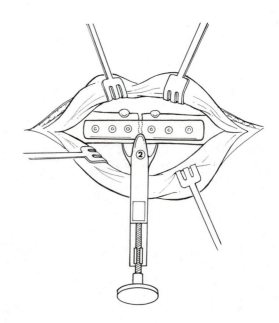

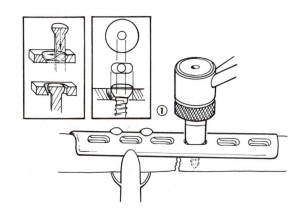

Plate fixation

The A.O. or A.S.I.F. technique of fixation is followed closely.

1. A neutral drill guide is used for the initial fixation of the plate to the bone. This guide is not marked by an arrow and it centers the chamfered screw at the bottom of the obliquely inclined screw hole. A 3.2 mm hole is drilled and tapped, and the first screw is inserted at least 1 cm from the fracture.

2. With the fracture anatomically reduced, the plate is pulled toward the upper fragment and a second hole is drilled with the load drill guide. This guide locates the hole 1.0 mm eccentrically from the geometric center of the hole. *The arrow of this eccentrically designed load drill guide must always point toward the fracture.*

3. As the screw is inserted eccentrically, it glides along the obliquely inclined edge of the screw hole toward the center, at the same time pushing or compressing the fracture.

4. The plate should be of adequate length to permit screw fixation of at least five cortices proximal and five cortices distal to the fracture. These remaining screw holes are drilled using the neutral drill guide.

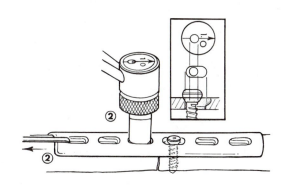

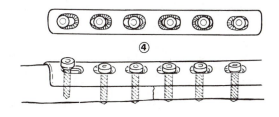

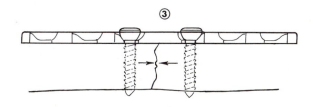

Postreduction X-Ray

Reduction of the radial fracture will usually also reduce the distal joint.

If the distal radioulnar joint remains unstable, temporary Kirschner wire fixation may be used.

1. Compression plating of the distal radial fracture with persistent radio-ulnar dislocation.

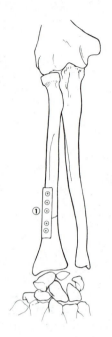

1. Compression plate is combined with

2. Radioulnar fixation to reduce the joint.

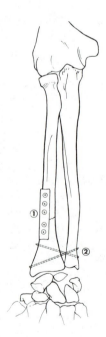

Postoperative Management

IMMEDIATE MANAGEMENT

1. Apply a compression dressing for three to five days.
2. The elbow is flexed 90 degrees.
3. The forearm is in midrotation.

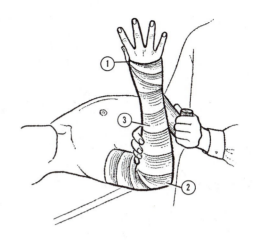

SUBSEQUENT MANAGEMENT

Immobilization should be individualized according to the type of fracture, the adequacy of the fixation, and the cooperation of the patient.

After initial postoperative swelling has subsided, external support may sometimes be discarded, although it is usually safer to employ a functional cast-brace.

If the fracture was unstable and pins were required to immobilize the distal radioulnar joint, postoperative immobilization should be continued for a month, or until the pins are removed.

During postoperative immobilization, the patient should actively exercise the shoulder, elbow, and fingers of the injured limb.

Remove the pins at one month and begin active range-of-motion exercises.

Follow-up Management

On the average, the fracture line will fill in by eight weeks and the external cast support can be discarded.

For active individuals, a protective splint should be continued for an additional two to three months.

Routine removal of the plate is not necessary except in athletic individuals who participate in contact sports or in patients in whom subcutaneous presence of the plate irritates overlying soft tissues.

Displaced Fractures of the Ulna
(in Adults)

REMARKS

Ulnar fractures do well when treated by closed methods and functional bracing (see page 906).

Indications for operative fixation of an ulnar fracture include associated dislocation of the proximal or distal radioulnar joint, delayed union, and nonunion.

Remember also that an ulnar fracture that persists on x-ray may be well-healed clinically. Be sure that the patient's symptoms and functional limitation warrant treatment for "ununited" ulnar fracture.

Frequently, nonunion of the ulna is due to extensive bone loss, as occurs in a gunshot fracture.

The ulna is analogous to the fibula in that a sizable defect may not cause pain symptoms or instability, whereas an undisplaced but unhealed fracture may well cause pain.

A good portion of the ulna is expendable, especially from the distal half toward the wrist. Keep this in mind before carrying out elaborate bone grafting procedures to heal nonunited ulnar fractures with large defects.

Prereduction X-Ray

1. Angulation of the ulnar fragments toward the radius.

2. The interosseous space is narrowed.

Note: This fracture can ordinarily be treated by closed methods. Operative fixation is indicated only when closed reduction is unsuccessful.

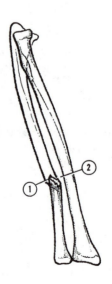

Operative Procedure

INCISION

1. Make a 13-cm incision over the crest of the ulna and centered over the site of the fracture.

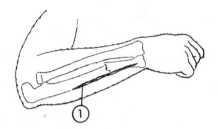

EXPOSURE AND REDUCTION

1. Expose both fragments by extraperiosteal dissection.

2. Apply a six-hole dynamic compression plate to the fracture. (A five-hole plate may be suitable if the fracture is not comminuted.)

3. A three-prong Lowman clamp is centered over the fracture.

4. Any bone fragments must be inserted under the plate, which is carefully aligned in the long axis of the bone to compress the fracture without angulation.

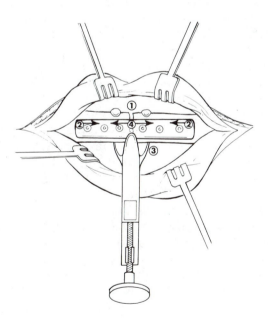

PLATE FIXATION

The A.O. or A.S.I.F. technique of fixation is followed closely.

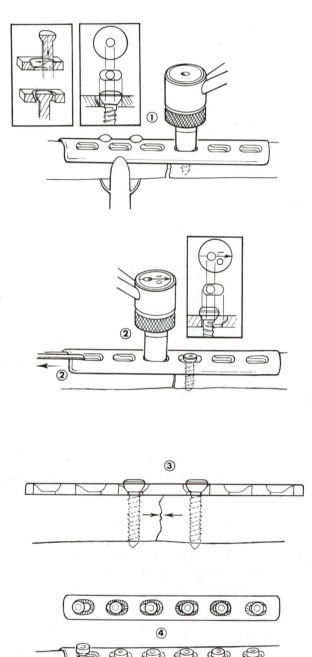

1. A neutral drill guide is used for the initial fixation of the plate to the bone. This guide is not marked by an arrow and it centers the chamfered screw at the bottom of the obliquely inclined screw hole. A 3.2 mm hole is drilled and tapped, and the first screw is inserted at least 1 cm from the fracture.

2. With the fracture anatomically reduced, the plate is pulled toward the upper fragment and a second hole is drilled with the load drill guide. This guide locates the hole 1.0 mm eccentrically from the geometric center of the hole. *The arrow of this eccentrically designed load drill guide must always point toward the fracture.*

3. As the screw is inserted eccentrically, it glides along the obliquely inclined edge of the screw hole toward the center, at the same time pushing or compressing the fracture.

4. The plate should be of adequate length to permit screw fixation of at least five cortices proximal and five cortices distal to the fracture. These remaining screw holes are drilled using the neutral drill guide.

Postoperative Management

Avoid closing fascia; tight closure over plates can produce compartmental syndrome and ischemic necrosis. Immobilization should be individualized according to the type of fracture, the adequacy of fixation, and the cooperation of the patient.

IMMEDIATE MANAGEMENT

1. Apply a circular cast.
2. The forearm is in neutral rotation.
3. The elbow is flexed 90 degrees.

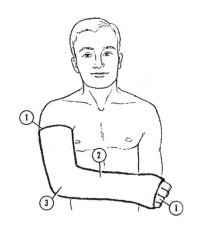

SUBSEQUENT MANAGEMENT

The cast is removed when the postoperative swelling subsides, usually by the third to fifth day, while the patient is still in the hospital to allow supervised range-of-motion exercises. The patient is encouraged to begin active finger and shoulder exercises immediately and also to work on forearm rotation.

If the fracture was unstable, a forearm sleeve (see page 906) may be applied when the initial swelling subsides.

The forearm sleeve may be discarded by six to eight weeks if healing of the fracture line is evident on x-ray.

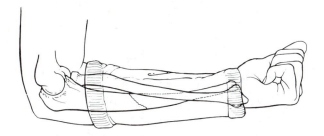

Follow-up Management

The patient should be cautioned to avoid any heavy lifting or reinjury to the forearm as it regains strength, and for active individuals a protective brace is useful during the third to fourth postoperative months.

Routine removal of the plate is unnecessary except in athletic individuals who wish to return to contact sports or in patients in whom the subcutaneous presence of the plate irritates overlying soft tissues.

937

Solitary Fractures of the Ulna with Large Defects: "The Three-Bone Forearm"

REMARKS

Frequently a gunshot injury or violent, direct trauma to the ulna will produce a large fracture defect in the ulna with no or minimal fracture of the radius.

After the soft tissue injury and the radial fracture (if it occurred) have healed, an extensive bone graft may be necessary to fill in the ulnar defect.

Before advising operative treatment of these defects, evaluate the patient's forearm function, which can be quite normal and pain-free in spite of the ulnar defect.

Operative grafting of the ulnar defect may actually worsen forearm rotation because of the associated scarring and prolonged immobilization.

Appearance Immediately After Injury

1. Gunshot fracture to the ulna has produced a large defect.

2. The ulnar nerve is also damaged.

3. The radius is intact.

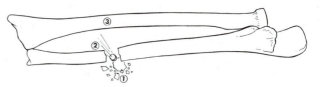

Range of Motion After Healing of Soft Tissue and Ulnar Nerve

1. Forearm rotation is minimally limited despite ulnar defect. This is essentially a "three-bone" forearm.

2. Occasionally with this instability the proximal or distal end of the defect will become prominent and can be treated by surgical excision.

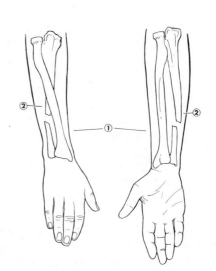

RESECTION OF THE DISTAL ULNA

Chronic dislocation of the distal ulna that causes wrist pain and limitation of motion is best treated by resection of the distal 2 cm of the bone.

Nonunited fractures of the distal 5 to 6 cm of the ulna may also be managed effectively by resection rather than internal fixation.

A surprising amount of the ulna may be resected without disability and without causing protrusion of the proximal ulna, provided that the interosseous membrane is stable.

The ulna is analogous to the fibula in that a good deal of the bone may be lost without causing a problem, except where it is necessary for joint stability.

Just as the entire proximal two-thirds of the fibula may be removed without affecting knee joint stability, a sizable proportion of the ulna may also be lost without detriment to forearm or wrist function.

Keep the expendability of the ulna in mind before performing elaborate bone grafting procedures to heal ulnar fractures or to fill large defects of the distal or middle third.

CAUTION:

Avoid resecting the ulna in conjunction with acute treatment of associated radial fracture (Galeazzi's fracture). The radial fracture must heal before the chronically dislocated ulna is resected.

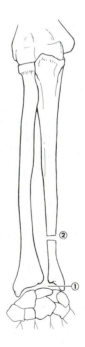

Indications for Ulnar Resection

1. Chronic symptomatic dislocation of the distal radioulnar joint with a healed fracture of the distal radius.

2. Chronic nonunion of the distal ulna with a fracture gap.

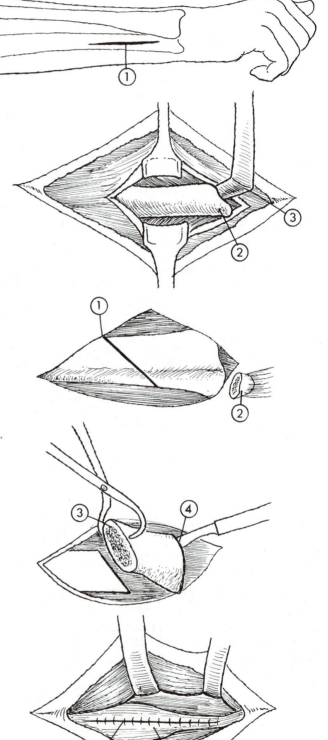

Operative Procedure

INCISION AND EXPOSURE

1. Make a 6-cm incision on the lateral aspect of the distal end of the forearm between the flexor carpi ulnaris and the extensor carpi ulnaris.

2. Divide the periosteum over the distal 5 cm of the ulna, and by subperiosteal dissection expose the ulna as far as the styloid process.

3. Isolate the end of the ulna with small reverse retractors.

RESECTION

1. With an electric saw, cut obliquely through the bone from the outer border to the inner border.

2. Osteotomize transversely the ulnar styloid process at its base and leave it attached to the lateral ligament.

3. Grasp the distal end of the ulna with a towel clip and

4. By sharp dissection excise the fragment.

5. Cover the ulnar stump with the surrounding muscle tissue.

6. Approximate the periosteal sleeve with fine sutures.

940

Displaced Fractures of Both Bones in the Proximal Half of the Forearm

REMARKS

Fractures of both bones that cannot be reduced by closed methods or that are comminuted enough to require grafting are best treated by plate fixation.

Exposure in this region is best via the Thompson dorsal approach in order to protect the radial nerve and to allow dorsal application of the plate to the radius so as not to block rotation.

The ulnar fracture is exposed by a second, separate incision.

Reduce both fractures prior to applying a plate and fix the stable, less comminuted fracture first; this is usually the ulnar fracture. Do not discard loose bone fragments, but insert them into the fracture directly under the plate.

If a bone gap remains because of comminution after the plate is applied, fill the defect with autogenous bone graft.

Ordinarily if more than one-third of the cortex is comminuted, bone grafting is necessary.

Be careful to avoid injury to the posterior interosseous nerve, which is close to the proximal portion of the plate. The nerve runs directly over the radius opposite the level of the bicipital tuberosity.

Prereduction X-Ray

1. The fragments are angulated and overriding.

2. The interosseous space is obliterated.

3. The proximal radial fragment is supinated and is displaced anteriorly.

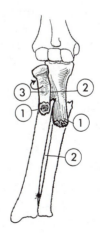

Operative Exposure of the Ulnar Fracture

1. Make a 13-cm incision over the crest of the ulna centered over the site of fracture.

2. Expose both fragments by subperiosteal dissection and then expose the radial fracture by a second posterior incision.

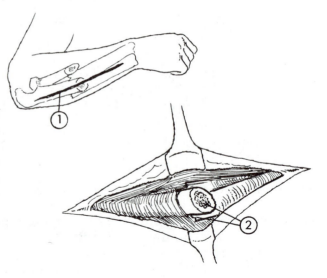

Operative Exposure of Radial Fracture by Thompson Approach

1. Incision runs posterior from the lateral epicondyle to the midforearm between the extensor digitorum communis and the extensor carpi radialis brevis, with the forearm pronated.

2. The fascia is opened, and dissection is continued carefully between the extensor digitorum communis and the extensor carpi radialis brevis.

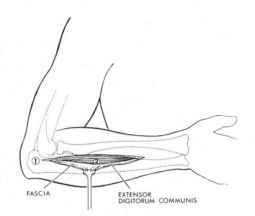

3. To protect the dorsal interosseous (radial) nerve exiting from the superior margin of the supinator, the forearm is supinated and the supinator muscle is detached from its radial insertion.

4. Additional exposure is obtained by reflecting the abductor pollicis longus while protecting the radial nerve.

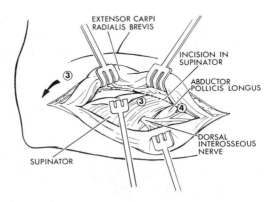

Reduce both fractures and fix the more stable one first with a dynamic compression plate (see page 935).

If a butterfly fragment is present, insert it into the fracture under the plate.

For a comminuted fracture with bone loss, fill the defect with cancellous bone from the iliac crest.

942

TECHNIQUE OF ILIAC CREST BONE GRAFTING

1. An incision is made directly down onto the iliac crest.

2. The iliac crest is split without disturbing the muscle attachments.

3. Small chips of cancellous bone are removed to fill the defect in the forearm.

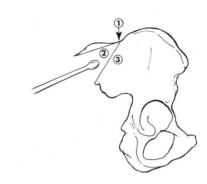

Postreduction X-Ray

1. The ulnar fracture is stabilized by a six-hole dynamic compression plate.

2. The radial fracture is held by a six-hole dynamic compression plate applied to the dorsal surface.

3. Bone graft has been added because of comminution of the radial cortex.

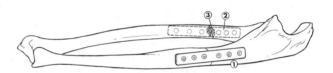

Postreduction Management

Avoid closure of the fascia; tight closure over the plate can produce compartmental syndrome and ischemic necrosis.

Immobilization should be individualized according to the type of fracture, the adequacy of fixation, and the cooperation of the patient.

IMMEDIATE MANAGEMENT

1. Apply a compression dressing for three to five days.

2. The elbow is flexed 90 degrees.

3. The forearm is in midrotation.

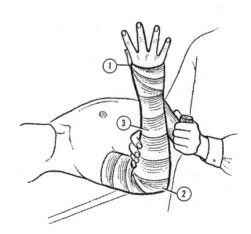

943

Postreduction Management
(Continued)

SUBSEQUENT MANAGEMENT

Apply a functional cast-brace for six weeks after initial postoperative swelling subsides.

Encourage free use of the patient's shoulder, elbow, and hand during the period of immobilization.

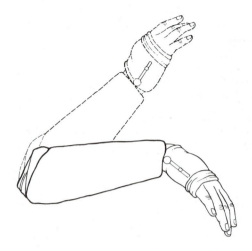

Follow-up Management

On the average, the fracture line will fill in by eight weeks and all external support can be discarded.

The patient should be cautioned to avoid heavy lifting or reinjury of the forearm as it regains strength.

In active individuals a protective brace is prudent during the third and fourth postoperative months, until union is complete on x-ray.

Routine removal of the plates is not necessary except in athletic individuals who participate in contact sports or in patients in whom the subcutaneous presence of the plates irritates overlying soft tissues.

Fracture of Both Bones of the Distal Half of the Forearm

REMARKS

Operative reduction and internal fixation should be done when a satisfactory closed reduction is not achieved for functional treatment or when the fracture is sufficiently comminuted to require bone grafting.

The radial fracture at this level is best approached anteriorly by Henry's exposure.

The fractures are exposed by separate incisions and are reduced prior to plate application.

The more stable or less comminuted fractures should be fixed first; this is usually the ulnar fracture.

Preoperative X-Ray (After Unsuccessful Closed Reduction)

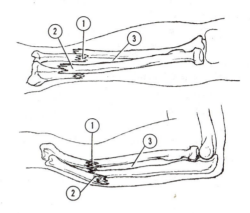

1. The fragments are angulated and the ends are comminuted.
2. The fragments are overriding.
3. The interosseous space is markedly narrowed.

Operative Reduction

EXPOSURE

1. Make a 13-cm incision over the crest of the ulna and centered over the site of fracture.
2. Expose both fragments by subperiosteal dissection. Then expose the radial fracture by a second incision.

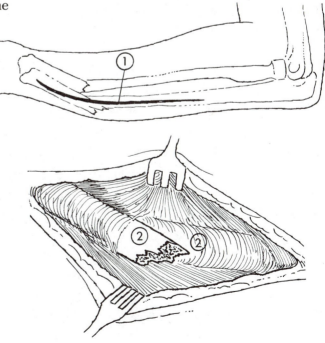

Operative Reduction (Continued)

THE EXPOSURE OF HENRY

1. Make an incision along the anterior margin of the brachioradialis beginning at the radial styloid process and extending proximally for the required distance.

2. Divide the deep fascia along a line slightly medial to the margin of the brachioradialis.

3. Identify the radial artery and vein between the brachioradialis (laterally) and the flexor carpi radialis (medially).

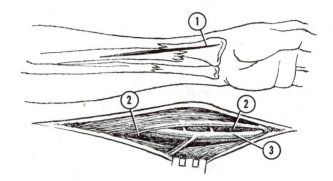

4. Identify and protect the sensory branch of the radial nerve. It lies beneath the brachioradialis.

5. Develop the interval between the brachioradialis and the extensor carpi radialis longus (laterally) and the flexor carpi radialis (medially).

6. Now the floor of the wound is composed of the pronator quadratus, the flexor pollicis longus, and the flexor digitorum sublimis.

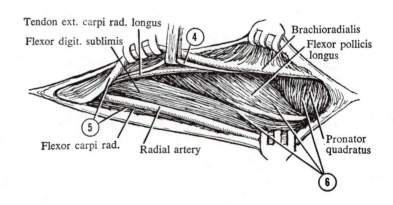

Tendon ext. carpi rad. longus
Flexor digit. sublimis
Brachioradialis
Flexor pollicis longus
Flexor carpi rad.
Radial artery
Pronator quadratus

1. Pronate the forearm.

2. Incise the tissue longitudinally on a line between the origin of the pronator quadratus and the flexor pollicis longus medially and the tendon of the extensor carpi radialis longus laterally.

3. Expose the shaft of both fragments by subperiosteal dissection.

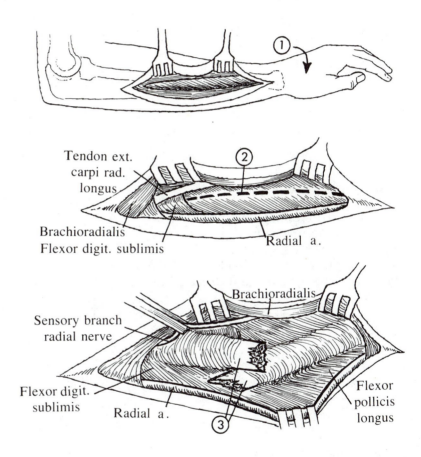

FIXATION WITH DYNAMIC
COMPRESSION PLATES (SEE PAGE 935)

1. The ulna and

2. The radius are fixed with dynamic compression plates.

3. Bone graft is used if fracture is comminuted.

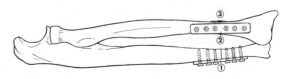

947

Postoperative Management

Avoid closing the fascia; tight closure over plates can cause compartmental syndrome and ischemic necrosis.

Immobilization should be individualized according to the type of fracture, the adequacy of reduction, and the cooperation of the patient.

IMMEDIATE MANAGEMENT

1. Apply a circular cast.
2. The forearm is in neutral rotation.
3. The elbow is flexed 90 degrees.

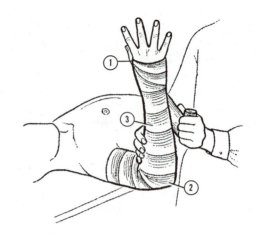

SUBSEQUENT MANAGEMENT

Apply a functional cast-brace after initial postoperative swelling subsides and maintain for six weeks.

Encourage free use of the patient's shoulder, elbow, and hand during immobilization.

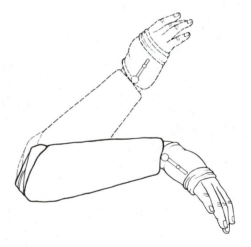

Follow-up Management

On the average, the fracture line will be filled in on x-ray by eight weeks and all external support can be discarded.

The patient should be cautioned to avoid heavy lifting or reinjury of the forearm as it regains strength.

In active individuals a protective brace is useful during the third and fourth postoperative months.

Routine removal of the plates is not necessary except in athletic individuals who participate in contact sports or in patients in whom the subcutaneous presence of the plates irritates overlying soft tissues.

Segmental Fractures of Both Bones of the Forearm

REMARKS

These lesions usually are the result of considerable violence, and the fragments may show extensive comminution.

There is usually soft tissue damage and other multiple injuries.

Because of the degree of fracture instability and the likelihood of malunion, open reduction and plate fixation, frequently supplemented by autogenous bone grafts, are the most effective treatment.

Treat each fracture of the segment with separate plate fixation rather than trying to fix the complex injury with one long plate.

Expose and reduce each fracture prior to plate application and then plate the least comminuted, most stable fracture first; this is usually in the ulna.

Do not discard loose bone chips, but insert them under the plate in order to fill any bone defects.

Apply supplemental cancellous graft if more than one third of the cortex is comminuted.

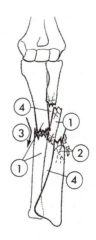

Prereduction X-Ray

1. Segmental fracture of the radius and fracture of the ulna.

2. The radial fragments are moderately comminuted.

3. There is marked angulation of the fragment.

4. The interosseous space is severely distorted.

Operative Reduction

1. Make a 10-cm incision over the crest of the ulna and centered over the site of the fracture.

2. Expose both fragments by subperiosteal dissection and then expose the radial fracture.

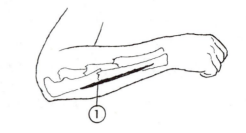

EXPOSURE OF HENRY

Note: Exposure of the radial fracture may be possible through one incision via the Henry approach, but frequently both dorsal and volar approaches are necessary in order to apply separate plates without blocking rotation.

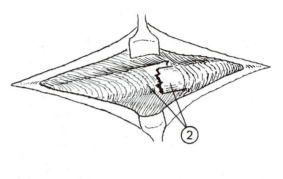

1. Make an incision along the anterior margin of the brachioradialis extending downward for a distance of 18 cm from the level of the lateral epicondyle.

2. Divide the deep fascia along the anterior margin of the brachialis for the entire length of the incision and expose the biceps tendon in the upper portion of the wound.

3. Identify, ligate, and cut the radial recurrent vessels.

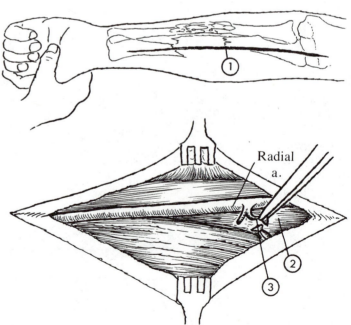

Radial a.

1. Displace the brachioradialis laterally and identify the superficial branch of the radial nerve.

2. Identify the pronator teres on the medial side of the wound, the supinator and radial artery on the medial side.

3. Develop the interval along the line of the junction of the supinator and the pronator teres. Expose the radius by subperiosteal dissection, reflecting the supinator laterally.

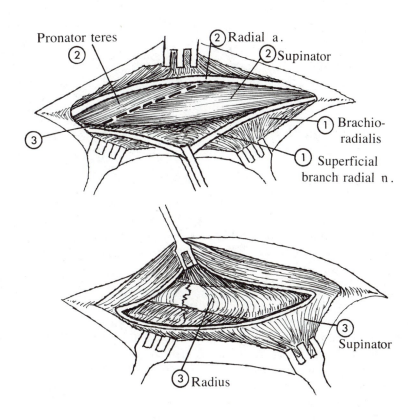

Operative Reduction (Continued)

REDUCTION

1. Extend the dissection proximally, exposing the tuberosity and neck of the radius; then pronate the radius and expose the distal segment of the shaft.

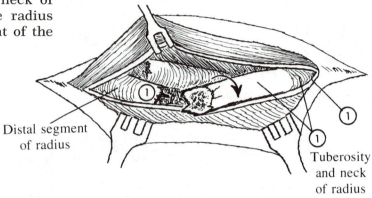

Distal segment of radius

Tuberosity and neck of radius

2. Stabilize the segmental radial fracture with bone-holding clamps.

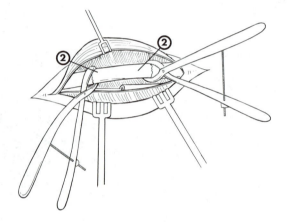

3. With the radius stabilized, fix the ulna using the dynamic compression plate technique (see page 935).
After fixing the ulna:

1. Fix the distal radial fracture with a dynamic compression plate applied to the volar surface.

2. Fix the proximal radial fracture with a dynamic compression plate applied to the dorsal surface.

3. Add supplemental bone graft for any comminution of more than one third of the cortex.

Note: Be careful to avoid placing bone near the interosseous border of the radius.

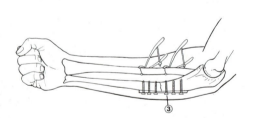

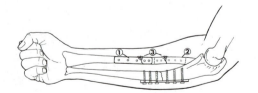

Postoperative Management

IMMEDIATE MANAGEMENT

1. Apply a circular cast from the axilla to the proximal crease of the hand.
2. The elbow is flexed 90 degrees.
3. The forearm is in midposition.
4. Mold the plaster on the volar surface of the radius.

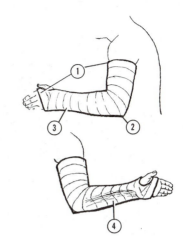

SUBSEQUENT MANAGEMENT

Apply a functional cast-brace after the initial swelling subsides and maintain for eight to twelve weeks.

Allow free use of the patient's shoulder, elbow, and hand.

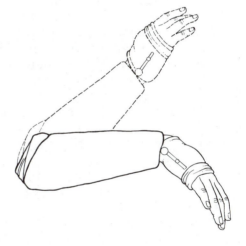

Follow-up Management

On the average the fracture line will fill in by eight to twelve weeks and all external support can be discarded.

The patient should be cautioned to avoid heavy lifting or reinjury of the forearm as it regains strength. In active individuals a protective brace is necessary during the third and fourth postoperative months.

Routine removal of the plates is not necessary except in athletic individuals who participate in contact sports or in patients in whom the subcutaneous presence of the plates irritates overlying soft tissues.

MANAGEMENT OF OPEN
FRACTURES OF THE
BONES OF THE FOREARM

REMARKS

Approximately 15 per cent of forearm fractures are open injuries requiring complete wound debridement.

The smallest wounds often prove the most treacherous, because fracture fragments may have been driven out through the wound to be contaminated by dirt, barnyard manure, or a variety of pathogens, and then have returned under the skin.

Avoid the inclination to debride only the superficial wound for fear of damaging underlying tendons or nerves. Too often this leaves the patient with a significant deep abscess at the fracture site and a strong chance for a tragic outcome.

All open forearm fractures, even with slight and seemingly insignificant puncture wounds, require complete operative cleansing of the bone ends as outlined on pages 125 and 130, including tetanus prophylaxis.

If the wound is explored surgically within six hours, before bacteria become firmly established in the traumatized tissues, and if the bone ends are found to be clean, the wound may be closed primarily.

All other wounds, especially wounds of an uncertain nature, should be left open to be reexplored and reirrigated within three days. Secondary closure may be performed at this time of reexploration but the edematous wound should never be closed under tension. If there is any doubt, the wound should be allowed to heal spontaneously by intussusception of the wound edges.

Undisplaced open fractures heal well when treated by functional cast-bracing.

Comminuted or segmental open fractures that are likely to require bone grafting respond best to compression plate techniques.

Special problems of open forearm fractures require adaptable approaches to the functional needs of the patient.

Open forearm fractures are more likely than closed fractures to be associated with vascular or neural injuries, especially when the mechanism of injury is direct violence, as in gunshot fracture. The artery injured at the forearm level should be repaired or replaced by autogenous graft at the time of initial debridement.

954

Injured nerves should be repaired promptly, but the neurorrhaphy can be done in conjunction with fracture fixation after the initial wound has healed without infection (usually within 10 to 14 days).

During the healing period of the primary wound, the fracture can usually be immobilized with a long arm plaster. External skeletal fixation or traction may be necessary for an unstable fracture.

Types of Open Fractures

PUNCTURE WOUND

1. Beware of small puncture wounds, which do not always reflect the degree of contamination.

2. Fragments may have been driven through the skin and into the ground or dirt and then returned beneath the skin.

Note: All open forearm fractures require complete wound debridement.

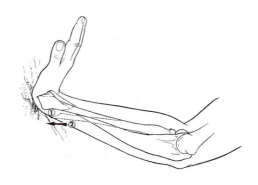

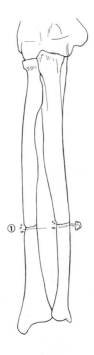

GUNSHOT FRACTURE

1. Undisplaced gunshot fracture may be treated by functional cast-brace. Low-velocity gunshot wound does not necessitate fracture exploration (see page 132).

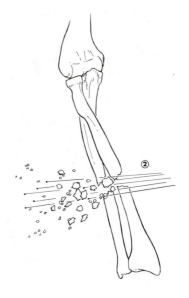

2. Comminuted gunshot fracture requires thorough debridement and secondary internal fixation with bone graft.

Note: Comminuted open fractures frequently damage adjacent arteries and nerves, which must also be repaired.

SKELETAL TRACTION FOR UNSTABLE OPEN FRACTURES OF BOTH BONES OF THE FOREARM

Prereduction X-Ray

After debridement, the wound was left open.

Fractures of both bones of the forearm are severely comminuted.

Note: Many open fractures may be treated by functional cast-bracing. Fractures with this much displacement require temporary traction to align the fragments until plating and bone grafting can be carried out.

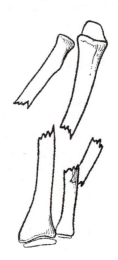

Skeletal Traction

1. Pass a threaded wire through the radius and ulna 2 cm above the wrist joint.

2. Pass another threaded wire through the distal end of the humerus 3 cm above the epicondyles of the humerus. Insert the pin from the ulna side to avoid impaling the nerve.

3. Apply 10 lb (4.5 kg) of traction to the forearm. The traction on the lower end of the humerus should be sufficient to keep the humerus in a plane parallel with the patient's trunk.

4. The forearm is held in neutral rotation to maintain the interosseous space in its widest position.

Note: Pins should fix the humerus and the distal radioulnar structures rather than the proximal forearm in order to avoid damaging any of the interosseous soft tissues. As soon as swelling subsides, the proximal and distal pins may be incorporated in plaster.

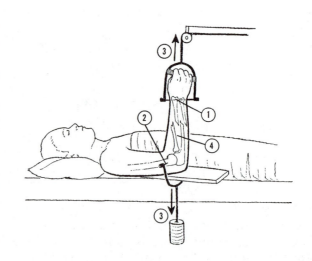

956

FRACTURE OF THE ULNA WITH DISLOCATION OF THE RADIAL HEAD (MONTEGGIA FRACTURE)

REMARKS

About 7 per cent of forearm fractures are a combination of fracture of the ulna at any level and dislocation of the radial head (Monteggia fracture).

Results from this injury in the past have been notoriously bad, because either the dislocation goes unrecognized or nonunion occurs. Awareness of this likely combination and use of adequate operative fixation techniques for Monteggia fractures in the adult have improved results significantly.

In contrast to Galeazzi's fracture (fracture of the distal radius and dislocation of the radioulnar joint), which rarely occurs in children, approximately 25 per cent of Monteggia fracture-dislocations are sustained by patients less than 15 years of age.

The angulation of the ulnar fracture consistently points in the direction of the radial head dislocation. Most commonly (70 to 85 per cent of cases) the angulation and dislocation are anterior. Less often (10 to 15 per cent of cases) they are posterior. Lateral angulation of the fracture with lateral dislocation of the radial head is the least common (5 to 10 per cent of cases); this lesion has been reported only in children, and generally the ulnar fracture is a greenstick type instead of a true fracture.

Occasionally, additional fracture of the radius or a dislocation of the distal radioulnar joint occurs in association with a Monteggia injury. Keep all these possible combinations in mind when evaluating any ulnar fracture at any level in a patient of any age.

Mechanisms of Injury

Although Monteggia fracture-dislocations may result from a direct blow to the ulnar aspect of the upper forearm, most patients sustain an indirect injury as the result of a fall on the outstretched hand.

When an individual falls, the forearm may be forced into any rotational position and the elbow into a variety of flexed or hyperextended positions.

To absorb the force of a fall forward, the forearm usually pronates and the elbow flexes slightly.

A fall backward generally requires the arm to supinate fully and the elbow to hyperextend. With the elbow hyperextended, the longitudinal force vectors and the associated violent reflex contraction of the elbow flexors result in the anterior Monteggia fracture (anterior dislocation of the radial head with anterior angulation of the ulnar fracture).

Another commonly described mechanism of injury is forceful internal rotation of the forearm with simultaneous external torsion of the arm and trunk. These opposing torsional forces are centered about the elbow, with the result being an anterior Monteggia fracture.

Should the torsional loading from arm and trunk rotation be parallel to the rotation of the forearm, the force with the wrist hyperextended would be absorbed by the distal radius and ulna and would produce a Galeazzi's fracture-dislocation in the adult (see pages 898 and 926).

The usual mechanism for the second most common Monteggia fracture, with posterior angulation and dislocation, is a fall on the arm with the elbow flexed. Ordinarily this would dislocate the elbow posteriorly, but the force vectors may occasionally produce a posterior Monteggia lesion.

The lateral Monteggia lesion is the least common and is restricted to young children. The primary mechanism is sudden adduction as the forearm absorbs the falling body weight. This produces a greenstick, laterally angulated ulnar fracture and either anterolateral or posterolateral dislocation of the radius. The direction of the radial dislocation depends on the rotational position of the forearm at the time of the primary adduction injury.

Understanding the mechanism of any fracture or dislocation is important for adequate reduction; quite often the fracture victim, if asked, can recall the position of the limb at the time of injury.

INDIRECT MECHANISMS

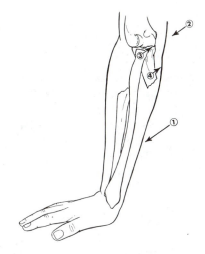

Anterior Monteggia Lesion from Elbow Hyperextension

1. A fall backward forces the forearm into supination.
2. The elbow is hyperextended.
3. Reflex contraction of the elbow flexors dislocates the radial head anteriorly.
4. Force of injury may be sufficient to cause an open fracture of the ulna through the flexor carpi ulnaris muscle.

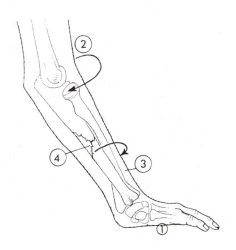

Anterior Monteggia Lesion from Torsional Injury

1. The hand is fixed to the ground.
2. The momentum of the body forces the humerus and elbow to rotate externally.
3. Floor reaction and muscle response cause the forearm to rotate internally while humerus and elbow rotate externally.
4. Fracture of the ulna results.

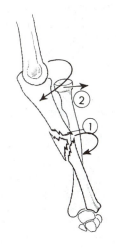

As the force continues,
1. The radius and the proximal fragment of the ulna come into contact.
2. The radial head is levered anteriorly out of the proximal radioulnar joint.

Posterior Monteggia Lesion with Elbow Flexion

The hand strikes the ground with
1. The forearm in supination and
2. The elbow flexed 45 degrees.
3. The axial force up the radius tends to dislocate the radius.
Simultaneously there occurs

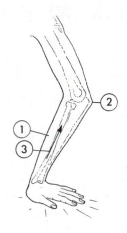

1. A comminuted fracture of the upper end of the ulna with posterior angulation and
2. Posterior fracture-dislocation of the head of the radius.
3. The dislocation may be posterior or posterolateral.

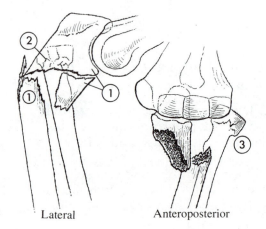

Lateral   Anteroposterior

Lateral Monteggia Lesion from Adduction Mechanism (in Children)

1. A fall on the outstretched arm causes
2. The force vector to pass medial to the ulna, resulting in
3. A greenstick fracture of the ulna and
4. Lateral dislocation of the radius.

Note: The final position of the radial head may be anterolateral or posterolateral depending on the rotational position of the forearm at the time of the primary adduction injury.

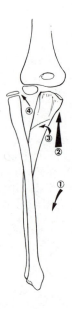

DIRECT MECHANISM

Anterior Monteggia Lesion

1. A blow to the posterior ulnar aspect causes an ulnar fracture with anterior angulation and

2. Anterior dislocation of the radial head.

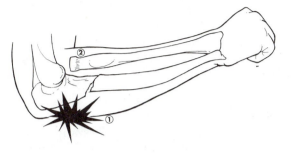

Closed Reduction Techniques

REMARKS

Reserve closed reduction almost entirely for Monteggia fractures in children. Monteggia fracture-dislocations in adults invariably require open reduction and plate fixation of the ulnar fracture.

The closed reduction technique should reverse the mechanism of injury.

Anterior hyperextension Monteggia fracture-dislocations are reduced in flexion.

Posterior flexion injuries are reduced and reversed by extension and adduction.

Lateral Monteggia fractures are reduced by abduction of the extended, supinated forearm.

Check the reduction of the radius carefully on the postreduction x-ray. The lines drawn on the x-ray through the anterior and posterior cortices of the radius should encompass the entire capitellum if the radius is reduced. Failure to reduce the radial dislocation may rarely be due to the radial head buttonholing through the capsule; this requires open reduction.

The usual tendency of the ulna after reduction is to angulate towards the radius. This can be anticipated and diminished by molding carefully along the lateral border of the ulna during cast application.

Should the dislocation of the radial head go unrecognized for 6 to 12 weeks, operative reduction should be carried out, combined with reconstruction of the annular ligament if necessary.

ANTERIOR MONTEGGIA LESION

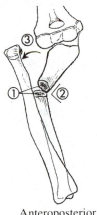

Prereduction X-rays (Child's Fracture)

ANTEROPOSTERIOR VIEW

1. Fracture of the ulna.
2. Radial angulation of the fragments. (This can be corrected by molding on the lateral border of the ulna with the arm in slight supination.)
3. The radial head is dislocated anteriorly and laterally.

Anteroposterior

LATERAL VIEW

1. Fracture of the ulna.
2. Anterior angulation of the fragments.
3. Anterior and lateral dislocation of the head of the radius.

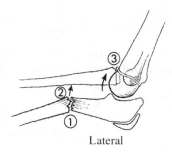

Lateral

Manipulative Reduction (Used Only in Children)

1. An assistant makes counter traction on the arm.
2. A second assistant grasps the forearm at the wrist and makes steady traction with the forearm supinated.
3. While traction is maintained, the operator first makes direct backward pressure over the distal end of the upper ulnar fragment and then direct backward pressure on the radial head.

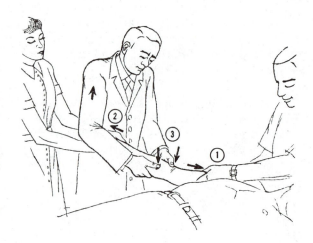

964

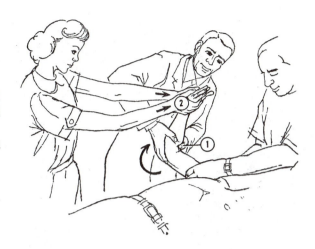

1. While pressure is maintained over the radial head and the proximal ulnar fragment,

2. The forearm is acutely flexed in the supinated position.

Postreduction X-Ray

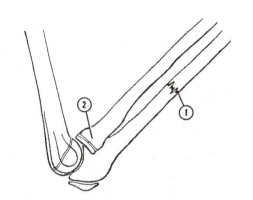

1. The ulnar fragments are in normal alignment and the volar angulation is corrected.

2. The radial head is in its normal anatomic position.

Note: Avoid pseudoreduction. If the relationship of the radius to the capitellum is not appreciated, dislocation or subluxation will persist after reduction. Evaluate radial reduction carefully on the x-ray using the Reckling-Cordell method.

X-Ray Determination of Radial Head Reduction (Reckling-Cordell Method)

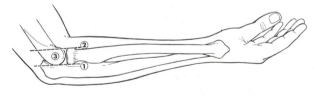

1. On a lateral x-ray taken with forearm supinated, draw a line tangential to the bicipital tuberosity.

2. Draw a second line along the other radial border.

3. If the radial head is reduced, the lines encompass the capitellum.

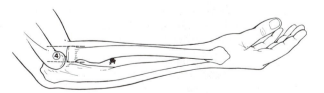

4. Failure to encompass the capitellum indicates a persistent subluxation or dislocation.

Note: If the radial head is not reduced, remanipulate or perform open reduction and internal fixation (see page 973).

Immobilization

To avoid the tendency of the ulnar fracture to develop a radial bow,

1. The forearm is placed in neutral or slight supination to allow molding over the ulna.

2. The cast is molded along the lateral border of the ulna.

3. The elbow is flexed beyond a right angle.

Note: As long as the elbow is flexed sufficiently, it is unnecessary to keep the forearm fully supinated to maintain the radial head reduction.

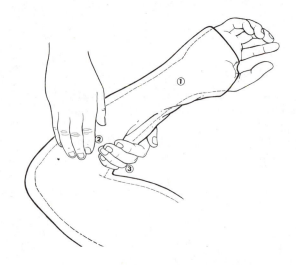

Postreduction Management

Observe the arm carefully for postoperative swelling, and bivalve the cast if indicated.

When swelling subsides, apply a cast that is molded well over the lateral ulna.

Remove the cast at the end of six weeks.

Apply a triangular sling for seven to ten days.

Allow the child free use of the arm.

Do not permit passive stretching of the elbow in a misguided attempt to improve motion. This only worsens the stiffness.

POSTERIOR MONTEGGIA LESION

Prereduction X-Ray

1. Fracture of the upper third of the ulna with posterior angulation of the fragments.

2. The head of the radius is dislocated posteriorly.

Closed Reduction

1. An assistant makes counter traction on the arm.

2. The operator makes steady traction on the extended forearm with one hand and

3. Makes direct forward pressure at the apex of the dorsal angulation of the ulna with the other hand.

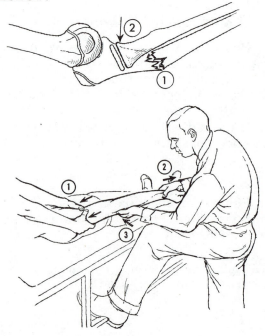

966

Postreduction X-Ray

1. The dorsal angulation is corrected.

2. The radial head is in its normal anatomic position.

Note: Be certain the radial head is reduced (see page 965).

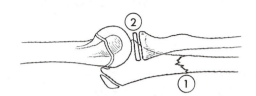

Immobilization

1. Apply a long arm cast.

2. Forearm is in neutral or slight supination to allow molding of the lateral ulna.

3. The elbow is fully extended.

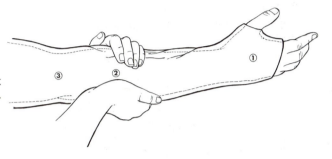

Postreduction Management

Elevate the limb and observe the arm carefully for any swelling after reduction. Bivalve the cast as indicated.

When swelling completely subsides, apply another cast, molding over the lateral ulna.

Remove the cast at the end of six weeks.

Apply a triangular sling for seven to ten days.

Allow the child free use of the arm.

Do not permit passive stretching of the elbow in a misguided attempt to improve motion. This only worsens the stiffness.

Note: If the radial head is unstable, the annular ligament is blocking reduction or the radial head is actually buttonholed through the capsule. Open reduction may be necessary to remove the soft tissue obstruction to reduction and to repair the ligament.

If the shaft of the ulna is extremely unstable (this is indeed rare), stabilize the fragments with an intramedullary pin passing through the olecranon.

Remove the pin through a hole in the cast at the end of three to four weeks.

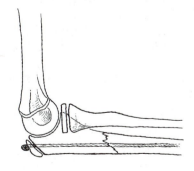

LATERAL MONTEGGIA LESION IN A CHILD

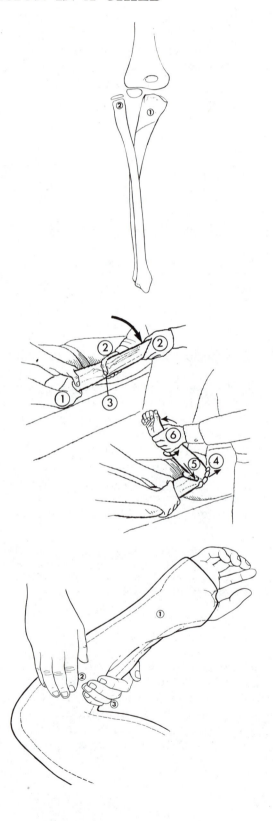

Prereduction X-Ray

1. A greenstick fracture of the upper ulna with lateral angulation.

2. Lateral displacement of the radial head.

Note: This lesion occurs exclusively in children.

Closed Reduction

1. An assistant makes counter traction on the arm.

2. The surgeon makes steady traction on the extended forearm with one hand and

3. Applies direct finger pressure over the angulated ulna and thumb pressure over the dislocated radius.

4. The forearm is then slightly abducted.

5. Firm pressure is continued over the upper end of the elbow.

6. The forearm is then supinated and flexed beyond a right angle.

Note: Evaluate reduction carefully on x-ray in both anteroposterior and lateral planes by the Reckling-Cordell method (see page 965).

Immobilization

If reduction is verified by x-ray,

1. Apply a long arm cast.

2. The forearm is in neutral or slight supination to allow molding of the lateral ulna.

3. The elbow is flexed beyond a right angle.

Postreduction Management

Observe the arm carefully for swelling after reduction. Bivalve the cast as indicated.

When swelling completely subsides, apply another cast, again molding over the lateral ulna.

Remove the plaster at the end of four weeks.

Apply a triangular sling for five to seven days.

Allow the child free use of the arm.

Do not permit passive stretching of the elbow in a misguided attempt to improve motion. This only worsens the stiffness.

Other Greenstick Fractures of the Upper End of the Ulna with Dislocation of the Radial Epiphysis

REMARKS

Greenstick fractures of the ulna must be carefully evaluated for associated dislocation of the radial head.

The upper end of the ulna, usually at the level of the superior radioulnar joint, suffers a greenstick fracture that may not displace or that may angulate anteriorly, posteriorly, medially, or laterally.

The radial epiphysis also dislocates in any direction.

Too often dislocation of the radial epiphysis in these injuries of young children is not recognized or is incompletely reduced and the result is restricted motion or angulatory deformity.

Because the position of the radial epiphysis may be difficult to evaluate on x-ray in young children, use the Reckling-Cordell method (see page 965).

If the injury is seen late, after healing has occurred, the deformity must be accepted. The radial head can be excised at the termination of growth if it is causing symptoms. Never excise the radial head in the growing child's elbow, because further deformity will result.

Chronic post-traumatic dislocation of the radial head should be distinguished from congenital dislocation. Usually, congenital dislocation is associated with underdevelopment of the capitellum.

969

TYPES OF FRACTURE

Undisplaced Fracture with Anterior Dislocation of the Radial Epiphysis

ANTEROPOSTERIOR VIEW

1. Fracture of the upper end of the ulna, which is not displaced.

LATERAL VIEW

2. Tangential lines drawn along the radius do not encompass the capitellum. This indicates dislocation of the radial head even though the ulnar fracture is undisplaced.

Note: Carefully evaluate the position of the radial epiphysis associated with any fracture of the ulna at this level whether displaced or undisplaced.

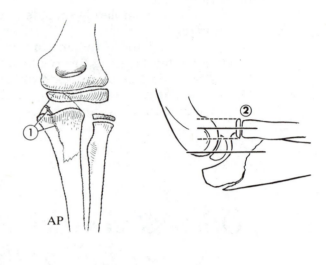

Hyperextension Fracture with Anterior Dislocation of the Radial Epiphysis

ANTEROPOSTERIOR VIEW

1. Fracture of the upper end of the ulna.

LATERAL VIEW

1. Extension deformity at the level of the radioulnar joint.
2. Anterior dislocation of the radial epiphysis.

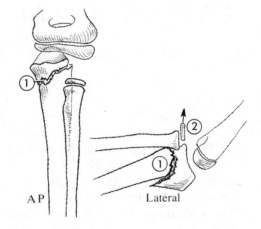

Lateral Angulation of Greenstick Fracture with Lateral Dislocation of the Radial Epiphysis

1. Fracture through the upper end of the ulna with lateral angulation.
2. Lateral dislocation of the radial epiphysis.

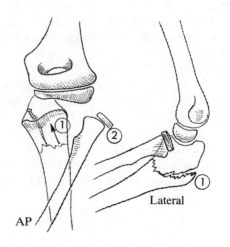

Medial Angulation of Greenstick Fracture with Medial Fracture Separation of the Radial Epiphysis

ANTEROPOSTERIOR VIEW

1. Fracture of the upper end of the ulna with medial displacement.
2. Fracture-separation of the radial epiphysis with some medial displacement.

LATERAL VIEW

1. Fracture of the upper end of the ulna.
2. Fracture-separation of the radial epiphysis.

Note: Medial lesions may be complicated by separation of the medial epicondyle.

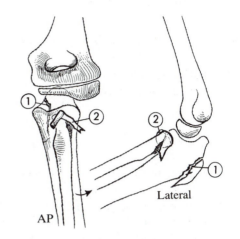

REDUCTION TECHNIQUES

For Laterally Angulated Fractures and Lateral Dislocation of the Radial Epiphysis

1. Make firm inward pressure over the radial head and with the arm extended and supinated,
2. Forcefully abduct the forearm, then
3. Flex the forearm to 90 degrees.

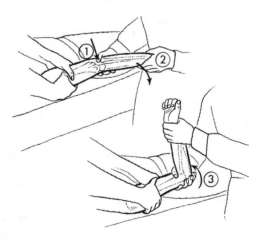

971

For Medially Angulated Fractures with Medial Displacement of the Radial Epiphysis

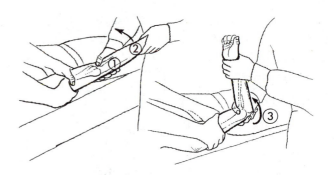

1. With the arm extended and supinated,
    2. Forcefully adduct the forearm.
    3. Flex the forearm to 90 degrees.

Postreduction Management

Apply a long arm cast with the forearm in slight supination.

Mold over the lateral border of the ulna to prevent angulation and flex the elbow (see page 968).

Support the limb in a sling.

After four weeks remove the cast and permit free use of the arm.

No other measures are needed in children. Avoid forceful stretching of the joint.

If the radial head cannot be reduced it may have buttonholed through the capsule, and open reduction may be necessary (see page 973).

Congenital Dislocation of the Radial Head and Unrecognized Monteggia Fracture in Children

REMARKS

The radial head may rarely be dislocated congenitally rather than from injury. Radiographically, congenital dislocation can be distinguished by marked underdevelopment of the capitellum. Operative treatment of a congenital dislocation is consistently unrewarding.

When the problem is an unrecognized Monteggia fracture more than three months old, the elbow is best left undisturbed until the child reaches skeletal maturity. Attempts to correct old deformities only worsen forearm function.

Should the appearance of the elbow be unacceptable to the family, it may be improved by radial head resection after the child reaches skeletal maturity. Radial head resection before growth is completed will lead to cubitus valgus deformity, prominence of the distal ulna, and radial deviation of the hand.

Management of Monteggia Fracture in Adults: Open Reduction and Fixation

REMARKS

Open reduction and rigid internal fixation of the ulnar fracture is the treatment of choice for Monteggia injury in adults.

Stabilization of the ulna permits reduction of the radial head.

Occasionally partial disruption of the annular ligament must also be repaired.

Rarely, the stabilizing annular ligament will be so disrupted that a reconstructive procedure is necessary.

The surgical approach to the combined ulnar fracture and radial head dislocation should not add to soft tissue trauma or deprive the ulnar fragments of their blood supply.

A lateral approach through the interval between the anconeous muscle and the extensor carpi ulnaris muscle offers the best exposure and causes the least additional trauma.

Operative Exposure via Lateral Anconeus Approach

1. Make an incision 2 cm proximal to the lateral condyle of the humerus at the lateral border of the tricep.

2. Extend the incision distally over the olecranon and the fracture site.

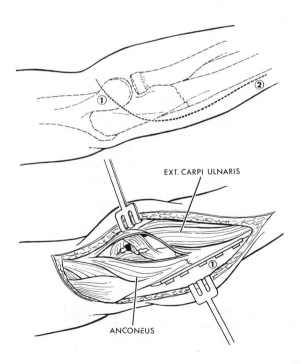

Fixation

Fix the ulna fracture by the most rigid fixation possible, using either

1. A dynamic compression plate applied to the radial surface of the ulna,

973

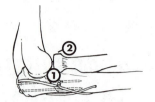

Fixation (Continued)

2. Tension band wirings, or,

3. For proximal oblique fractures, two lag screws.

Note: Avoid excising the olecranon in this unstable injury.

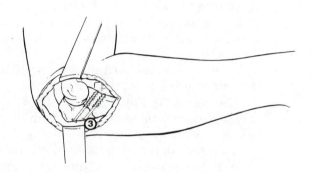

Repair of Annular Ligament Disruption

After the ulnar fracture is fixed

1. Retract the skin flaps and develop the interval between the

2. Anconeus and

3. The extensor carpi ulnaris to demonstrate

4. The radiocapitellar joint.

5. Repair any tears in the annular ligament.

Note: Occasionally the annular ligament will be completely disrupted and must be completely reconstructed.

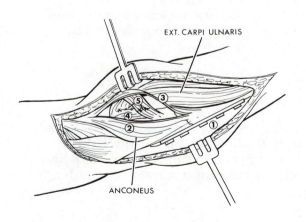

974

Complete Reconstruction of the Annular Ligament

Note: Reconstruction of the annular ligament may be necessary for reduction and stabilization of unrecognized radial head dislocation associated with an ununited ulnar fracture.

1. Dissect from the muscles of the forearm a strip of fascia 1.5 cm wide and 10 cm long; the proximal end remains attached to the elbow.

2. Pass the strip between the radius and the ulna and then around the neck of the radius. (Do not suture the ligament at this time.)

3. Fix the ulnar fracture with plate and bone grafting as necessary. Then suture the reconstructed annular ligament back down to the proximal ulna.

Excision of the Radial Head

If the radial head is comminuted, it may be excised provided that the annular ligament is intact.

1. Place a small reverse retractor around the neck of the radius.

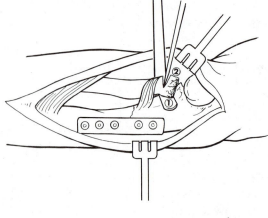

2. With a thin sharp osteotome, cut the bone at the junction of the head and neck.

Note: Excision of ulnar fracture fragments should be avoided in the Monteggia fracture because elbow instability may result.

Immobilization

Postoperatively, apply a circular cast from the axilla to the distal crease.

1. The elbow is flexed 90 degrees.
2. The forearm is in neutral rotation.

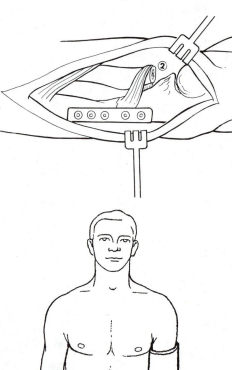

Postoperative Management

Bivalve the cast and surround the elevated limb with ice bags.

Watch the fingers for evidence of circulatory embarrassment.

When swelling has subsided, begin guarded range-of-motion exercises to the elbow but continue cast or splint immobilization until there is radiographic evidence of healing, which usually requires at least six weeks.

When clinical and bony union are assured, remove the cast or splint and use a sling support.

Continue a program of active exercises to restore range of motion to the elbow.

Avoid forceful physical therapy and passive stretching exercises.

Internal fixation devices, either plate or screws, need not be routinely removed.

Prevention and Management of Complications of Monteggia Fracture

REMARKS

In the past, Monteggia fracture has been associated with more problems, difficulties, and general failure of treatment than almost any other skeletal injury.

The most common complication has been persistent loss of elbow motion and forearm rotation.

Failure to recognize the radial head dislocation associated with ulnar fracture is a common hazard and a common cause of functional loss. Radial head dislocation is especially likely to go unrecognized in a child.

Carefully evaluate the alignment of the radius on x-ray using the Reckling-Cordell method (see page 965).

Nonunion is a frequent sequela of this injury, especially if the fracture is comminuted. Rigid dynamic compression fixation supplemented by autogenous bone graft for comminution gives the best chance for successful fracture union in the adult.

If compression cannot be achieved successfully, the internal fixation should be protected by external immobilization for at least six weeks after injury.

Closed reduction is usually successful in children, but the radial head must be completely reduced. If the radial head does not line up anatomically with the capitellum, there may be interposed capsule, which should be removed in conjunction with annular ligament repair.

The majority of these injuries do not completely disrupt the proximal radioulnar articulation. Stabilizing the ulnar fracture usually reduces the radial head. If the annular ligament is significantly disrupted it should be repaired or reconstructed as necessary to stabilize the radius.

Radial nerve injury occurs both before and after reduction of the Monteggia fracture-dislocation. Check frequently for nerve function.

INJURY OF THE RADIAL NERVE ASSOCIATED WITH MONTEGGIA FRACTURE

Damage to the radial nerve occurs in 15 to 20 per cent of Monteggia fractures, either as a result of injury or secondary to reduction.

Most often the neural injury is transitory and clears within ten weeks. Persistent radial nerve loss after twelve weeks that is evident clinically and is confirmed by electromyography indicates the need for surgical decompression.

Usually the posterior interosseous nerve is found to be entrapped by the arcade of Frohse, a fibrous arch through which the nerve enters the supinator muscle. This must be approached anteriorly, so it is usually not visualized by the posterior exposure of the Monteggia fracture.

1. Posterior interosseous nerve may be scarred down by

2. The arcade of Frohse on the

3. Superior border of the supinator muscle.

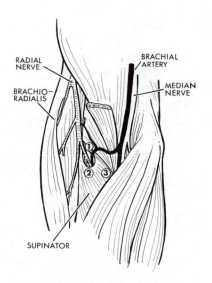

FRACTURES OF THE BONES OF THE FOREARM IN CHILDREN

REMARKS

Forearm fractures are common injuries in children and most often involve both bones, particularly in the lower third of the forearm. The only more common site of fracture in children is the hand.

Children less than 12 years old have an impressive capacity to remodel most forearm fracture deformities, particularly those close to joints and growth centers.

The remodeling capacity diminishes in teenagers, in whom the healing response becomes more like that of adults.

Bayonet apposition of the forearm fracture, which would be unacceptable in adults, is quite acceptable in children because it remodels promptly.

Rotational malalignment or angulation of more than 10 degrees in the midshaft region will persist as a permanent deformity and will limit forearm rotation.

Keep these factors in mind in deciding whether to "accept" a reduction. The child's arm must heal straight to be acceptable. When in doubt, look at the arm. Clinical appearance is frequently of greater value in estimating the reduction than radiographic appearance.

The majority of children's forearm fractures are either simple torus or incomplete greenstick fractures.

The torus fracture is unique to childhood because of the structural weakness of a child's incompletely mineralized bone to compressive loading. The bone simply buckles inward on itself.

The greenstick fracture results from sudden twisting of the forearm, usually by hypersupination as the child falls backward on the outstretched hand. The injury produces a compression failure on the dorsal side and a tensile failure on the volar side. The fracture then angulates volarly.

The greenstick deformity is corrected by a quick hyperpronation to convert the compression fracture of the dorsal surface to a tensile fracture. If this is not done the initial volar angulation is likely to recur even in plaster.

Because of the virtually unlimited ability of growing bones to remodel, open treatment is unjustified in children less than 12 years of age.

Surgical treatment may rarely be necessary in young teenagers to correct irreducible angulation of a midshaft fracture.

Before resorting to operative treatment or repeated closed reductions for a fracture that seems to defy reduction, try fixed finger traction. This frequently maintains length and satisfactory alignment for the few weeks required for the fracture to become "sticky."

Although growth may remodel many deformities, try to reduce the fracture as anatomically as possible.

Recheck the position on x-ray within one week after reduction to insure that displacement does not occur within the cast.

Occasionally remanipulation may be necessary to improve position. Advise the child's parents of this possibility. Attempts to remanipulate after 7 to 10 days are generally inadvisable because the fracture will already have started to heal.

MECHANICS OF FOREARM FRACTURE DEFORMITIES IN CHILDREN

Torus Fracture

1. Relative undermineralization of the child's radius and ulna causes the bones to fail with compressive loading. The result is a buckle or torus fracture, the most common childhood forearm fracture.

Note: This fracture does not displace further, and treatment by two to three weeks of cast immobilization serves mainly to relieve pain symptoms.

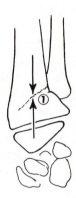

Greenstick Fractures

Greenstick fractures are produced typically by torsional or twisting loading combined with axial loading. Torsional loading combines tensile, compressive and shear forces with the failure occurring first through the plane of maximum tensile loading.

The direction of failure after torsional loading is consistently dependent on the direction of the twist.

External rotation or supination twist creates maximum tensile forces on the volar surface so that the fracture angulates volarly.

Internal rotation or pronation twist concentrates the maximum tension loading on the dorsal surface of the forearm bones and the fracture angulates dorsally.

These fractures can be reduced most simply by reversing the torsional mechanism, i.e., pronating the fracture with volar angulation or supinating the fracture with dorsal angulation.

1. A fall on the outstretched arm produces a combination of torsional and axial loading.

2. This causes compression failure on one cortical surface of the bone and

3. Tensile failure on the opposite cortical surface.

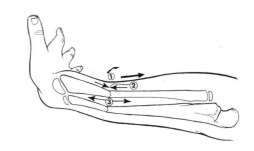

SUPINATION INJURY

1. Force vectors from hypersupination cause

2. A greenstick fracture with volar angulation.

The greater angulation of the radius indicates the torsional mechanisms as this bone rotates around the ulna.

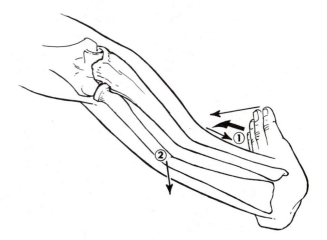

PRONATION INJURY

1. Force vectors from hyperpronation mechanism cause

2. Greenstick fracture with dorsal angulation.

Note: Greenstick fractures with volar angulation are reduced by supination, and those with dorsal angulation are corrected by pronation (see page 996).

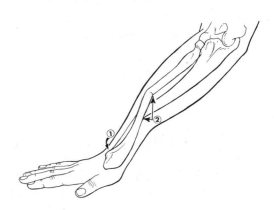

981

Fractures of the Distal Radius and Ulna

REMARKS

This injury may consist of either an incomplete greenstick fracture or a complete two-bone fracture with dorsal displacement.

The fracture should be reduced promptly, because a delay of a few days makes reduction difficult.

The technique of reduction consists of applying traction and increasing and then decreasing the fracture deformity.

After reduction, allow the hand to rotate into its natural pronated position. Avoid hyperpronation, which tends to accentuate the deforming pull of the brachioradialis muscle.

To neutralize the pull of the brachioradialis, immobilize the elbow in flexion.

Operative treatment is not justified for this fracture because the child's remodeling capacity is extensive at this level.

Redisplacement after reduction is fairly common with this fracture owing to the pull of the brachioradialis muscle and a tendency to use short arm casts. Immobilize this fracture in a long arm cast to neutralize the deforming tendency of the mechanical and muscle forces, and follow progress closely.

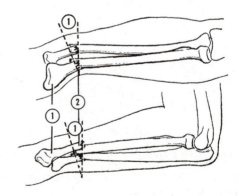

Prereduction X-Rays

1. Dorsally displaced fractures of both bones.
2. Overriding is moderate.

MANIPULATIVE REDUCTION

Reduction is performed with the patient under general or regional intravenous anesthesia (see page 909).

1. Apply steady but gentle traction to restore length to the forearm.

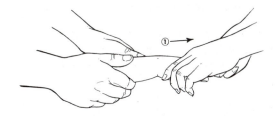

Then,
1. Hyperextend the fracture to "hook" the fragments together and
2. Depress the distal fragment to correct dorsal displacement.

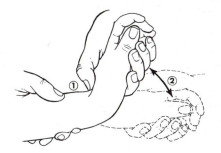

Postreduction X-Ray

1. The dorsal displacement of the distal fragments is corrected.
2. The lateral displacement is corrected.
3. Length has been restored.

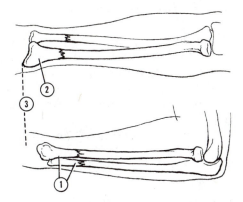

Cast Immobilization

Avoid a loose short arm cast.
1. The pull of the brachioradialis may reangulate this distal fracture unless the elbow is immobilized.
2. Failure to neutralize the mechanical torsional forces on the fracture may reproduce or accentuate the volar angulation of the fracture.

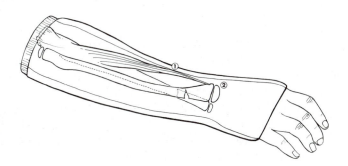

Cast Immobilization (Continued)

The operator should apply a long arm cast, molding plaster firmly on

1. The dorsum of the distal fragment and

2. The volar and

3. The dorsal surfaces of the proximal fragment.

4. The long arm cast neutralizes the pull of the brachioradialis as well as the rotational forces acting on the distal fracture.

Note: Careful molding and three-point fixation are essential. Since the cast is firmly applied, the child's arm should be elevated after reduction and circulation should be checked closely. Ischemic muscle necrosis can occur with overvigorous manipulation of fractures in this area.

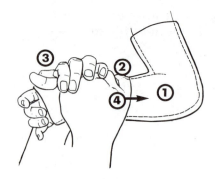

Postreduction Management

Immediately after application of the cast and for 24 to 48 hours, elevate the arm and apply ice bags to the forearm.

Check regularly for any evidence of circulatory embarrassment of the forearm.

Take x-rays within one week and check for displacement or angulation of the fragments.

If the cast becomes loose after swelling of the limb subsides, the cast must be replaced.

Plaster immobilization is maintained for 6 to 8 weeks. Check x-rays for evidence of union.

Allow the child free use of the arm. Physical therapy is not essential.

ALTERNATE METHOD: FIXED TRACTION

REMARKS

Fixed traction can be employed when manipulative maneuvers fail to achieve or maintain reduction.

End-to-end apposition of the fragments is not necessary, but fracture angulation and rotational malalignments should be corrected.

Operative intervention is not indicated to improve reduction in children younger than 12 years. However, if the fracture is opened in the process of wound debridement, transcutaneous pin fixation of the fracture fragments can be very helpful and is usually indicated (see page 986).

Prereduction X-Ray

Manipulative reduction failed in this case.

1. Some angulation of the distal fragments is still present.

2. The fragments are overriding.

3. Some lateral displacement is present.

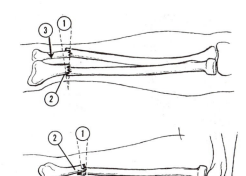

Alignment by Fixed Traction (Blount)

1. Apply a circular cast from the axilla to the wrist: the forearm is in pronation.

2. Incorporate a banjo splint made of coat-hanger wire into the cast.

3. Apply skin traction to all fingers by rubber bands.

Note: Traction is maintained for three weeks.

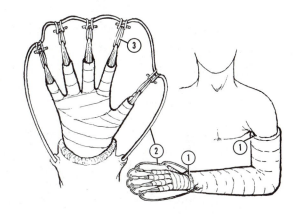

Post-traction X-Ray

1. Alignment is restored.

2. The amount of overriding is reduced.

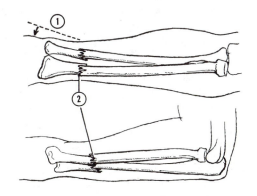

Immobilization

1. After the traction apparatus is removed, apply a circular cast from the axilla to the midpalmar crease.

2. The elbow is flexed 90 degrees.

3. The forearm is pronated.

4. The wrist is in a neutral position.

5. Mold the plaster well on the volar surface of the radius.

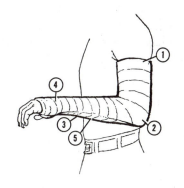

Subsequent Management

The plaster immobilization is continued for three to four additional weeks. The cast may be removed after this period if clinical and radiographic union is evident.

Allow the child free use of the arm. Physical therapy is not essential.

Management of Open Forearm Fractures in Children

REMARKS

The most common open fracture in the child's forearm occurs with the volarly angulated fracture in the distal third. The force of this injury may drive the proximal fracture fragment out through the skin.

These wounds can be quite treacherous: the bone may be extremely contaminated by dirt but the skin may appear to be merely punctured.

All open fractures, particularly fractures in this area, require operative exploration and thorough cleansing of the fracture, as described in Chapter 1 (pages 125 and 130).

The open forearm fracture is frequently quite unstable, and transcutaneous Steinmann pin fixation for two to three weeks is usually indicated while the soft tissues heal.

1. Beware of small puncture wounds that do not reflect the degree of contamination with fractures in the distal forearm.

2. The fragments may have been driven through the skin and into the ground or dirt and then returned beneath the skin.

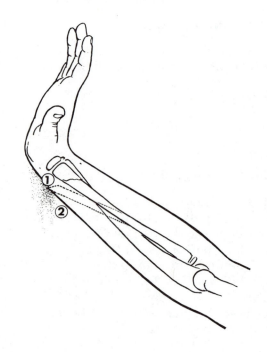

Operative Management

1. The fracture should be exposed by an S-shaped incision that includes and excises the puncture wound.

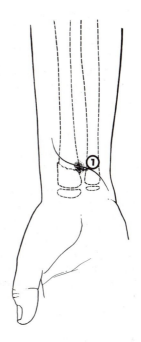

2. The flexor tendons and median nerves are identified and protected.
3. The fracture fragments are visualized and curetted as well as washed thoroughly.

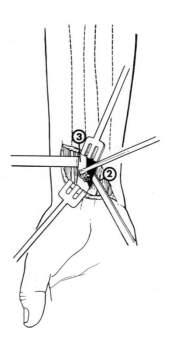

987

Operative Management
(Continued)

1. These fractures are generally unstable and should be supported by transcutaneous Steinmann pin fixation for three weeks while the soft tissues heal.

2. The wound is drained with a Penrose drain and is not closed primarily. Use loose wire sutures.

Note: Antibiotic treatment for presumed Staph infection of these wounds should be started in the emergency room after cultures have been taken. Continue broad-spectrum antibiotics for five to seven days, depending on the healing of the wound and the absence of pathogens on reculturing. Reinspect and redebride the fracture site in the operating room within three to five days.

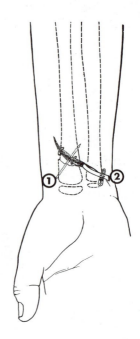

Subsequent Management

The transcutaneous Steinmann pins are removed after three weeks, when soft tissue healing is adequate and swelling has subsided.

The fracture may then be immobilized in a long arm cast with the forearm in pronation (see page 985).

Cast immobilization is continued for at least eight weeks since these open fractures tend to be slower to heal than the usual fracture in the child.

Growth Remodeling of Fracture Deformities

REMARKS

Although one should strive for anatomic reduction, keep in mind the significant capacity of certain fractures in children to remodel.

The capacity for spontaneous correction with growth is greatest in the distal metaphyseal region of the radius and ulna.

Högström and coworkers showed that children younger than ten demonstrate a greater ability to remodel than do older children but that this can vary considerably from child to child.

Repeated manipulation or surgical treatment can be avoided if the physician appreciates the type of fracture deformity that will remodel with growth.

FRACTURE DEFORMITIES THAT MAY NOT REMODEL AND SHOULD BE CORRECTED

1. This fracture appears to be satisfactorily corrected but there is rotational malalignment.

2. The end-to-side apposition is satisfactory.

3. The asymmetric widths of the cortices in the proximal and distal fragments indicate that rotational reduction should be improved or limitation of forearm rotation may result.

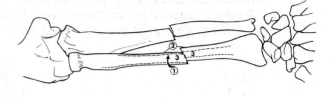

1. Angulation of more than 10 degrees in the diaphyseal region should be corrected, since it is cosmetically unsatisfactory and is likely to restrict forearm rotation significantly.

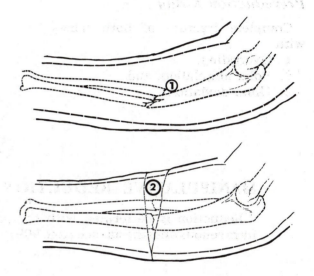

2. The angulation is corrected by an opening wedge on the volar surface of the cast rather than by remanipulation.

Fractures of the Bones of the Middle Third of the Forearm with Displacement

REMARKS

Fractures of the radius or the ulna or of both bones occur relatively frequently in children.

Most often in two-bone fractures, the lesion is a greenstick fracture with volar angulation caused by hypersupination.

Angulation and rotational deformities at this level cannot be accepted. The key to reduction is to correct rotational alignment.

991

Greenstick fractures should be completely fractured by reversing the rotational mechanism of injury. If this is not done the volar angulation is likely to increase even after plaster application.

Normal anatomic reduction is not essential, but alignment must be straight and angulation and rotational deformity must be eliminated.

Bayonet apposition or corner-to-corner reduction will give satisfactory healing with good function and no deformity.

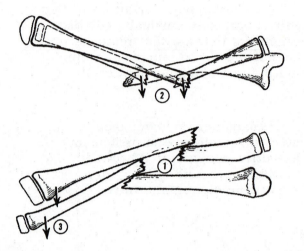

Prereduction X-Ray

Complete fracture of both bones with
1. Overriding,
2. Volar angulation, and
3. Ulnar deviation.

MANIPULATIVE REDUCTION

Reduction is performed with the patient under general or regional intravenous anesthesia (see page 909).

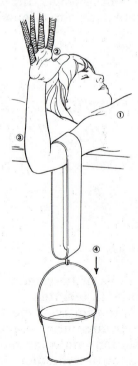

1. The patient is supine with the injured arm suspended over the edge of the table.

2. The hand is supported by finger-traps.

3. The forearm is in neutral rotation.

4. Counter traction is applied with weight attached to a felt pad or sling — a water bucket works very well for traction.

While the traction is maintained

5. The surgeon palpates along the borders of the ulna and radius.

6. By rotation of the patient's hand and forearm the fracture cortices are "hooked."

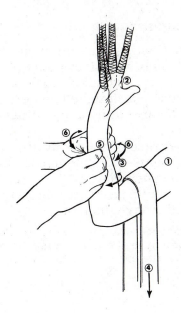

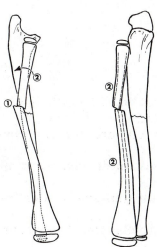

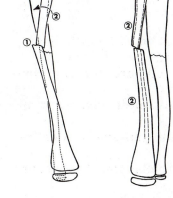

Postreduction X-Rays

UNACCEPTABLE REDUCTION

1. Volar angulation persists.

2. Inadequate rotational realignment is evident as the result of pronation of the distal fragment. This is evident from the asymmetric cortical widths in the proximal and distal fragments.

ACCEPTABLE REDUCTION

1. The fragments are in slight bayonet apposition.

2. The volar angulation is corrected.

3. Rotational alignment of the distal fragment is satisfactory as indicated by symmetric cortical widths.

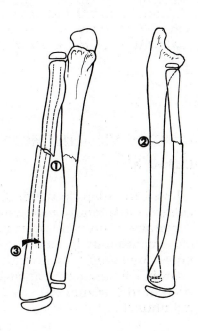

Cast Immobilization

1. While traction is maintained, the surgeon applies a long arm cast from the axilla to the midpalmar crease.

2. The elbow is flexed 90 degrees.

3. The forearm is held in neutral position.

4. The surgeon molds firmly between the radius and ulna to maintain the interosseous space.

5. The wrist is placed in slight flexion and ulnar deviation.

Note: Remove water-bucket traction from the arm after the forearm cast is set and continue the cast above the elbow.

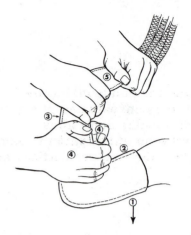

Postreduction Management

Immediately after application of the cast and for 24 to 48 hours, elevate the arm and apply ice bags to the forearm.

Check regularly for any evidence of circulatory embarrassment of the forearm.

Take x-rays on the 3rd and 14th days and check for displacement or angulation of the fragments.

If the cast comes loose after swelling of the limb subsides, it must be replaced.

Plaster immobilization is maintained for 6 to 8 weeks. Check x-rays for evidence of union.

Allow the child free use of the arm. Physical therapy is not essential.

ALTERNATE METHOD: FIXED TRACTION

REMARKS

Fixed traction is helpful when manipulative maneuvers fail to achieve satisfactory correction of angulation or rotational deformities.

Operative intervention is not indicated in children less than 10 years old. Occasionally in a child older than 12 years, when closed reduction proves impossible, open reduction is useful.

Ordinarily, anatomic apposition of fragments is not essential, provided that the alignment is satisfactory and the interosseous space is maintained.

Prereduction X-Ray

Manipulative reduction failed in this case.

1. The fragments are overriding.

2. Volar angulation is not corrected.

3. The fragments are displaced medially.

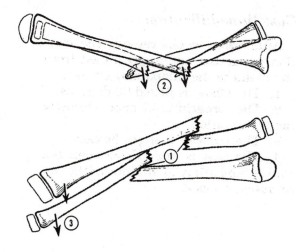

Alignment by Fixed Traction (Blount)

1. Apply a circular cast from the axilla to the wrist; the forearm is in midposition.

2. Incorporate a banjo splint made of coat-hanger wire into the cast.

3. Apply skin traction to all fingers by rubber bands.

Note: Traction is maintained for three weeks.

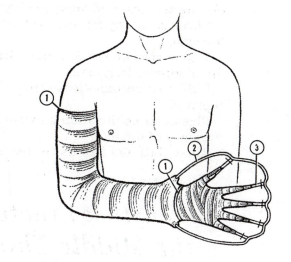

Post-traction X-Ray

1. Volar angulation has been corrected.

2. Overriding is reduced.

3. Rotational realignment has been achieved by rotating the distal fragment so it lines up with the proximal fragment, as judged by the widths of the fragments.

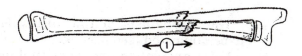

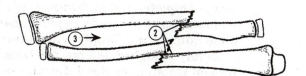

Cast Immobilization

After three weeks remove the traction apparatus and apply a cast from the axilla to the midpalmar crease.

1. The elbow is flexed 90 degrees.
2. The forearm is in approximately neutral rotation.
3. The wrist is in slight flexion.
4. The cast is molded between the radius and ulna to maintain the interosseous space.

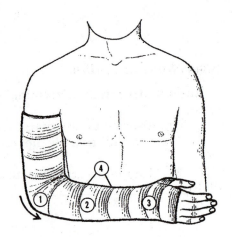

Postreduction Management

Immediately after application of the cast and for 24 to 48 hours, elevate the arm and apply ice bags to the forearm.

Check regularly for any evidence of circulatory embarrassment of the forearm.

Take x-rays on the 3rd and 14th days and check for displacement or angulation of fragments.

If the cast becomes loose after swelling of the limb subsides, it must be replaced.

Plaster immobilization is maintained for 6 to 8 weeks. Check x-rays for evidence of union.

Allow the child free use of the arm. Physical therapy is not essential.

Greenstick Fractures of the Bones of the Middle Third of the Forearm

REMARKS

The mechanism of this injury is usually a fall with the forearm hypersupinated (see page 981).

Volar angulation and rotational deformity are not acceptable at this level.

In order to prevent recurrence of the deformity in a greenstick fracture, complete tensile failure must be achieved. To do this, reverse the mechanism of injury by hyperpronating the forearm. This can usually be done quickly and simply with intravenous anesthesia.

Merely straightening out the bone is not sufficient. The cortex must be broken through, or the deformity may recur even in plaster.

Typical Deformity

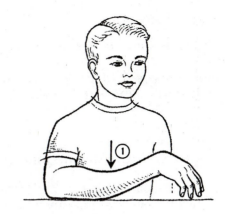

1. Volar angulation centered over the middle third of the forearm. (Soft tissues obscure the severity of the bone deformity.)

Prereduction X-Ray

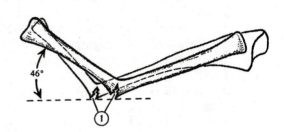

1. Greenstick fractures of both bones in the middle third of the forearm.
2. Volar angulation deformity measures 46 degrees; indicates a supination mechanism.

Manipulative Reduction to Complete the Fracture

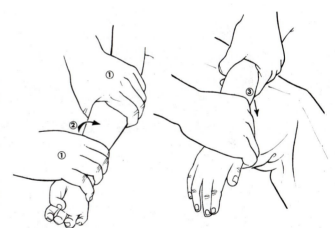

1. The surgeon grasps the forearm with one hand above and one hand below the fracture site.
2. While quickly pronating the distal fragment, the surgeon levers the fracture over his knee.
3. When the fracture is complete, the surgeon supports the limb to avoid displacement.

Cast Immobilization

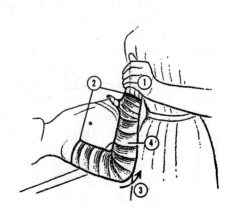

1. An assistant suspends the arm by the patient's fingers and thumb.
2. A circular cast is applied from the axilla to the midpalmar crease.
3. The elbow is flexed 90 degrees.
4. The forearm is held in neutral rotation while the surgeon molds along the interosseous space.

Postreduction X-Ray

1. The angulatory deformity is corrected.

2. The bones are in normal alignment with both cortices fractured.

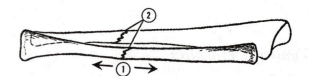

Postreduction Management

Immediately after application of the cast and for 24 to 48 hours, elevate the arm and apply ice bags to the forearm.

Check regularly for any evidence of circulatory embarrassment of the forearm.

Take x-rays on the 3rd and 14th days and check for displacement or angulation of the fragments.

If the cast becomes loose after swelling of the limb subsides, the cast must be replaced.

Plaster immobilization is maintained for 6 to 8 weeks. Check x-rays for evidence of union.

Allow the child free use of the arm. Physical therapy is not essential.

Fractures of the Bones of the Proximal Third of the Forearm

REMARKS

Angular and rotational deformities at this level must be corrected.

Normal alignment is essential for good function.

Side-to-side position (bayonet apposition) with overriding is acceptable provided that alignment is good.

Failure to achieve reduction by traction and manipulation is not an indication for operative intervention; fixed traction is sufficient to achieve the desired alignment of the fragments.

These fractures are reduced and immobilized by supinating the distal fragment to align with the proximal fragment as judged by the position of the bicipital tuberosity. Avoid extreme supination, which tends to narrow the interosseous space.

Operative intervention is justified only in the case of irreducible angulation in a child older than 12 years, which is indeed rare.

998

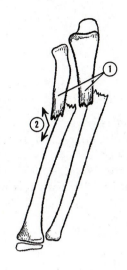

Prereduction X-Ray

In a child 7 years of age, there is
1. Fracture of both bones in the proximal third of the forearm.
2. The fragments are overriding and angulated.

MANIPULATIVE REDUCTION

Reduction is performed with the patient under general or regional intravenous anesthesia (see page 909).

1. The child is in a supine position with the arm supported over the edge of the table.

2. The fingers are supported in a finger-trap apparatus.

3. Counter traction is applied by a felt sling over the arm. (A water bucket is an excellent means of applying weight for counter traction.)

4. The forearm is rotated into supination.

After traction is maintained for at least 10 minutes,

5. The surgeon feels along the cortex of the ulna and radius to evaluate reduction and

6. Presses with the thumb and fingers on the soft tissue between the bones to widen the interosseous space.

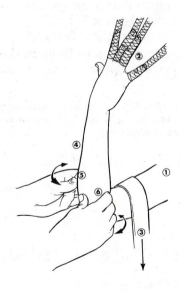

Postreduction X-Ray

1. Overriding is corrected.
2. Angulation is corrected, restoring normal alignment.
3. The interosseous space is restored to normal width throughout.

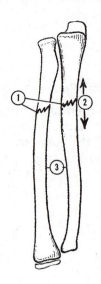

Cast Immobilization

1. While traction is maintained, the circular cast is applied from the axilla to the midpalmar crease.
2. The elbow is flexed 90 degrees.
3. The forearm is supinated, but extreme supination is avoided.
4. The wrist is in slight flexion.
5. The cast is molded well along the dorsal and volar aspect between the bones.

Note: Remove water-bucket traction after the forearm cast is set and continue the cast above the elbow.

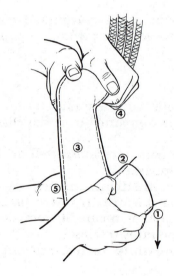

ALTERNATE METHOD: FIXED TRACTION

REMARKS

Fixed traction (Blount) is employed if traction and manipulation fail to reduce the fracture or to restore normal alignment.

Bayonet apposition of fragments is acceptable provided that alignment is good.

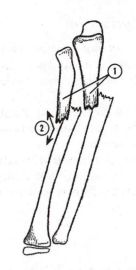

Prereduction X-Ray

Traction and manipulation failed in this case.
1. The fragments are overriding.
2. Angulation is present.

Alignment by Fixed Traction (Blount)

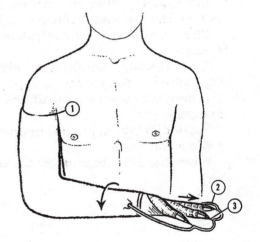

1. Apply a circular cast from the axilla to the wrist; the forearm is in complete supination.
2. Incorporate into the cast a banjo splint made of coat-hanger wire.
3. Apply skin traction to all fingers with rubber bands.

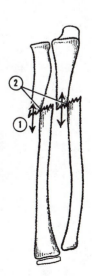

Postreduction X-ray

1. Alignment is end-to-side.
2. Overriding is minimal.

Cast Immobilization

After three weeks remove the traction apparatus and apply a circular cast from the axilla to the midpalmar crease.

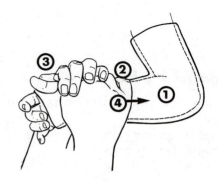

1. The elbow is flexed 90 degrees.
2. The forearm is in neutral rotation or slight supination.
3. The wrist is in neutral position.
4. The cast is molded well along the entire volar aspect between the radius and ulna.

Postreduction Management

Immediately after application of the cast and for 24 to 48 hours, elevate the arm and apply ice bags to the forearm.

Check regularly for any evidence of circulatory embarrassment of the forearm.

Take x-rays on the 3rd and 14th days and check for displacement or angulation of fragments.

If the cast becomes loose after swelling of the limb subsides, it must be replaced.

Plaster immobilization is maintained for 6 to 8 weeks. Check x-rays for evidence of union.

Allow the child free use of the arm. Physical therapy is not essential.

SUMMARY: COMPLICATIONS AND PITFALLS OF FOREARM FRACTURES

REMARKS

Among the most common diagnostic errors in forearm fractures is failure to appreciate disruption of either the proximal or distal radioulnar joint in association with a one-bone or two-bone fracture. All x-rays of forearm fractures must include true anteroposterior and lateral views of the elbow and the wrist to evaluate for radial or ulnar dislocation.

Another judgmental pitfall is underestimating the significance of an open forearm fracture. Even though these wounds may frequently be small, the contamination of the bone ends may be great. Complete surgical exploration and cleansing of the open forearm fracture are critical to prevent tragic results, even limb loss, from infection.

Avoidable complications of fracture management may result from overtreatment as well as undertreatment. Isolated fractures of the ulna heal well by closed methods and unite clinically prior to radiographic evidence of union. Fractures of the ulna should be considered analogous to fibular fractures. Prolonging immobilization or recommending bone grafts because of persistent radiographic defects in a clinically asymptomatic ulnar fracture is a fairly frequent example of overtreatment.

When an ulnar fracture is associated with a dislocation of the radius, prompt and adequate internal fixation is necessary to permit adequate healing. Attempted closed treatment of a Monteggia fracture in an adult represents undertreatment, which leads consistently to nonunion and frequently to a significant loss of elbow and forearm function.

Distal radial fractures also frequently require internal fixation to stabilize an associated radioulnar dislocation. However, those fractures produced by a direct blow are usually undisplaced and can be treated effectively by closed, functional methods.

Closed, functional treatment is desirable for the majority of forearm fractures not associated with proximal or distal radioulnar instability or fracture comminution. Prolonged immobilization of the wrist and elbow with closed treatment has been proven unnecessary. Prolonged cast immobilization in forced pronated or supinated positions may actually add to the complications by promoting excessive scarring and muscle contracture within the interosseous space.

Children's forearm fractures are subject occasionally to both over-treatment and undertreatment. The basic objective should be to reduce and hold the child's forearm straight. Forearm fractures in children frequently cause some loss of rotation even with ideal treatment. However, the patient and the family are more dissatisfied with appearance of a malunited forearm fracture than they are affected by functional loss. Loss of forearm rotation, particularly pronation, can be accommodated in most instances by shoulder motion.

Effective management of these common forearm fractures depends on the physician's anticipating both the diagnostic and the therapeutic pitfalls in order to minimize complications for the patient.

REFERENCES

Anderson, L. D., Sisk, T. D., Tooms, R. E., et al.: Compression-plate fixation in acute diaphyseal fractures of the radius and ulna. J. Bone and Joint Surg., 57A:287, 1975.

Bado, J. L.: The Monteggia lesion. Clin. Orthop., 50:71, 1967.

Bagby, G. W.: Compression bone-plating: historical considerations. J. Bone and Joint Surg., 59A:625, 1977.

Blount, W. P.: Fractures in Children. Baltimore: Williams & Wilkins Company, 1955, pp. 76–112.

Bruce, H. E., Harvey, J. P., and Wilson, J. C.: Monteggia fractures. J. Bone and Joint Surg., 56A:1563, 1974.

Castle, M. E.: One-bone forearm. J. Bone and Joint Surg., 56A:1223, 1974.

Du Toit, F. P., and Gräbe, R. P.: Isolated fractures of the shaft of the ulna. S. Afr. Med. J., 56:21, 1979.

Elstrom, J. A., Pankovich, A. M., and Egwele, R.: Extra-articular low-velocity gunshot fractures of the radius and ulna. J. Bone and Joint Surg., 60A:335, 1978.

Evans, E. M.: Fractures of the radius and ulna. J. Bone and Joint Surg., 33B:548, 1951.

Gandhi, R. K., Wilson, P., Brown, J. J., et al.: Spontaneous correction of deformity following fractures of the forearm in children. Brit. J. Surg., 50:5, 1962.

Gordon, J. L.: Monteggia fracture: a combined surgical approach employing a single lateral incision. Clin. Orthop., 50:87, 1967.

Högström, H., Nilsson, B. E., and Willner, S.: Correction with growth following diaphyseal forearm fracture. Acta Orthop. Scand., 47:299, 1976.

Mikic, Z. D.: Galeazzi fracture-dislocations. J. Bone and Joint Surg., 57A:1071, 1975.

Mullick, S.: The lateral Monteggia fracture. J. Bone and Joint Surg., 59A:543, 1977.

Nilsson, B. E., and Obrant, K.: The range of motion following fracture of the shaft of the forearm in children. Acta Orthop. Scand., 48:600, 1977.

Reckling, F. W., and Cordell, L. D.: Unstable fracture-dislocations of the forearm: the Monteggia and Galeazzi lesions. Arch. Surg., 96:99, 1968.

Sarmiento, A., Cooper, J. S., and Sinclair, W. F.: Forearm fractures. Early functional bracing — a preliminary report. J. Bone and Joint Surg., 57A:297, 1975.

Sarmiento, A., Kinman, P. B., Murphy, R. B., et al.: Treatment of ulnar fractures by functional bracing. J. Bone and Joint Surg., 58A:1104, 1976.

Schiller, M. G.: Intravenous regional anesthesia for closed treatment of fractures and dislocations of the upper extremities. Clin. Orthop., 118:25, 1976.

Spinner, M.: Injuries to the Major Branches of Peripheral Nerves of the Forearm. Philadelphia: W. B. Saunders Company, 1972, pp. 29–62.

REFERENCES

Stein, F., Grabias, S. I., and Deffer, P. A.: Nerve injuries complicating Monteggia lesions. J. Bone and Joint Surg., 53A:1432, 1971.

Steindler, A.: Kinesiology of the Human Body. Springfield, Illinois: Charles C Thomas, Publisher, 1955, pp. 490–508.

Stewart, T. D.: Nonunion of fractures in antiquity, with descriptions of five cases from the New World involving the forearm. Bull. N.Y. Acad. Med., 50:875, 1974.

Tompkins, D. G.: The anterior Monteggia fracture: observations on etiology and treatment. J. Bone and Joint Surg., 53A:1109, 1971.

INDEX